Clinical Oral Science

Clinical Oral Science

Edited by

Malcolm Harris MD, FDSRCS, FFDRCSI
Department of Oral and Maxillofacial Surgery,
Eastman Dental Institute, University of London,
UK

Michael Edgar DDSc, PhD, FDSRCS
Oral Biology Group,
Department of Clinical Dental Sciences,
University of Liverpool,
Liverpool, UK

Sajeda Meghji BSc, MPhil, PhD
Department of Oral and Maxillofacial Surgery,
Eastman Dental Institute, University of London,
UK

wright

Wright
An imprint of Butterworth-Heinemann
Linacre House, Jordan Hill, Oxford OX2 8DP
225 Wildwood Avenue, Woburn, MA 01801-2041
A division of Reed Educational and Professional Publishing Ltd

A member of the Reed Elsevier plc group

OXFORD BOSTON JOHANNESBURG
MELBOURNE NEW DELHI SINGAPORE

First published 1998

British Library Cataloguing in Publication Data
A catalogue record for this book is available from the British Library

Library of Congress Cataloguing in Publication Data
A catalogue record for this book is available from the Library of Congress

ISBN 0 7236 1059 2

Composition by Scribe Design, Gillingham, Kent, UK
Printed and bound in Great Britain by The Bath Press, Somerset

Contents

Errata

On page v the authors of Chapter 11 should read:
Gavin McKay, Robert Yemm and Samuel W. Cadden

page vii should include:

Dr Samuel W. Cadden
Dundee Dental School
Dundee

On page 141 the chapter heading should read:
11 The structure and function of the
temporomandibular joint
Gavin McKay, Robert Yemm and Samuel W. Cadden

Contributors

Dr Behnam Aghabeigi
Department of Oral Maxillofacial Surgery
Eastman Dental Institute
London

Andrew William Barrett
Department of Oral Pathology
Eastman Dental Institute
London

Dr St John Crean
Departments of Oral and Maxillofacial Surgery
Eastman Dental Institute
London

Dr C. W. Ian Douglas
Department of Oral Pathology
Sheffield School of Clinical Dentistry
Sheffield

Professor Michael Edgar
Oral Biology Group
Department of Clinical Dental Sciences
University of Liverpool
Liverpool

Dr Patrizia Ferretti
Developmental Biology Unit
Institute of Child Health
London

Dr Christopher Franklin
Department of Oral Pathology
School of Clinical Dentistry
Sheffield

Mohammed F. Haque
Department of Oral and Maxillofacial Surgery
Eastman Dental Institute
London

Professor Jeremy Hardie
Department of Oral Microbiology
London Hospital Dental Institute
London

Professor Macolm Harris
Department of Oral and Maxillofacial Surgery
Eastman Dental Institute
London

Professor Brian Henderson
Department of Oral Maxillofacial Surgery
Eastman Dental Institute
London

G. R. Holland
Department of Cariology, Restorative Science and Endontology
University of Michigan
Ann Arbor
Michigan

Dr Nigel Hunt
Department of Orthodontics
Eastman Dental Institute
London

Dr Nicholas J. Lench
Department of Molecular Genetics
St James Hospital
Leeds

Dr Roger W. A. Linden
Clinical Craniofacial Biology Research Unit
Kings College School of Medicine and Dentistry
London

Dr Douglas Luke
Department of Anatomy
UMDS
London

Dr Gavin McKay
Dundee Dental School
Dundee

Dr Sajeda Meghji
Department of Oral and Maxillofacial Surgery
Eastman Dental Institute
London

Dr Sean Nair
Department of Oral and Maxillofacial Surgery
Eastman Dental Institute
London

Professor Stephen R. Porter
Department of Oral Medicine
Eastman Dental Institute
London

Professor Peter P. Robinson
Department of Oral and Maxillofacial Surgery
School of Clinical Dentistry
Sheffield

Dr Jonathan R. Sandy
Department of Child Health
Bristol Dental School
Bristol

Professor Crispian Scully
Department of Oral Medicine
Eastman Dental Institute
London

Dr Mamta Shah
Department of Plastic Surgery
University Hospital of South Manchester
West Didsbury
Manchester

Dr Alan I. Thexton
Department of Physiology
UMDS
London

Professor Peter Thorogood
Developmental Biology Unit
Institute of Child Health
London

Dr Susan Wright
Department of Anaesthetics
The Middlesex Hospital and University College London Hospitals
London

Professor Robert Yemm
Dundee Dental School
Dundee

Foreword

This book is an augmented and revised revival of a series of applied basic science papers published in the *British Dental Journal* 5 years ago. That series and this book are an attempt to translate the complexities of new science, especially molecular genetics and molecular biology, into a digestible form for orofacial clinicians. An equally important stimulus has been the radical revision of postgraduate training in all disciplines of dentistry and medicine; this has created an assessment hurdle placed between a basic training period of 2–3 years and subsequent higher or specialist training. The structure of these examinations, regardless of specialism, has been designed to fuse basic science and clinical practice, which has also been the aim in the presentation of each subject in this book.

We are very grateful for the authors' patience in awaiting publication and their willingness to revise their work.

Malcolm Harris, Michael Edgar,
Sajeda Meghji

1

Cytokines and related intercellular signals in tissue pathology

Brian Henderson and Sean Nair

Introduction

It is self-evident that the maintenance of bodily and tissue homeostasis in multicellular organisms requires cell-to-cell communication. Claude Bernard (1957)[1] created the concept of the maintenance of the *milieu intérieur* (i.e. homeostasis) and suggested that the system of ductless glands, the endocrine system, performed an integrating function to help maintain homeostasis. Bayliss and Starling in 1902[2] demonstrated that an acid extract of the duodenum when injected into dogs induced a marked flow of pancreatic juice. The substance was named secretin and Starling subsequently coined the term hormone (from the Greek word meaning 'I excite') for such intercellular messengers. From this study the concept developed of hormones as molecules produced by specific glands, secreted directly into the blood and by this means conveyed to selected organs or tissues where they exerted their effect. The medical and scientific discipline of endocrinology developed from these pioneering studies and is still growing healthily.

During the past four decades scientists and clinicians from a range of disciplines have demonstrated the presence of an additional system of intercellular signalling. It has been revealed that a large and rapidly growing number of peptide and protein factors are produced by a wide range of cells and that these have potent actions on probably all cells, barring erythrocytes. Unlike the endocrine hormones, these factors, termed cytokines, are not produced by specific tissues and do not have selected target cells. While they can have systemic effects, it is believed that their major role is as local paracrine (*para* nearby) and autocrine factors. However, they have one major similarity to endocrine hormones in that they bind to high-affinity cell surface receptors to induce cellular activation. In addition to directly stimulating cells, cytokines can induce cells to produce and/or release additional cell-to-cell signals such as vascular adhesion molecules, eicosanoids and nitric oxide (NO). The cytokines and the signals they induce are now seen to be crucially involved both in normal homeostatic interactions and in the pathology of many disease states. In the field of dentistry cytokines have been implicated in the pathology of periodontal disease and associated bone destruction in oral cancer, wound healing and in the bone response in orthodontic treatment.

The aim of this review is to give a brief introduction to the nature and biological actions of the cytokines with particular reference to their involvement in tissue pathology. The therapeutic use of cytokines or of agents capable of inhibiting cytokine synthesis or action will also be considered (reviewed by Henderson and Poole[3]). In this review the term cytokine will have a broad definition and will include growth factors, interferons and related peptides.

History

Our current understanding of cytokines can be traced back to a handful of individuals who were intrigued by the relationship between inflammation and fever. The 19th century saw the first attempts to bring science to bear on the study of pyrexia. The findings from the newly developing disciplines such as physiology, pathology and microbiology were synthesized by the American pathologist William Welch, who hypothesized that fever resulted from a disturbance of the normal regulation of body temperature in the brain caused by 'ferments' produced by the action of microbes (or their products) on host cells (Welch, 1888, in Atkins[4]). However, it was not until the 1950s that the pioneering work of Bennett and Beeson[5] and Atkins and Wood[6] demonstrated that mammalian cells produced a proteinaceous substance that caused fever when injected into animals. This activity was variously called granulocyte pyrogen, leukocytic pyrogen (LP) or endogenous pyrogen (EP) and later leukocyte endogenous mediator (LEM[7]).

In 1972 Gery and coworkers[8] described a soluble mediator which was released by human adherent leukocytes and which augmented the proliferative response of mouse thymocytes to lectins (a group of plant-derived proteins capable of binding to the surface of animal cells, e.g. concanavalin A). This activity was termed lymphocyte-activating factor (LAF) and was not thought to be related to the various EP molecules previously described. This activity was just one of a vast number of undefined factors (termed lymphokines) which had been described by immunologists since the mid-1960s. In 1979 LAF was renamed interleukin-1 (IL-1) and with the cloning of the gene for this molecule it was shown that IL-1 was equivalent to LAF and to the various other activities that had been described previously (Table 1.1).

Interleukin-1 is now known to be two distinct proteins (IL-1α and IL-1β) but which bind to the same receptors. Thus IL-1 was the first cytokine to be discovered (see Bomford and Henderson[13] for general reviews of IL-1). The term interleukin means between leukocytes and originally was meant to define the known immunological role of molecules such as LAF (IL-1) and T-cell growth factor (TCGF: IL-2), i.e. molecules produced by macrophages and lymphocytes respectively involved in stimulating lymphocyte proliferation. Unfortunately, IL-1 and most other cytokines have multiple activities and are produced by many cell types in addition to leukocytes. Thus, at the very inception of our understanding of cytokines, an inappropriate

Table 1.1 History of interleukin-1 (IL-1) research

Experimental findings		*Synonym for IL-1*
Peritoneal cells release substance producing fever[9]	(1948)	Granulocyte pyrogen
Injection of endotoxin into rabbits produces a circulating pyrogenic protein	(1953–1955)	Endogenous pyrogen (EP)
Proteinaceous material from leukocytes mediates acute-phase response[7]	(1969)	Leukocyte endogenous mediator (LEM)
Stimulation of thymocyte proliferation	(1972)	Lymphocyte activating factor (LAF)
International Lymphokine Workshop (1979) IL-1		
Monocyte factor stimulating prostaglandin E_2 and collagenase production by synovial cells[10]	(1979)	Mononuclear cell factor (MCF)
Synovial factor stimulating articular cartilage breakdown[11]	(1980)	Catabolin
Cloning of IL-1α and IL-1β[12]	(1984)	
Cloning of the third member of this family – IL-1ra	(1990)	

nomenclature was introduced. This problem has dogged the development of cytokine research and has given rise to much confusion. It should therefore be borne in mind that the name given to any particular cytokine (as an example: tumour necrosis factor or TNF), will only describe one of its varied activities. Similarly, transforming growth factor (TGF)-β acts as a growth factor for some cells but as a growth inhibitor of others and recently has been shown to be the most potent chemotactic factor for polymorphonuclear leukocytes.[14]

The reader is referred to a number of recent books which review the field of cytokine biology in detail.[13,15–17]

Definition

The term cytokine was introduced to describe any soluble substance produced by cells which exerted specific effects on other target cells. This original definition would also include the prostaglandins, steroid and peptide hormones, etc. The present definition of a cytokine is that it is an inducible protein of molecular weight greater than 5000 (or 5 kDa) which produces specific receptor-mediated effects on target cells or on the producer cell. At present, cytokines can be grouped into six overlapping families of molecules which are shown in (Table 1.2). This classification is rather artificial but is done to produce some order for further discussion. The various cytokines can be subdivided into the families: interleukins, cytotoxic factors, interferons, colony-stimulating factors, growth factors and chemokines.[16,18] It must be appreciated that all of these molecules have a plethora of biological actions.

To further define the nature of cytokines their characteristics have been compared with those of classic endocrine hormones (Table 1.3). It is now clear that, with the exception of erythrocytes, most cells in the body are

Table 1.2 Cytokine families

Family	*Examples*
Interleukins (IL)	IL-1 to IL-17
Cytotoxic cytokines	Tumour necrosis factor (TNF)
Colony-stimulating factors (CSF)	IL-3, granulocyte-CSF
Interferons (IFN)	IFN-α, -β, -γ
Growth factors (GF)	Fibroblast GF, platelet-derived GF
Chemokines	IL-8

For more details see Ibelgaufts[16]

Table 1.3 Comparison of endocrine hormones with cytokines

Endocrine hormones	*Cytokines*
Peptides, proteins, glycoproteins or steroids, or derivatives of aromatic amino acids	Proteins, glycoproteins (mol. wt $>$ 5000)
Synthesized by specialized gland cells, released into blood to act on target cells in other tissues	Normally produced by many distinct cells to act locally in paracrine or autocrine manner (exceptions: interleukin-2 and interferon-γ). Some cytokines have systemic actions e.g. (erythropoietin, interleukin-1)
Restricted range of biological actions with little overlap between hormones	Widespread overlap of biological actions
Receptors (high-affinity) found in relatively large numbers on target cells	Very high-affinity receptors found in small numbers on many cell populations

capable of synthesizing at least one cytokine and many cells, e.g. macrophages and fibroblasts, can synthesize a number of distinct cytokines. Likewise, most cells in the body are capable of responding to various cytokines. For example, osteoblasts in bone can respond to a wide range, including IL-1α and -β, TNF-α and -β, IL-6, leukaemia-inhibitory factor (LIF), interferon-γ (IFN-γ). In general, especially with the interleukins, the cellular response to cytokines is transduced by low numbers of very high affinity cell surface receptors.[16] One of the curious facets of cytokine biology is the finding that many of these molecules share the same activities. For example, both forms of IL-1, both forms of TNF, IL-6 and IFN-γ are EPs capable of inducing fever.[19]

Functions of cytokines

Cytokines and cytokine-generated messengers are not only important in tissue pathology they also play a major role in tissue, organ and body homeostasis (see Meager[15] and Ibelgaufts[16]). The complete list of functions played by cytokines remains to be defined. However, at the present time it is clear that cytokines interact with cells to cause:

1. Activation (of metabolism, cellular synthesis, etc).
2. Proliferation or inhibition of proliferation.
3. Apoptosis.
4. Differentiation.
5. Chemotaxis.

These actions may overlap, as a dividing or differentiating cell is, by definition, in an activated state. In terms of maintaining homeostasis, cytokines are involved in haematopoiesis, the process whereby stem cells in bone marrow differentiate into mature circulating leukocytes, erythrocytes and platelets. Colony-stimulating factors, erythropoietin, IL-1 and possibly other cytokines are involved in this process. Many cytokines are growth and activation factors for lymphocytes and it is presumed that the normal functioning of the immune system is dependent upon the production and action of these cytokines. Our host defence response is obviously dependent upon the cytokines involved in haematopoiesis and the immune response. Other cytokines are also involved, including the so-called inflammatory cytokines, IL-1, IL-6, IL-8 and TNF, which can stimulate production of liver acute-phase proteins, alter plasma ions and induce fever. The antiviral interferons are also important in the response to viral infections. Wound healing involves an inflammatory and a reparative phase. Both require the participation of cytokines such as IL-1 and TNF and growth factors such as TGF-β or fibroblast growth factor (FGF). The large family of bone morphogenetic proteins (BMPs) are examples of growth factors/cytokines which play a role in bone remodelling and are important in bone repair.[20]

Table 1.3 compares and contrasts the actions of endocrine hormones and cytokines. By definition, the former are produced in specialized glands and act at a distance on their target cells. Certain cytokines, such as erythropoietin also act in an endocrine manner; others such as IL-1 or TNF have systemic actions such as inducing fever in, for example, septic shock. Most cytokines tend to act in a paracrine or autocrine manner (Fig.1.1). Paracrine action means that cytokines act locally, binding to and activating cells close to the cytokine-synthesizing cell. Autocrine stimulation describes the condition in which a cell secretes

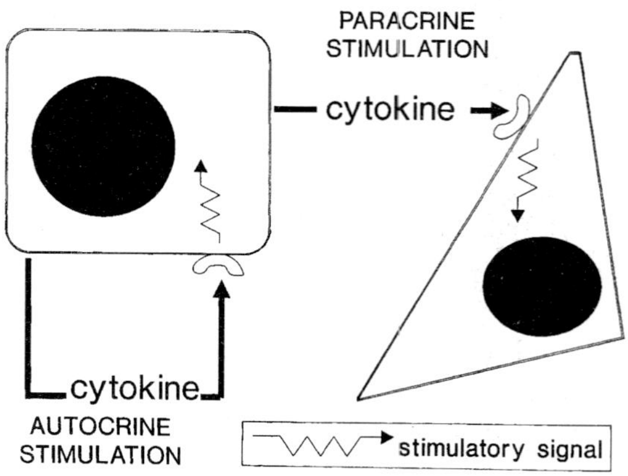

Fig. 1.1 Schematic definition of autocrine and paracrine signalling by cytokines. In autocrine stimulation the cell producing the cytokine is also stimulated by that cytokine. In paracrine stimulation the cytokine produced by one cell interacts with a nearby cell to cause stimulation.

a cytokine which then binds to receptors on that same cell, causing cellular activation. It has even been suggested that cytokines may act within the cell that is synthesizing them.

The cytokine network

Both in normal, and particularly in inflamed tissues, cells are exposed not to single cytokines but to a cocktail of such proteins. This is assumed to be the case for normal lymphoid tissues in which a large number of cytokines act as growth and differentiation factors for the various lymphoid cell populations. A large number of cytokines have been found in the rheumatoid joint[21] and there are a growing number of these molecules reported in crevicular fluid and gingival tissues of patients with chronic inflammatory periodontal disease (CIPD).[22] The response of cells to this mixture of cytokines, which probably changes both in composition and in the concentration of individual molecules in the course of any particular pathological state, is extremely complex. This complexity is compounded by the finding that cytokines act in an autocrine manner (Fig. 1.1). The classic example of this is the activation of T lymphocytes to produce IL-2 and the IL-2 receptor. The IL-2 produced by activated cells can then bind to the receptor on the same cell and stimulate it to divide and also produce additional cytokines. Cytokines can act on cells to upregulate the synthesis of other cytokines or of the activating cytokine. For example, IL-1 can stimulate cells to produce IL-1.[23] Cytokines can act additively or synergistically. It has been demonstrated that the injection of IL-1 and TNF into rabbit knee joints induces the accumulation of three times as many polymorphonuclear leukocytes as does the additive effects of injecting these cytokines alone.[24] Cytokines can also act in an antagonistic fashion. For example, TGF-β is a potent inhibitor of IL-1-induced protease synthesis by chondrocytes and of IL-1-induced cartilage breakdown.[25] Cytokines can also interact with other mediators, e.g. prostaglandins, or with endocrine hormones. For example, IL-1 and parathyroid hormone have been shown to interact in a synergistic manner in stimulating bone resorption *in vitro*.[26]

Cytokines and tissue pathology

While it is clear that cytokines have a role in the maintenance of cellular homeostasis, it has become evident over the past two decades that the overproduction of cytokines is associated with the induction and maintenance of tissue pathology. In addition, the absence of particular cytokines can also result in tissue pathology. The best example of the latter is the anaemia associated with chronic renal failure. This is caused by the failure to produce the cytokine erythropoietin, which is the principal regulator of erythrocyte production. Anaemia can now be corrected by replacement of erythropoietin.[27] However, at the present time most pathological states associated with cytokines are due to elevations in cytokine production.

The disease areas in which cytokine overproduction have been implicated are listed in Table 1.4. These include acute inflammation, septic shock and chronic inflammatory diseases such as rheumatoid arthritis, periodontal disease and asthma.[13,15,21,22] These diseases are associated with tissue damage which is believed to be due to cytokines. Septic shock is now clearly associated with the production of cytokines such as IL-1 and TNF which indirectly stimulate hypotension and end-organ failure.[28] Cell growth-promoting cytokines are implicated in the pathology of fibrotic diseases

Table 1.4 Pathogenic cytokines in human diseases

Disease	*Cytokines implicated*
Malaise, fever associated with infections	IFN-α, -β, -γ, IL-1, IL-6, TNF
Septic shock	IL-1, IL-6, TNF-α
Malaria	TNF-α
Cerebral malaria	IL-3, GM-CSF
Rheumatoid arthritis	IL-1, TNF, growth factors, etc.
Chronic inflammatory periodontal disease	IL-1, TNF
Scleroderma	Growth factors
Psoriasis	IL-2, IL-8
Atherosclerosis	Growth factors
Cancers	Growth factors, TNF-α

IFN = Interferon; IL = interleukin; TNF = tumour necrosis factor; GM-CSF = granulocyte–macrophage colony-stimulating factor.

such as scleroderma, liver fibrosis and oral submucous fibrosis.[29] The past two decades have seen oncogenes, which include many growth factors or their receptors, strongly implicated in the process of oncogenesis.[30]

This review will concentrate on IL-1 as more is known about its role in tissue pathology than any other cytokines. IL-1 is also a key mediator of the induction of other intercellular signalling systems such as vascular adhesion molecules, eicosanoids and NO. The reader is referred to Bomford and Henderson[13] for a detailed review of the structure and functions of IL-1.

Table 1.5 Inducers and suppressors of IL-1 synthesis

Inducers of synthesis	*Inhibitors of synthesis*
Lipopolysaccharides	Dexamethasone
Peptidoglycans	Prednisolone
Exotoxins	Prostaglandin E_2
Complement components (C5a)	Retinoic acid
Phorbol esters	IFN-γ
Zymosan	IL-2
Calcium ionophores	TGF-β
Cytokines	IL-4
IL-1	
TNF	
IFN-γ	
GM-CSF	
LTB_4	

IFN = Interferon; IL = interleukin; TGF = transforming growth factor; TNF = tumour necrosis factor; GM-CSF = granulocyte–macrophage colony-stimulating factor; LTB_4 = leukotriene B_4.

The role of IL-1 in tissue pathology

The synthesis and release of IL-1

IL-1 exists as two distinct molecules, termed IL-1α and IL-1β, with only about 25% homology (similarity in amino acid sequence) between them. Both forms are synthesized initially as non-glycosylated precursors (or proforms) which are then proteolytically cleaved to produce the active form of the molecule, although the proform of IL-1α does have some biological activity. In common with most cytokines, IL-1 is not believed to be constitutively produced but requires cell activation to induce synthesis, although there may be exceptions in certain neural tissues and in skin. The cell most active in synthesizing IL-1 is the monocyte and many factors have been shown to stimulate IL-1 synthesis by this cell (Table 1.5). Probably the most potent activator of IL-1 synthesis is lipopolysaccharide (LPS) from the cell walls of Gram-negative bacteria. As little as 10 pg/ml of endotoxin can stimulate human blood monocytes to synthesize IL-1. Exposure of human monocytes to LPS rapidly induces messenger RNA (mRNA) synthesis. This message is then translated into the proform of IL-1. Human monocytes make predominantly IL-1β, mouse monocytes mainly IL-1α and pig monocytes produce equal amounts of both. Human keratinocytes preferentially produce IL-1α. Once the IL-1 proforms are synthesized, they must be exported from the cell and cleaved to generate the active form. The mechanism by which IL-1 is released from cells is still unclear and may involve a novel process (the same pathways may be involved in the release of other cytokines such as FGF).[31] The cleavage of IL-1β proform into the active molecule has now been shown to be due to the action of a unique heterodimeric (containing two distinct protein subunits) cysteine protease termed IL-1β convertase.[32]

Once active IL-1 has been released from the monocyte, or from the many other cells now known to be capable of synthesizing it (neutrophils, keratinocytes, fibroblasts, T and B lymphocytes, etc.), it can then act to stimulate cells by binding to the IL-1 receptor. Two receptors, termed type I and type II, are now recognized. The type I receptor is found on T cells, fibroblasts, endothelial cells, chondrocytes and hepatocytes and belongs to the so-called immunoglobulin superfamily because it contains three extracellular domains which show homology with immunoglobulin domains.[33] The type II receptor has been found expressed on B cells, neutrophils and bone marrow cells. Strangely, binding to this type II receptor appears to have no effect on the cell and it has been suggested that this receptor has some function in downregulating cellular responses to IL-1 by binding to and thereby inactivating IL-1. Most cells contain only a few hundred to a few thousand type I receptors, depending on the cell, but these receptors have a very high affinity for IL-1. This contrasts with endocrine hormone receptors which are normally present in high numbers on the surface of target cells (thousands to tens of thousands).

Table 1.6 Biological effects of IL-1

In vitro	*In vivo*
Stimulates prostaglandin E_2 synthesis	Produces fever
Stimulates metalloproteinase synthesis	Induces acute-phase response
Stimulates fibroblast proliferation	Local injection produces inflammation
Thymocyte proliferation	Stimulates bone resorption
Macrophage stimulator	High doses induce hypotension
Stimulates endothelial cells	Potent inducer of hyperalgesia
Induces hepatocyte acute-phase protein synthesis	Accelerates wound healing
Tumoricidal (limited)	Stimulates neuropeptide release
Stimulates keratinocyte proliferation	
Cytotoxic to β islet cells	

Proinflammatory activity of IL-1

IL-1 demonstrates a wide range of activities which contribute to the inflammatory process (Table 1.6). The systemic and local effects of IL-1 will be considered in turn.

The systemic inflammatory effects of IL-1

It has been known for some years that the intravenous administration of IL-1 to animals induces systemic acute-phase responses including fever, hepatic acute-phase protein synthesis, neutrophilia, changes in serum metal ion content and increased levels of hormones. With higher doses of IL-1 it is possible to induce a hypotensive shock-like state. In more recent years IL-1 has been administered to humans in various clinical trials. Intravenous administration of 10–100 ng/kg IL-1 was associated with side-effects including fever, generalized myalgias and arthralgias and headaches[34,35]

Fever

Recombinant IL-1 induces a monophasic fever when injected into rabbits, mice or humans. This fever is blocked by non-steroidal anti-inflammatory drugs (NSAIDs) such as aspirin. Surprisingly, IL-1 does not enter the brain as it appears unable to cross the blood–brain barrier. It is postulated that IL-1 stimulates the specialized endothelial cells of the periventricular organs where the blood–brain barrier is interrupted and that these cells release the prostaglandins, causing fever.

Acute-phase protein synthesis

Acute-phase proteins are largely synthesized by the liver and are released into the blood where they have a wide range of activities, including opsonization, enzyme inhibition and free radical scavenging. IL-1 stimulates the synthesis of some acute-phase reactants such as α_1-acid glycoprotein, serum amyloid A (SAA) and serum amyloid P (SAP). Other cytokines, notably IL-6 and TNF-α, also stimulate liver acute-phase protein synthesis and, like IL-1, contribute to the acute-phase response, which is our important first line of defence against the pathogenic microorganisms in our environment.

Alterations in hormone levels

Exposure to bacterial endotoxins has long been known to stimulate the release of hormones from the anterior pituitary. Intravenous administration of IL-1 to mice results in the release into the blood of corticotrophin-releasing factor, adrenocorticotrophic hormone, vasopressin and somatostatin. It is believed that IL-1-induced corticosteroid release, which occurs via release of adrenocorticotrophic hormone, represents a biological feedback loop to inhibit the inflammatory actions of IL-1. Indeed, IL-1 at low levels is lethal to adrenalectomized animals.

Effects on circulating leukocytes

Systemic injection of IL-1 causes a transient neutrophilia due to rapid margination of these cells. After 4–6 h there is an increase in circulating neutrophils due to increased release from the bone marrow. This activity is shared by TNF-α and TNF-β. IL-1 has complex actions on haemopoiesis, including induction of colony-stimulating factors and synergizing with these cytokines. IL-1 has been given to cancer patients and shown to increase circulating numbers of both neutrophils and platelets.[34]

Effects on the immune system

IL-1 was discovered (or rediscovered) as LAF, a molecule which stimulated the proliferation of murine thymocytes exposed to suboptimal concentrations of the mitogen phytohaemagglutinin. It was accepted for many years that IL-1 was an important cofactor in immune responses. However, in recent years this role in immune responsiveness has been questioned. The use of the natural antagonist of the IL-1 receptor (IL-1ra)[36] has allowed the importance of IL-1 in immune responses to be investigated. It has therefore been surprising to find that, although IL-1ra can block many of the actions of IL-1, it does not appear to inhibit human T-cell responses *in vitro*. For example, this antagonist did not inhibit the proliferation of human peripheral blood T cells produced when these cells are activated by mitogen or soluble antigens.[36]

Tissue breakdown

Systemic administration of IL-1 to animals induces hypercalcaemia similar to that seen in a proportion of patients with cancer.[37]

Local inflammatory effects of IL-1

During the past decade the availability of recombinant IL-1 has enabled investigations to be made of the effects of local administration of this cytokine. It has been found that such administration can give rise to the cardinal signs of inflammation (rubor, calor, dolor and functio laesa).[38]

Leukocyte emigration

The local accumulation of leukocytes is the hallmark of both acute and chronic inflammation. Local injection of IL-1α or -β causes the accumulation of polymorphonuclear leukocytes and monocytes. In rabbit skin the injection of as little as 10^{-15} mol/site IL-1 produces leukocyte infiltration. However, it is now firmly established that IL-1 is not a chemoattractant in its own right. The attraction of leukocytes to sites of IL-1 injection is now believed to be due to two processes. The first is the activation of vascular endothelial cells to express so-called adhesion molecules on their luminal surface and the second is the stimulation of local cells to synthesize chemotactic cytokines such as IL-8. This combination of events is now believed to account for the potent leukocyte-accumulating actions of IL-1. The relationship between cytokines and adhesion molecules will be discussed in more detail in the next section.

Vascular permeability

Many mediators which induce polymorphonuclear infiltration, such as the bacterial chemotactic peptide, *N*-formyl-Met-Leu-Phe (FMLP), leukotriene B_4 or the complement component C5a, also increase vascular permeability, leading to oedema formation, by a neutrophil-dependent mechanism.[39] Although IL-1 is a potent inducer of leukocyte infiltration in the rabbit, it does not increase vascular permeability. It is assumed that the reason for this is that the IL-1 does not activate the infiltrating leukocytes.

Pain

Inflammation is normally associated with the phenomenon of hyperalgesia. This is an increased sensitivity of nociceptors to mechanical, chemical or thermal stimuli.[40] A common example of this phenomenon is experienced with sunburn. The inflamed skin is not overtly painful until it is stimulated by touch, heat or chemical means. The prostaglandins are well-known hyperalgesic mediators and the analgesic actions of aspirin-like drugs is due to their inhibition of the enzyme cyclooxygenase which is responsible for prostaglandin synthesis. IL-1β has recently been shown to be the most potent hyperalgesic agent discovered with doses as low as 5×10^{-15} g (5 fg) inducing a rapid and long-lasting hyperalgesia in rats.[41] This hyperalgesia is not due to prostaglandins as it is not inhibited by administration of indomethacin but it is inhibited by the neuropeptide α-melanocyte-stimulating hormone (α-MSH).[42] Other cytokines, such as TNF-α and IL-8, have also been shown to possess hyperalgesic properties.[43] The possibility that cytokines contribute to pain in conditions where these mediators are known to be produced, such as arthritis and cancer, is currently under active investigation.

Tissue injury

Progressive destruction of alveolar bone is found in periodontal disease and of articular cartilage and subchondral bone in rheumatoid and osteoarthritis. The pathogenesis of these diseases is believed to be due to the action of cytokines and, in particular, IL-1 and TNF-α. Addition of IL-1 or TNF to explants of articular cartilage from young animals or fetal rodent bone induces resorption of the extracellular matrices of these tissues.[44] Local injection of IL-1 into rabbit knee joints stimulates cartilage matrix destruction[45] and systemic injection of IL-1 to rodents induces bone breakdown.[37] However, recombinant IL-1 does not stimulate significant breakdown of adult articular cartilage but instead inhibits the synthesis of cartilage matrix.[46] The role of cytokines in diseases involving tissue loss may therefore be due to the activation of tissue breakdown and inhibition of tissue synthesis.

Fibrosis

Tissue and organ pathology is often due to the overproduction of connective tissue matrix components. This is seen in idiopathic diseases such as scleroderma, in drug-induced lesions such as oral submucous fibrosis or gingival hyperplasia or in association with inflammation in rheumatoid arthritis. IL-1 is a potent stimulator of fibroblast proliferation. This appears to be an indirect activation, with IL-1 inducing fibroblasts to synthesize and secrete the platelet-derived growth factor (PDGF) which then acts in an autocrine fashion to cause fibroblast division.[47] Other cytokines, such as TNF-α and TGF-β, are also implicated in fibrotic lesions.[29]

It should be emphasized that a number of cytokines share many of the activities of IL-1 (Table 1.7) and are implicated in those pathological states in which IL-1 has been proposed as a pathological mediator.

Table 1.7 Common biological action of cytokines

Biological activity	*IL-1*	*TNF*	*IL-6*
Hepatic acute-phase protein synthesis	+	+	+
Fever	+	+	+
Slow-wave sleep	+	+	−
T- and B-cell activation	+	+	+
Fibroblast proliferation	+	+	−
Endothelial cell activation	+	+	−
Metalloproteinase induction	+	+	−

IL = Interleukin; TNF = tumour necrosis factor.

Intercellular signalling systems induced by cytokines

Cytokines are potent, promiscuous, intercellular signalling molecules and in the past decade it has been found that they also induce the appearance of additional intercellular signalling systems of importance in both homeostasis and tissue pathology. These signalling systems lie at opposite ends of the molecular mass range. Weighing in at around 100 kDa are the growing family of cell adhesion molecules and, in particular, those molecules associated with cytokine-activated vascular endothelial cells. The other signalling molecules are of low-molecular-weight eicosanoids and the gas NO which has a molecular mass of only 30 D.

Cytokine-activated vascular adhesion molecules

It is obvious that cells adhere to each other in tissues and organs and that such adherence is specific. Thus, liver cells stick only to other liver cells and they do not adhere to cells in other tissues or to cells in the blood. In the past decade the molecular complexities underlying cell-to-cell and cell-to-extracellular matrix adhesion have begun to be deciphered. The greatest advances have been in understanding the nature of the molecules responsible for the selective and short-term adherence of blood-borne leukocytes to vascular endothelium and to the extracellular matrix. This network of interactions is important in the regulation of leukocyte recirculation, in the acute phase response to infections, in chronic inflammation and in wound healing.

Table 1.8 Leukocyte/vascular adhesion molecules

Adhesion molecule	*Cells expressing adhesion molecules*	*Counter-receptor*
Selectin family		
E-selectin (ELAM-1)	Cytokine-activated vascular endothelial cells	Sialyl-Lewis^x antigen
L-selectin (Mel 14)	PMNs, monocytes, lymphocytes	Carbohydrate
P-selectin (GMP-140)	Activated endothelial cells, platelets	Sialyl-Lewis^x antigen
Integrin family		
LFA-1 (CD11a/CD18)	All leukocytes	ICAM-1
Mac-1 (CD11b/CD18)	PMN, monocytes, some lymphocytes	ICAM-1, iC3b
P150, 95 (CD11c/CD18)	PMN, monocytes	iC3b
VLA-1-6	Lymphocytes, leukocytes	Lamin, collagen fibronectin, (VLA4-VCam)
IgG superfamily		
CD2	T lymphocytes	LFA-3
LFA3	Widespread	CD2
ICAM-1	Cytokine-activated endothelial cells, leukocytes	LFA-1, MAC1
ICAM-2	Endothelial cells	LFA-1
VCAM-1	Cytokine-activated endothelial cells	VLA-4

PMN = Polymorphonuclear.

The first clues to this rapidly growing arena of leukocyte adhesion molecules came from the description of patients with a rare inherited condition termed leukocyte adhesion deficiency (LAD). Sufferers have a clinical syndrome characterized by recurrent bacterial infections, generally involving the skin and subcutaneous tissues, middle ear and oropharyngeal mucosa, delayed separation of the umbilical cord and poor healing of surgical or traumatic wounds, and abnormal leukocyte function.[48] Infections appear to be due to the inability of neutrophils to leave the blood vessels and move to sites where bacteria are present. The neutrophils from patients with LAD do not adhere to endothelial cells and have deficiencies in cell aggregation, phagocytosis and antibody-dependent cytotoxicity. A large proportion of LAD patients die of overwhelming sepsis despite antibiotic therapy.

We now know that there are at least three families of adhesion molecules which are responsible for the control of leukocyte emigration (Table 1.8). These are:

1. The selectins or lectin–epidermal growth factor–complement-related cell adhesion molecules (LECCAMs) which include E-selectin, also known as ELAM-1 (endothelial leukocyte adhesion molecule) and P-selectin.
2. The heterodimeric integrins (e.g. lymphocyte function-associated antigen-1 or LFA-1).
3. Members of the immunoglobulin superfamily such as ICAM (intercellular adhesion molecule)-1. (see reviews[49–52]).

The potential interactions between these various adhesive proteins is shown in Figure 1.2. The adherence, transendothelial migration and retention of leukocytes at site of inflammation and wound healing are now seen to involve these various families of molecules and require the upregulation of certain of the receptors by cytokines.

Cultured human vascular endothelial cells when exposed to inflammatory cytokines such as IL-1 or TNF-α or to LPS are induced to synthesize the immunoglobulin-like adhesive proteins ICAM-1 and VCAM-1, reaching maximal levels within 6 h. Interferon-γ also stimulates ICAM-1 but not VCAM-1 expression. Likewise, IL-1 and TNF-α stimulate vascular endothelial cells to synthesize E-selectin. Certain cytokines, notably TNF-α and IL-8, can also act on leukocytes and increase their adhesiveness, by acting conformationally to change the integrin CD11b/CD18 or Mac-1. The consequence of the local production of cytokines in an inflammatory site is that it stimulates endothelial cells and leukocytes to become more sticky and adhere to each other (Fig. 1.3). This is the key first step in a complex set of events that results in the appearance of leukocytes at sites of inflammation and infection.[49–52]

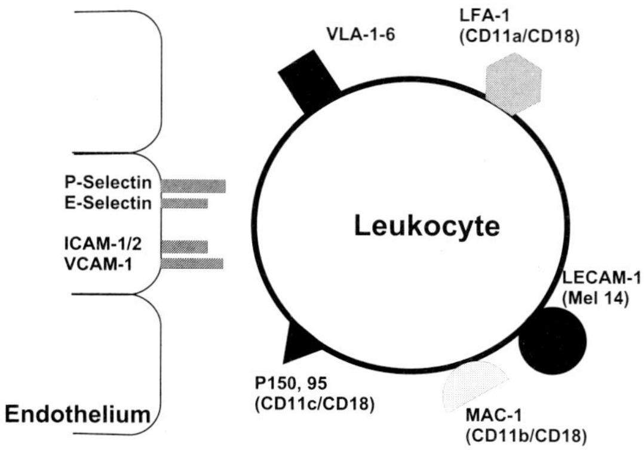

Fig. 1.2 Schematic diagram to show the interactions between leukocytes and vascular endothelial cells via the various families of cellular adhesion molecules described in Table 1.8. The pairing of adhesion receptors is defined in this table. The leukocytes express members of the β_1- and β_2-integrin families. For example, VLA-1-6 are β_1-integrins which bind to connective tissue macromolecules, while LFA-1, p150,95 and MAC-1 are members of the β_2-integrin family and bind to ICAM or VCAM on the activated endothelial cell surface. The vascular endothelial cell normally does not express adhesion receptors. However, exposure to lipopolysaccharide or interleukin-1/tumour necrosis factor activates the endothelial cells to synthesize the selectins (E- and P-) and members of the immunoglobulin superfamily adhesion receptors (ICAM and VCAM).

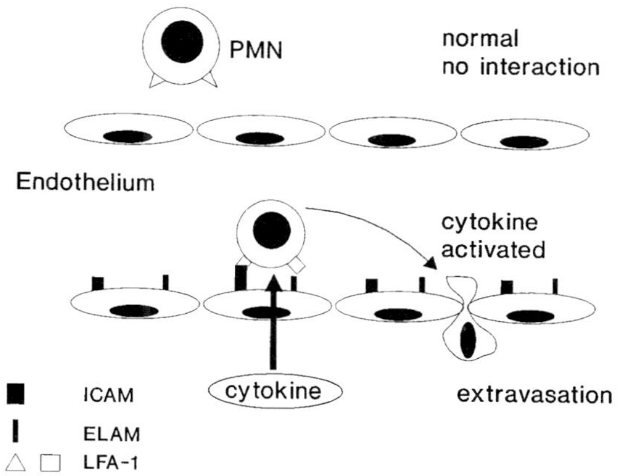

Fig. 1.3 Schematized mechanism of recruitment of leukocytes to sites of inflammation induced by the action of locally produced cytokines. In the normal state the leukocytes (which express integrins) move through the blood vessels without adherence to the vascular endothelial cell layer. If cytokines (e.g. interleukin-1 (IL-1), tumour necrosis factor (TNF), IL-8, etc.) are produced in the extravascular space due to, for example, infection or injury, this will cause the endothelial cells to synthesize and express (i.e upregulate expression) the endothelial adhesion molecules ICAM-1, VCAM-1 and E-selectin. Cytokines such as TNF-α can also upregulate the binding affinity of integrin receptors for vascular adhesion molecules by altering the conformation of the integrin (shown here as a change in receptor shape). The result of this upregulation of adhesion molecules is the binding of leukocytes to the vascular endothelial cell layer followed by extravasation of the cells to the site of infection or injury. In slightly more detail, the function of E- and P-selectin (which bind to carbohydrates on leukocytes) is to slow down the rapidly moving leukocytes so that they can be finally halted by interaction between the β_2-integrins and ICAM/VCAM. This is then followed by the passage of the leukocyte through the vascular endothelial barrier.

Briefly, the selectins on the surface of vascular endothelial cells act to bind to carbohydrate antigens, such as Sialyl-Lewis^x on the surface of circulating leukocytes. These low-affinity interactions slow down the leukocytes and cause them to roll along the vascular cell wall at sites of inflammation. The leukocytes are caused to stop rolling by the binding of the β_2-integrins on the leukocyte membrane to ICAM or VCAM on the endothelial cell. This then starts the process by which leukocytes cross the vascular cell barrier in the process known as diapedesis. Once in the underlying connective tissue, leukocytes are trapped by the binding of another set of receptors called β_2-integrins, which have an affinity for the proteins of the connective tissue matrix, for example collagen.

Cytokine-stimulated eicosanoid synthesis

In the 1930s it was reported that human semen and extracts of ovine seminal vesicular glands contracted smooth muscle. Von Euler identified the active component as a fatty acid and, because of the similarity of the vesicular gland to the human prostate, coined the term prostaglandin for the active principle.[53] However, it was not until the 1960s that the structure of the prostaglandins was elucidated and they were shown to be 20-carbon fatty acids containing a cyclopentane ring[54,55] (Fig. 1.4). The prostaglandins are synthesized by enzymatic metabolism of fatty acids (and in particular, arachidonic acid,[54] which, as it contains 20-carbon atoms and four double bonds, is termed eicosatetraenoic acid) present in the phospholipids which form the cell

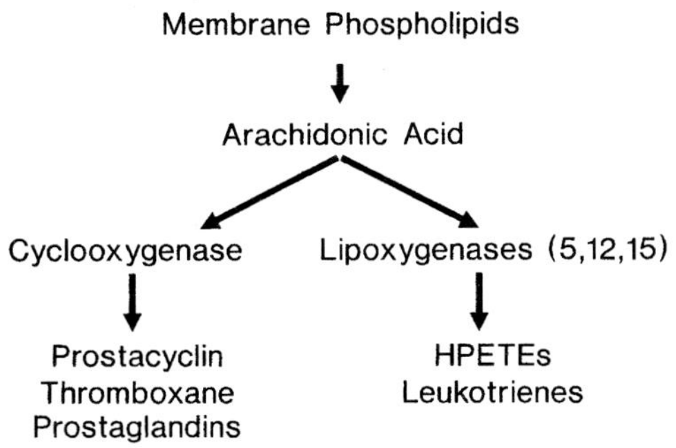

Fig. 1.4 Pathways of arachidonic acid metabolism. The cyclooxygenase pathway (which is inhibited by aspirin-like drugs) produces the prostanoids. The 5-lipoxygenase pathway generates 5-hydroperoxyeicosatetraenoic acid (HPETE) and the leukotrienes.

membranes. Arachidonic acid is acted upon by the enzyme cyclooxygenase, to generate the prostaglandins and the related lipid mediators, prostacyclin and thromboxane.[57] These lipid products are collectively termed the prostanoids. Cyclooxygenase is inhibited by the non-steroidal anti-inflammatory class of drugs, such as aspirin and ibuprofen, and this action accounts for their therapeutic efficacy (Fig. 1.4).

A second family of enzymes, termed the lipoxygenases, also metabolize arachidonic acid to produce a family of lipid metabolites.[58] The best known family of compounds are the leukotrienes, produced by the action of the enzyme 5-lipoxygenase (Fig. 1.4). Other lipoxygenases acting at the 12 or 15 position in arachidonic acid are known and their products are known to have important biological functions. Products of the action of cyclooxygenase and the lipoxygenases are collectively termed eicosanoids.

The eicosanoids have a wide range of actions and much of the pioneering work on these molecules was concerned with their proinflammatory activities. For example, prostaglandin E_2 and prostacyclin are potent vasodilators, being responsible for the erythema seen at sites of inflammation. Prostaglandins also enhance the action of inflammatory mediators which cause vascular permeability, such as bradykinin and histamine, and are therefore responsible for inflammatory swelling. The hyperalgesic activity of prostaglandins and prostacyclin has already been mentioned. The anti-inflammatory and analgesic activity of non-steroidal drugs is due to their inhibition of cyclooxygenase which prevents the synthesis of prostanoids at sites of inflammation. Unfortunately, these drugs do not inhibit the lipoxygenase pathways, which may account for their limited value in chronic painful hyperalgesic states.

The leukotrienes have a wide range of actions, including contraction of bronchial smooth muscle and stimulation of vasodilation in most blood vessels. Leukotriene B_4 is a potent chemoattractant for polymorphonuclear leukocytes. Products of the action of 12- and 15-lipoxygenases are also believed to contribute to tissue pathology. For example, 15-hydroperoxyeicosatetraenoic acid (15-HPETE) can induce a state of prolonged hyperalgesia, not associated with inflammation or tissue damage, by sensitizing peripheral nociceptors (see Chapter 23).

In addition to their proinflammatory actions, prostaglandins have long been known to effect bone remodelling. In more recent years, work from this laboratory has shown that leukotrienes are potent effectors of bone turnover. The role of eicosanoids in bone remodelling has been reviewed in Chapter 7. Eicosanoids are not produced constitutively but require cellular activation for their generation. Inflammmatory cytokines, such as IL-1 and TNF-α, are probably the most potent stimuli for the generation of prostanoids at sites of inflammation. In turn, prostaglandins can inhibit the synthesis of IL-1 and TNF by monocyte/macrophages. This suggests that there is a homeostatic feedback loop between inflammatory cytokines and prostanoids for regulating the synthesis of these two classes of potent inflammatory mediators (reviewed by Bomford and Henderson[13]).

One of the potentially most exciting developments in the field of eicosanoid metabolism has been the finding that mammals have two genes for cyclooxygenase (Cox). It now appears that Cox-1 is a constitutive enzyme crucially important in the maintenance of the blood flow in the stomach. The second form, Cox-2, is an inducible enzyme whose synthesis is regulated by LPS and proinflammatory cytokines (IL-1 and TNF).[59] This has engendered great excitement in the world's pharmaceutical companies because of the possibility of designing selective inhibitors of Cox-2, which would be free of the severe gastric side-effects which accompany administration of conventional NSAIDs such as ibuprofen. These drugs inhibit Cox-1 and -2, thus inhibiting inflammation but at the price of affecting stomach blood flow such that gastritis occurs. Selective Cox-2 inhibitors, in theory, should be anti-inflammatory but have no gastric side-effects.[60]

Cytokine-stimulated nitric oxide production

While botanists have known for some years about the importance of simple gases (e.g. ethylene $CH_2{=}CH_2$) in plant physiology, it is only in the last decade that the fascinating discovery has been made that the diatomic gas NO acts as an intercellular signalling molecule. This gas mediates a growing number of important biological functions in the mammal, including:

1. The bactericidal and tumoricidal activity of macrophages.[61–63]
2. Maintenance of normal vascular tone.[64]
3. Neuronal transmission.[65]

NO is synthesized from the essential amino acid arginine by the action of enzymes termed nitric oxide synthases (NOS). These enzymes generates NO and citrulline from arginine. Activated macrophages are major producers of NO. LPs and cytokines such as IFN-γ, IL-1 and TNF-α stimulate the expression of a calcium-independent NOS in these cells. The NO produced is cytotoxic for bacteria and this is believed to be a major pathway for host-defence killing of infectious agents. T-lymphocyte-derived lymphokines can induce NOS production in macrophages in the process of macrophage-induced tumour cell killing. It has also been reported that cytokines such as TNF-α, IL-6 and IL-2 have a negative inotropic effect due to their stimulation of the activity (but not synthesis) of myocardial NOS.[66]

The therapeutic potential of cytokine administration or inhibition

The dramatic growth of the biotech industry has been fuelled to a large extent by the therapeutic promise of the administration of certain cytokines and the inhibition of others. Indeed, the sheer complexity of the activities of certain cytokines has led some companies to argue that they can be used therapeutically while other companies are seeking to block the synthesis or action of the same cytokines. A classic example is IL-1. It is argued that IL-1 can be of therapeutic benefit in wound healing, protection from infections or as a radioprotectant (due to its ability to stimulate bone marrow progenitor cell growth). Equally, the case for blocking IL-1 synthesis or action is being pursued by a number of companies for the treatment of chronic inflammatory diseases in which there is tissue destruction, such as periodontal disease and rheumatoid arthritis.

Table 1.9 Therapeutic potential of cytokines

Cytokine	*Therapeutic activity*
IL-1	Wound healing, radioprotection, immune stimulant
IL-2	Stimulates tumour cell killing, vaccine adjuvant
IL-4	Similar to IL-2
IL-6	Antitumour, septic shock
TNF-α/β	Antitumour, wound healing
TGF-β	Wound healing
Interferons	Antiviral, anticancer
GM-CSF	Treatment for cancer patients undergoing chemo-/radiotherapy
Erythropoietin	Anaemia associated with kidney failure

IL = Interleukin; TNF = tumour necrosis factor; TGF-β = transforming growth factor-β; GM-CSF = granulocyte–macrophage colony-stimulating factor.

A list of cytokines which are in clinical use, undergoing clinical trials or of suggested clinical efficacy for various diseases is given in Table 1.9. The most successful of these to date has been the cytokine-like hormone erythropoietin which is in clinical use for the treatment of the debilitating anaemia which occurs in patients with kidney failure.

The inhibition of the inflammatory cytokines IL-1 and TNF is seen as a major therapeutic target for a range of inflammatory/destructive diseases and septic shock. There have been a number of distinct approaches taken to block the activity of these cytokines. At the present time the most promising are neutralizing antibodies; soluble receptors and natural antagonists. It has recently been shown that monocytes and other cells produce a protein with the property of antagonizing the binding of IL-1 to its receptors on cells. This molecule, termed IL-1ra, binds to IL-1 receptors on cells but fails to trigger any cellular response. Because IL-1ra has a similar affinity for binding to the IL-1 receptors as does IL-1, it antagonizes binding and thus blocks the activity of IL-1. IL-1ra has been in clinical trial for septic shock, rheumatoid arthritis and inflammatory bowel disease but has not shown its expected therapeutic benefit.[17] However, the use of a chimeric neutralizing antibody to TNF-α has shown substantial clinical benefit in patients with rheumatoid arthritis.[67,68]

Conclusions

The study of cytokines is in its infancy and we are still finding 5–10 new cytokines a year. It is clear that these variegated molecules play pivotal roles in body homeostasis and are prime movers in tissue pathology, ranging from infections to cardiovascular and cerebral diseases and cancers. The key to understanding cytokines lies in comprehending how they interact with cells to form the networks of interactions which correspond to health or disease.

Cytokines or inhibitors/antagonists of cytokines will be found in increasing numbers in the clinic in years to come. In dentistry, the clinical problems of wound healing, of inflammation and of cancer require a better understanding of the biology of cytokines to appreciate the biological mechanisms underlying these pathological processes and the potential of the new pro- or anticytokine therapeutics.

Acknowledgements

We are grateful to the Arthritis and Rheumatism Council for Research for financial support.

References

1. Bernard C. *An Introduction to the study of Experimental Medicine* (trans;ated by H. C. Breen). New York: Dover Publications, 1957.
2. Bayliss WB, Starling EH. On the causation of the so called 'peripheral reflex secretion of the pancreas' *Proc R Soc Lond* (Biol.) 1902; **69**: 325.
3. Henderson B, Poole S. Modulation of cytokine function: therapeutic applications. *Adv Pharmacol* 1994; **25**: 53–115.
4. Atkins E. Fever: Historical aspects. In Bomford R. & Henderson B. (eds). *Interleukin-1, Inflammation and Disease*, pp. 3–15. Amsterdam: Elsevier, 1989.
5. Bennett IL, Beeson PB. Studies on the pathogenesis of fever I and II. *J Exp Med* 1953; **98**: 477–508.
6. Atkins E, Wood WB. Studies on the pathogenesis of fever. I. The presence of transferable pyrogen in the blood stream following the injection of typhoid vaccine. *J Exp Med* 1955; **101**: 519–528.
7. Kampschmidt RF, Upchurch HF. Lowering of plasma iron concentration in the rat with leukocytic extracts. *Am J Physiol* 1969; **216**: 1287–1291.
8. Gery I, Gershon RK, Waksman BH. Potentiating of the T-lymphocyte response to mitogens. I. The responding cell. *J Exp Med* 1972; **136**: 128-142.
9. Beeson PB. Temperature-elevating effect of a substance obtained from polymorphonuclear leukocytes. *J Clin Invest* 1948; **27**: 524 (abstract).
10. Dayer J-M, Breard J, Chess L, Krane SM. Participation of monocyte-macrophages in the production of a factor that stimulates collagenase and prostaglandin release by rheumatoid synovial cells. *J Clin Invest* 1979; **64**: 1386-1392.
11. Saklatvala J, Dingle JT. Identification of catabolin, a protein from synovium which induces degradation of cartilage in organ culture. *Biochem Biophys Res Commun* 1980; **96**: 1225–1231.
12. Lomedico PT, Guebler U, Hellmann CP *et al.* Cloning and expression of murine interleukin-1 cDNA in *Escherischia coli. Nature* 1984; **312**: 458–461.
13. Bomford R, Henderson B (eds) *Interleukin-1, Inflammation and Disease.* Amsterdam: Elsevier, 1989.
14. Reibman J, Meixler S, Lee TC *et al.* $TGF\beta_1$, a potent chemoattractant for human neutrophils, bypasses classic signal transduction pathways. *Proc Natl Acad Sci USA* 1991; **88**: 6805–6809.
15. Meager A. *Cytokines.* Milton Keynes: Open University Press,1990.
16. Ibelgaufts H. *Dictionary of Cytokines.* Weinheim: VCH Press, 1995.
17. Henderson B, Bodmer M. *Therapeutic Modulation of Cytokines.* Boca Raton: CRC Press, 1996.
18. Oppenheim JJ, Zachariae COZ, Mukaida N, Matsushima K. Properties of the novel proinflammatory supergene 'intercrine' cytokine family *Annu Rev Immunol* 1991; **9**: 617–648.
19. Dinarello C. Fever. In: Bomford R, Henderson B (eds) *Interleukin-1, Inflammation and Disease*, pp. 175–190. Amsterdam: Elsevier, 1989.
20. Rosen V, Thies RS. The BMP proteins in bone formation and repair. *Trends in Genetics* 1992; **8**: 97–102.
21. Henderson B, Edwards JCW, Pettipher ER. *Models and Mechanisms in Rheumatoid Arthritis.* Academic Press: London, 1995.
22. Kjeldsen M, Holmstrup P, Bendtzen K. Marginal periodontitis and cytokines: a review of the literature. *J Periodontol* 1993; **64**: 1013–1022.
23. Dinarello CA, Ikejima T, Warner SJC *et al.* Interleukin-1 induces interleukin-1. *J Immunol* 1987; **139**: 1902–1910.

24. Henderson B, Pettipher ER. Arthritogenic actions of recombinant IL-1 and TNF-α in the rabbit: evidence for synergistic interactions between cytokines *in vivo*. *Clin Exp Immunol* 1989; **75**: 306-310.
25. Chandrasekhar S, Harvey AK. Transforming growth factor β is a potent inhibitor of IL-1 induced protease activity and cartilage proteoglycan degradation. *Biochem Biophys Res Commun* 1988; **157**: 1352-1359.
26. Dewhirst FE, Ago JM, Peros WJ, Stashenko P. Synergism between parathyroid hormone and interleukin-1 in stimulating bone resorption in organ culture. *J Bone Min Res* 1987; **2**: 127.
27. Oster W, Herrmann F, Lindemann A, Mertelsmann R. Experimental and clinical evaluation of erythropoietin. In Habenicht A (ed) *Growth Factors, Differentiation Factors and Cytokines*, pp. 232–242. Berlin: Springer-Verlag, 1990.
28. Glauser MP, Heumann D, Baumgartner JD, Cohen J. Pathogenesis and potential strategies for prevention and treatment of septic shock: an update. *Clin Infect Dis* 1994; **18**: S205–S216.
29. Kovacs EJ. Fibrogenic cytokines: the role of immune mediators in the development of scar tissue. *Immunol Today* 1991; **12**: 17–23.
30. Carney D, Sikora K (eds) *Genes and Cancer*. Chichester: Wiley, 1990.
31. Rubartelli A, Sitia R. Interleukin-1β and thioredoxin are secreted through a novel pathway of secretion. *Biochem Soc Trans* 1991; **19**: 255–259.
32. Thornberry NA, Bull HG, Calaycay JR *et al.* A novel heterodimeric cysteine protease is required for interleukin-1β processing in monocytes. *Nature* 1992; **356**: 768–774.
33. Sims JE, March CJ, Cosman D *et al.* cDNA expression cloning of the IL-1 receptor, a member of the immunoglobulin superfamily. *Science* 1988; **241**: 585–589.
34. Tewari A, Buhles WC, Fletcher Starnes H. Preliminary report: effects of interleukin-1 on platelet counts. *Lancet* 1990; **ii**: 712–714.
35. Iizumi T, Sato S, Iiyama T *et al.* Recombinant human interleukin-1β analogue as a regulator of haematopoiesis in patients receiving chemotherapy for urogenital cancers. *Cancer* 1991; **68**: 1520–1523.
36. Arend WP. Interleukin-1 receptor antagonist: a new member of the interleukin-1 family. *J Clin Invest* 1991; **88**: 1445–1451.
37. Boyce BR, Yates AJP, Mundy GR. Bolus injection of recombinant human interleukin-1 causes transient hypercalcaemia in normal mice. *Endocrinology* 1989; **125**: 2780–2783.
38. Pettipher ER, Henderson B. Inflammatory activities of locally or systemically administered interleukin-1. In: Bomford R, Henderson B (eds) *Interleukin-1, Inflammation and Disease*, pp. 217–228. Amsterdam: Elsevier, 1989.
39. Wedmore CV, Williams TJ. Control of vascular permeability by polymorphonuclear leukocytes in inflammation. *Nature* 1981; **289**: 646–650.
40. Ferreira SH, Nakamura M. Pathogenesis and pharmacology of pain. In: Weissmann G, Samuelsson B, Paoletti R (eds) *Advances in Inflammation Research*, pp. 317–329. New York: Raven Press, 1979.
41. Ferreira SH, Lorenzetti BB, Bristow AF, Poole S. Interleukin-1β as a potent hyperalgesic agent antagonized by a tripeptide analogue. *Nature* 1988; **334**: 698–700.
42. Follenfant RL, Nakamura-Craig M, Henderson B, Higgs GA. Inhibition by neuropeptides of interleukin-1β-induced prostaglandin-independent hyperalgesia. *Br J Pharmacol* 1989; **98**: 41-43.
43. Cunha FQ, Lorenzetti BB, Poole S, Fereirra SH. IL-8 as a mediator of sympathetic pain. *Br J Pharmacol* 1991; **104**: 765–767.
44. Saklatvala J. Interleukin-1 and connective tissue. In: Bomford R, Henderson B (eds) *Interleukin-1, Inflammation and Disease*, pp. 143–162. Amsterdam: Elsevier, 1989.
45. Pettipher ER, Higgs GA, Henderson B. Interleukin-1 induces leukocyte infiltration and cartilage proteoglycan degradation in the synovial joint. *Proc Natl Acad Sci USA* 1986; **83**: 8749–8753.
46. Tyler J. Influence of interleukin-1 and insulin-like growth factor on the integrity of cartilage matrix. In: Glauert AU (ed) *The Control of Tissue Damage*, pp. 197-219. Amsterdam: Elsevier, 1988.
47. Raines EW, Dower SK, Ross R. IL-1 mitogenic activity for fibroblasts and smooth muscle cells is due to PDGF-AA. *Science* 1989; **243**: 393–394.
48. Todd RF, Freyer DR. The CD11/CD18 leukocyte glycoprotein deficiency. *Haematol/Oncol Clin North Am* 1988; **2**: 13–31.
49. Pardi R, Inverardi L, Bender JR. Regulatory mechanisms in leukocyte adhesion: flexible receptors for sophisticated travellers. *Immunol Today* 1992; **13**: 224–230.
50. Shimuzu Y, Newman W, Tanaka Y, Shaw S. Lymphocyte interactions with endothelial cells. *Immunol Today* 1992; **13**: 106–112.
51. Harlan JM, Liu DY (eds). *Adhesion: its role in Inflammatory Disease*. New York: Freeman, 1992.
52. Kishimoto T, Rothlein R. Integrins, ICAMs, and selectins: role and regulation of adhesion molecules in neutrophil recruitment to inflammatory sites. *Adv Pharmacol* 1994; **25**: 117–169.
53. Von Euler US. On the specific vaso-dilating and plain muscle stimulating substance from accessory genital glands in man and certain animals (prostaglandin and vesiglandin). *J Physiol* 1937; **88**: 213–220.
54. Bergstrom S, Sjovall J. The isolation of prostaglandin F from sheep prostate glands. *Acta Chem Scand* 1960; **14**: 1693–1700.
55. Bergstrom S, Sjovall J. The isolation of prostaglandin E from sheep prostate glands. *Acta Chem Scand* 1960; **14**: 1701–1708.
56. Van Dorp DA. Aspects of the biosynthesis of prostaglandins. *Prog Biochem Pharmacol* 1967; **3**: 71–82.

57. Samuelsson B, Goldyne M, Granstrom E, Hamberg M, Hammarstrom S, Malmsten C. Prostaglandins and thromboxanes. *Annu Rev Biochem* 1978; **47**: 997–1029.
58. Parker CW. Lipid mediators produced through the lipoxygenase pathway. *Annu Rev Immunol* 1987; **5**: 65–84.
59. Hla T, Neilson K. Human cyclooxygenase-2 cDNA. *Proc Natl Acad Sci USA* 1992; **89**: 7384–7388.
60. Vane JR, Botting RM. New insights into the mode of action of anti-inflammatory drugs. *Inflamm Res* 1995; **44**: 1–10.
61. Liew FY. Role of cytokines in killing of intracellular pathogens. *Immunol Lett* 1991; **30**: 193–197.
62. Nathan C. Mechanisms and modulation of cytokine activation. *Behring Inst Mitt* 1991; **88**: 200–207.
63. Li LM, Kilbourn RG, Adams J, Fidler IJ. Role of nitric oxide in lysis of tumor cells by cytokine-activated endothelial cells. *Cancer Res* 1991; **51**: 2531–2535.
64. Lowenstein CJ, Dinerman JL, Snyder SH. Nitric oxide: a physiologic messenger. *Ann Int Med* 1994; **120**: 227–237.
65. Bredt DS, Snyder SH. Nitric oxide, a novel neuronal messenger. *Neuron* 1992; **8**: 3–11.
66. Finkel MS, Oddis CV, Jacob TD, Watkins SC, Hattler BG, Simmons RI. Negative inotropic effects of cytokines on the heart mediated by nitric oxide. *Science* 1992; **257**: 387–389.
67. Elliott MJ, Maini RN, Feldmann M *et al.* Randomized double-blind comparison of chimeric monoclonal antibody to tumour necrosis factorα (cA') versus placebo in rheumatoid arthritis. *Lancet* 1994; **344**: 1105–1110.
68. Henderson B. Therapeutic modulation of cytokines. *Ann Rheum Dis* 1995; **54**: 519–523.

2

The application of molecular genetics to orofacial and dental disorders

Nicholas J. Lench

Introduction*

One of the most important advances in clinical science has been the application of molecular genetics which offers new insights into the mechanisms of dental, oral and facial development. These complex events involve many cell types and the coordinated expression of multiple genes. The study of genetic disorders in which developmental defects occur as a consequence of single-gene mutations, enables the dissection of the molecular events that produce the complex biological structures of the head and face. The techniques used to identify and isolate genes involved in selected developmental disorders and tumour growth are reviewed. A glossary of terms used in molecular genetics is provided at the end of this book to help those unfamiliar with this field.

The central dogma of molecular biology is that the deoxyribose nucleic acid (DNA) of the cell nucleus produces ribonucleuic acid (RNA) which in turn produces the vast number of proteins present both within cells and in the extracellular matrices of the body. The genetic information in all eukaryotic cells (i.e those containing a nucleus) is contained within the biomolecule DNA. DNA is a double-stranded helical molecule consisting of a sugar and phosphate backbone to which are linked four different ring-shaped molecules called bases: adenine (A), cytosine (C), guanine (G) and thymine (T), which project into the centre of the double helix (Fig. 2.1).

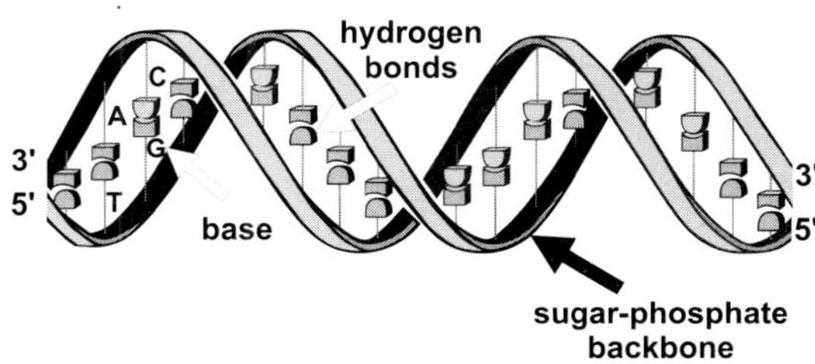

Fig. 2.1 Diagrammatic representation of the DNA double helix. Complementary base-pairing occurs between bases adenine (A) and thymine (T) and cytosine (C) and guanine (G). The deoxyribose sugars forming the DNA backbone are covalently joined to each other by phosphodiester bonds.

It is these bases that facilitate storage and transmission of the genetic information coded by the DNA. The two DNA chains in the double helix are held together by hydrogen bonds and hydrophobic interactions. The bases on opposite strands have a precise relationship in which A is always paired with T (by two hydrogen bonds) and G is always paired with C (joined by three hydrogen bonds). Accurate copying of these so-called complementary base pairs during DNA synthesis and replication, ensures that genetic information is faithfully inherited by daughter cells from parent cells.

Cellular DNA is packed very tightly into structures called chromosomes and human cells contain 23 pairs of chromosomes which vary in size, and therefore, DNA content. Each chromosome is essentially a single continuous molecule of double-stranded DNA that contains functional gene sequences

*The Glossary (p. 330) might be helpful.

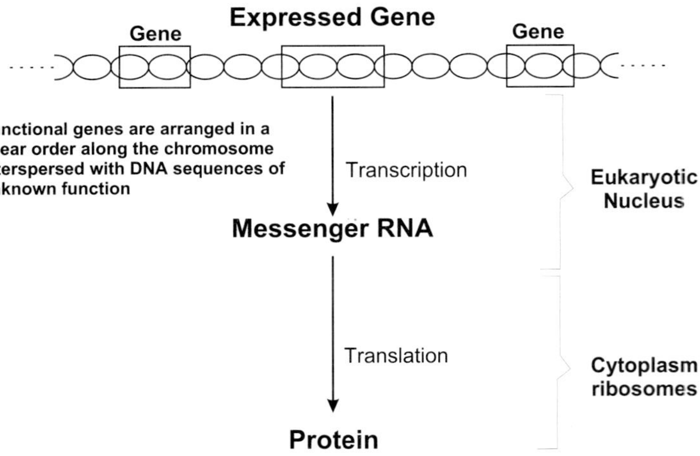

Fig. 2.2 Genes are arranged in a linear order along the chromosome, interspersed with DNA sequences of unknown function. Individual genes are expressed via transcription of the DNA template to form single-stranded messenger RNA molecules. These are translocated to the cytoplasmic ribosomes where they are translated into proteins.

arranged along its length, interspersed with DNA of unknown function. The genes specify the individual proteins that are made by cells but, as stated, DNA is not the direct template for protein synthesis. The templates for protein synthesis are molecules of ribonucleic acid (RNA). Several types of RNA exist in cells, the major species being: 1) messenger RNA (mRNA), 2) transfer RNA (tRNA), and 3) ribosomal RNA (rRNA). Messenger RNA is copied from the nuclear DNA sequences by enzymes called RNA polymerases in a process known as transcription. The mRNA is then used as a template for protein synthesis in the cytoplasm of the cell. This translation of the mRNA into protein is mediated by transfer RNA molecules. tRNAs translocate specific amino acids to the cytoplasmic ribosomes where they are incorporated into the growing protein molecule (Fig. 2.2).

Thus, the genetic code is determined by the sequence of bases in the DNA of a gene (or its mRNA transcript) which in turn is translated into the sequence of amino acids in the protein. This code, which is similar in all organisms, is made up of a series of triplets of bases known as codons. Each codon specifies one of the 20 amino acids used to form all of the proteins in a cell. Therefore, the gene and its transcribed mRNA can be viewed as a collection of sequential bases arranged in groups of three. Each triplet can bind to a complementary tRNA which, in turn carries the amino acid coded for by that triplet. The ribosomal RNA ensures that each new amino acid is bonded to the preceding amino acid to form a linear sequence of amino acids that constitutes the primary protein structure determined by the gene. It has been estimated that there are approximately 100 000 functional gene sequences in the human haploid genome, representing a mere 5% of the total genome size. The haploid genome is present in the germ (egg and sperm) cells and contains approximately 3×10^9 DNA base pairs (bp). During fertilization, an egg cell and sperm cell fuse to form a zygote and the resulting diploid genome contains 46 chromosomes (22 pairs of autosomes and one pair of sex chromosomes: X X – females; XY – males).

There are many agents that cause damage to DNA, including exposure to ionizing radiation and chemical carcinogens. If the damage is not repaired, and the DNA sequence is altered, a mutation is said to have occurred. If the mutation occurs in the germ cells it can be stably inherited and passed on from generation to generation. The majority of mutations are point or frameshift mutations (Fig. 2.3). In point mutations a base pair is changed so that the genetic code is altered. Due to the triplet nature of the genetic code, this can change the

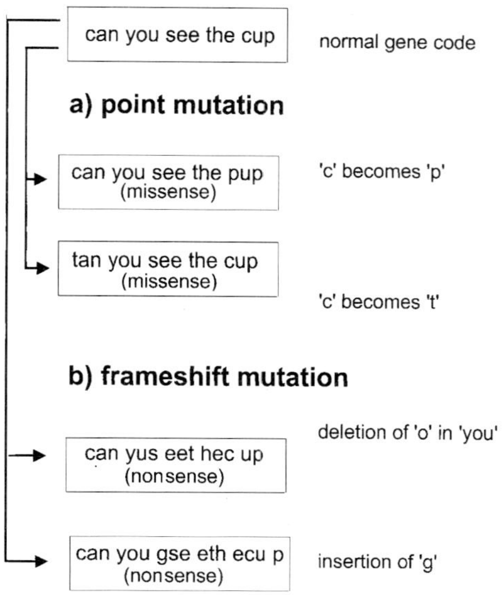

Fig. 2.3 Most genetic aberrations arise from point mutations or frameshift mutations.

amino acid specified by the codon. Frameshift mutations occur when one or more base pairs are deleted or inserted in a gene sequence so that the code is read in the wrong frame. Therefore, the amino acid content of the protein produced is completely different and cannot function properly. Occasionally, the DNA sequence of a functional gene is altered by mutation, and as a result, the function of the protein is impaired or abolished. If the protein is essential for cell viability then the consequences for the cell – and indeed the entire organism – can be catastrophic.

Molecular genetics enables the identification and isolation of genes responsible for inherited disorders, the characterization of the causative mutation(s) and an understanding of the function of the normal and abnormal proteins. Recent advances in molecular genetics now make it possible to identify and clone gene loci on the basis of their chromosomal location in the human genome. This technique, known as positional cloning, can be used to identify genes that are involved, for example, in orofacial development and inherited cancers.

Recombinant DNA technology

Recombinant DNA technology has revolutionized biochemistry by providing a powerful means of analysing and altering genes and their protein products. The molecular biologists' 'tool-kit' contains many enzymes that are used to manipulate DNA. Of these, the most important are the enzymes that cut (restriction enzymes), join (ligases) and replicate (polymerases) DNA and RNA. A brief description of some of the fundamental tools and techniques[6] used in gene mapping follows.

Restriction enzymes

Restriction enzymes, also known as restriction endonucleases, are enzymes that recognize and cleave at specific base sequences in double-helical DNA molecules. These enzymes occur naturally within bacteria, where their function is to protect the bacterium by degrading 'foreign' DNA carried into the cell by infecting viruses. The bacterium's own DNA is chemically modified to protect it from degradation by endogenous restriction enzymes. Many restriction enzymes have now been purified from different bacteria and are available commercially. Restriction enzymes cut at specific DNA sequences called restriction sites, and each enzyme has its own unique restriction site. This is usually between four to six bp in length. A particular restriction enzyme will cut a double-stranded DNA molecule into a series of discrete restriction fragments of different sizes. Depending on where the enzyme cuts within the restriction site, the resulting restriction fragments will have cohesive ends or blunt ends. Restriction fragments with cohesive ends can be joined to any DNA fragment that has a cohesive end generated by digestion with the same restriction enzyme. This process is facilitated by complementary base-pairing between the two fragments. Similarly, a blunt-ended DNA fragment can be joined to any other blunt-ended DNA fragment. Thus, recombinant DNA molecules can be made by joining different DNA restriction fragments.

DNA cloning

The basic steps in cloning DNA are shown in Figure 2.4:

1. The construction of a recombinant molecule. DNA molecules can be inserted into the

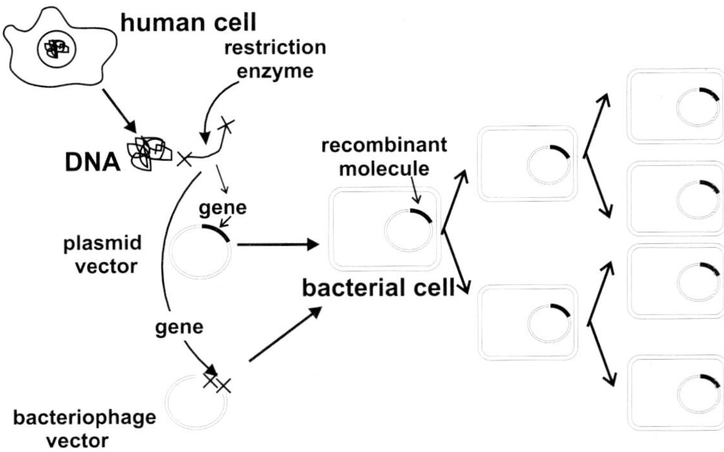

Fig. 2.4 A simplified diagram representing the basics of cloning a human gene. Genomic DNA is isolated, purified and cut into small pieces using restriction endonucleases. Recombinant DNA molecules are then constructed by the ligation of insert and vector DNA fragments and introduced into bacterial cells by transformation.

genomes of self-replicating, extra-chromosomal genetic elements (cloning vectors). A recombinant molecule is formed when a DNA restriction fragment (insert) is covalently joined (ligated) to a vector. Many different cloning vectors are available.[1–5] The major difference between them is their cloning capacity. This refers to the length of insert DNA that can be ligated to the vector. This can range from < 100 base pairs to more than 3×10^6 bp DNA. Bacterial plasmids are the most commonly used cloning vector. These genetic elements occur naturally and are responsible for conferring antibiotic resistance to bacteria. Other vectors include bacteriophages (viruses which infect bacteria), cosmids and bacterial, yeast and mammalian artificial chromosomes.

2. The recombinant DNA molecule is introduced into host cells. Many bacterial and eukaryotic cells can be induced to take up recombinant DNA molecules capable of independent replication within the host cell. This process is known as transformation. A clone of bacteria containing the recombinant DNA molecule serves as a factory for the production of unlimited amounts of the recombinant DNA fragment. In this way multiple copies of the DNA sequence of interest are produced. Bacterial colonies containing recombinant DNA clones can be identified. Recombinant DNA molecules are then selectively isolated from the bacteria and used for gene analysis.

DNA libraries

In order to identify and isolate a specific gene or DNA sequence from a complex mixture of DNA (e.g. total genomic DNA from a whole cell) it is necessary to construct an appropriate DNA library. A DNA library is a collection of all the DNA (both genes and non-coding DNA of unknown function) of the cell's genome. By analogy with a conventional library, one can think of the total genome as a collection of 24 encyclopaedias of DNA (one for each chromosome). Each encyclopaedia will have millions of letters (A,C,G,T) spread over many thousands of pages representing the unique DNA sequence of each chromosome. A single gene may only be present on one page of an encyclopaedia demonstrating the difficulty of finding single gene sequences. The magnitude of the task can be reduced if the starting material for library construction is DNA from a single chromosome. It would then only be necessary to search one volume of an encyclopaedia. Alternatively, a complementary DNA (cDNA) library can be constructed. This consists of every gene sequence that is actively expressed by a given cell type (i.e. only those genes that are being transcribed). In this way, all the non-coding 'junk' DNA is excluded from the library. The encylopaedia will then contain many fewer pages. Of the 100 000 genes present in the human genome, only a small proportion are transcribed at any one time by any particular cell type. To obtain this cDNA library, total RNA is extracted from the cells of interest and mRNA selectively isolated. The mRNA is then converted into cDNA by a special enzyme called reverse transcriptase which synthesizes DNA from a RNA template.

The DNA from which the library is made, is digested with restriction enzymes and cloned into an appropriate vector. Conditions are optimized to favour the formation of enough recombinant molecules to represent the entire starting DNA at least once. The vectors containing the multitude of DNA fragments are then introduced into the host bacteria by transformation. The next problem is to recognize the bacterial colony containing the gene of interest. The library is screened for the DNA sequence of interest by hybridization to an appropriate DNA probe. The DNA probe is able to recognize the gene sequence of interest (target sequence) by complementary base-pairing. If the DNA probe is radioactively labelled with ^{32}P-phosphorus, then positively hybridizing bacterial clones (i.e. those containing the gene of interest) can be identified by autoradiography. Other screening protocols involve the use of specific antibodies that bind to the recombinant proteins produced by the bacteria in the library. Here one uses a modification of immunocytochemical techniques to detect the colony containing the DNA sequence of interest.

Gel electrophoresis and blotting of nucleic acids

DNA fragments can be separated by size using gel electrophoresis. In general, polyacrylamide gels are used to analyse DNA fragments less than 1000 bp in size, and agarose gels are used for DNA fragments greater than 1000 bp. The gel is submerged in an electrolyte buffer and a current passed across the gel. DNA is negatively charged and therefore, migrates towards the anode, the smaller molecules migrating fastest. Following electrophoresis, DNA is stained with ethidium bromide, a fluorescent dye, and viewed under ultraviolet (UV) light. A stable 'copy' of the gel is made by transferring the DNA to a nylon or nitrocellulose membrane. These membranes have a high affinity for single-stranded DNA and RNA. DNA is denatured to single strands by soaking the gel in alkali and then neutralized. During blotting, osmotic pressure of a salt solution is used to draw transfer buffer through the gel and moves the DNA out of the gel and on to the membrane. The DNA is then irreversibly bound to the membrane by baking or exposure to UV light. This transfer of DNA is commonly known as Southern blotting (Fig. 2.5); the same process with RNA is known as northern blotting.

Nucleic acid hybridization (Fig. 2.5)

Double-stranded DNA is denatured by heating to 100°C or by exposure to very high pH (>13). The resulting complementary single strands of DNA are able to reassociate in aqueous solution at 65°C, a process known as nucleic acid hybridization. This hybridization will occur between any two single strands of nucleic acids (e.g. DNA:DNA, RNA:RNA, DNA:RNA) provided they have complementary nucleotide sequences. Specific DNA or RNA sequences can be analysed in this way. For example, a Southern blot of digested genomic DNA containing a gene sequence present in only one copy per haploid genome can be detected by hybridization with a complementary labelled DNA sequence (DNA probe) (Fig. 2.5). The DNA probe hybridizes by complementary base-pairing with the corresponding DNA sequence immobilized on the membrane. Following hybridization, non-specifically-bound DNA is washed off the membrane and the genomic DNA fragment complementary to the DNA probe is detected by autoradiography.

Other nucleic acid hybridization techniques are available that identify the location of complementary mRNA within tissues (tissue RNA hybridization) or the location of gene sequences on metaphase chromosome spreads (*in situ* hybridization).

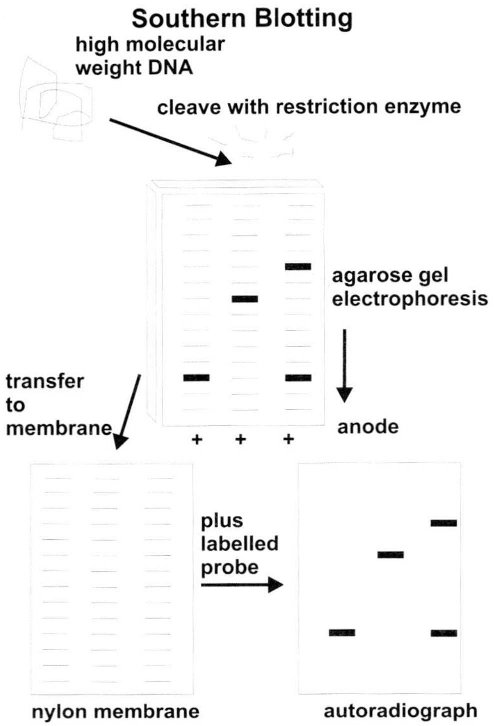

Fig. 2.5 To determine if a particular stretch of DNA is present in the genomic DNA of a particular organism (or individual) the procedure known as Southern blotting is used. The DNA is cleaved into small pieces by restriction endonucleases and these are separated on the basis of their molecular mass (i.e. size) by electrophoresis in agarose gels. A characteristic pattern of DNA bands (restriction fragments) is produced which represent a restriction map of the DNA. To determine if the DNA of interest is present in this large collection of restriction fragments, the DNA is transferred (blotted) on to nitrocellulose or nylon membranes and incubated with a radioactively tagged piece of complementary DNA or RNA. After appropriate washings the membrane is then exposed to a photographic film. If there has been specific binding of the labelled DNA, by the process termed hybridization, then a dark line (or in this example, lines) will be seen on the film.

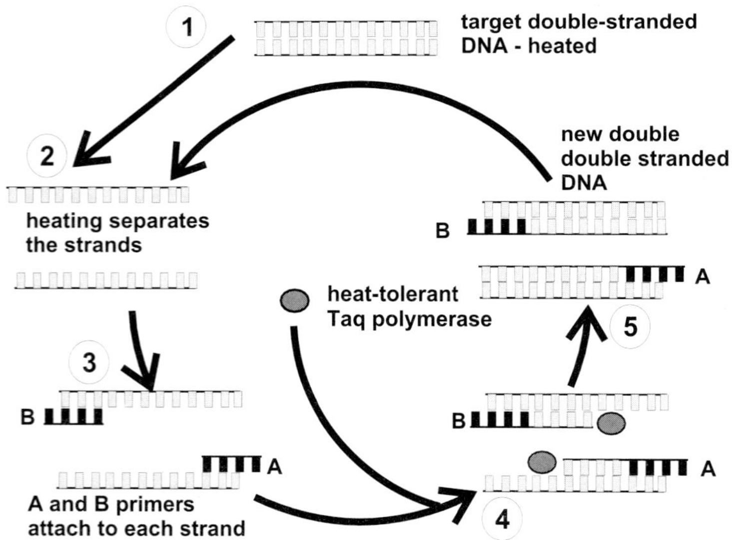

Fig. 2.6 The polymerase chain reaction (PCR) begins with the denaturation of DNA to form two single strands. This is followed by the addition of two short strands of complementary DNA known as primers, which bind (anneal) to complementary bases, here shown as A and B. Once bound, the enzyme Taq. DNA polymerase can then add bases to synthesize (extend) a double strand of DNA beginning from the primer. The end-result is two double strands of DNA. The process is repeated many times (usually 35–40).

The secret of the PCR methodology is that the polymerase used is heat-stable. This is essential, as once the polymerase has made a segment of double-stranded DNA beginning from the primer, the DNA needs to be heated to make further single-stranded DNA, thus allowing the primers to rebind, beginning a new cycle in which the DNA is replicated. The procedure becomes one in which there is denaturation of the DNA, binding of the primers and synthesis (extension) of new DNA. In practice, this is performed in an automated heating block which can heat and cool rapidly.

Polymerase chain reaction

The polymerase chain reaction (PCR)[7] is an *in vitro* method for producing many thousands of copies (amplification) of a DNA sequence (Fig. 2.6). This is achieved by heat denaturation of a target DNA sequence producing two single-stranded DNA molecules. Short, synthetic oligonucleotide primers (single-stranded DNA moleucules about 20 bases in length) are able to anneal (bind) to their DNA complement by specific base pair interactions. DNA synthesis is then directed from these annealed primers using a heat stable enzyme, *Taq* DNA polymerase. The resultant products serve as templates for further primer annealing and DNA synthesis, and so by cycling the PCR through three basic steps of DNA denaturation, DNA primer annealing and DNA synthesis, it is possible to obtain an exponential increase in the amount of target DNA sequence produced. The intrinsic DNA sequence-specificity of the reaction (i.e. A-T and G-C base pairing) makes PCR an exquisitely sensitive technique. Provided sufficient DNA sequence data are available to design oligonucleotide primers, single copy sequences can be amplified from genomic DNA, cloned DNA and mRNA via a cDNA intermediate produced by reverse transcriptase. Amplification can be achieved from multiple copies of template as well as from single copies present in complex mixtures of molecules. PCR has revolutionized biology – it is now a commonly used technique that has many applications in diverse disciplines such as molecular biology, molecular genetics, pathology, medicine, forensic science, evolutionary biology and archaeology.

Gene mapping

The isolation of a disease gene proceeds through a series of well-defined steps[8] (Fig 2.7). The disease locus is first localized to a specific human chromosome and then genetic and physical mapping techniques are used to narrow the physical limits of the DNA region likely to contain the gene. Numerous inherited disorders with oral–facial–dental anomalies have already been mapped to specific human chromosomes and, in certain cases, the underlying gene mutation(s) characterized (Table 2.1).[9,10]

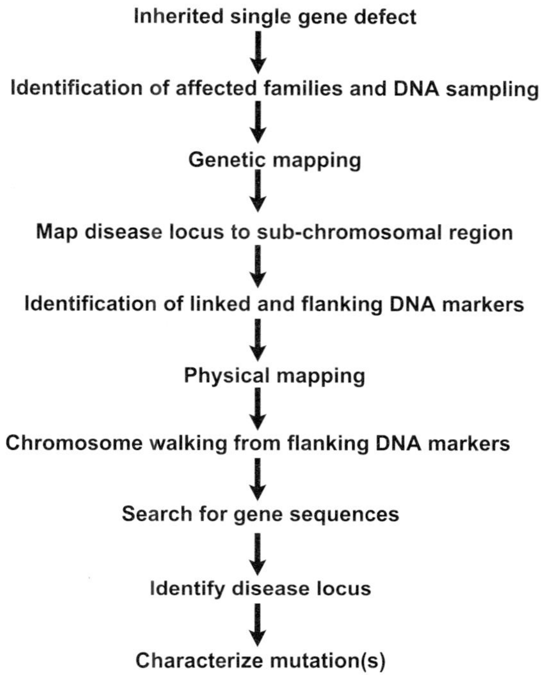

Fig. 2.7 Flow chart outlining the major steps involved in gene isolation using positional cloning techniques.

Genetic linkage mapping

Genetic linkage mapping is the determination of the linear arrangement of genes and DNA markers along a chromosome. During meiotic cell division homologous chromosomes pair with one another and allow the physical exchange of chromosomal material to occur. This is the mechanism by which genetic diversity is produced. Not all DNA sequences on the same chromosome are inherited together, although the closer two loci are, the more likely they are to be co-inherited. The further apart two genes are along the chromosome, the more likely it is that a physical exchange will occur in the region between them. This is known as a genetic cross-over, or recombination event. By estimating the relative frequency of recombination between gene loci, it is possible to determine their linear order along the chromosome (Fig. 2.8). Genes or DNA sequences on different chromosomes segregate independently during meiosis.

Linkage mapping in humans is hampered by the infeasibility of controlling matings, small

Table 2.1 Selected genetic disorders with oral–facial–dental anomalies for which gene localization is available

*Anomaly/Disease**	*Mode of inheritance*	*Chromosomal defect location**	*Gene*
Achondrogenesis	AR	12q14.3	COL2A1
Amelogenesis imperfecta	XL	Xp22.1-22.3	AMGX
Cleft lip and palate 1	A	2p	
Cleft lip and palate 2	A	10q23	
Cleft palate and ankyloglossia	XL	Xq21.3-22	
Coffin-Lowry syndrome	XL	Xp22	
Dentinogenesis imperfecta type I	AD	17q21.3-q22	COL1A1
		7q21.3-q22.1	COL1A2
Dentinogenesis imperfecta type II	AD	4q12-q23	
Dentinogenesis imperfecta type III	AD	4q12-q23	
Epidermolysis bullosa dystrophica	AR	11q21-q22	
Gardner syndrome	AD	5q21-q22	
Gorlin syndrome	AD	9q22.3-q31	patched
Gorlin–Goltz syndrome	XL	Xp22.31	
Hypohydrotic ectodermal dysplasia	XL	Xq12.2-q13.1	
Hypophosphatasia	A	1p36.1-p34	
Orofacial cleft	A	6pter-p21.3	
Stickler syndrome	AD	12q14.3	COL2A1
Treacher Collins	AD	5q23-q34	treacle
Van der Woude syndrome 1	AD	1q32-q41	
Van der Woude syndrome 2	AD	2q34-q36	
Zellwegger syndrome	AR	7q11.23	

*Detailed descriptions of these conditions and information regarding genetic localization can be found in reference 9.
A = Autosomal; D = dominant; R = recessive; XL = X-linked.
COL1A1 = proα-1 chain collagen type I; COL1A2 = proα-2 = chain collagen type I; COL2A1 = proα-2 chain collagen type II; AMGX = amelogenin.

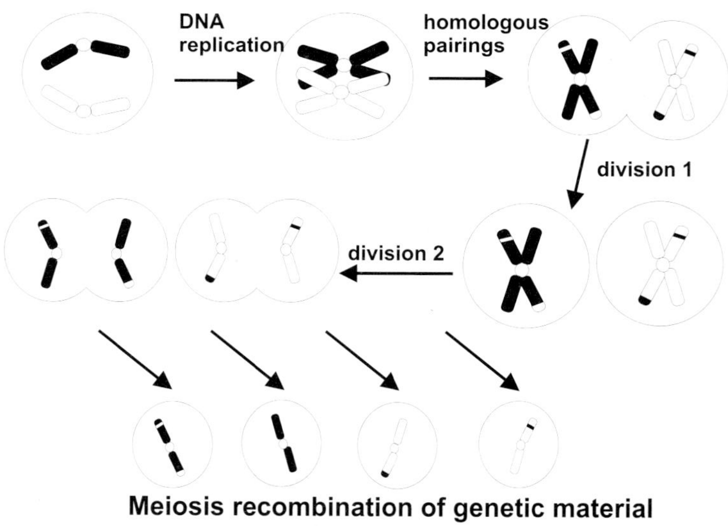

Fig. 2.8 Meiosis showing recombination of genetic material

numbers of offspring, and the large generation times required. Extended, multigeneration families are the most effective resource for human genetic linkage studies. However, two-generation family data are often all that is available, and so the number and size of families available will determine the outcome of the genetic linkage study. During a genetic linkage study, blood samples are collected from all the family members and DNA is isolated from the white blood cells. This genomic DNA is hybridized to the DNA markers under study and genotypings obtained. The results are analysed to determine the ratio of recombinants to non-recombinants, and a linkage map constructed.

DNA markers

Using recombinant DNA technology it is possible to isolate specific DNA sequences from known regions of the human genome. These cloned DNA sequences are called DNA markers, and are used as landmarks from which a complete genetic and physical map of each chromosome can be established. Ideally, a physical map consists of a set of overlapping DNA markers stretching from one end of the chromosome to the other. This is one of the goals of the Human Genome Project and already, overlapping clones have been isolated for the entire long arm of human chromosome 21[11] and a large region of the Y chromosome.[12]

Restriction fragment length polymorphisms

Double-stranded DNA is cut at specific sequences by restriction enzymes. The variation of natural DNA sequences within the population (polymorphism) means that occasionally the number of restriction sites for a particular enzyme will differ from individual to individual. A given site for a restriction enzyme will be present in one person's DNA, but absent in another's. Consequently, the resulting restriction fragments produced following digestion of the DNA with the restriction enzyme will differ in size from person to person. This is called a restriction fragment length polymorphism (RFLP). To visualize a RFLP, it is necessary to use a DNA probe that is contained on, or overlaps with, one of the restriction fragments whose length is altered by the polymorphism. The variant restriction fragments identified by the DNA probe represent different alleles of the RFLP (Figs 2.9 and 2.10). Polymorphic DNA markers are an essential tool of gene mapping because they can be used to study the pattern of inheritance in families with a certain disease, and to determine if the gene causing that disease is in the same chromosomal region as the polymorphic DNA marker (Fig. 2.11).

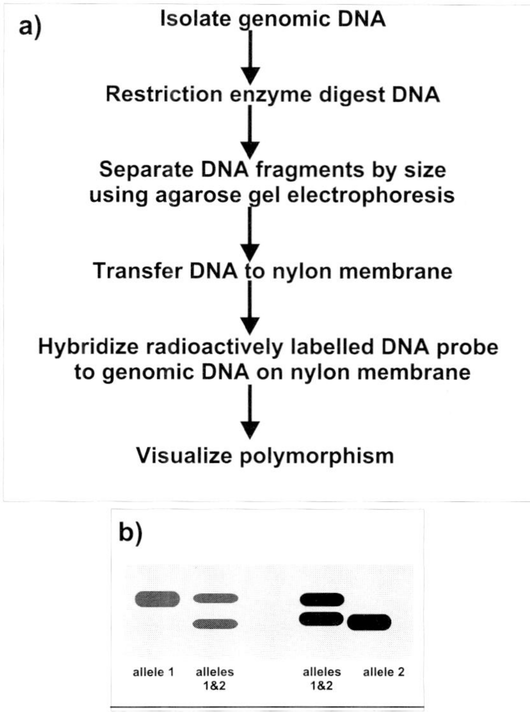

Fig. 2.9 (a) Flow chart outlining experimental techniques involved in restriction fragment length polymorphism (RFLP) detection. (b) Human genomic DNA samples following restriction enzyme digestion and agarose gel electrophoresis. Polymorphic restriction fragments are visualized following hybridization and autoradiography.

In general, most RFLPs exhibit two alleles with only two variant forms within the population; allele 1 and allele 2 (representing the absence and presence of the polymorphic restriction site respectively). Consequently the possible combinations of the two alleles are the genotypes 1/1, 1/2 and 2/2 (analogous to –/–, –/+, +/+). This hinders genetic linkage analysis because it is not always possible to determine the parental origins of each allele inherited by the affected individual. This is important because it is necessary to establish which parental chromosome carries the gene(s) causing the disease. By using DNA markers that detect multiple alleles, it is likely that one will be able to determine the parental origin of a given allele. This problem has been overcome by the development of highly polymorphic DNA markers that detect multiple alleles (microsatellites markers, VNTR

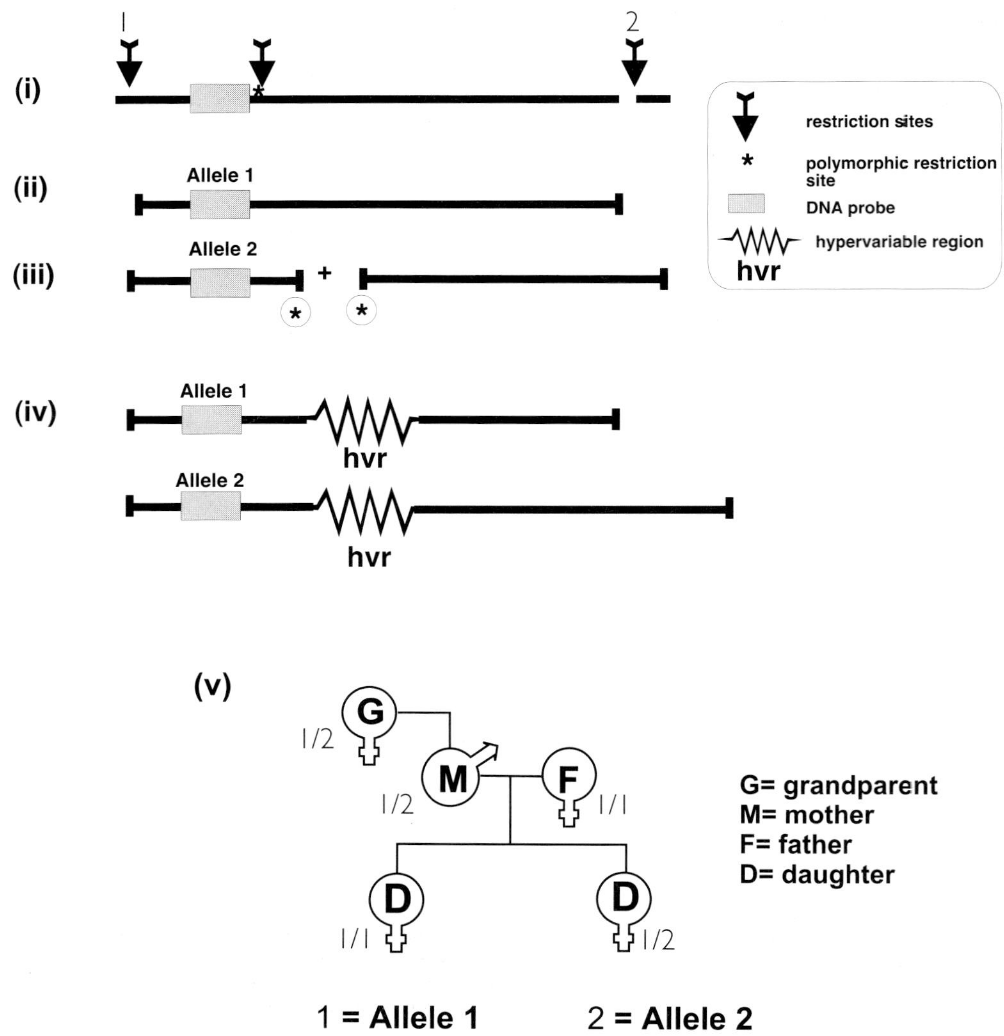

Fig. 2.10 In some individuals, additional restriction sites (*) will be present on one or both chromosomes, These are called polymorphic restriction sites. This can be seen in:

(i) Region of genomic DNA containing polymorphic restriction site (*).
(ii) Restriction fragment produced by cutting at sites 1 and 2. The entire fragment will hybridize to the DNA probe, and this represents allele 1 of the restriction fragment length polymorphism (RFLP).
(iii) Restriction fragments produced by cutting at sites 1 and 2 when the polymorphic site is present on the chromosome. Note that only the smaller of the two fragments will hybridize to the DNA probe; this represents allele 2 of the RFLP.
(iv) A polymorphism may also arise through the occurrence of tandem pairs of silent bases called hypervariable regions. Note that the restriction sites remain the same.
(v) Hybridization of a radioactively labelled DNA probe to restriction enzyme digested genomic DNA from a family allows visualization of the polymorphic bands using autoradiography. Normal Mendelian inheritance of polymorphic DNA marker alleles is demonstrated.

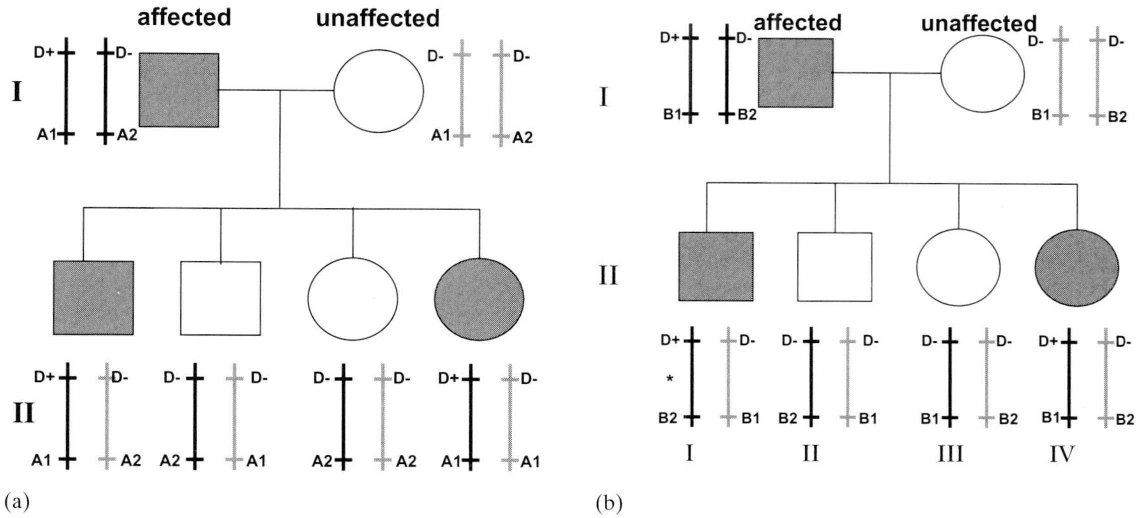

Fig. 2.11 Genetic linkage mapping.
(a) Genetic analysis of marker A in family 1. If a dominant disease locus (D) is flanked by two DNA markers A and B, which have alleles A1, A2 and B1, B2 respectively, it is possible to determine which of the two markers is closer to the disease locus by using genetic linkage mapping.
Where D+ is the dominant disease allele, and D– the normal non-disease allele, then the corresponding genotypes and phenotypes will be:

Genotype	Phenotype
D+/D+	affected
D+/D–	affected
D–/D–	unaffected

There are no recombination events between marker A and the disease locus.
(b) Genetic analysis of marker B in Family 1. A recombination event* has occurred between marker B2 and the disease locus D+ in individual II-I. Allele B2 is co-segregating with the disease allele D+ and not allele B1 as is the case in the affected father I-I, and affected sibling II-III. It can be concluded that marker A is closer to the disease locus than marker B, because marker A does not show a recombination event with the disease locus.

markers).[13–15] Thousands of polymorphic DNA markers are now available that cover large regions of the 22 autosomes and sex chromosomes.[16] Genetic linkage maps are available for each individual human chromosome which facilitate the positioning of new loci within the framework of existing genetic maps. Thus, these maps can be used for navigation of the human genome by molecular geneticists.

Physical mapping – isolation of the chromosomal region of interest

Having established the genetic linkage of a DNA marker to a disease locus at a specific chromosomal location (Fig. 2.12), it is necessary to move from the marker to the gene itself. This can be established by various means. The principle is to isolate closer and closer DNA markers from a known starting point(s). The isolation of an ordered set of overlapping DNA markers is called chromosome walking (Fig. 2.13). It is advantageous to have flanking DNA markers, thereby having a reference point on either side of the gene of interest and a definition of the physical limit (i.e. size of DNA fragment in base pairs) in which the gene must reside. The correlation between genetic and physical distance varies from chromosome to chromosome, as well as between different regions of the same chromosome. However, for

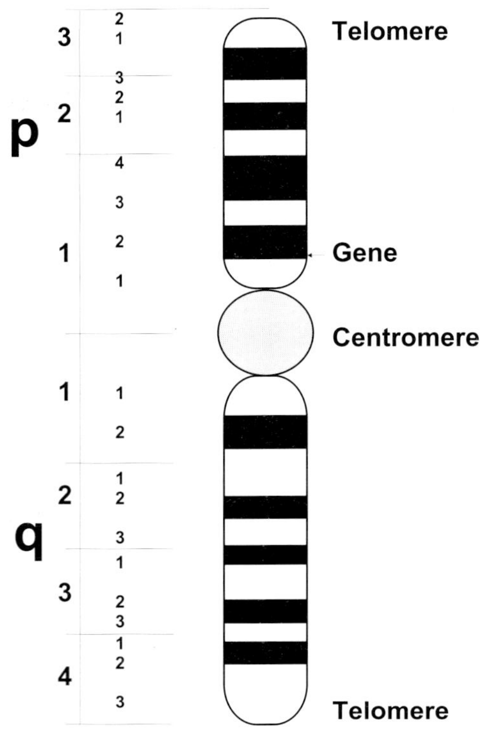

Fig. 2.12 Schematic diagram of a human chromosome. p is the short arm of the chromosome and q is the long arm. Each chromosome can be divided into regions, which in turn can be subdivided into bands. These provide internationally standardized cytogenetic map coordinates for the localization of genes and DNA markers. For example, the gene locus marked Gene is at p12 – where p is the short arm, region 1 band 2.

DNA markers also have a standardized nomenclature system. Each DNA segment is assigned a D number.For example, DXS17 represents a DNA segment D, on the X chromosome, S segment, number 17 (the 17th anonymous DNA marker isolated from the X chromosome). As new markers are isolated they are assigned the next D number in sequence. At the Human Gene Mapping Conference HGM11 (1991), 727 anonymous DNA segments had been reported on the human X chromosome.

most purposes one can assume that 1% recombination is equal to approximately one million base pairs of DNA. Construction of physical maps of specific chromosomal regions is possible using pulsed-field gel electrophoresis.[17] This technique allows the separation of very large fragments of DNA ($50\,000 - 5 \times 10^6$ bp) that are produced by restriction enzymes that cleave the DNA double helix very infrequently. The identification of a number of large restriction fragments that include the linked DNA markers enables the assembly of a restriction fragment map of the area containing the gene of interest.

Although the isolation of genetically linked markers can substantially limit the amount of DNA to be analysed, the distances involved may still be extremely large. Therefore, to reduce the complexity of the DNA sequences to be analysed, a hybrid somatic cell line[18,19] is produced that contains the chromosomal region of interest. In general, these cell lines contain a single human chromosome, or a region of chromosome, maintained in a rodent cell. This means that a normal rodent cell line is capable of accepting a foreign human chromosome as though it was its own genetic material. This cellular manipulation can be used to produce a 'panel' of somatic cell hybrids each containing a different human chromosome. This can be extended further, by producing cell lines with progressively smaller regions of a given chromosome. Each cell line is tested for the presence or absence of DNA markers linked to the gene of interest, which delineates the area encompassed by the DNA markers to a specific chromosomal region or sub-region. From these cell lines, DNA can be used to construct genomic DNA libraries representing the chromosomal region containing the gene. Having established the physical boundaries of the chromosomal region, one can then 'chromosome walk' from both ends by isolating new DNA markers from the libraries. The markers are genetically and physically mapped and the whole process repeated until a region containing the gene is selected.

Identification of gene sequences

Once DNA markers have been isolated that are linked genetically and physically to the gene under investigation, it is necessary to search that region of DNA for coding gene sequences. The DNA sequences that code for proteins can be recognized by numerous methods.

1. Genomic DNA clones can be used to screen complementary DNA libraries (cDNA) constructed from messenger RNA isolated from tissues known to express the genetic defect.

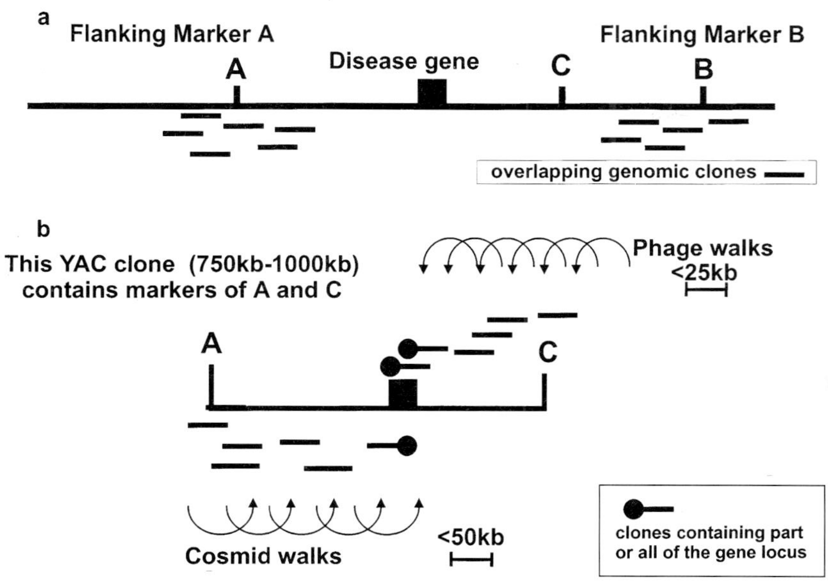

Fig. 2.13 Chromosome walking using different cloning vectors to locate a disease locus. (a) Genetic linkage mapping is first used to determine that markers A and B flank the gene locus. Chromosome walking from markers A and B using short overlapping walks isolates DNA markers that are closer to the disease locus.
(b) Using yeast artificial chromosomes (YAC) cloning vectors carrying large inserts of DNA (e.g. 150–1500 kb), it is possible to isolate the marker C that is located on the opposite side of the gene locus from A. Therefore, this large DNA insert contains the actual gene locus. A new round of shorter chromosome walking can now begin from A (cosmid walks) and backwards from C (phage walks) until a region small enough to search for gene sequences is isolated.

2. Coding sequences can also be identified by cross-species homology. This involves hybridization of genomic DNA sequences to 'zoo blots' containing DNA from diverse animal species. If a protein has been functionally conserved throughout evolution, then homology between species will be detected at the DNA sequence level. For example, all eukaryotic species contain the skeletal protein actin. Actin genes have been highly conserved throughout evolution and actins from diverse species such as yeast and chicken display 90% DNA sequence homology.
3. Many genes are associated with regions of DNA that are unusually rich in the dinucleotide CpG clustered together in structures called 'HTF-islands';[20] so called, because digestion with the restriction enzyme *HpaII* produces *t*iny *f*ragments. Therefore, HTF islands can be regarded as flags that mark the precise location of gene sequences within the genome. By cutting DNA with restriction enzymes that only recognize these HTF-islands it is possible to screen genomic DNA for the presence of gene sequences.

Having identified a DNA sequence, it is then necessary to prove that this gene is causal in the pathology of the disease under investigation. This is by no means a simple task, and many complementary approaches are used. Cells known to express the genetic defect are tested for expression of the 'candidate gene sequence'. Cells from disease-affected tissues are examined for qualitative and quantitative alterations in gene expression. The candidate gene DNA sequence is analysed for causative mutations – point mutations, deletions, insertions, duplications and inversions. If such a mutation is found, it is then necessary to demonstrate that it is inherited in a Menedelian manner. Many sophisticated experimental techniques have been developed to identify and analyse DNA mutations.[21] In general, these methods serve to identify the DNA region containing the mutation. DNA sequencing, the elucidation of the linear order of DNA bases, is used to confirm the exact nature of the mutation.

Recent advances in mapping and identification of genes involved in human orofacial and dental anomalies

The methods described above can be applied to the investigation of genetic syndromes involving craniofacial and dental structures, and the following examples demonstrate the usefulness and importance of such techniques.

Cleft palate

Cleft palate and cleft lip are the most common congenital facial abnormalities. They can occur independently or together, and display sex-linked or autosomal inheritance. They are developmentally different, spatially, temporally and with respect to their developmental cell lineage. Cleft lip occurs as a result of non-fusion of the upper lip and anterior part of the maxilla, while cleft palate is caused by failure of fusion of the palatine processes. These events occur during weeks 5–7 and 7–12 of development respectively. The aetiology of these disorders is complex and both polygenic and multifactorial inheritance patterns have been proposed. Polygenic inheritance is due exclusively to the additive effects of more than one gene whereas multifactorial traits result from the additive effects of genetic and environmental factors. Analysis of these diseases by normal genetic linkage analysis is very difficult. At present the most practical approach of addressing the problems is to analyse pedigrees in which the complex disease phenotype is due to a single gene defect. To date, five pedigrees have been described in which cleft palate is unequivocally an X-linked trait. These include a single large Icelandic pedigree with over 280 individuals exhibiting X-linked secondary cleft palate and ankyloglossia (tongue-tie) CP + A.[22–25] The large size of the pedigree and the availability of many accurately mapped X chromosome polymorphic DNA markers, have facilitated mapping of the gene defect to the CP + A locus at Xq21.3–q22, between the markers DXYS12 and DXS17, a distance of approximately 5 million bp.[26,27]

It has been suggested that the cleft palate gene may be a member of a multigene family involved in embryonic development. These are genes with related functions whose coordinated expression give rise to a complex phenotype and may be clustered on one chromosome region as a supergene family. Cloning of the gene for X-linked cleft palate will therefore represent an important step towards understanding one of the processes controlling embryonic development.

Treacher Collins syndrome

Treacher Collins syndrome (TCS), also known as mandibulofacial dysostosis, is an autosomal dominant disorder of craniofacial development.[28] The major clinical features of TCS include abnormalities of the external ears, hypoplasia of the facial bones, particularly the mandible and zygomatic complex, downward slanting of the palpebral fissures and cleft palate. Genetic analysis of TCS is hindered by reduced penetrance of the gene and a high *de novo* mutation rate accounting for approximately 60% of all cases. Using 12 TCS families the TCS gene has been localized to chromosome 5q31–34, between the anonymous DNA marker D5S22 and the glucocorticoid receptor gene, a distance of approximately 9 million bp.[29]

The tissues affected in TCS are derived from the first and second branchial arches, therefore, it has been proposed that the condition may arise from abnormal neural crest cell migration[30] (see Chapter 3). Facial development involves the interaction of growth factors and extracellular matrix proteins, and anomalies in either of these molecules could play a role in the molecular pathology of TCS.[31] It is noteworthy that the genes for the glucocorticoid receptor,[32,33] platelet-derived growth factor receptor,[34] acidic fibroblast growth factor[35] and osteonectin[36] map to this region of chromosome 5 and are candidate genes for the Treacher Collins syndrome. A candidate gene is defined as one in which there is a biochemical, genetic or epidemiological reason to believe that mutation of its DNA sequence may cause or contribute to the genetic component or clinical phenotype of the disease. In a linkage analysis using polymorphic gene probes, one would expect to see absolute linkage between the candidate gene probe and the disease allele(s). If the chromosomal location of a disease locus is known, and the candidate gene profile also maps to the same chromosome, then the argument for involvement of the candidate gene is increased. Restriction fragment length polymorphisms identified by the glucocorticoid and osteonectin receptors were analysed in TCS families. However, recombination events were detected between each of these genes and the TCS locus, thus excluding them as the defective genes in TCS. The subsequent isolation of new polymorphic DNA markers allowed the region containing the TCS locus to be narrowed even further. The isolation of gene sequences from this region led to the identification of a new gene of unknown function called treacle. DNA analysis of the treacle gene in five unrelated TCS patients revealed the presence of different mutations causing premature truncation of the treacle protein. Therefore, this is compelling evidence that treacle is causal in the molecular pathology of Treacher Collins syndrome.[37]

Hereditary defects of tooth enamel and dentine

Amelogenesis imperfecta

Amelogenesis imperfecta (AI) represents a heterogeneous collection of human genetic disorders causing both hypoplastic and hypomineralized enamel formation that display autosomal dominant, autosomal recessive or X-linked inheritance.[38,39] Amelogenins are heterogeneous extracellular matrix proteins of dental enamel that are transiently, but abundantly expressed during tooth development. The amelogenin protein comprises approximately 90% of the entire enamel matrix and plays a major role in enamel biomineralization. Human, mouse and bovine amelogenin cDNA clones have been isolated and characterized.[40–42] In humans, two amelogenin genes have been cloned and mapped to the X and Y chromosomes – AMGX and AMGY. Both genes show extensive DNA and protein homology with each other, and also with the mouse and bovine sequences, again showing conservation of function of the amelogenin protein throughout evolution.

In X-linked hypoplastic amelogenesis imperfecta, affected males exhibit uniformly thin and smooth enamel, whereas females have alternating bands of hypoplastic and near normal enamel. By contrast, in the X-linked hypomineralized form, enamel thickness lies within normal limits but is soft and mottled in appearance. In both cases the enamel wears away quickly and easily, causing severe dental attrition if early interventive treatment is not administered. The penetrance of the disease in clinically affected females varies significantly between individuals of the same family and also between individuals from different families. Also, it is apparent that enamel hypoplasia and hypomaturation are not always mutually exclusive. Both phenotypes can occur within the same individual but with one condition predominating.

Initial studies of two X-linked AI families using 11 polymorphic X chromosome DNA markers demonstrated linkage of the disease locus to the marker DXS85 at Xp22.[43] Subsequently, the human amelogenin gene AMGX was cloned and localized to Xp22.1–p22.3, suggesting that this gene was defective in patients exhibiting X-linked forms of amelogenesis imperfecta.[44] A deletion of approximately 5 kb, removing exons 3–6 and intervening intron sequences, was identified in a family with hypomineralized X-linked AI following hybridization with an AMGX gene probe. However, a second family exhibiting hypoplastic XAI did not have the deletion.[45] This implies the existence of genetic heterogeneity. Indeed, mutations in the AMGX gene have been described in different families with concurrent features of enamel hypoplasia and hypomineralization.[46,47] In general, these mutations cause the introduction of a premature stop codon leading to production of a shortened, non-functional (or only partially functional) amelogenin protein. Further genetic linkage studies have also provided evidence of a second amelogenin locus at Xq22–28.[48]

Dentinogenesis imperfecta

Dentinogenesis imperfecta (DI) is an inherited defect of dentine affecting both primary and secondary dentition. DI can be associated with osteogenesis imperfecta, DI type I, or can occur as an independent trait, DI type II, also known as hereditary opalescent dentine. A third form of the disease, DI type III, is classified by a rare condition known as the 'Brandywine isolate'. This is thought to be an allelic variant of DI type II (i.e. a different mutation occurring in the same gene). All forms of DI are inherited as autosomal dominant traits. DI is characterized by opalescent or translucent teeth that discolour with age. The teeth have short roots and show obliteration of the pulp chambers and canals shortly after eruption. The enamel tends to chip away from the underlying dentine at an early stage and the teeth are prone to severe attrition.[49] Histologically, the dentine has a laminated appearance, with the bulk of circumpumpal dentine consisting of short segments of abnormally shaped tubules distributed in an atypical granular basophilic dental matrix. The dentine, though mineralized, has a low inorganic content when compared to normal teeth.[50]

DI type I

Osteogenesis imperfecta (OI) is a heterogeneous group of inherited disorders characterized by bone fragility and connective tissue abnormalities with highly variable degrees of severity.[51] The condition affects approximately 1/10 000 individuals and autosomal dominant OI almost always results from mutations in the genes that encode the chains of type I collagen – the major structural protein of bone and dentine.[52] Collagen gene expression is tissue-specific; precisely how expression is controlled by odontoblasts during dentine development is poorly understood. It is predicted that mutations altering type I collagen synthesis will affect normal dentine development. The genes for the collagen type I α-1 and α-2 chains have been identifed, cloned and mapped as COL1A1 on chromosome 17 and COL1A2 on chromosome 7. To date, over 70 mutations have been identified in these two genes, all of which adversely affect the assembly or processing and secretion of the collagen triple helix.[53]

DI type II

Patients exhibiting DI type II show no signs of a generalized connective tissue disorder. Initial linkage studies have shown the DI-II locus to be located on the long arm of chromosome 4, being linked to the group-specific component Gc (vitamin D-binding protein).[54] Deletion mapping and *in situ* hybridization studies with the cloned Gc cDNA probe placed the locus at 4q11–q21.1.[55,56] It is possible that defects of non-collagenous proteins of the dentine extracellular matrix such as dentine phosphoprotein (DPP; dentine phosphophoryn) may contribute to the disease phenotype. DPP is the major non-collagenous protein of dental extracellular matrix and histological studies indicate that teeth from DGI-II patients lack phosphophoryns.[57,58] However, it has been shown that DPP does not map to chromosome 4, excluding it as the defective gene in DI-II.[59]

Tumour suppressor genes

The retinoblastoma – susceptibility gene Rb

The existence of tumour suppressor genes was predicted by Knudson[60] over 20 years ago during his studies of retinoblastoma, a syndrome characterized by retinal tumours. Knudson noted that retinoblastomas could be inherited, or occur sporadically, but clinically and histologically the tumours were indistinguishable. The inherited tumours were often multiple, pathologically more aggressive, and on average, occurred earlier. Knudson proposed that these tumours developed when both chromosomal copies of an antiretinoblastoma (tumour supressor) gene were lost from retinal cells. Therefore, in patients with the inherited form of the disease, one initial loss is inherited as a mutation in the germ cell line (e.g. point mutation) and every cell is affected

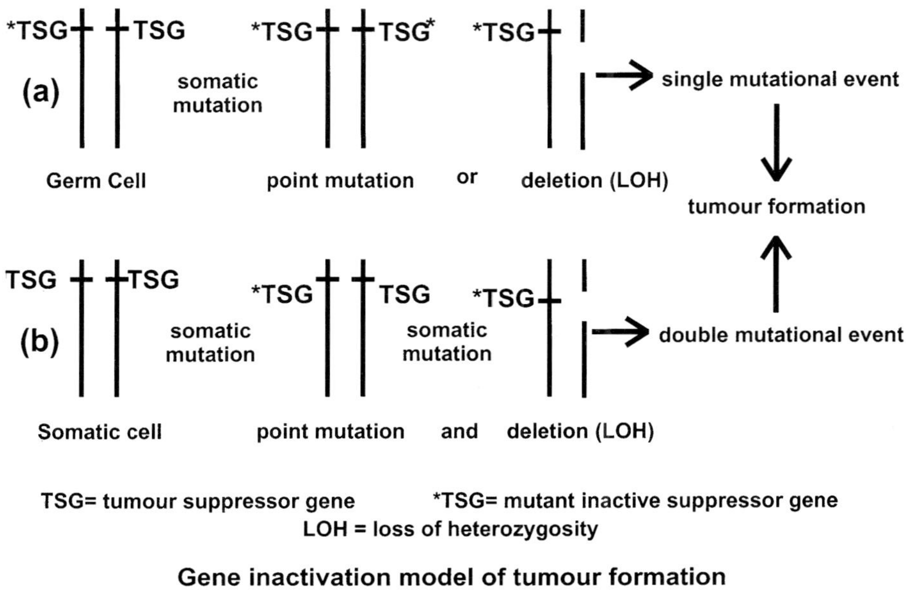

Fig. 2.14 Knudson's tumour suppressor gene (TSG) theory.
In its normal state, the TSG acts as an antioncogene by regulating cell growth and differentiation. If both alleles are inactivated by mutation (*), then tumour formation ensues. In hereditary forms of the disease, a pre-existing gene mutation is passed on through the germ cell line. Therefore, only one somatic cell mutational event is required for tumour formation. In spontaneous tumours, two independent mutational events are required.

in the target tissue. Consequently, only one further mutational event (e.g. a chromosomal deletion) is required to inactivate the second copy of the gene, thus making the cell homozygously inactivated for the tumour suppressor gene (Fig 2.14). Cell growth is then deregulated and tumour formation ensues. In sporadic cases, two consecutive independent events are required to inactivate both copies of the tumour suppressor gene in the same target cell. Rb gene inactivation is also associated with bone and soft-tissue sarcomas, breast, lung, prostate, bladder and various lymphomas.

The identification and diagnosis of oral carcinomas are particularly important to the oral pathologist. At present, the multistep processes involved in tumour development and progression are poorly understood. However, significant progress has been made in elucidating the role of the p53 tumour suppressor gene in human neoplasms, and in the identification of a gene on human chromosome 9 that is implicated in Gorlin syndrome.

Gorlin syndrome

Gorlin syndrome (also known as naevoid basal cell carcinoma syndrome) is an autosomal dominant disorder that predisposes to tumours, in particular basal cell carcinomas (BCCs) of the skin.[61] Multiple BCCs occur following brief exposure to ionizing radiation and appear relatively early compared to sporadic tumours of the same type. Other prominent features of the disease include recurrent multiple jaw keratocysts and congenital malformations (calcification of the corpus callosum, spine abnormalities, bifid ribs). Clearly, the complex varied forms of this syndrome suggests that under normal circumstances, the causative genes play an important role in early embryonic development and continued cell growth and differentiation. Cancer predisposition observed in Gorlin syndrome patients has led to the suggestion that the defective gene involved may be a tumour suppressor gene, i.e antioncogene. Under normal circumstances, the presence of a particular tumour suppressor gene product is

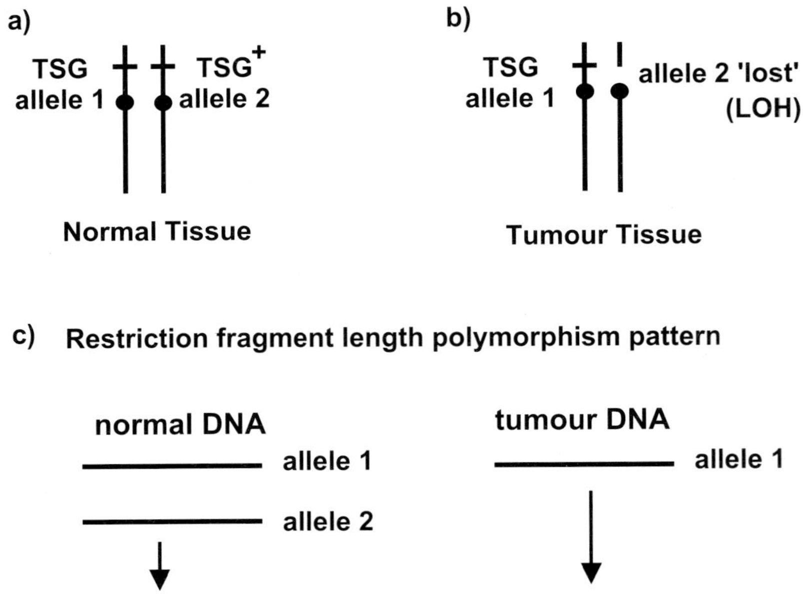

Fig. 2.15 Identification of a tumour suppressor gene (TSG) by demonstration of loss of heterozygosity for a closely linked polymorphic DNA marker, shown as a filled circle (●). (a) Allele 2 of the polymorphic DNA marker is lost due to deletion of a region of the chromosome containing the DNA marker and the normal copy of the tumour suppressor gene (TSG+)
(b) Using restriction fragment length polymorphisms of known chromosomal location in normal tissue, it is possible to analyse tumour DNA for loss of allele 2.

essential to maintain control of normal growth and differentiation of a particular cell type.

Genetic linkage studies have localized the gene for Gorlin syndrome to human chromosome 9q22.3–q31, closely linked to the DNA markers D9S12 and D9S5359[62,63] – an interval of approximately 6 million bps. In normal, non-cancerous cells, both copies of the Gorlin syndrome gene will be present and functional. However, if one copy of the gene is inactivated by a mutation, and the second copy of the gene is then deleted, homozygous inactivation will occur (Fig. 2.14). Deletion of the normal allele of the Gorlin gene can be detected using RFLPs known to map to the same chromosomal region as the Gorlin syndrome locus (9q22.3–q31). DNA from non-tumour cells, such as circulating blood lymphocytes, is genotyped with polymorphic DNA markers to localize alleles 1 and 2 (Fig. 2.15). Markers that detect these heterozygous alleles are then used to type the tumour cell DNA. If the region of one chromosome containing the polymorphic DNA markers is deleted, then this is detected by loss of the allele, and only the remaining chromosome allele is observed. This is referred to as loss of heterozygosity (LOH) for a given DNA marker. It is important that when tumours are used for DNA analysis, surrounding stromal tissue is not included. Otherwise genetic alterations in tumour cell DNA will be masked by the presence of DNA from admixed normal tissues.

Tumour DNA obtained from hereditary and sporadic basal cell carcinomas from Gorlin and non-Gorlin patients, was screened for LOH using 33 RFLPs from 22 autosomes.[64] Allelic loss of heterozygosity for 5 RFLP mapping to chromosome 9 was found in 72% of tumours analysed. The area of overlap for these markers included the DNA marker D9S29 located at 9q22.3 and all the hereditary tumours studied showed allelic loss of heterozygosity at this locus. Loss of heterozygosity at 9q22.3, implies that the Gorlin gene is homozygously inactivated, particularly in hereditary tumours, and normally functions as a tumour suppressor gene. In contrast, multiple congenital malformations caused by defective early embryonic development could be due to hemizygous germ cell line mutations of the gene. It is clear that the region 9q22.3 plays a critical role in normal cell development, growth and differentiation. Identification and isolation of genes from this region may be crucial to the understanding of early embryonic development and the mechanisms of carcinogenesis. Indeed, a gene from chromosome 9q22.3 has recently been identified called patched that is altered in DNA from Gorlin patients as well as in DNA isolated from sporadically occurring basal cell carcinomas.[65]

p53

The tumour suppressor gene p53 is implicated in the majority of human malignancies, both spontaneous and inherited.[66] About 50% of all human cancers contain a mutation in p53. It is postulated that uncontrolled cell proliferation and dedifferentiation in cancers follow a common pathway and altered p53 function is a possible cause. p53, so called because it is a 53 kDa, acts as a transcription factor (i.e. switches certain genes on), and binds to genes responsible for inhibiting cell growth. p53 is a potent inhibitor of oncogenic transformation and, under normal circumstances, is able to suppress cell growth in response to DNA damage by ionizing radiation and/or chemotherapeutic reagents, and can even induce programmed cell death (apoptosis). Inactivation of both p53 alleles by point mutations and/or chromosomal deletions has been observed in numerous tumours. The p53 gene contains four regions that are especially prone to mutation. Resulting mutant forms of p53 protein are unable to bind to p53 binding sites efficiently and the transcription of growth inhibitory genes is reduced or abolished. Certain viral proteins (e.g. from the *Herpes* virus) can induce cervical cancers by interacting with p53 protein. In this manner, transcription of growth-inhibitory genes by p53 is blocked. It is important to identify the genes that are transcriptionally activated by p53 protein in tumours cells of all types, and to identify pre-disposing genetic lesions. In this way, it will be possible to screen the population for individuals at risk of developing cancer.

Conclusions

It is clear that significant progress has already been made towards the isolation and identification of genes involved in facial clefting, facial development and tooth organogenesis. The concerted effort currently underway to map the entire human genome means that many more gene sequences will soon be available for analysis (currently 20 000 genes have been mapped to specific chromosomal locations). The characterization of gene products and definition of their structure and function will ultimately lead to a detailed understanding of the complex series of biological events that lead to the beautifully designed and exquisitely adapted orofacial structure. Analysis of the function of tumour suppressor genes and isolation of growth inhibitory genes will help dissect the multistep processes involved in tumorigenesis, with important consequences for cancer diagnosis and prognosis.

References

1. Cohen SN, Chang ACY, Boyer HW *et al.* Construction of biologically functional bacterial plasmids *in vitro*. *Proc Natl Acad Sci USA* 1973; **70**: 3240–3244.
2. Hohn B, Murray K. Packaging recombinant DNA molecules into bacteriophage particles *in vitro*. *Proc Natl Acad Sci USA* 1977; **74**: 3259–3263.
3. Collins J, Hohn B. Cosmids: a type of plasmid gene-cloning vector that is packageable *in vitro*. in bacteriophage λ heads. *Proc Natl Acad Sci USA* 1978; **75**: 4242–4246.
4. Sternberg N. Cloning high molecular weight DNA fragments by the bacteriophage P1 system. *Trends in Genetics* 1992; **8**: 11–16.
5. Schlessinger D. Yeast artificial chromosomes: tools for mapping and analysis of complex genomes. *Trends in Genetics* 1990; **6**: 248–258.
6. Sambrook J, Fritsch EF, Maniatis T (eds). *Molecular cloning: a laboratory manual* (2nd edition). New York: Cold Spring Harbor Laboratory Press, 1989.
7. Saiki RK, Gelfand DH, Stoffel S *et al.* Primer-directed enzymatic amplification of DNA with a thermostable DNA polymerase. *Science* 1988; **239**: 487–491.
8. Wicking C, Williamson R. From linked marker to gene. *Trends in Genetics* 1991; **7**: 288–293.
9. Gorlin RJ, Cohen MM, Levin LS (eds). *Syndromes of the Head and Neck (3rd edition)*. New York: Oxford University Press, 1990.
10. Solomon E, Rawlings Ch (eds). Human Gene Mapping 11. Switzerland: Karger, 1991.

11. Chumakov I, Rigault P, Guillou S *et al.* Continuum of overlapping clones spanning the entire human chromosome 21q. *Nature* 1992; **359**: 380–387.
12. Foote S, Vollrath D, Hilton A *et al.* The human Y chromosome: overlapping DNA clones spanning the euchromatic region. *Science* 1992; **258**: 60–66.
13. Jeffreys AJ, Wilson V, Thein SL. Hypervariable 'minisatellite' regions in human DNA. *Nature* 1985; **314**: 67–73.
14. Nakamura Y, Leppert M, O'Connell P *et al.* Variable number tandem repeat (VNTR) markers for human gene mapping. *Science* 1987; **235**: 1616–1622.
15. Litt M, Luty JA. A hypervariable microsatellite revealed by *in vitro* amplification of a dinucleotide repeat within the cardiac muscle actin gene. *Am J Hum Genet* 1989; **44**: 397–401.
16. Dib C, Faure S, Fizames C *et al.* A comprehensive genetic map of the human genome based on 5,264 microsatellites. *Nature* 1996; **380**: 152–154.
17. Schwartz DC, Cantor CR. Separation of yeast chromosome-sized DNAs by pulsed field gel electrophoresis. *Cell* 1984; **37**: 67–75.
18. Goss SJ, Harris H. New method for mapping genes in human chromosomes. *Nature* 1975; **255**: 680–684.
19. Ruddle FH. A new era in mammalian gene mapping: somatic cell genetics and recombinant DNA methodologies. *Nature* 1981; **294**: 115–119.
20. Bird AP. CpG islands as gene markers in the vertebrate nucleus. *Trends in Genetics* 1987; **3**: 342–347.
21. Landegren U. (ed) Laboratory protocols for mutation detection. Oxford: Oxford University Press, 1996.
22. Lowry RB. Sex-linked cleft palate in a British Columbian Indian family. *Paediatrics* 1970; **46**: 123–128.
23. Rushton AR. Sex-linked inheritance of cleft palate. *Hum Genet* 1979; **48**: 179–181.
24. Bjornsson A, Arnason A, Tippet P. X-linked cleft palate and ankyloglossia in an Icelandic family. *Cleft Palate J* 1988; **26**: 3–8.
25. Rollnick BR, Kaye CI. Mendelian inheritance of isolated non-syndromic cleft palate. *Hum Genet* 1979; **48**: 179–181.
26. Moore GE, Ivens A, Chambers J *et al.* Linkage of an X-linked cleft palate gene. *Nature* 1987; **326**: 91–92.
27. Ivens A, Moore GE, Chambers J *et al.* X-linked cleft palate: the gene is localised between polymorphic DNA markers DXYS12 and DXS17. *Hum Genet* 1988; **78**: 356–358.
28. Fazen LE, Elmore J, Nadler HL. Mandibulo-facial dysostosis (Treacher Collins syndrome). *Am J Dis Child* 1967; **113**: 405–410.
29. Dixon MJ, Read AP, Donnai D *et al.* The gene for Treacher Collins syndrome maps to the long arm of chromosome 5. *Am J Hum Genet* 1991; **49**: 17–22.
30. Poswillo D. The pathogenesis of the Treacher Collins syndrome (mandibulofacial dysostosis). *Br J Oral Surg* 1975; **13**: 1–26.
31. Herring SW, Rowlatt UF, Prozansky S. Anatomical abnormalities in mandibulofacial dysostosis. *Am J Med Genet* 1979; **3**: 225–259.
32. Giuffra LA, Kennedy JL, Castiglione CM *et al.* Glucocorticoid receptor maps to the distal long arm of chromosome 5. *Cytogenet and Cell Genet* 1988; **49**: 313–314.
33. Theriault A, Boyd E, Harrap SB *et al.* Regional chromosomal assignment of the human glucocorticoid receptor gene to 5q31. *Hum Genet* 1989; **83**: 289–291.
34. Yarden Y, Escobedo JA, Kuang WJ *et al.* Structure of the receptor for platelet-derived growth factor helps define a family of closely related growth factor receptors. *Nature* 1986; **323**: 226–232.
35. Jaye M, Howk R, Burgess W *et al.* Human endothelial cell growth factor: cloning, nucleotide sequence, and chromosomal localization. *Science* 1986; **233**: 541–545.
36. Swaroop A, Hogan BLM, Francke U. Molecular analysis of the cDNA for human SPARC/osteonectin/BM-40: sequence, expression, and localization of the gene to chromosome 5q31–q33. *Genomics* 1988; **2**: 37–47.
37. The Treacher Collins Syndrome Collaborative Group. Positional cloning of a gene involved in the pathogenesis of Treacher Collins syndrome. *Nature Genet* 1996; **12**: 130–136.
38. Witkop CJ, Rao S. Inherited defects in tooth structure. In Bergsma E (ed). *The clinical delineation of birth defects Part XI orofacial structures. Birth Defects Original Article Series* 1971; **7**(7): 153–184.
39. Witkop CJ. Amelogenesis imperfecta, dentinogenesis imperfecta and dentin dysplasia revisited: problems in classification. *J Oral Path* 1988; **17**: 547–553.
40. Nakahori Y, Takenaka O, Nakagome Y. A human X–Y homologous region encodes 'amelogenin'. *Genomics* 1991; **9**: 264–269.
41. Snead ML, Lau EC, Zeichner-David M *et al.* DNA sequence for cloned cDNA for murine amelogenin reveals the amino acid sequence for enamel-specific protein. *Biochem Biophys Res Commun* 1985; **129**: 812–818.
42. Shimokawa H, Sobel ME, Sasaki M *et al.* Molecular cloning of bovine amelogenin cDNA. *Adv Dent Res* 1987; **1**: 293–297.
43. Lagerstrom M, Dahl N, Iselius L *et al.* Mapping of the gene for X-linked amelogenesis imperfecta by linkage analysis. *Am J Hum Genet* 1990; **46**: 120–125.
44. Lau EC, Mohandas TK, Shapiro LJ *et al.* Human and mouse amelogenin gene loci are on the sex chromosomes. *Genomics* 1989; **4**: 162–168.
45. Lagerstrom M, Dahl N, Nakahori Y *et al.* A deletion in the amelogenin gene (AMG) causes X-linked amelogenesis imperfecta. *Genomics* 1991; **10**: 971–975.
46. Aldred MJ, Crawford PJ, Roberts E *et al.* Identification of a nonsense mutation in the amelogenin gene (AMELX) in a family with X-linked amelogenesis imperfecta (AIHI). *Hum Genet* 1992; **90**: 413–416.
47. Lench NJ, Winter GB. Characterization of molecular defects in X-linked amelogenesis imperfecta (AIH1). *Hum Mutation* 1994; **5**: 251–259.
48. Aldred MJ, Crawford PJ, Roberts E *et al.* Genetic heterogeneity in X-linked amelogenesis imperfecta. *Genomics* 1992; **14**: 567–573.

49. Pindborg JJ. Dental aspects of osteogenesis imperfecta. In *Pathology of the dental hard tissues.* pp. 81–84. Copenhagen: Munksgaard, 1970.
50. Kerebel B, Daculsi G, Menenteau J *et al.* The inorganic phase in dentinogenesis imperfecta. *J Dent Res* 1981; **60**: 1707–1709.
51. Sillence DO, Senn A, Danks DM. Genetic heterogeneity in osteogenesis imperfecta. *J Med Genet* 1979; **16**: 101–116.
52. Sykes B, Ogilvie D, Wordsworth P *et al.* Consistent linkage of dominantly inherited osteogenesis imperfecta to the type I collagen loci: COL1A1 and COL1A2. *Am J Hum Genet* 1990; **46**: 293–307.
53. Kuivaniemi H, Tromp G, Prockop DJ. Mutations in collagen genes: causes of rare and some common diseases in humans. *Faseb J* 1991; **5**: 2052–2060.
54. Ball SP, Cook PJL, Mars M, Buckton KE. Linkage between dentinogenesis imperfecta and Gc. *Ann Hum Genet* 1982; **46**: 35–40.
55. Mikkelsen M, Jacobsen P, Henningsen K. Possible localization of Gc-system on chromosome 4: loss of long arm 4 material associated with father-child incompatibility within the Gc-system. *Hum Hered* 1977; **27**: 105–107.
56. McCombs JL, Yang F, Bowman BH *et al.* Chromosomal localization of group-specific component by in situ hybridization. *Cytogenet and Cell Genet* 1986; **46**: 62–64.
57. Takagi Y, Sasaki S. Histological distribution of phosphophoryn in normal and pathological human dentins. *J Oral Path* 1986; **15**: 463–467.
58. Takagi Y, Veis A, Sauk JJ. Relation of mineralization defects in collagen matrices to non-collagenous protein components. *Clin Orthop Rel Res* 1983; **176**: 282–290.
59. McDougall M, Zeichner-David M, Murray JC *et al.* Dentin phosphoprotein gene locus is not associated with dentinogenesis imperfecta types II and III. *Am J Hum Genet* 1992; **50**: 190–194.
60. Knudson AG Jr, Hethcote HW, Brown BW. Mutation and childhood cancer: a probabilistic model for the incidence of retinoblastoma. *Proc Natl Acad Sci USA* 1975; **72**: 5116–5120.
61. Gorlin RJ. Nevoid basal-cell carcinoma syndrome. *Medicine* 1987; **66**: 98–113.
62. Farndon PA, Del Mastro RG, Evans DGR *et al.* Location of the gene for Gorlin syndrome. *Lancet* 1992; **339**: 581–582.
63. Reis A, Kuster W, Gebel E *et al.* Localization of gene for the naevoid basal-cell carcinoma syndrome. *Lancet* 1992; **339**: 617.
64. Gailani MR, Bale SJ, Leffell DJ *et al.* Developmental defects in Gorlin syndrome related to a putative tumour suppressor gene on chromosome 9. *Cell* 1992; **69**: 111–117.
65. Hahn H, Wicking C, Zaphiropoulous PG *et al.* Mutations of the human homolog of Drosophila patched in the nevoid basal cell carcinoma syndrome. *Cell* 1996; **85**: 841–51.
66. Vogelstein B, Kinzler KW. p53 function and dysfunction. *Cell* 1992; **70**: 523–526.

3

Craniofacial development

Peter Thorogood and Patrizia Ferretti

Introduction

In the last few years, our understanding of the complex series of events governing the format of the head and face (craniofacial morphogenesis) has significantly increased. A variety of experimental approaches, such as cell lineage marking, monoclonal antibodies, organ culture and recombinant DNA techniques, have enabled this progress to take place. The neural crest contribution to the head and face of the embryo has been mapped, epithelial–mesenchymal interactions are better understood and a number of regulatory molecules, which are likely to be involved in the morphogenesis of the different craniofacial regions, have been identified. Although the information presently available is far from complete, and needs further refinement, the existence of specific gene codes (the so-called homeobox-containing gene code) has become evident. These findings are invaluable to our understanding of the mechanisms underlying craniofacial development, and of certain syndromes affecting craniofacial structures in humans, caused by teratogenic insult or as a result of genetic mutation. For many years, embryologists avoided analysing the mechanisms of craniofacial morphogenesis, largely because of the three-dimensional complexity of the final form. However, there has recently been a renaissance of interest in the underlying mechanisms. This is due in part to new science in related fields such as molecular and cell biology and also to significant technical advances which have provided the means to answer long-standing questions and pose new ones. In this chapter we review briefly some of these advances in order to provide an insight into what is now possible and what will be possible in the future. A glossary of terms can be found at the end of the book.

Background

The face itself is formed from a number of protrusions or swellings that grow out ventrolaterally at the rostral (cephalic) end of the embryonic axis, from the fourth week of embryonic life onwards. The most rostral of these, and in a virtually terminal location, is a single midline process called the frontonasal mass. Flanking this, and first distinguishable during the fifth week, is a pair of olfactory placodes, areas of thickened ectoderm which will invaginate to give rise to much of the olfactory organs. The medial and lateral edges of these placodes will grow into the paired, bilateral medial and lateral nasal processes respectively, followed by the maxillary swellings or processes (Fig. 3.1). By a coordinated process of growth and fusion, these primordia will collectively form the upper and mid-face. Thus, the medial nasal processes and frontonasal mass-derived tissue will form the midline structures including the philtrum, the lateral nasal process and the alae of the nostrils, and the maxillary swellings develop into the cheek and upper jaws. Moving back

This chapter is based largely on an article entitled ‘Heads and tales: recent advances in craniofacial development’ by Peter Thorogood and Patrizia Ferretti, which appeared in *British Dental Journal*, 1992; **173**, 301–306

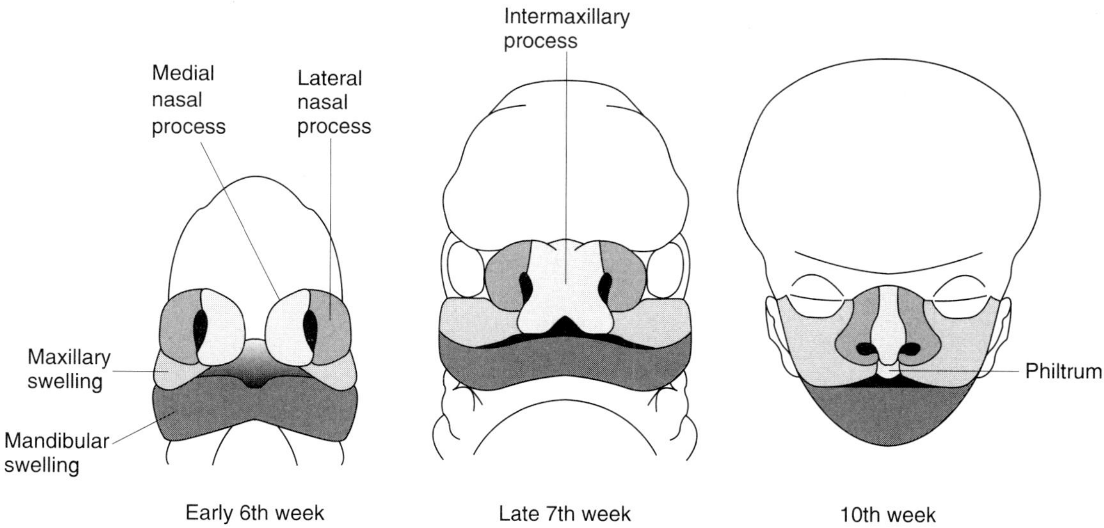

Fig. 3.1 Frontal view of the human embryonic face between 5 and 10 weeks, displaying the derivation of the face from the facial processes and primordia. From Thorogood[30] and modified from Larsen.[31].

along the axis, there are a series of paired ventrolateral processes called branchial arches, each separated from its neighbouring arches fore and aft by a groove in the surface ectoderm termed the branchial groove and matched by an internal branchial or pharyngeal pouch. The maxillary swelling or process forming the cheek and upper jaw is generally regarded as a projection from the first or mandibular arch which itself forms the lower jaw. Thus, derivatives of the first arch enclose the primitive mouth or stomodeum.

Proximally, tissue derived from the first two arches is involved both in jaw articulation and in forming the conductive bones of the middle ear. The mandibular arch together with some tissue from the second (hyoid) arch will thus give rise to the lower jaw (Fig. 3.1) and the groove between these two arches will deepen and sink inwards to form the auditory meatus of the external ear (the pinna of the ear is formed by the fusion of small swellings of first and second arch tissue around the forming meatus). Within the primitive oropharynx, the tongue is derived from arches 1, 2 and 3, together with a proximal tissue contribution from the occipital somites. The medial surfaces of the maxillary processes project initially downwards into the oropharynx as the palatal shelves which then rotate through 90° and fuse in the midline to form the secondary palate. The eustachian tube is the remnant of the first branchial pouch. Derivatives from the remaining arches contribute to the neck with the pouches themselves giving rise to the palatine tonsils (second pouch), parathyroids (third and fourth pouches), ultimobranchial bodies (fifth pouch) and making an essential contribution to the thymus (third pouch), all of which is completed by the eighth week of embryonic life.

Craniofacial development, despite this apparent anatomical complexity, has to be explained in molecular and genetic terms. We should start by asking ourselves what we expect to find in our genome (our individual genetic inheritance) which might explain the effect of mutational genetic change, ethnic phenotypes (the expression of racial genetic characteristics) and the inheritance of family facial form. As the genome is often described as a genetic blueprint, we might expect the relevant genes to provide a description of facial form. Since genes only act as codes for proteins in a one-dimensional series of nucleotide base sequences, it is difficult to imagine how this might constitute a three-dimensional description. Instead we should think in terms of assembly rules. Developmental biologists sometimes use the analogy of an origami construction to illustrate this point.

Origami is the Japanese art of constructing shapes such as flowers or animals, from folded paper. A literal description of an origami swan will be long and rather detailed since it is an object of complex topography with its many planes, corners, crevices and cavities. In contrast, the rules for folding the paper to create this paper swan will be relatively simple and will not contain any description of the final form. It is simply generated by the implementation of the assembly rules. Thus, we can more accurately regard our genome, or at least those genes involved in embryogenesis, as a set of assembly rules whose implementation (gene expression) and interaction determine the transition from the one-dimensional information of the genotype to the three-dimensional complexity of the phenotype.

Developmental biologists seeking to understand how an embryo is created need to disturb embryonic systems in some way by disassembly, reassembly and the study of the component parts in isolation. In this way knowledge can move beyond simple descriptive embryology to an understanding of how the embryo builds a head and face. Also, by working at successively finer levels of organization, from organ to tissue, cell to the molecule, these crucial assembly rules can be gradually defined. We can then begin to understand what happens when they are incorrectly specified or wrongly interpreted and congenital abnormality results.

As such analyses depend almost entirely on the use of model systems, we must ask ourselves if it is appropriate to extrapolate from other vertebrate species to humans. Since evolution is a conservative process, in that it retains and refines successful morphogenetic (form-shaping) mechanisms, the answer is basically 'yes'. Just as the mechanisms operating very early in the development of a limb appear to be largely equivalent in a human, mouse, bird or amphibian, so too are the mechanisms involved in early craniofacial development. Causal mechanisms are conserved over millions of years because they generate a phenotype which is successful in its terms of adaptive value and its selection by environmental pressure. Although mechanisms may become progressively refined in later development to produce different phenotypes, this interpretation still holds for the events of early ontogeny (the development of the individual).

Armed with these two concepts, that embryologically significant genes are assembly rules, and that extrapolation from animal model systems is a valid strategy of analysing the human face formation, let us now look at the current state of understanding. Many advances have been made recently, of which three areas have been selected.

Epithelia – fate mapping and morphogenesis

Two fundamental issues for a developmental biologist are:

1. Cell lineage – What are a cell's antecedents? In effect, what is a cell's family tree?
2. Cell fate – To what does a cell or its progeny give rise?

This is because of the need to know if there is a constant relationship between certain embryonic cell populations and units of anatomical organization. It is also important

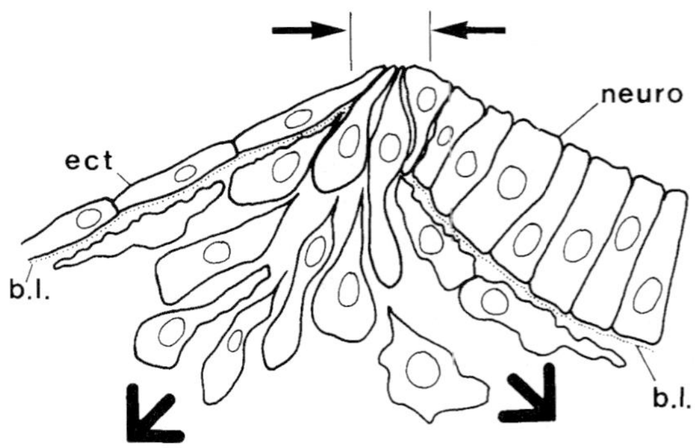

Fig. 3.2 Diagrammatic representation of neural crest origin. The interface between the neuroectoderm (neuro) and ectoderm (ect), during early formation of the neural tube, is depicted in a section plane transverse to the embryonic axis (the dorsiventral midline is off to the right). At this interface, within the region defined by the small arrows, the cells lose their epithelial organization, due to changes in adhesive relationships between neighbouring cells and the dissolution of the basal lamina (b.l.). The liberated neural crest cells proceed to migrate (large arrows) throughout the body of the forming embryo. The migration of neural crest cells before completion of neural tube closure, as illustrated here, is characteristic of the anterior or cranial crest. More posteriorly, the trunk crest originates at completion of, or shortly after, neural tube closure.

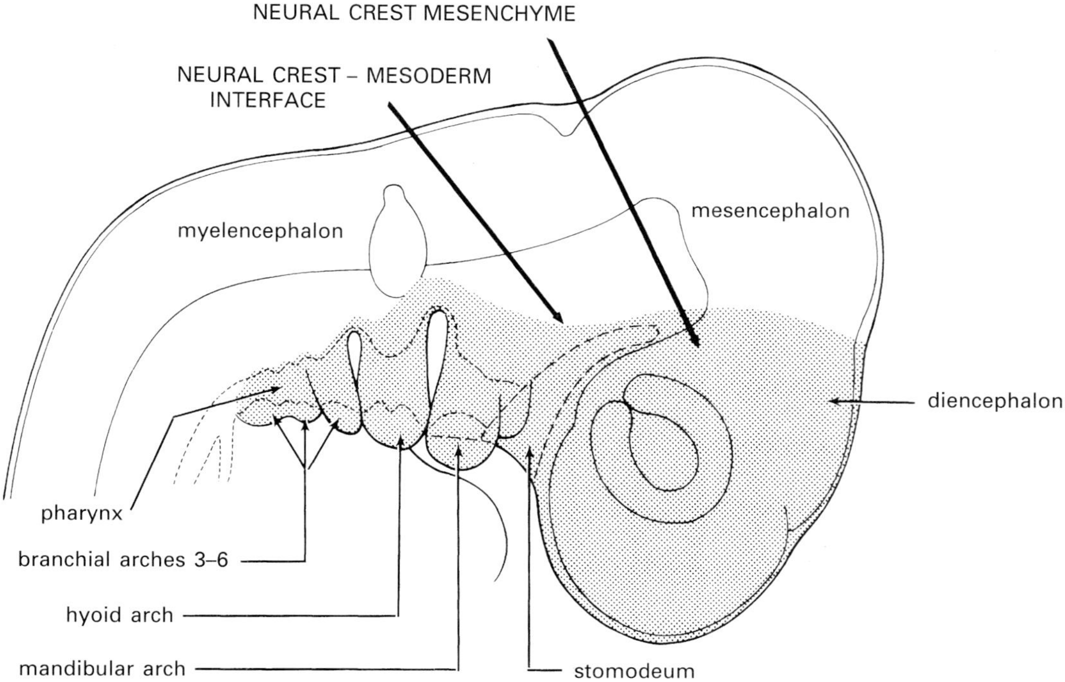

Fig. 3.3 This shows the distribution of crest-derived mesenchyme in the embryonic head. The ventrolateral distribution of crest-derived mesenchyme in the region of the forming face has a well-defined interface with the distribution of the dorsolateral mesoderm-derived mesenchyme (the remaining unshaded area). Evidence to date suggests that this is a pattern generally applicable to all vertebrates, including mammals. From Noden[3] with permission.

because what a cell and its progeny do is determined by its developmental history as well as its present circumstances. Such considerations are important in craniofacial development where much of the facial mesenchyme (embryonic connective tissue) arises from the neural crest, that is, the population of cells which originates at the interface of the neuroectoderm and the ectoderm during the formation of the neural tube[1,2] (Fig. 3.2). Because this is a migratory cell population, many of the crucial events involving their specific fate take place long before the cells' final position is established, perhaps even before they migrate. In recent years the full extent of the neural crest contribution to the embryonic head and face has been mapped and catalogued using a marker technique that enables experimentalists to trace neural crest derivatives. The relative contributions of host and donor cells can be mapped out by creating what are called interspecific chimeric embryos[2] (Fig. 3.3). Such embryos are composed of cells derived from two closely related avian species, chick and quail, which can be histologically distinguished from one another. Tracing the fate of grafted neural crest cells has demonstrated the full extent to which they contribute to craniofacial development. This has revealed their contribution to the sensory and autonomic nervous systems, much of the facial connective tissues, corneal fibroblasts, much of the cartilage and bone in the head, smooth muscle of the major blood vessels of the head and neck, the septation of the outflow tract of the heart, and the connective tissue which patterns the facial musculature.[2–4]

Similarly, by grafting small fragments of tissue between donor and hosts, Couly and Le Douarin have been able to map the fate of the epithelial primordium (primitive structure) of the forebrain, with surprising results.[5,6] It appears that the anterior neural folds give rise to much of the epidermal covering of the forehead and frontonasal regions, the epithelium of the primary palate and of the nasal cavities. Furthermore, the more posterior

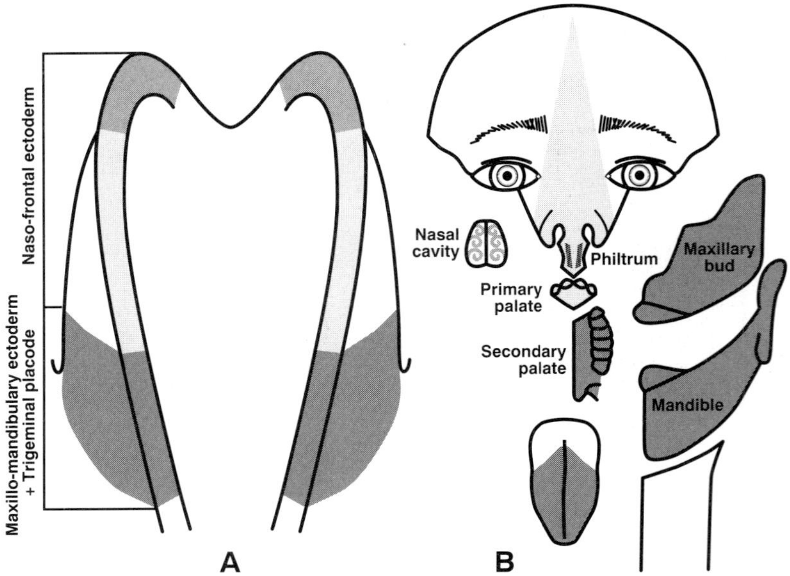

Fig. 3.4 (A) This shows the the embryo at the open neural plate stage. The origins of various epithelia from the (a) fore- and (b) midbrain primordia are displayed as a fate map (plotted from the analysis of interspecific chimeric avian embryos). Note that a significant proportion of the facial ectoderm (and epidermis in the adult) is derived from within the neural folds themselves. (B) Extrapolation from (A) to the human face, indicating that the epithelia of the nasal cavities are derived from the very anterior forebrain folds, and that progressively more posteriorly the folds give rise to the epidermis of the frontonasal region and the epithelia covering the primary palate, and the epithelia covering the dorsum of the tongue and the oral surface of secondary palate, and the epidermis of the maxillary and mandibular regions. Adapted from Figure 3, reference 27, after an original supplied by Professor Nicole Le Douarin.

(midbrain) neural folds contributed to the epidermis of the maxillary and mandibular regions, the secondary palate and the dorsum of the tongue. This result is surprising as it had long been assumed that ectoderm lying lateral to the neural plate and neural folds gives rise to the epidermis of the facial region. Extrapolation from this to the component parts of the human face is depicted in Figure 3.4. Thus, during craniofacial morphogenesis, there is not only considerable rearrangement of the mesenchyme cells due to neural crest migration, but also of the epithelia, especially the superficial epithelium which flows over subjacent mesenchyme to establish the integumentary (covering surface) domains of the face.

During early morphogenesis of the head (the fourth and fifth weeks of development in humans), epithelia derived in this way cover the surface of the facial primordia, which themselves then undergo fusion and remodelling to build the face. At sites of contact between adjacent facial processes, such as the lateral and medial nasal processes and the maxillary process, and at the midline between the palatal shelves, these epithelia fuse and refashion, creating continuity between the mesenchymal populations (Fig. 3.5). Such events are the result of carefully coordinated adhesive changes occurring at particular loci at specific times. There are almost certainly changes in the range of adhesion molecules displayed by the cells at sites destined to contact and fuse but, to a large extent, these changes remain relatively unexplored territory, despite their importance in relation to facial clefting. One exception is the fusion of the secondary palate which has over the years attracted a great deal of attention.

By studying murine palatal shelves *in vivo*, and organ-cultured palatal shelves *in vitro*, Dixon *et al.*[7] and Ardinger *et al.*[8] have begun to identify and catalogue the molecular landmarks of palatal shelf fusion.[7,8] Changes in the composition of the extracellular matrix are clearly correlated with shifts in the various

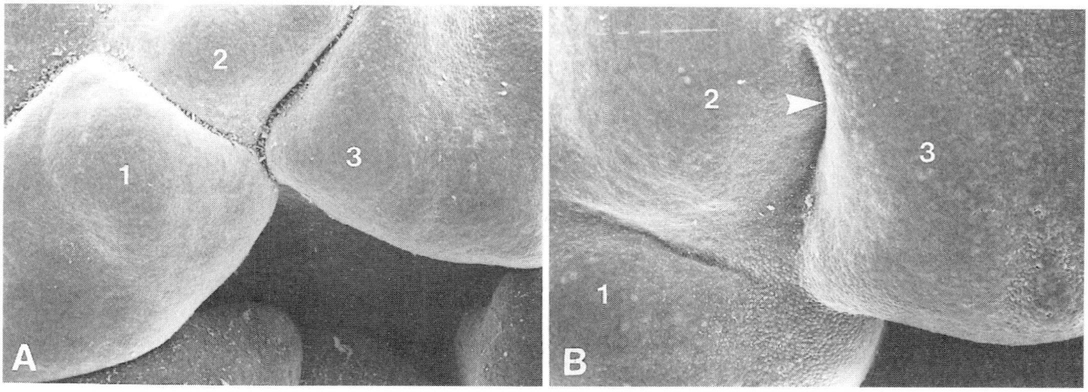

Fig. 3.5 (A) and (B) are scanning electron micrographs of the maxillary (1), lateral nasal (2) and medial nasal (3) processes during avian craniofacial morphogenesis. In (A), the facial processes have just contacted and fine cell extensions can be distinguished within the grooves between adjacent processes. (B) Subsequently, these grooves or seams will disappear as fusion progresses, so that epithelial continuity across the forming face is established and various later morphogenetic events, such as the formation of the external nares (arrowhead), ensue.

growth factors and their receptors. These are low-molecular-weight polypeptides with mitogenic activity which can elicit certain differentiative responses from cells. Degeneration of the midline epithelial seam, formed by the fused medial edge epithelia, is correlated with significant increases in transforming growth factor-α (TGF-α) amongst the epithelial cells and a parallel increase in the epidermal growth factor (EGF) receptor in both epithelia and mesenchyme.[7] These changes are clearly developmentally regulated since they occur in precise site and time (spatiotemporal) patterns within the tissues of the palatal shelves. Other changes still remain to be identified. However, it has been independently shown that mutational changes at the human TGF-α gene locus are associated with an increased incidence of facial and palatal clefting in Caucasians.[8]

Many of the epithelial changes involved in shelf fusion are likely to be the consequence of signalling from the underlying palatal mesenchyme. Culture techniques have proved invaluable in understanding the precise role of such epithelial–mesenchyme interactions. One significant step forward has been the recent development of techniques whereby palatal shelf epithelia can be cultured in isolation and protein markers for various oral, nasal and medial edge domains have been identified.[9] Exploitation of these techniques is likely to be important in the further analysis of palatal morphogenesis and its 'assembly rules'. If the fusion and remodelling of palatal shelves are equivalent to similar changes undergone by the facial processes then similar experimental strategies might be employed to investigate this neglected area and thereby expand our understanding of the broader issue of orofacial clefting.

Mesenchyme – genes and pattern

Recently there has been a revolution in our understanding of the organization of the crest-derived head mesenchyme in the branchial arch region. This has come from two parallel strategies, one a neurobiological approach analysing the organization of the hindbrain and the other resulting from the identification of families of regulatory genes which are expressed in precise patterns within the developing head.

Lumsden and Keynes, using avian model systems, have demonstrated that the embryonic hindbrain is segmented.[10] The periodic bumps or bulges in the neural tube at this region, long known to neuroanatomists as rhombomeres, reflect a metameric or segmental distribution of proliferation centres in the neuroepithelium. Furthermore, there is a corresponding segmental pattern of neuronal differentiation.[10] From an early stage in hindbrain development, the rhombomere boundaries are sites of a periodic pattern of cell lineage restriction that is a progressive reduction in the cells' differentiative potential so that the cells of each rhombomere become committed to forming a specific part of the nervous system.[11]

Meanwhile, molecular biologists have identified genes which are primary candidates for establishing regional identity, that is, the patterning and differentiation which characterize different parts of the embryonic head. To explain this, we have to sidetrack briefly to the geneticists' favourite model system, *Drosophila melanogaster*, the fruitfly. Within this species, developmental mutants frequently arise with body parts which are transformed into identifiable but inappropriate structures – a phenomenon termed homeosis by the geneticist Bateson in the last century. For example, the second thoracic segment, which normally bears a pair of balancing organs called halteres, may be transformed into an extra first thoracic wing-bearing segment, thus producing a mutant phenotype (bithorax) with two pairs of wings rather than one. This is termed a homeotic transformation. Similarly, antennae can be transformed into legs (the mutant antennapedia), and so on. Clearly at some critical stage in the sequence of genetic 'decision-making' that takes place within a cell lineage and specifies cell fate, an inappropriate decision has been made regarding the differentiation and morphogenesis of a discrete group of cells at one particular point in the early embryo. It transpires that these homeotic transformations are due to single-gene mutations. By analysing these and other homeotic mutants, groups of genes have been identified as being involved in the normal specification of regional identity within the *Drosophila* embryo.[12] Mutation within these genes switches the fate of the concerned cells into one that is inappropriate for that site in the embryo. In other words, the mutation changes a particular assembly rule.

Each of these genes concerned with homeotic transformation has been found to be a regulatory gene, that is a gene whose function is to control the function of other genes by either upregulating or downregulating their expression. This is achieved by a regulatory gene product, a protein with a specific DNA-binding activity such that particular downstream genes are targeted to alter their messenger RNA expression, or transcriptional activity. Each of these homeotic genes has been found to contain a region of 180 nucleotide bp. This is the so-called homeobox, which is the DNA genetic code (encodes the DNA domain) for the protein in question. It has emerged that homeobox-containing genes have a very widespread distribution from yeasts to humans and that the homeobox has been very highly conserved over millions of years (see later).

Recombinant DNA technology[13] enables the production of 'probes' composed of specific nucleic acid sequences which are complementary to fragments of the homeobox-containing gene. In this way, labelled probes can be used to identify the localization of such a gene on a chromosome, or to detect the presence of its messenger RNA, which indicates if the gene is transcriptionally active. Such probes can be constructed from sequences of the *Drosophila* homeobox-containing genes and these can then be used to explore the genomes of other species with the objective of identifying homologous genes. These are detectable because evolution has preserved their identical structure, that is, their highly conserved base sequence homology.

Precisely how such regulatory genes may be deployed during development varies. For example, they can be expressed as a feature of tooth development,[14] of neuronal differentiation, and during wound healing and regeneration. Therefore, genes homologous to those in *Drosophila* are not only found in vertebrates, but are expressed in the same precise spatial patterns during early development and appear to be responsible for the specification of anatomical form. A major group of homeobox-containing regulatory genes, the *Hox* genes, are expressed along the anterior–posterior axis of the embryo but with segmental differences in their expression.[15,16] In the developing head, this spatially ordered pattern of gene expression is seen initially in the hindbrain region and the anterior limits of expression correspond to the rhombomere boundaries mentioned earlier. This pattern of gene expression is also seen in the crest-derived mesenchyme of the forming branchial arches. Thus, each segment (rhombomere) of the hindbrain expresses a particular and unique combination of *Hox* genes which are specific for each axial level (Fig. 3.6). This is transmitted to the corresponding arches by the neural crest cells which migrate from the

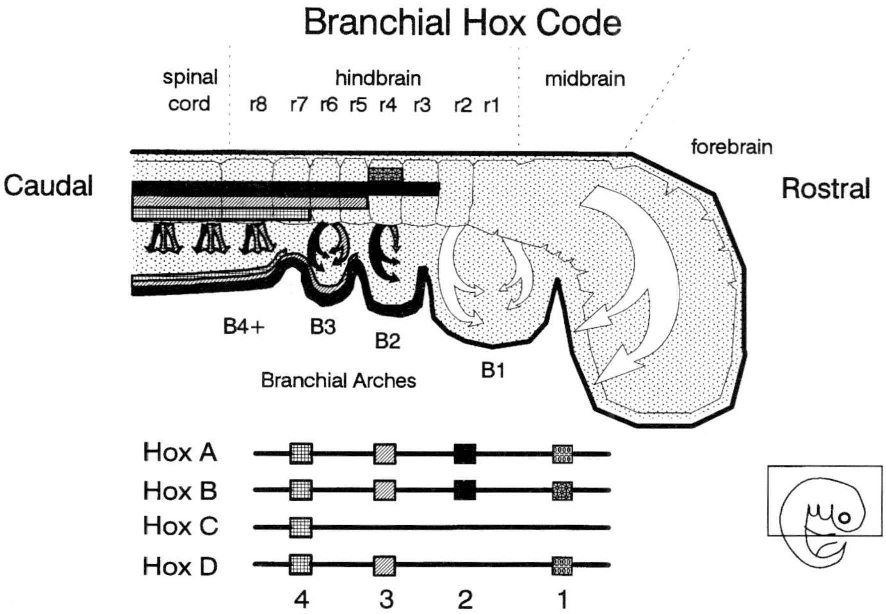

Fig. 3.6 Diagram showing the relationship between *Hox* gene expression in the hindbrain and the migrating neural crest cells and branchial arches. *Hox* genes exist in four clusters A–D, each on different chromosomes; those in the branchial region are depicted in the lower half of the diagram. Each group of *Hox* genes, numbered 1–4, is identified by the type of hatching in order to display their expression within the rhombomeres, the migrating crest cells (depicted by the arrows) and branchial arches. Note the correlations between the *Hox* gene expression in the hindbrain rhombomeres (r1–r8) and the specific axial level expression by the crest cells as they migrate in an orderly fashion into their particular arches (B1–B4+). Note also the lack of *Hox* gene expression, depicted as white arrows, in cells migrating from rhombomeres 1 and 2 into the first (mandibular) arch and in the crest cells migrating from the midbrain rostrally into the future upper face. The region of the embryo is indicated by the lower right plan diagram. (Figure supplied by Paul Hunt.)

neural tube and continue to express a combination of *Hox* genes appropriate to their level of origin (Fig. 3.7).

The chromosomal organization of the *Hox* genes also displays a direct relationship to their patterns of phenotypic expression. Thus, in both mice and humans, *Hox* genes are organized into four clusters, each cluster on a

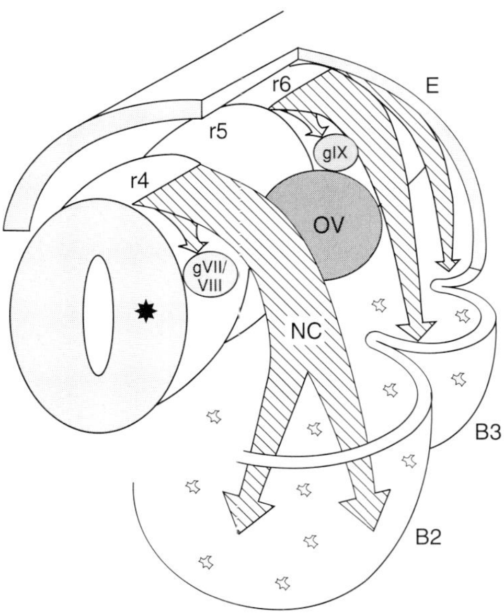

Fig. 3.7 Exploded diagram illustrating the migration of neural crest cells from discrete axial levels of the segmented hindbrain into the forming branchial arches. Migration from rhombomere 4 (r4) into the second arch (B2), and from rhombomere 6 (r6) into the third arch (B3) are depicted. The hindbrain is shown transected at the level of the anterior border of rhombomere 4 (r4); the transected surface is marked with an asterisk and the more anterior parts of the embryonic head are not shown. OV = Otic vesicle; gVII/VIII, gIX = the seventh, eighth and ninth cranial ganglia; E = the ectoderm covering the dorsolateral surface of the embryo. (Figure supplied by Paul Hunt.)

different chromosome, and within each cluster the gene sequence along the chromosome is in the same order as their expression along the long axis of the embryo.

Hox genes: transgenes and abnormality

Two important conclusions can be drawn from these observations. First, there is a *Hox* gene 'code' with different and characteristic patterns of *Hox* genes for each of the branchial arches 1–4 (Fig. 3.6). The precise pattern of these regulatory genes is now assumed to be the means of specifying form in different regions of the head during craniofacial development. In other words, these genes determine the morphogenetic fate of the cells concerned, as do the homologous counterparts of those in *Drosophila*.[17]

The *Hox* code is probably incomplete since other families of regulatory genes almost certainly remain to be discovered. None the less, there does appear to be a combinatorial code and the key question is whether it is causally involved in specifying different regions of the head and face. Can we test this hypothesis experimentally? One strategy is to create animals in which exogenous DNA (e.g. a modified gene) is incorporated into the genome of that individual and inherited by all of its progeny.[18] In such transgenic animals, the expression of the gene of interest can be eliminated, a so-called gene knock-out or expressed at an ectopic site or overexpressed. The normal expression pattern for *Hox* A7 during development is in the spinal ganglia, neural tube and sclerotomes. By creating a transgenic mouse in which *Hox* A7 expression was no longer controlled in this orderly manner, a number of craniofacial anomalies were generated.[19] These included cleft palate, open eyes at birth (normally closed) and ear abnormalities. More recently, disruption of *Hox* A3 expression in a transgenic mouse line produced an array of abnormalities in the face, heart and thymus reminiscent of the Di George syndrome.[20] Strategies based upon experimental embryology and involving ablation of neural crest, or rotation of the neural tube to confront neural crest cells with inappropriate axial environments, confirm the relationship between *Hox* gene expression and morphogenetic specification of the fate of the cells concerned.[21] Furthermore, the recent definition of the human branchial *HOX* code not only demonstrates its conservation, but through this, validates the use of the mouse as an experimental system to develop morphogenetic models of craniofacial development and dysmorphogenesis.[22]

Although such experimental strategies indicate that these regulatory genes are important, it is difficult to define the precise causal relationship between the altered expression of a regulatory gene and the dysmorphogenesis observed. This is partly because the identity of the related downstream genes is unknown. Undoubtedly, as more controlled molecular manipulation becomes possible, further characterization of the genes involved in craniofacial morphogenesis will be achieved. Indeed, recent reports indicate that not only mutations in regulatory genes can be responsible for craniofacial dysmorphic syndromes[23] but also in the putative downstream targets of regulatory genes such as genes encoding adhesion molecules[24] and growth factor receptors.[25]

Conclusions

Regulatory genes containing a base sequence which produces crucial regulatory proteins, called a homeodomain, operate within the genetic hierarchy of facial development. This hierarchy appears to be sequence of interactions from upstream to homeobox to downstream genes. A major challenge is cataloguing all such genes involved in craniofacial development and the identification of both the upstream and downstream genes within the hierarchy. The downstream genes are likely to include genes encoding for molecules such as growth factors and their receptors, cytoskeletal proteins, extracellular matrix molecules and cell adhesion molecules, including receptors for matrix components. It is the fine spatial and temporal control of their synthesis and action that builds form and pattern during embryogenesis. The upstream controlling genes are a matter for speculation, but may involve the retinoids, that is, vitamin A and its metabolites.

Retinoids are indispensable for normal vision and skin differentiation, and are important signalling molecules during normal embryogenesis. Elevated levels of retinoids have long been known to be potent craniofacial teratogens (reviewed by Lammer and Chen[26]) and have recently been shown to alter patterns of *Hox* gene expression in cultured cells in an ordered and concentration-dependent manner.[27] In the developing vertebral column of early mouse embryos, retinoids can act by changing the trunk *Hox* code, resulting in the transformation of individual vertebrae to a morphology characteristic of other axial levels, i.e. equivalent to a homeotic transformation.[28]

The *Hox* codes that are emerging indicate fundamental differences between the head and trunk, and even between parts of the head, in terms of the genes which specify regional identity and particular tissue structures. These differences probably reflect the evolution of our body plan over many millions of years.[29] Thus, the analysis of the underlying assembly rules is now proceeding to the point where it is likely to clarify how the head evolved in time, as well as how it develops embryologically.

Acknowledgements

We wish to thank our colleagues Paul Speight and Jim Hanken for their comments on draft forms of this article, Paul Hunt for supplying Figures 3.6 and 3.7 and Sanjukta Sakar for photographic assistance. Professor Nicole Le Douarin kindly provided Figure 3.4. The work of the authors is supported by grants from the Medical Research Council, the Wellcome Trust, European Union, Birth Defects Foundation and Child Health Appeal Trusts.

References

1. Hall BK, Horstadius S. *The Neural Crest*, 2nd edn. Oxford: Oxford University Press, 1988.
2. Le Douarin N. *The Neural Crest*. Cambridge: Cambridge University Press, 1982.
3. Noden D. Craniofacial development: new views on old problems. *Anat Rec* 1984; **208**: 1–13.
4. Thorogood P, Tickle C. (eds) Craniofacial development. *Development* 1988; **103** (suppl).
5. Couly G, Le Douarin N. Mapping of the early neural primordium in quail-chick chimeras. II. The prosencephalic neural plate and neural folds: implications for the genesis of cephalic human congenital abnormalities. *Dev Biol* 1987; **120**: 198–214.
6. Couly G, Le Douarin N. Head morphogenesis in embryonic avian chimeras: evidence for segmental pattern in the ectoderm corresponding to the neuromeres. *Development* 1990; **108**: 543–558.
7. Dixon MJ, Garner J, Ferguson MJW. Immunolocalization of epidermal growth factor (EGF), EGF receptor and transforming growth factor alpha (TGFα) during murine palatogenesis *in vivo* and *in vitro*. *Anat Embryol* 1991; **184**: 83–91.
8. Ardinger HH, Buetow KH, Bell GI, Bardach J, Van der Mark DR, Murray JC. Association of genetic variation of the transforming growth factor-alpha gene with cleft lip and palate. *Am J Hum Genet* 1989; **45**: 348–353.
9. Carette MJM, Lane EB, Ferguson MWJ. Differentiation of mouse embryonic palatal epithelium in culture: selective cytokeratin expression distinguishes between oral, medial edge and nasal epithelial cells. *Differentiation* 1991; **47**: 149–161.
10. Lumsden A, Keynes R. Segmental patterns of neuronal development in the chick hindbrain. *Nature* 1989; **337**: 424–428.
11. Fraser S, Keynes R, Lumsden A. Segmentation in the chick embryo hindbrain is defined by cell lineage restrictions. *Nature* 1990; **344**: 431–435.
12. De Robertis EM, Oliver G, Wright CVE. Homeobox genes and the vertebrate body plan. *Sci Am* 1990; **263**: 26–32.
13. Sofaer J. Dentistry and the new genetics. *Br Dent J* 1989; **167**: 209–212.
14. Mackenzie A, Leeming GL, Jowett AK *et al.* The homeobox gene *Hox* 7.1 has regional and temporal expression patterns during early murine craniofacial embryogenesis, especially *in vivo* and *in vitro*. *Development* 1991; **111**: 269–285.
15. Hunt P, Wilkinson D, Krumlauf R. Patterning the vertebrate head: murine *Hox*2 genes mark distinct subpopulations of premigratory and migrating cranial neural crest. *Development* 1991; **112**: 43–50.
16. Hunt P, Krumlauf R. Deciphering the *Hox* code: clues to patterning branchial regions of the head. *Cell* 1991; **66**: 1075–1078.
17. Hunt P, Gulisano M, Cook M *et al.* A distinct *Hox* code for the branchial region of the vertebrate head. *Nature* 1991; **353**: 861–864.
18. Jaenisch R. Transgenic animals. *Science* 1988; **240**: 1468–1474.
19. Balling R, Mutter G, Gruss P, Kessel M. Craniofacial abnormalities induced by ectopic expression of the homeobox gene *Hox* 1.1 in transgenic mice. *Cell* 1989; **58**: 337–347.
20. Chisaka O, Capecchi MR. Regionally restricted developmental defects resulting from targeted disruption of the mouse homeobox gene *Hox* 1.5. *Nature* 1991; **350**: 473–479.

21. Hunt P, Ferretti P, Krumlauf R, Thorogood P. Restoration of normal Hox code and branchial arch morphogenesis after extensive deletion of hindbrain neural crest. *Dev Biol* 1995; **168**: 584–597.
22. Vieille-Grosjean I, Hunt P, Gulisano M, Boncinelli E, Thorogood P. Branchial HOX gene expression and human craniofacial development. *Dev Biol* 1997; **183**: 49–60.
23. Jabs EW, Muller U, Xiang L *et al.* A mutation in the homeodomain of the human MSX2 gene in a family affected with autosomal dominant craniosynostosis. *Cell* 1993; **75**: 443–450.
24. Duke VM, Winyard PJD, Thorogood P, Soothill P, Bouloux PMG, Woolf AS. *KAL*, a gene mutated in Kallmann's syndrome, is expressed in the first trimester of human development. *Mol Cell Endocrin* 1995; **110**: 73–79.
25. Reardon W, Winter R. The molecular pathology of syndromic craniosynostosis. *Moi Med Today* 1995; **1**: 432–437.
26. Lammer EJ, Chen DT, Hoar RM *et al.* Retinoic acid embryopathy. *N Engl J Med* 1985; **313**: 832–841.
27. Boncinelli E, Simeone A, Acampora D, Mavilio F. *Hox* gene activation by retinoic acid. *Trends Genet* 1991; **7**: 329–334.
28. Kessel M, Gruss P. Homeotic transformations of murine vertebrae and comcomittant alteration of *Hox* codes induced by retinoic acid. *Cell* 1991; **67**: 89–104.
29. Thorogood P, Hanken J. Body building exercises: segmentation along the body axis. *Curr Biol* 1992; **2**: 1–4.
30. Thorogood P. (ed) *Embryos, Genes and Birth Defects*. Chichester: John Wiley, 1997.
31. Larsen WJ. *Human Embryology*. New York: Churchill Livingstone, 1993.

4

Chromosomes, genes and oral cancer

Crispian Scully

Introduction

Oral squamous cell carcinoma arises as a consequence of multiple molecular events induced by the effects of various habits such as tobacco and alcohol use, influenced by environmental factors, possibly viruses in some instances, against a background of inherited resistance or susceptibility. Other cancers have a similar aetiology, especially those affecting the upper aerodigestive tract. Damage affects many chromosomes and genes, particularly oncogenes and tumour suppressor genes, and it is the accumulation of such genetic damage and the consequent disturbed cell growth and control which in some instances appears to lead to carcinoma.

This chapter reviews our understanding of this complex and rapidly developing area of research.

Growth-signalling pathways

One fundamental problem in growth control is to understand how growth signals are transmitted from the cell surface to the nucleus (Fig. 4.1). Molecules inducing cell signals bind initially to cell surface receptors. Those molecules signalling growth are termed growth factors, and they bind to growth factor receptors (Fig. 4.2). Many growth factors have been identified, the most relevant being epidermal growth factor (EGF) and transforming growth factors (TGF). These growth factors may influence the growth of adjacent cells (paracrine effect) or even the cell actually producing the factor (autocrine effect). These are the first messengers in the activation pathway.[1]

There are many different cell surface receptors. Some of these cell receptors contain proteins that bind guanosine triphosphate

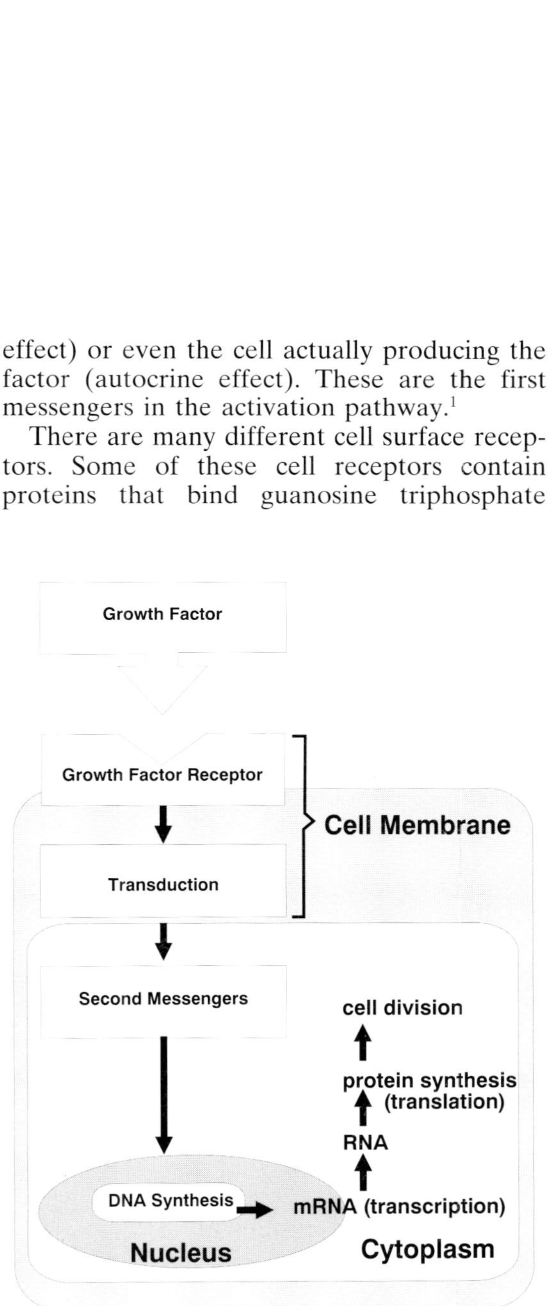

Fig. 4.1 Transmission of growth signal to cell division. mRNA = Messenger RNA.

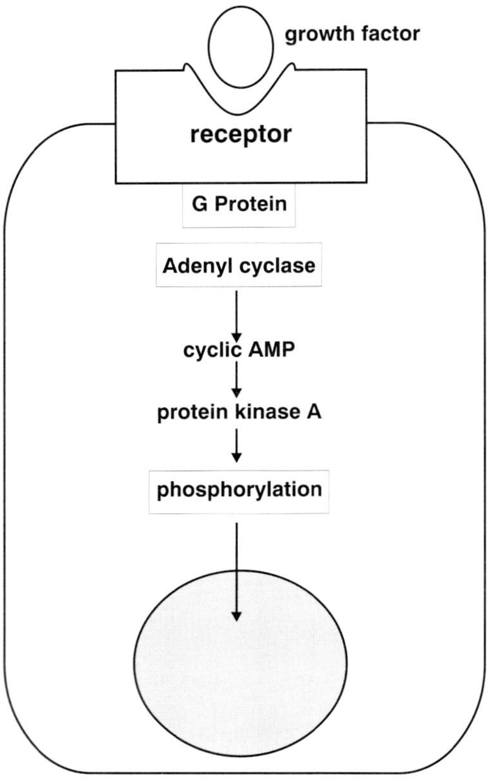

(a)

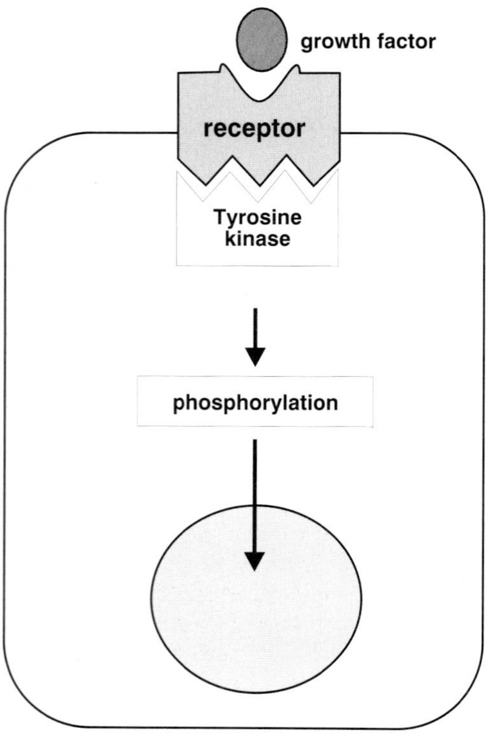

(b)

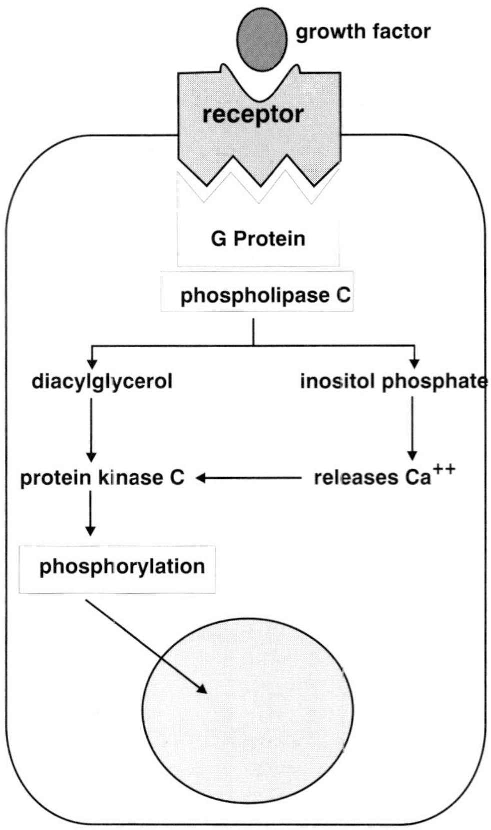

(c)

Fig. 4.2 Diagrammatic representation of growth factor interaction showing pathways for: (a) cyclic adenosine monophosphate (AMP); (b) tyrosine kinase; (c) phospholipase C via inositol phosphate and diacylgycerol.

Table 4.1 Cell signal transduction

Location	*Signal transducer*
Cell membrane	Growth factors
	Growth factor receptors
	Tyrosine kinases
	G proteins
Cytoplasm	Serine-threonine kinases
	Hormone receptors
Nucleus	DNA-binding proteins
	Other factors

(GTP)–hence G proteins. These then activate ion channels, e.g. sodium or calcium ions, or phospholipases or the enzyme adenylate cyclase (see also Chapter 7).

Growth factor activation of phospholipase C results in the hydrolysis of inositol glycolipids

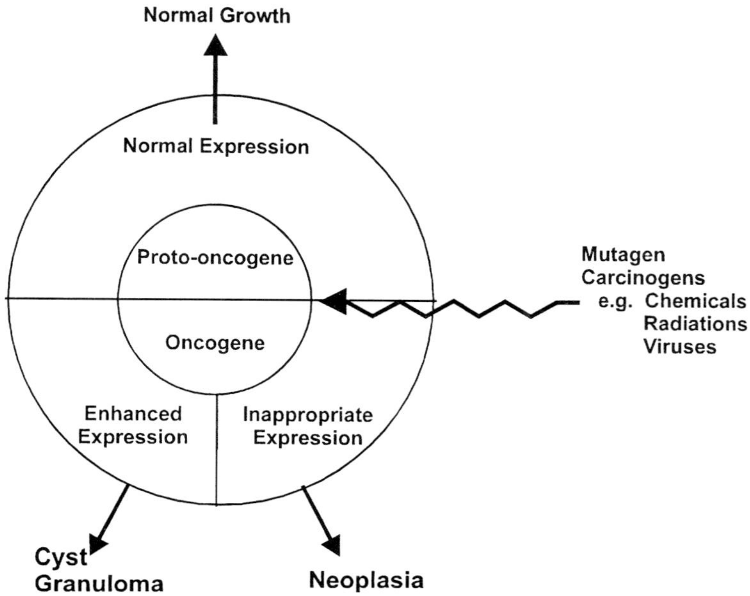

Fig. 4.3 Proto-oncogenes and oncogenes in cell growth and neoplasia.

to two second messengers, diacylglycerol and inositol phosphate, both of which then activate many cell functions. Similarly, the activation of adenylate cylase produces cyclic adenosine monophosphate (cAMP), another second messenger.

In this way, a growth signal arrives at the nucleus from the cell surface and binds to DNA to promote the transcription of messenger RNA and the production of cell-specific proteins. Other agents can also bind to DNA and influence replication. For instance, the steroid hormone receptors, after interacting with their relevant glucocorticoid, sex, thyroid, vitamin D or retinoid hormones, move to the nucleus where they bind to DNA, and cause changes in DNA expression.

By this complex pathway signals arrive at the nucleus, indicating that a growth factor has been encountered by the cell and that cell proliferation should start (Table 4.1). However, the proliferation must be controlled to maintain health. Thus, growth-inhibitory mechanisms are also required in order to prevent cell proliferation from proceeding indefinitely.

The precise regulation of this positive and negative signalling is essential to maintain normal cell growth and health, and any disturbance of such regulation can lead to disease, including hyperplasia and neoplasia (Fig. 4.3).

Proto-oncogenes and oncogenes

Proto-oncogenes

Proto-oncogenes (cellular oncogenes: e.g. c-*onc*) are genes in normal cells that control cell growth, proliferation and differentiation (Fig. 4.4). They are the normal counterparts to the oncogenes carried by some viruses.[1] Such oncogenes are genes that have the ability to transform cells. Proto-oncogenes and the oncogenes seen in tumour cells are designated by curious three-letter abbreviations (such as *ras*) based on the animal or tumour in which they were first identified (Tables 4.2 and 4.3).

The protein products of proto-oncogenes typically control growth at one or more steps in the growth-signalling pathway. Some of these proteins are growth factors, while others are cell receptors for growth factors. Proto-oncogene proteins can also regulate the production of messenger RNA from adjacent genes (gene transcription).

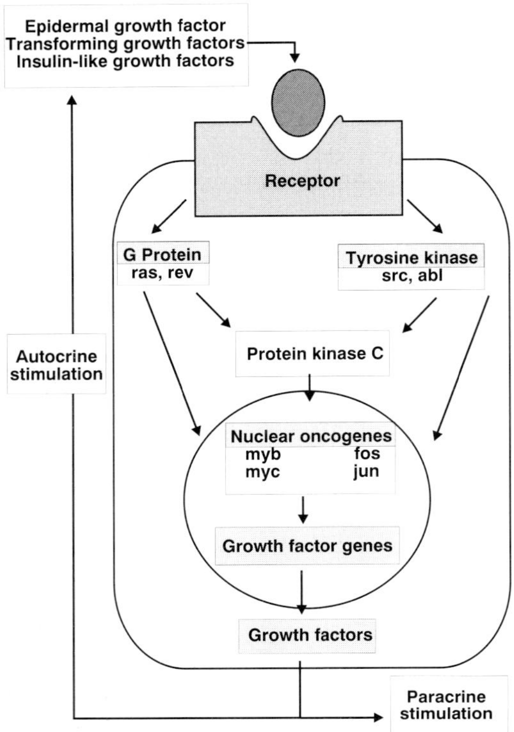

Fig. 4.4 Diagrammatic representation of some of the various proto-oncogenes involved in cell growth regulation.

Table 4.2 Examples of proto-oncogenes and growth regulation

	Signal transducer	*Proto-oncogene*
Cell membrane	Growth factors	*sis* *hst/int*-2
	Growth factor receptors	*erb*-B
	Tyrosine kinases	*src* *abl*
	G proteins	*ras*
Cytoplasm	Serine-threonine kinases	*raf* *mos*
Nucleus	DNA-binding proteins	*fos* *myc* *myb*
	Other factors	*jun*

When cells re-enter the cell division cycle, many genes become involved, particularly the proto-oncogenes c-*fos*, c-*jun* and c-*myc*. The c-*fos* and c-*jun* proteins appear to regulate DNA transcription, whereas the action of c-*myc* protein on DNA is unclear.

Table 4.3 Oncogene associations with various malignant neoplasms

Oncogene	*Associated neoplasm*
abl	Chronic myelogenous leukaemia
erb-B-1	Squamous carcinoma Glioblastoma
erb-B-2 (*neu*)	Adenocarcinoma of breast and ovary
myc	Burkitt's lymphoma Small-cell carcinoma of lung Carcinoma of the breast and cervix
L-*myc*	Small-cell carcinoma of lung
N-*myc*	Neuroblastoma Retinoblastoma Small-cell carcinoma of lung
K-*ras*	Carcinomas of colon, lung and pancreas
N-*ras*	Acute myelogenous and lymphoblastic leukaemia Some carcinomas
H-*ras*	Carcinomas of genitourinary tract and thyroid
bcl-1	B-cell lymphoma
bcl-2	Follicular lymphoma

Other proto-oncogenes, particularly the c-*ras* gene family, appear to be important in terminal cell differentiation. There is thus a highly complex system in place to control cell growth, proliferation and differentiation.

Oncogenes

Oncogenes (viral oncogenes: v-*onc*) are genes present in human cells but which were originally identified in retroviruses, hence the nomenclature v-*onc*. Oncogenes are very closely related to proto-oncogenes but they have mutated to produce abnormal products, or the cell control mechanisms have altered to allow gene overexpression (protein overproduction) and thus they have lost the normal constraints on their activity.[2]

Carcinogenic agents can convert proto-oncogenes to oncogenes in one of four main ways:

1. Point mutations, where a different base has been introduced into a gene. For example, *ras* mutations are found in some colon, breast and oral cancers.
2. Insertional mutagenesis and transduction. For example, some retroviruses can integrate adjacent to a proto-oncogene and

can cause DNA mutations which will activate transduction or transcription.

3. Chromosomal rearrangements and chromosome translocations. In many haematological malignancies, such as Burkitt's lymphoma, parts of chromosomes can be rearranged or translocated to other chromosomes.
4. Amplification, producing many extra copies of the proto-oncogene protein. For example, c-*myc* and c-*erb* B are amplified in some breast and oral carcinomas. This is often accompanied by chromosome abnormalities, leading to poor prognosis, and resistance to cytotoxic drugs.

However, even though oncogene activation is not uncommon, it only rarely results in malignancy.[3] Other factors are also involved, such as host inhibitory mechanisms which may control disturbed cell function for a time. For example, at least three identifiable steps are needed for Burkitt's lymphoma to develop:

1. Infection of B lymphocytes with Epstein–Barr virus enhances their growth.
2. The c-*myc* oncogene translocates and comes to lie adjacent to, and activates, an immunoglobulin gene.
3. The *ras* oncogene is activated.

Multiple steps are also involved in colon carcinogenesis where there are changes involving chromosome 5 so that K-*ras* is activated, and inactivation of the p53 suppressor gene (see below), and a gene on chromosome 18.[3]

To date, more than 50 oncogenes have been identified that are associated with neoplasia (Table 4.3).[4] Initial evidence that an oncogene is associated with a neoplasm depends on finding that the oncogene is amplified or mutated. However, stronger support is the detection of increased amounts of the oncogene protein (oncoprotein) with increased messenger RNA levels since this indicates that the oncogene is not only present, but also active.

Therefore (Fig. 4.5; Table 4.3):

1. *Oncogenes may result in abnormal cell-signalling proteins*. The normal *ras* proto-oncogene produces a protein which binds alternately to guanosine diphosphate (GDP) to switch the cell on or to GTP, which then switches the cell off. Unfortunately, the protein coded by the mutant *ras* oncogene is locked into the active GTP-bound form and continually signals cell division.

   The *ras* oncogene protein first binds to GTP and activates a kinase called RAF. This phosphorylates (adds phosphate) to another kinase, MEK, which results in a kinase cascade in which phosphate is added to a series of proteins, all kinases, which activates them in turn. This phosphorylation is then repeated until it leads to cell replication (Fig.

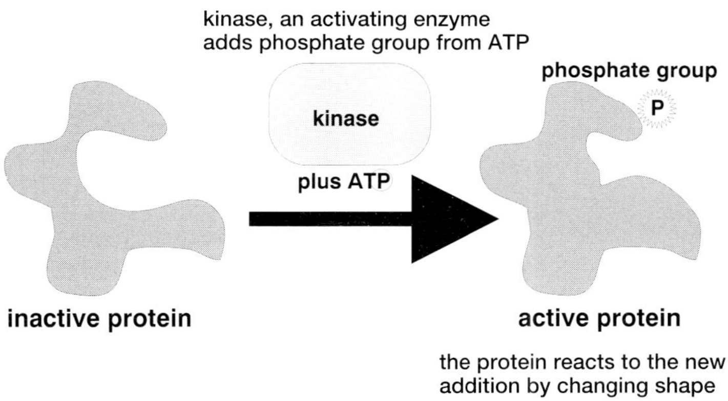

Fig. 4.5 Kinases add phosphate groups to proteins. This phosphorylation activates the protein by changing its shape. Phosphatase enzymes can reverse this process by removing the phosphate group. This addition and subtraction of phosphate is one way of turning protein activity on and off within the cell. ATP = Adenosine triphosphate.

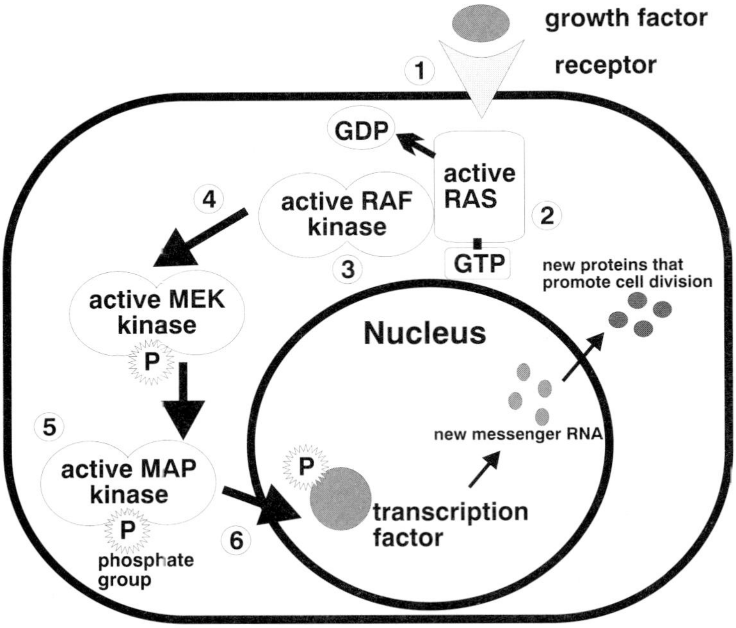

Fig. 4.6
1. The normal cell divides in response to a growth factor acting on the receptor protein.
2. RAS protein is activated to release its guanosine diphosphate (GDP) and bind to the guanosine triphosphate (GTP).
3. The GTP-bound RAS then binds to and activates RAF kinase.
4. MEK kinase is activated.
5. MAP kinase is activated.
6. Cell proliferation is activated.

RAS usually reverts to its inactive GDP-bound form when growth factor stimulation ceases. The mutant RAS oncogene produces a protein which is permanently bound into the active GTP form resulting in a continual kinase cascade. This may also result from mutant forms of RAF and MEK becoming oncogenes.

4.6). *Ras* oncogenes are often active early in formation of chemically induced carcinomas and in some tobacco-related oral cancers. The *ras* oncogene family, which produce such abnormal oncoproteins, includes Harvey *ras* (Ha-*ras*), Kirsten-*ras* (K-*ras*) and N-*ras*.

2. *Oncogenes may act as growth factor receptors*. Oncogene c-*erb*-B1 identifies (has homology) with EGF receptors and is expressed in some oral cancers. c-*erb*-B2 oncogene is associated with breast adenocarcinoma as well as some oral carcinomas.
3. *Oncogenes may act as protein kinases (see point 1 above)*. The *src* oncoprotein, for example, acts as a protein kinase in the cytoplasmic membrane and may be involved in tumour promotion. It phosphorylates tyrosine and also may affect vinculin, a molecule responsible for cell-to-cell adhesion.
4. *Oncogenes may influence DNA replication or transcription*. Oncogene *fos*, for example, appears to be a master switch, upregulating other genes. The *myc* oncoprotein, also termed p62, is a regulator of cell proliferation, and is involved in a number of neoplasms, including oral carcinoma and Burkitt's lymphoma.

Tumour suppressor genes (oncosuppressors or TSGs)

Genes involved in tumorigenesis do not always stimulate cell growth and proliferation. Some

Table 4.4 Neoplasms in some autosomal recessive syndromes

Syndrome	*Leukaemias*	*Carcinomas*	*Others*
Ataxia telangiectasia	+	Gastric Ovarian	Brain tumours Lymphomas
Bloom's syndrome	+	Oral	
Fanconi's anaemia	+	Oesophagus Skin	Hepatomas
Werner's syndrome	+	Breast Thyroid	Hepatomas Sarcomas
Xeroderma pigmentosum	+	Skin Oral	Melanoma

have an effect of suppressing carcinogenesis.[5] Experimental work has shown that the tumorigenicity of some cancer cells can be suppressed if the neoplastic cells are hybridized with normal cells, suggesting that the normal cell contains a gene that suppresses cancer development. These tumour suppressor genes (antioncogenes), which are present at least on chromosomes 3, 9, 13 and 17, may regulate oncogenes or antagonize the effects of oncoproteins. Mutations or deletions in these tumour suppressor genes or blockade of their activity may then result in a defective suppressor protein and consequently a lack of tumour suppression.[6]

Two main suppressor genes, Rb (retinoblastoma suppressor gene) and p53 (so called because of its molecular size), have been studied in some depth and have provided insight as to how some cancers are inherited as gene abnormalities. Some are recessively inherited, and are associated with defects in DNA repair (Table 4.4), whereas others are dominantly inherited and involve the total loss of the tumour suppressor gene (Table 4.5). Retinoblastoma is the best known example to illustrate these features.

Table 4.5 Tumour suppressor gene loss associated with tumours

Tumour	*Chromosome involved*
Multiple endocrine neoplasia type 2	1
Familial adenomatous polyposis	6
Multiple endocrine neoplasia type 2A	10
Multiple endocrine neoplasia type 1	11
Wilm's tumour	11
Retinoblastoma	13
Bilateral acoustic neurofibromatosis	22
Multiple basal cell naevus syndrome	9

The retinoblastoma gene (Rb protein)

Deletions or mutations in the Rb gene on chromosome 13 result in inactivation of the Rb protein, which may give rise to the development of several human malignant neoplasms, including retinoblastoma, osteosarcoma, breast carcinoma and lung cancer. If these genetic changes involve the germ cell, the tendency for tumour formation is inherited. Proteins from DNA viruses, such as some adenoviruses and papillomaviruses, also appear to bind to the retinoblastoma gene product (Rb) in somatic cells and block this oncosuppressor and so these viruses may be sporadically oncogenic (see Chapter 2).

p53

The gene on chromosome 17 is so called because it produces a 53 kDa nuclear phosphoprotein. The protein product of p53 normally binds to DNA and suppresses cell growth and division. If cell repair is impossible, p53 triggers apoptosis (programmed cell death). Mutations or deletions in the p53 gene that give rise to an altered p53 protein are seen in a wide range of malignant neoplasms, including oral, colon, lung and breast cancer and brain tumours. Indeed, p53 mutations are the most common genetic alterations in cancers.

There are p53 mutations in up to 60% of oral dysplastic lesions and carcinomas[7–11] and, according to some workers, the more frequent the p53 mutations, the worse the prognosis.[8,12–17] The detection of p53 mutations at the margins of resected tumours may herald future recurrence. Also, p53 mutations can be detected in salivary cells from patients with head and neck cancer and this may prove to be a useful screening test for oral carcinoma.

The expression of p53 may be altered by mutation or deletions or by degradation by viral or other proteins. Viral proteins such as human papillomavirus (HPV) type 16, E6 protein may be significant in this respect, although HPV is by no means consistently found in tumours with p53 mutations.[14–16]

Aberrations in p53 are clearly a major and early event in oral carcinogenesis but p53 is not the sole gene responsible and many other molecular events occur. One very interesting recent study suggesting possible future directions is the introduction of wild-type (normal) p53 into carcinoma cells which led to growth arrest in the cell lines and reduced tumorigenicity.[17]

Other tumour suppressor genes are also mutated, including some on chromosome 3 and on chromosome 9 (MTS-1) – the multiple tumour suppressor gene. This latter tumour suppressor gene is associated with Gorlin's syndrome.

Chromosomal aberrations may be primary, that is to say, essential to the malignant process, whereas others may be secondary and appear during the tumour progression. Such aberrations may be random events that occur throughout the genome, and are thus sometimes termed noise. Certain chromosomal sites are especially liable to mutations and are termed fragile sites and these are increased in frequency in persons who chew or smoke tobacco.[18,19]

There is also increasing evidence for an underlying inherited susceptibility to cancer.[20,21] Assays using bleomycin to detect chromosomal fragility in lymphocyte cultures have shown an increased susceptibility to breakage in patients with head and neck cancers,[22–25] a trait which correlates with a positive family history.[26] There is also clear evidence of cellular DNA damage in some patients with oral cancer, which is greater than that in persons with no tumour but with similar tobacco and/or alcohol habits.[19,27–30]

Chromosomal aberrations reported in oral cancer have been seen both on the short arms (p) and on the long arms (q) of several chromosomes. Studies have been facilitated by recent advances in DNA technology including restriction fragment length polymorphism (RFLP) and polymeric microsatellite markers (see Chapter 2), both of which enable the loss of crucial gene alleles to be examined. The DNA molecule normally has two copies (alleles) of every sequence. If these alleles are different, the sequence is termed polymorphic in the population, and heterozygous in the individual. The total loss of an important tumour suppressor gene will produce a change from the heterozygous state to a hemizygous state. This is termed loss of heterozygosity (LOH). Losses on several chromosomes suggest that there is a pathway of progression of allelic loss in oral carcinogenesis similar to that seen in colonic and other cancers. Some 70% of head and neck cancers have allelic loss on 9p, and 50% have losses on chromosomes 3q, 11q, 13q and 17p.[31] Similarly chromosomal aberrations have been detected in oral leukoplakias, and were prognostic of premalignancy[32] (Table 4.6). Recently interest has focused on chromosome 9, in view of the high frequency of allelic loss found, and the presence there of MTS-1.

Geographical and racial variations are also beginning to emerge. H-*ras* mutations have been found in oral cancers from patients in the developing world, particularly in advanced tumours in India.[33–35] Whereas H-*ras* mutations have been very uncommon in intraoral carcinomas from western patients,[36–38] this oncogene is often mutated in lip carcinomas from the West.[39]

There is considerable interest in the possible role in carcinogenesis arising from H-*ras* changes due to HPV, which have potentially oncogenic genes such as E6 and E7. H-*ras* is mutated in about one-quarter of oral squamous carcinomas, and half of these

Table 4.6 Chromosome, oncogene and tumour suppressor gene changes reported in oral cancer

Chromosome	*Oncogenes*	*TSG*
3		D8 ACY1 PTP
9		MTS-1
11	H-*ras* PRAD-1 *Int*-2 *hst*-2 *bcl*-1	
13		Rb
17		p53
18		DCC

samples contained HPV. A quarter of verrucous carcinomas were also positive for both H-*ras* mutations and the presence of HPV;[40] this raises the possibility that the virus protein may interfere with the normal *ras* gene protein.

Summary

Multiple tumour-associated genetic aberrations are seen in oral dysplastic and malignant epithelium. The aberrations are seen on many different chromosomes, particularly on 3, 9, 11, 13 and 17. Genetic changes may involve tumour suppressor genes and oncogenes. Tumour suppressor genes may be activated but produce abnormal proteins. Oncogenes may be mutated, amplified or overexpressed. There are differences between carcinomas from the west and those from the developing world, presumably related to the somewhat different aetiological factors for oral cancer implicated in different regions.

Clinical applications

There are several examples in which oncogene amplification in cancer has been shown to be related to a poor prognosis, and there have also been attempts at blocking various sites in the disordered growth pathway in neoplasia. For example, inhibition of tyrosine kinase in squamous carcinoma cell culture has been shown to be able to block cell proliferation. Monoclonal antibodies against some oncogenes can reverse the phenotypic changes in tumour cells. Some tumour inhibitory factors, for example the interferons and interleukin-2, are now being used therapeutically. Undoubtedly, there will be gene therapy and many other advances in the near future.

References

1. Druker BJ, Mamon HJ, Roberts TM. Oncogenes, growth factors and signal transduction. *N Engl J Med* 1989; **321**: 1383–1391.
2. Malcolm S. Oncogenes in malignancy. *Arch Dis Child* 1988; **63**: 1099–1103.
3. Weinberg RA. Oncogenes, antioncogenes and the molecular bases of multistep carcinogenesis. *Cancer Res* 1989; **49**: 3713–3721.
4. Studzinski GP. Oncogenes, growth and the cell cycle: an overview. *Cell Tissue Kinetics* 1989; **22**: 405–424.
5. Friend SH, Dryja TP, Weinberg RA. Oncogenes and tumor-suppressing genes. *N Eng J Med* 1988; **318**: 618–622.
6. Levine AJ, Momand J, Finlay CA. The p53 tumour suppressor gene. *Nature* 1991; **351**: 453–456.
7. Scully C, Field J. Genetic aberrations in squamous cell carcinoma of the head and neck (SCCHN) with reference to oral carcinoma. *Int J Oncol* 1997; **10**: 5–21.
8. Field JK. Oncogenes and tumour-suppressor genes in squamous cell carcinoma of the head and neck. *Oral Oncol Eur J Cancer* 1992; **28B**: 67–76.
9. Johnson NW, Ranasinghe AW, Warnakulasuriya KAAS. Potentially malignant lesions and conditions of the mouth and oropharynx: natural history – cellular and molecular markers of risk. *Eur J Cancer Prevention* 1993; **2** (suppl 2): 31–51.
10. Somers KD, Schechter GL. Genetic alterations in head and neck cancer. *Otolaryngol Clin North Am* 1992; **25**: 1065–1071.
11. Scully C. Oncogenes, tumour suppressors and viruses in oral squamous carcinoma. *J Oral Pathol Med* 1993; **22**: 337–347.
12. Gluckman JL, Stambrook PJ, Pavelic ZP. Prognostic significance of p53 protein accumulation in early stage T1 oral cavity cancer. *Oral Oncol, Eur J Cancer* 1994; **30B**: 281.
13. Field JK, Pavelic ZP, Spandidos DA, Stambrook PJ, Jones AS, Gluckman JL. The role of the p53 tumor suppressor gene in squamous cell carcinoma of the head and neck. *Arch Otolaryngol Head Neck Surg* 1993; **119**: 1118–1122.
14. Burns JE, Baird MC, Clark LJ *et al.* Gene mutations and increased levels of p53 protein in human squamous cell carcinomas and their cell lines. *Br J Cancer* 1993; **67**: 1274–1284.
15. Thomas S, Brennan J, Martel G *et al.* Mutations in the conserved regions of p53 are infrequent in betel-associated oral cancers from Papua New Guinea. *Cancer Res* 1994; **54**: 3588–3593.
16. Brachman DG, Graves D, Vokes E *et al.* Occurrence of p53 gene deletions and human papilloma virus infection in human head and neck cancer. *Cancer Res* 1992; **52**: 4832–4836.
17. Liu T-J, Zhang W-W, Taylor DL, Roth JA, Goepfert H, Clayman GL. Growth suppression of human head and neck cancer cells by the introduction of a wild-type p53 gene via a recombinant adenovirus. *Cancer Res* 1994; **54**: 3662–3667.
18. Kao-Shan CS, Fine RL, Whang-Peng J, Lee EC, Chabner BA. Increased fragile sites and sister chromatid exchanges in bone marrow and peripheral blood of young cigarette smokers. *Cancer Res* 1987; **47**: 6278–6282.
19. Adhvaryu SG, Dave BJ, Trivedi AH. Cytogenetic surveillance of tobacco-areca nut (mava) chewers, including patients with oral cancers and premalignant conditions. *Mutat Res* 1991; **261**: 41–49.

20. De Vries N, De Lange G, Drexhage HA, Snow GB. Immunoglobin allotypes in head and neck cancer patients with multiple primary cancers. *Acta Otolaryngol (Stockh)* 1987; **104**: 187–191.
21. De Vries N, De Waal LP, De Lange G, Drexhage HA, Snow GB. HLA antigens and immunoglobulin allotypes in head and neck cancer patients with and without multiple primary tumors. *Cancer* 1987; **60**: 957–961.
22. Cloos J, Braakhuis BJM, Steen I *et al.* Increased mutagen sensitivity in head-and-neck squamous-cell carcinoma patients, particularly those with multiple primary tumors. *Int J Cancer* 1994; **56**: 816–819.
23. Schantz SP, Spitz MR, Tsu TC. Mutagen sensitivity in patients with head and neck cancers: a biologic marker for risk of multiple primary malignancies. *J Natl Cancer Inst* 1990; **22**: 1773–1775.
24. Spitz MR, Fueger JJ, Beddingfield NA *et al.* Chromosome sensitivity to bleomycin-induced mutagenesis, an independent risk factor for upper aerodigestive tract cancers. *Cancer Res* 1989; **49**: 4626–4628.
25. Spitz MR, Fueger JJ, Halabi S, Schantz SP, Sample D, Hsu TC. Mutagen sensitivity in upper aerodigestive tract cancer: a case-control analysis. *Cancer Epidemiol Biomark Prevent* 1993; **2**: 329–333.
26. Bondy ML, Spitz MR, Halibi S *et al.* Association between family history of cancer and mutagen sensitivity in upper aerodigestive tract cancer patients. *Cancer Epidemiol Biomark Prev* 1991; **2**: 103–106.
27. Bazopoulou-Kyrkanidou E, Garas J, Angelopoulos AP. SCE in lymphocytes of patients with oral carcinoma. *Cancer Genet Cytogenet* 1986; **20**: 35–38.
28. Trivedi AH, Bhavana JD, Adhvaryu SG. Monitoring of smokeless tobacco consumers using cytogenetic endpoints. *Anticancer Res* 1993; **13**: 2245–2250.
29. Popp W, Schell C, Kraus R *et al.* DNA stand breakage and DNA adducts in lymphocytes or oral cancer patients. *Carcinogenesis* 1993; **14**: 2251–2256.
30. Popp W, Wolf R, Vahrenholz C *et al.* Sister chromatid exchange frequencies in lymphocytes of oral cancer patients seem to be influenced by drinking habits. *Carcinogenesis* 1994; **15**: 1603–1607.
31. Nawroz H, van der Riet P, Hruban RH, Koch W, Ruppert JM, Sidransky D. Allelotype of head and neck squamous cell carcinoma. *Cancer Res* 1994; **54**: 1152–1155.
32. Lee JS, Kim SY, Hong WK *et al.* Detection of chromosomal polysomy in oral leukoplakia, a premalignant lesion. *J Nat Cancer Inst* 1993; **85**: 1951–1954.
33. McDonald JS, Jones H, Pavelic ZP, Pavelic LJ, Stambrook PJ, Gluckman JL. Immunohistochemical detection of the H-*ras*, K-*ras*, and N-*ras* oncogenes in squamous cell carcinoma of the head and neck. *J Oral Pathol Med* 1994; **23**: 342–346.
34. Saranath D, Bhoite LT, Deo MG. Molecular lesions in human oral cancer: the Indian scene. *Oral Oncol Eur J Cancer* 1993; **29B**: 107–112.
35. Saranath D, Pachal RG, Nair R *et al.* Oncogene amplification in squamous cell carcinoma of the oral cavity. *Jpn J Cancer Res* 1989; **80**: 430–437.
36. Rumsby G, Carter RL, Gusterson BA. Low incidence of *ras* oncogene activation in human squamous cell carcinomas. *Br J Cancer* 1990; **61**: 365–368.
37. Sheng ZM, Barrois M, Klinanienko J, Micheau C, Richard JM, Riou G. Analysis of the c-Ha-*ras*-1 gene for deletion, mutation, amplification and expression in lymph node metastases of human head and neck carcinomas. *Br J Cancer* 1990; **62**: 398–404.
38. Yeudall WA, Torrance LK, Elsegood KA, Speight P, Scully C, Prime SS. *Ras* gene point mutation is a rare event in premalignant tissues and malignant cells and tissues from oral mucosal lesions. *Oral Oncol Eur J Cancer* 1993; **29B**: 63–67.
39. Milasin J, Pujic N, Dedovic N, Nikolic Z, Petrovic V, Dimitrijevic B. High incidence of H-*ras* oncogene mutations in squamous cell carcinoma of lip vermilion. *J Oral Pathol Med* 1994; **23**: 298–301.
40. Anderson JA, Irish JC, McLachlin CM, Ngan BY. H-*ras* oncogene mutation and human papillomavirus infection in oral carcinomas. *Arch Otolaryngol Head Neck Surg* 1994; **120**: 755–760.

5

Haemostasis

St John Crean

Wounds bleed, but not for very long. Evolution has equipped the body with mechanisms which both limit the amount of blood lost and attempt to maintain the patency of the vasculature. As a result of injury, blood vessels demonstrate increased microvascular permeability with extravasation of plasma, fibrinogen, fibronectin, platelets and other cellular components of the blood. Clotting occurs not only within the vessels but also in the extravasated plasma. This results in a fibrin clot which provides a provisional matrix for cell migration, which is further enhanced by the degradation products of the fibrin clot, which are chemotactic to the various cells involved in wound healing.

Blood is normally separated from the activators of haemostasis by the endothelial cell lining. Injury will expose these constituents to collagen and initiate a series of events that will lead to haemostasis.

The major events in the haemostatic process are:

1. The interaction between platelets and the vessel wall results in the formation of a cellular plug from the adhesion and aggregation of circulating platelets, known as primary haemostasis.
2. The generation of an insoluble fibrin network, the end-product of the coagulation enzyme cascade, is known as secondary haemostasis.
3. There then follows a fibrin degradation process known as fibrinolysis.

Primary haemostasis

Vessel wall

In the uninjured state the normal endothelial platelet relationship is maintained by a balance between the production of two important products of the prostaglandin synthesis pathway.[1] Prostacyclin (PGI_2) is normally produced by the vascular endothelium. Its production leads to vasodilatation and an increase in the level of cyclic AMP, which results in the prevention of platelet aggregation on the normal endothelium, as well as limiting the formation of platelet plugs as a result of injury. PGI_2 works in direct opposition to another product of the prostaglandin synthesis pathway called thromboxane A_2 (TxA_2). TxA_2 is produced by platelets as a result of activation and acts as a powerful vasoconstrictor, lowering the levels of cAMP and leading to the platelet release reaction and platelet aggregation.

An injured vessel will reflexly vasoconstrict and thereby reduce the blood flow to the affected area. Damage to the endothelium will result in a reduced local PGI_2 production and the release of serotonin and TxA_2 from activated platelets; this will augment the local

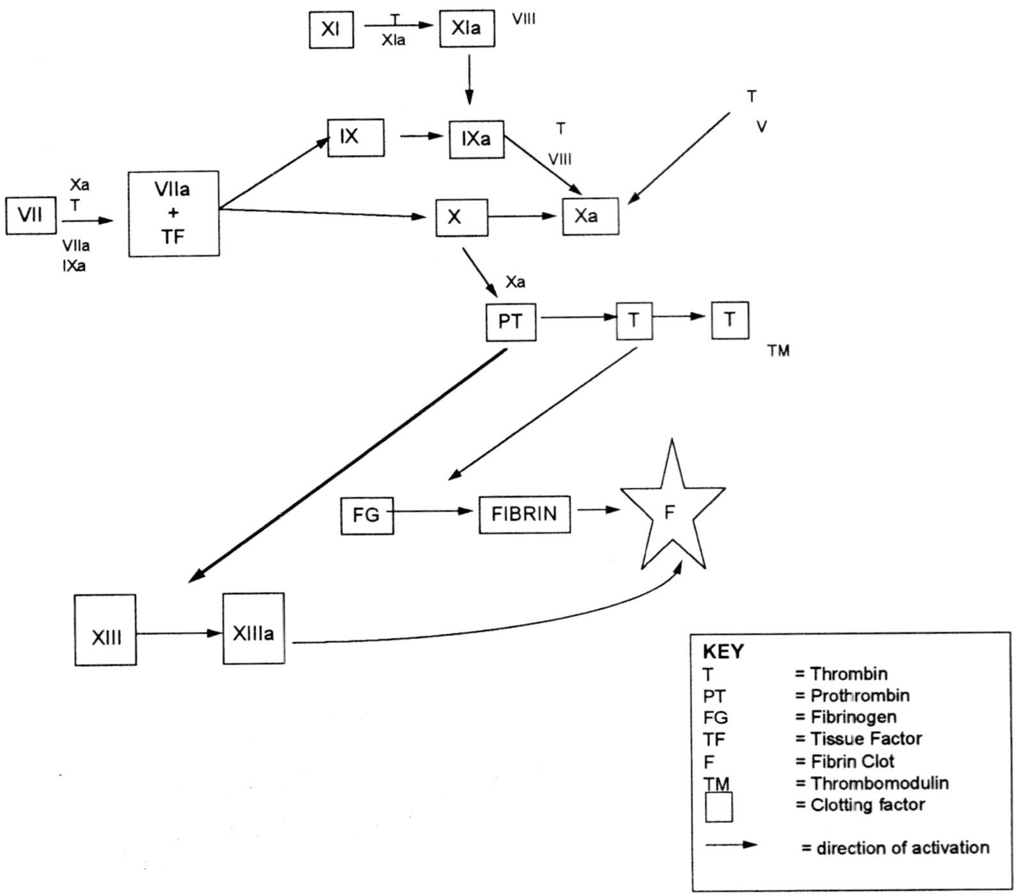

Fig 5.1 The blood coagulation cascade begins with the interaction between VIIa and tissue factor (TF) and ends with the cross-linking of fibrin into clots under the influence of transglutaminase factor XIII.

vasoconstriction and promote subsequent platelet aggregation.

Platelets

Platelets are anucleate discoid fragments, formed by the disintegration of megakaryocytes as they pass through the lung. They contain several important storage organelles. These include:

1. The α-granule, which is a storage site for several platelet-specific proteins and adhesive glycoproteins.[2]
2. The dense body, which is the main storage site for biogenic amines, e.g. serotonin. They also store adenine nucleotides, calcium and pyrophosphate.
3. Lysosomes, which contain several neutral and acid hydrolases.

Platelets will undergo aggregation, adhesion and the release of several factors. Their role in haemostasis and coagulation is reviewed by George *et al.*[3] They will adhere to collagen as a result of the interaction of their surface receptors, glycoprotein Ia (GPIa) binding to exposed collagen and glycoprotein Ib (GPIb), which will bind to von Willebrand factor (VIII:vWF) in the plasma, which in turn binds to collagen. Subsequent to this adhesion the platelets undergo a shape change from a disc to a sphere and spread out along the exposed subendothelium. This aggregate forms the initial plug, after which the platelets become further activated by platelet-activating factor (PAF), collagen, microfibrils and complement.

As a result of the shape change there follows the release from α-granules of several adhesion glycoproteins. These include fibrinogen, fibronectin, vWF and thrombospondin. Thrombospondin, a glycoprotein, is primarily found in the platelets but is also a biosynthetic product of endothelial cells, smooth-muscle cells and monocytes. These glycoproteins bind to other platelets and to the vessel wall, promoting plug formation. This process is known as primary haemostasis. These proteins need to interact with the platelet cell surface. Fibrinogen, fibronectin and vWF bind to the thrombin-activated platelets but require the presence of adenosine diphosphate (ADP) and divalent cations. The platelet membrane glycoprotein (GPIIb–GPIIIa) may act as a common receptor for fibronectin, fibrinogen and vWF. As a result of the binding to this receptor, further platelet release will occur.[4]

Platelets further contribute to primary haemostasis by providing their phospholipid membrane for the prothrombinase complex assembly and by releasing from the dense granules their stores of serotonin and ADP. Serotonin is a potent vasoconstrictor of the microvessels and the ADP will lead to the further exposure of the GPIIb–IIIa complex. As a result of the exposure of coagulation-promoting receptors, whose activity is called platelet factor 3 (PF-3), the clotting cascade is initiated and the production of thrombin will lead to the formation of fibrin to stabilize the plug and to further platelet fusion.

Secondary haemostasis

Coagulation

The coagulation cascade, which forms the basis of secondary haemostasis, is a series of enzymatic reactions which will result in the conversion of soluble plasma fibrinogen to a fibrin clot. Apart from factor XIII all the factors involved are enzyme precursors (factors XIII–XI) or cofactors (V and VIII). The enzymes are serine proteases which will hydrolyse peptide bonds. Once the cascade is activated, each factor or activated enzyme will activate the succeeding factor. Classically the coagulation pathway is thought of as consisting of two independent arms and a common pathway – the intrinsic and extrinsic pathway.[5]

The intrinsic pathway

Hageman factor (factor XII), prekallikrein and high-molecular-weight kininogen act as the initiating factors, in the presence of a negatively charged surface. Activated factor XII (HF) converts factor XI into factor XIa, which in turn converts factor IX into factor IXa in the presence of calcium ions. Activated HF also converts prekallikrein into kallikrein, which will digest kininogen to liberate bradykinin. This acts as a potent vasoactive mediator that will induce a rise in vascular permeabilty and so result in the extravasation of clotting proteins in and around the site of injury. Factor IXa will, in the presence of factor VIII, calcium ions and a phospholipid surface, convert factor X into factor Xa.

The extrinsic pathway

This is classically thought to be initiated by tissue thromboplastin, which will activate the coagulation cascade by converting factor VII into factor VIIa, which in the presence of calcium and a phospholipid surface will also result in the formation of factor Xa, independently of the intrinsic pathway.

Current theory

More recently, however, the coagulation cascade has ceased to be thought of as two separate pathways, but rather as being linked by the combining of tissue factor (formerly thromboplastin) with factor VIIa. Recent evidence has shown that the upper part of the intrinsic pathway, which includes kallikrein, kininogen and factors XI and XII, has little importance in *in vivo* haemostasis. Tissue factor is released by fibroblasts, smooth muscle and endothelial cells, especially after an injury, which in combination with factor VIIa will convert factor IX into factor IXa, which results in the activation of factor X into factor Xa. This is now thought to represent the main activation point of the clotting cascade, demonstrating an important link between the two pathways (Fig 5.1). Factor XI only makes an important contribution after major trauma. There also exists a natural inhibitor of tissue factor known as tissue factor plasma inhibitor, which also inhibits factors VII and Xa.[6]

Factor VIII is a heterodimeric (i.e. it is made up of two unequally sized units) complex protein consisting of a small coagulant molecule

(VIII:C) and a larger vWF (VIII:vWF) which is associated, as previously mentioned, in its multimeric form with platelet adhesion.

Common pathway

Factor Xa, also in the presence of calcium, a phospholipid surface and factor Va, will generate prothrombinase which cleaves prothrombin to form thrombin (factor II), which will subsequently lead to the conversion of fibrinogen to fibrin and further activation of factors V, VIII, XI and XIII.

The coagulation pathway terminates with the formation of cross-linked fibrin. Thrombin cleaves two of the chains of fibrinogen to release fibrinopeptides A and B, which undergo polymerization to form fibrin. The stability of the clot is conferred by the cross-linking of chains of adjacent fibrin strands, by the transglutaminase factor XIII. Fibrin will also cross-link to fibrinonectin and together they form a provisional stroma for macrophages, fibroblasts and endothelial cells to migrate along.

Inhibitors of coagulation

The coagulation process is inhibited by a number of factors released at the periphery of the damaged area. These include:

1. Antithrombin III, which inactivates serine proteases by forming stable complexes with them. Its action is greatly enhanced by heparin.[7]
2. Protein C is formed from a vitamin K-dependent precursor under the influence of thrombin. This conversion is enhanced when thrombin is bound to the endothelial cell receptor, thrombomodulin. Protein C destroys factor V and factor VIII so reducing further thrombin generation.[8,9]
3. Protein S, a cofactor for protein C, facilitates the binding of activated protein C to the activated protein surface.
4. Other natural inhibitors include α_2-macroglobulin, α_1-antitrypsin, α_1-antiplasmin and heparin cofactor II.

Fibrinolysis

This is the process of fibrin degradation, which commences with the formation of the clot. In other words, coagulation and fibrinolysis interact dynamically. Various cells contain tissue plasminogen activator, which rapidly converts plasminogen to plasmin, which in turn degrades fibrin. The most potent stimulator of its release is the presence of thrombin. Other natural plasminogen activators include urokinase, which is synthesized in the kidney and then released into the urogenital tract. Less important activators of plasminogen include factor XII and kallikrein. Damaged endothelial cells, neutrophils and macrophages are some of the sources of plasminogen activator which can localize at the surface of the clot. Plasminogen contains a binding site for fibrin which in turn has specific binding sites for plasminogen activators so both enzyme and substrate can interact and the resultant plasmin degrades the fibrin clot. This destruction of fibrin results in the production of several fragments which are collectively known as fibrin degradation products. Plasmin will also break down coagulation factors V and VIII.[10]

There exists a natural inhibition of this fibrinolytic pathway via plasminogen activator inhibitor 1 which is in turn inactivated by protein C. Protein C therefore has a role in the inhibition of both the coagulation and the fibrinolytic pathways. Drugs such as tranexamic acid and aprotonin exhibit purely antifibrinolytic activity and do not interfere with the coagulation cascade. Plasmin is also inactivated by plasma factors such as α_2-antiplasmin.

Bleeding disorders and their investigation

Much of the important information regarding a bleeding disorder may be obtained from a thorough history and investigation. Important points to elucidate are:

1. Is there evidence of a generalized defect with multiple bleeding sites?
2. Is there any family history?
3. Is there any current medication which may promote bleeding?
4. Is the defect in the vascular, platelet or coagulation part of haemostasis?

Vascular and platelet disorders are marked by easy bruising and bleeding into the skin and mucous membranes, whereas coagulation defects are associated with haemarthroses and muscle haematomas.

The following points discovered in the history and examination should alert the clinician to a potential bleeding disorder:

1. Bruising, purpura and telangiectasia.
2. Epistaxes, gastrointestinal bleeding, haematuria and menorrhagia.
3. Haemarthroses, arthropathy.
4. Prolonged or secondary haemorrhage after laceration, intramuscular injections, dental extractions, operations such as circumcision, tonsillectomy, appendicectomy and childbirth.
5. Blood product transfusion.
6. Drug ingestion, especially aspirin.
7. Family history.
8. Other diseases, especially hepatitic.

In the laboratory the following are the most useful tests in the search for the cause of a bleeding disorder:

1. *Full blood count and film* will identify the structure and number of platelets.
2. *Bleeding time* measures platelet plug formation *in vivo*. Abnormalities will indicate a reduced number of platelets, thrombocytopenia or an impaired platelet function. Pure coagulation defects give a normal result. The test is performed by measuring the time taken for two small arm skin incisions to stop bleeding. Any result greater than 8 min is taken as abnormal. Abnormalities will become evident at platelet counts less than 80×10^9/l. This is known as the Ivy method but a less frightening Dukes test, in which the earlobe is pricked with a stylet, has become more popular.
3. *Coagulation tests*. These use citrated blood that has had the calcium ions neutralized.
   (a) *Partial thromboplastin time with kaolin (PTTK)* is also known as the activated PTT (APTT). It is determined by the addition of a surface activator, kaolin, phospholipid (as a platelet substitute) and calcium to the patient's plasma. The normal is 30–50 s and any abnormality detected will indicate an abnormality in the intrinsic or common pathways.
   (b) *Prothrombin time (PT)* is measured by the addition of animal brain extract and calcium to the patient's plasma. Any result above 18 s is abnormal and indicates a defect in the extrinsic or common pathways.
   (c) *Thrombin time* is determined by the addition of thrombin to the patient's plasma. The normal is 12 s and any increase signifies a defect due to fibrinogen deficiency, fibrinogen function or interference by pharmacological agents such as heparin.
   (d) To differentiate between a coagulation deficiency and drug-induced abnormal coagulation test results, normal plasma is added to the patient's plasma. This will correct a deficiency but not the drug-induced problem.
   (e) *Special tests* include:
      (i) Fibrin degradation products and fibrinogen estimation.
      (ii) Assays of coagulation factors.
      (iii) Platelet function tests, such as platelet aggregometry.
      (iv) Fibrinolysis tests, such as the tissue plaminogen activator assays.

Use of tests in clinical medicine

Vascular disorders

Vascular disorders are characterized by easy bruising and bleeding into the skin. The bleeding is rarely severe and laboratory investigations, including the bleeding time, will be normal. The disorders include:

1. *Congenital*: hereditary haemorrhagic telangiectasia (Osler–Weber–Rendu) and connective tissue disorders (Ehlers–Danlos syndrome, osteogenesis imperfecta, Marfan's syndrome).
2. *Acquired*: severe infections such as septicaemia and meningococcal infections.
3. Allergic: Henoch–Schönlein purpura and connective tissue diseases such as systemic lupus erythematosus and rheumatoid arthritis.
4. Drugs: steroids and sulphonamides.
5. Other: senile purpura and scurvy.

Platelet disorders

Platelets may show reduced number (thrombocytopenia) or impaired function. The main clinical features are bleeding from the mucous membranes and purpura. Severe and spontaneous bleeding will manifest itself when the platelet count reaches less than 20 $\times 10^9$/l.

Reduced platelet number (thrombocytopenia)

This may result from reduced platelet production or increased platelet destruction. An essential part of the investigation includes a bone marrow biopsy to assess the megakaryocyte production. Causes of thrombocytopenia include:

1. *Impaired production*:
(a) impaired bone marrow function: leukaemia, aplastic anaemia, myeloma and marrow infiltration by solid tumours.
(b) selective reduction in megakaryocytes: viral infections and drugs such as co-trimoxazole.
2. *Increased destruction*:
(a) immunological: autoimmune thrombocytopenia, secondary immune thrombocytopenia.
(b) coagulation: disseminated intravascular coagulation, thrombotic thrombocytopenic purpura, haemolytic–uraemic syndrome.
3. *Others:* hypersplenism and transfusion of large quantities of stored blood.

The essential abnormality detected in the blood is a low platelet count and exclusion of other causes by the elucidation of a full and thorough history. Bone marrow biopsy in autoimmune thrombocytopenic purpura may be normal but will otherwise will give an indication as to the source of the problem.

Impaired platelet function

This will present with excessive bruising and bleeding. The platelet count is normal and the bleeding time is prolonged. More detailed investigation includes the platelet aggregation and VIII:vWF assays. Acquired forms include myeloproliferative disorders, uraemia, liver disease, paraproteinaemias and drugs such as aspirin and dipyridamole.

Treatment includes the withdrawal of the drug, platelet transfusion or infusion of desmopressin (DDAVP).

Coagulation disorders

These disorders can be acquired or inherited. Acquired defects are usually of more than one factor, whereas the inherited problems usually involve one factor only.

Inherited coagulation disorders

The most common disorders are:

1. Haemophilia A.
2. Haemophilia B.
3. von Willebrand's disease.

Haemophilia A is characterized by a reduction in the level of factor VIII:C with a normal level of VIII:vWF. It has an incidence of 1 in 5–10 $\times$ 1000 and is inherited as an X-linked recessive. The genetic defects may result from deletions, point mutations and insertions. The features of the disease are related to the level of the factor VIII:C and in general with factor VIII:C levels above 25%, the disease is mild and the patient can lead a relatively normal life with prolonged bleeding only after trauma or surgery. Levels of between 5 and 25% will result in persistent bleeding after even minor trauma. The most severe cases normally have levels of less than 5% with severe intramuscular haematomas, haemarthroses and spontaneous bleeding episodes, especially at levels less than 1%.

For major surgery like orthognathic procedures, the factor VIII:C levels should be raised to 100% at the time of surgery and maintained at 50–60% until healing has occurred. This may involve a postoperative stay in hospital of up to 2 weeks with regular APTT measurements and daily factor VIII:C infusions. Procedures such as simple dental (forceps) extractions or suturing of lacerations require a level of 50% with a concurrent injection of an antifibrinolytic agent such as tranexamic acid. Primary closure of the socket with sutures, with or without a small oxidized cellulose pack, is an essential aid to haemostasis. A soft diet is recommended for the rest of the next week. A full 10 days of tranexamic acid (1 g q.d.s.) is also recommended for all cases.

Table 5.1 demonstrates the blood changes associated with all the main inherited and acquired coagulation defects, including haemophilia A. Bleeding is treated by the administration of factor VIII concentrate and the conservation of clotting factors with antifibrinolytic agents. The production of recombinant factor VIII:C should avoid the

Table 5.1 Coagulation test results of the main inherited and acquired coagulation disorders

	Haemophilia A	*von Willebrand's disease*	*Vitamin K deficiency*
Bleeding time	Normal	↑	Normal
PT/INR	Normal	↑	↑
PTTK	↑+	↑+/–	↑
VIII:C	↓++	↓	Normal
VIII:vWF	Normal	↓	Normal

PT = Prothrombin time; INR = international normalized ratio; PTTK = partial thromboplastin time with kaolin; vWF = von Willebrand factor.

production of antibodies to the human factor VIII:C which occurs in up to 10% of recipients of the factor; currently this can only be managed by giving porcine factor VIII, recombinant factor VII or activated factor X in the hope of bypassing the inhibited step in the clotting pathway. An alternative method of raising factor VIII:C levels is to infuse intravenous desmopressin. This stimulates the release of bound factor VII:C. This has the advantage of avoiding the complications of blood product transfusion which, as well as antibody production, include the high risk of acquiring transfusion-transmitted infections such as hepatitis B, C and human immunodeficiency virus.

Haemophilia B (Christmas disease), also an X-linked inherited disease, is caused by a reduction in factor IX. It is treated in a similar fashion to haemophilia A, except that concentrates of factor IX are infused.

Von Willebrand's disease (vWD) is a deficiency of factor VIII:vWF. The role of this factor is to facilitate platelet adhesion to damaged subendothelium and the stabilization of factor VIII:C. So, not only will there be a prolongation of the bleeding time, but also the reduction factor VIII:C will lead to a haemophilia A-type picture with a prolongation of the PTTK. The disorder is inherited as an autosomal dominant with numerous mutations recognized on chromosome 12. The disease fluctuates in any individual from mild to severe, with the clinical symptoms of bleeding reflecting the severity of the problem and for this reason may not be discovered until the subject is an adult. Blood test results are shown in Table 5.1. Treatment will depend on the severity but includes DDAVP infusion and factor VIII concentrates for major surgery.

Acquired coagulation disorders

These include:

1. *Vitamin K deficiency*. Vitamin K is required for the γ-carboxylation of glutamic acid residues on factors II, VII, IX and X as well as proteins S and C. The lack of these side groups prevents the binding of Ca^{2+}, preventing the normal function of these clotting factors. The main causes of a lack of this vitamin are:
   (a) *Malabsorbtion*, e.g. cholestatic jaundice, as vitamin K is one of the fat-soluble vitamins and requires bile for its absorption;
   (b) *Malnutrition and inadequate stores*, e.g. haemorrhagic disease of the newborn;
   (c) *Oral anticoagulant drugs* which are vitamin K antagonists, e.g. warfarin.
   Table 5.1 shows the typical blood results. Treatment is by the administration of intravenously administered vitamin K (phytomenadione). Clinicians should be aware that anaphylactic reactions can occur with these injections and adrenaline should be available at all times. Haemorrhagic disease of the newborn can be prevented by 1 mg intramuscular administration of vitamin K at birth.
2. *Liver disease*. This may lead to bleeding problems as a result of vitamin K deficiency; reduced synthesis of clotting factors; secondary hypersplenism, leading to an increased platelet destruction, and, very rarely, in fulminant acute liver failure.
3. *Disseminated intravascular coagulation*. A wide variety of factors, such as Gram-negative septicaemia, metastatic malignant disease, amniotic fluid embolism, extensive burns, falciparum malaria and snake bites,

may all lead to this condition which involves the activation of the clotting cascade and generalized platelet aggregation. As a result there is a reduction in the available clotting factors and platelets, as well as an activation of the fibrinolytic pathway leading to the production of fibrin degradation products. This may result in widespread haemorrhage from many different sites, as well as fibrin and platelet plugs occluding vessels to important structures such as the kidney and the skin. All the coagulation tests are prolonged and the fibrinogen levels are extremely reduced. High levels of fibrin degradation products are found as well as a concurrent thrombocytopenia.

Treatment is based on the administration of an antifibrinolytic agent such as tranexamic acid and the replacement of the missing factors, which include platelet transfusion, fresh frozen plasma, cryoprecipitate and red cell concentrates. The use of heparin to prevent any further intravasular coagulation is no longer encouraged.

A more common disorder, called excessive fibrinolysis, may occur during prolonged surgical procedures, such as head and neck cancer resections with reconstruction and will give a similar blood picture to disseminated intravascular coagulation, without any thrombocytopenia. It is prevented or arrested by the administration of inhibitors of fibrinolysis such as tranexamic acid as well as by replacement therapy.

4. *Massive transfusion* can disrupt the haemostatic process due to the fact that stored blood contains very few platelets and has reduced levels of factors V and VIII. As a consequence, the PTTK and the PT should be checked at regular intervals during the transfusion. Stored blood also contains:

   (a) Citrate, which may lead to hypocalcaemia in individuals unable to metabolize the citrate;
   (b) increased levels of potassium;
   (c) increased levels of lactic acid;
   (d) if not warmed, it will lead to the development of hypothermia.

5. *Anticoagulant medication*:
   (a) *Heparin* exerts its main action through the potentiation of the formation of irreversible complexes between the naturally occurring cofactor antithrombin III and activated serine protease coagulation factors (thrombin, XIIa, Xa, IXa and VIIa). It therefore acts at various stages of the coagulation cascade. Control of heparin is unnecessary for 12-hourly subcutaneous prophylactic doses of 5000 U or for the low-molecular-weight heparins, given 24-hourly, as they have very little effect on the overall coagulation pathway, which is indicated by no measurable changes in the APTT levels. However, full heparinization by intravenous infusions will require an APTT after 6–8 h and adjustments to the rate of infusion made accordingly. Longer courses should be monitored because of the very real danger of haemorrhage. Continuous pump infusion provides the ideal delivery and its effects should be measured using the APTT and the thrombin time (TT) tests. They should be performed every 12 h. If required, then heparin can be reversed with titrated doses of protamine sulphate after stopping the heparin as an initial measure.[11]
   (b) *Oral anticoagulants (e.g. warfarin)* have an effect by competing with vitamin K and so reduce the levels of factors II, VII, IX and X. Monitoring is by the measurement of the PT. This is performed by the addition of a tissue thromboplastin and calcium to the patient's plasma in comparison to a control. The thromboplastin is derived from a variety of sources. To provide reproducible results around the world, the local thromboplastin is calibrated with a World Health Organization standard. This will provide a ratio called the international normalized ratio or INR. The onset and offset of warfarin action is slow – approximately 36 h – and may vary with the individual, therefore reversal of warfarin therapy requires early withdrawal if there is no emergency. As the half-lives for the production of factors II, VII, IX and X are a minimum of 48 h, then immediate results require the provision of fresh frozen plasma.[12]

For oral surgical procedures on patients currently taking warfarin then the following regimen is recommended: as a general rule patients *should not* have their medication stopped.

(i) Simple single or multiple extraction can be quite safely performed as long as the INR is not greater than 2.5. The sockets should be sutured and packed with oxidized cellulose if necessary. The avoidance of non-steroidal anti-inflammatory analgesics is essential. Any need to lower the level of the INR should be done in conjunction with the patient's coagulation physician, who should be told of the intended procedure and can then adjust the dose accordingly. On the day of extraction the INR should be checked to ensure that it is safe to proceed.

(ii) Major surgical procedures should be undertaken in a hospital environment, especially on those patients with a history of a prosthetic heart valve, in whom intravascular coagulation is a serious risk, or recurrent deep vein thrombosis. Such a patient is started on an infusion of heparin preoperatively and when the APTT has reached 2–2.5 times normal, then the warfarin can be stopped. Due to the long half-life of warfarin, the surgeon may need to wait 2–3 days before it has worn off. This is assessed by daily measurement of the INR. When the INR is below 1.5 and the APTT is above 2.0, then the surgery can proceed. Severe bleeding may now be controlled by reducing or stopping the heparin immediately before surgery and performing local haemostatic measures. Failing this, then protamine sulphate may be infused; this immediately reverses the effect of heparin. This is the major advantage of changing patients from warfarin to heparin. After completion of surgery, the warfarin may be restarted but the heparin infusion should not be stopped until the INR has once again stabilized at therapeutic levels for at least 24 h.

References

1. Salmon JA, Higgs GA. The eicosanoids: generation and actions. In *Textbook of Immunopharmacology*, 3rd edn, pp. 131–142. Oxford: Blackwell Scientific Publications, 1993.
2. Kaplan KL. Platelet granule proteins: localization and secretion. In *Platelets in Biology and Pathology*, vol 2, pp. 77–90. Amsterdam: Elsevier, 1981.
3. George JN, Nurden AT, Phillips DR. Molecular defects in interactions of platelets with the vessel wall. *N Engl J Med* 1984; **311**: 1084–1098.
4. Harker LA. Platelets and vascular thrombosis. *N Eng J med* 1994; **330**: 1006–1007.
5. Kumar PJ, Clark ML. Bleeding disorders. In *Clinical Medicine*, 3rd edn, pp. 336–341. London: Bailliere Tindall, 1994.
6. Bazan JF. Big rigs in blood coagulation. *Nature* 1996; **380**: 21–23.
7. Weitz JI, Hirsch J. Antithrombins: their potential as antithrombotic agents. *Ann Rev Med* 1992; **43**: 9–16.
8. Furie B, Furie BC. Molecular and cellular biology of blood coagulation. *N Eng J Med* 1992; **326**: 800–806.
9. Clouse LH, Comp PC. The regulation of haemostatis. The protein C system. *N Engl J Med* 1987; **314**: 1298–1304.
10. Heckman CA, Loskutoff DJ. Fibrinolytic pathways and the endothelium. *Semin Thromb Hemost* 1987; **13**: 514.
11. Hirsh J. Heparin. *N Engl J Med* 1991; **324**: 1565–1574.
12. Hirsh J. Oral anticoagulant drugs. *N Engl J Med* 1991; **324**: 1865–1873.

6

Wound healing

Mamta Shah

A wound may be defined as loss of tissue integrity and its restoration occurs by a complex process involving cellular and extracellular events. This includes migration, proliferation and differentiation of cells, along with synthesis and remodelling of the extracellular matrix. Healing by either primary intention, when the wound edges are held in apposition, or by secondary intention, when the wound edges are not apposed, involves all of the above events in varying degrees. This review will describe cutaneous wound healing as an example of the healing process. For descriptive purposes, the events involved in wound healing can be grouped into the following interrelated phases, which will be seen to cover all the major connective tissue processes in the body:

1. Haemostasis.
2. Inflammation.
3. Fibroplasia and neovascularization.
4. Re-epithelialization.
5. Extracellular matrix formation and remodelling.
6. Regeneration or scar formation.

Haemostasis (see Chapter 5 for a detailed description)

Evolution has equipped the body with mechanisms which both limit the amount of blood lost and attempt to maintain the patency of the vasculature. However, the formation of the blood clot is an important early stage in wound healing. As a result of injury, blood vessels demonstrate increased microvascular permeability with extravasation of plasma fibrinogen, fibronectin, platelets and other cellular components of the blood. Clotting occurs not only within the vessels but also in the extravasated plasma. This results in a fibrin clot which provides a provisional matrix for cell migration, which is further enhanced by the degradation products of the fibrin clot, which are chemotactic to the various cells involved in wound healing.

The major events in the haemostatic process are first, the formation of a cellular plug from the adhesion and aggregation of circulating platelets, known as primary haemostasis, and second, the generation of an insoluble fibrin network, the end-product of the coagulation enzyme cascade. This is known as secondary haemostasis. There then follows a fibrin degradation process known as fibrinolysis.

Inflammation (Table 6.1)

The inflammatory response is characterized by increased vascular permeability and cellular infiltration of the wound site. Platelets are among the first cells to be involved in the inflammatory response following tissue injury. Activated platelets release many inflammatory mediators. These include serotonin, which modulates the vascular tone and permeability, transforming growth factor-β (TGF-β), which attracts more inflammatory cells, and platelet-derived growth factor (PDGF),[1] which initiates

Table 6.1 Inflammatory cells and wound healing

Inflammatory cells	*Function*
Neutrophils	Phagocytosis, free oxygen radical production, bacterial and tissue destruction, production of growth factors
Lymphocytes	Growth factor/cytokine production, modulates fibroplasia and collagen production
Monocytes/macrophages	Tissue debridement, production of collagenases, tissue remodelling, extracellular matrix production, production of growth factors

wound repair by mitogenic effects on the connective tissue.[2] In the rabbit corneal system, implantation of autologous thrombin-activated platelets is sufficient to induce angiogenesis, fibroplasia and new collagen production.[3]

Neutrophils

Neutrophils, along with platelets, are amongst the first cells to accumulate at the site of tissue injury. They are attracted by chemotactic factors generated by extravasated blood and coagulation, platelet aggregation and complement activation. These factors include kallikrein, fibrinopeptides, complement 5a, leukotriene B_4 and released platelet products. The process of neutrophil migration from the blood stream into the wound involves a complex process influenced by many factors.

Initially, the emigrating neutrophil adheres to the microvascular endothelium adjacent to the wound. This adhesion is facilitated by inflammatory mediators and both the neutrophil and the endothelial cell participate. Recent studies have defined the role of specific leukocyte surface adhesion molecules. These adhesive glycoproteins include the Mac-1 glycoprotein family which is composed of three structurally and functionally related glycoproteins: Mac-1 (the C3bi complement receptor), LFA-1 (lymphocyte function-associated antigen) and the p150,95 glycoprotein.[4,5] Neutrophils from patients with a genetic deficiency of the Mac-1 glycoprotein family have leukocyte adhesion deficiency (LAD), and exhibit strikingly diminished adherence *in vitro* to cultured human endothelial cells compared with normal control neutrophils stimulated with chemotactic peptides. Patients with LAD are characterized by their inability to mobilize neutrophils (and monocytes) to injured and infected tissues, resulting in recurrent or progressive soft-tissue infections and impaired wound healing.[6] These patients are cured by bone marrow transplants, suggesting that neutrophil adhesion enhanced by inflammatory mediators plays a primary role in neutrophil emigration and accumulation at sites of injury. This adhesiveness of neutrophils is also increased by endothelial cells activated by certain cytokines, such as interleukin-1 and tumour necrosis factor-α, as well as by lipopolysaccharides.[7]

After adhesion to the endothelium, the neutrophils migrate through the vascular endothelium into the wounded tissue. Ultrastructural studies of the rat mesentery and rabbit lung[8] showed that neutrophils migrate between endothelial cells, first extending pseudopodia and then passing through the intercellular junctions close to the endothelial cell plasma membrane. The intercellular junctions reform immediately behind the emigrating cells. The passage of the neutrophils through the vascular basement membrane and the extracellular matrix to the site of tissue injury is possibly accomplished by proteolytic digestion.

Neutrophils form the first line of defence against infection by phagocytosis and intracellular killing of microorganisms. However, neutrophils do not appear to be essential for the process of wound repair in the absence of infection. Simpson and Ross[9] demonstrated that there were no differences in the fibroblast invasion, capillary formation and connective tissue formation in neutrophil-depleted guinea-pigs compared with normal wounded controls, although the rate of infection was higher in the former. Studies by Andersen *et al.*[10] showed no difference in the rate of re-epithelialization of oral wounds in neutrophil-depleted or normal guinea-pigs. Neutrophil-depleted animals, however, had a higher rate of deep wound infection. Recent studies have shown that in healing fetal wounds there is a marked reduction of neutrophil infiltration compared to adult wounds.[11] Neutrophils, however, can modulate the wound-healing process. Alexander *et al.*[12] noted an increase in wound connective tissue if neutrophil stimuli were added to the wound. Activated neutrophils release oxygen radicals, neutral proteases and lipid mediators, which may contribute to further tissue injury.

Monocytes and macrophages

Monocytes follow neutrophils at the site of tissue injury. Resident macrophages provide a first line of defence, which is reinforced by recruitment from the circulating blood monocytes.[13] The process of monocyte migration is a selective, time-dependent process which involves cell–cell and cell–matrix interactions; the endothelial cells play a role through the LFA-1 receptors. This influx of monocytes is influenced by various chemotactic mediators present in the wound. These include platelet releasates, thrombin,[14] complement products C5a, collagen,[15] elastin,[16] the proteolytic fragments of fibronectin[17] and certain cytokines released in the wound. TGF-β and PDGF are the most potent chemotactic factors for monocytes.[18,19]

After infiltrating the wound, monocytes rapidly differentiate into inflammatory macrophages. A possible mechanism for this differentiation from monocyte to macrophage in the wound is the binding of monocytes to insolubilized fibronectin. Circulating monocytes express a magnesium and energy-dependent plasma membrane receptor for surface-bound fibronectin. In the presence of interferon α, β or γ, the inflammatory macrophage is converted to a primed macrophage which is then capable of being converted into an activated macrophage by a triggering stimulus such as TGF-β and lipopolysaccharide. Inflammatory macrophages are characterized by the increased secretion of collagenase, elastase and plasminogen activator as well as increased intracellular products such as lysosomal acid hydrolases.[20]

Unlike neutrophils, monocytes appear to be essential for wound healing. Using steroids to produce monocytopenia and antimacrophage serum to eliminate resident tissue macrophages, Leibovitch and Ross[13] reported delayed debridement and reduced fibroplasia and fibrosis of incisional wounds in guinea-pigs. Conversely, peritoneal macrophages applied locally to cutaneous wounds in old mice accelerate wound closure.[21]

Tissue debridement

Monocytes continue with the debridement initiated by neutrophils. Macrophages secrete abundant quantities of collagenase, elastase and plasminogen activator, which generates plasmin.[22] These enzymes degrade the connective tissue matrix extracellularly. *In vivo* studies have shown macrophages to be actively engaged in phagocytosis of stromal collagen fibres.[23] These studies suggest that the macrophage-dependent degradation is a two-staged process. The enzymes secreted by macrophages initiate the degradation of connective tissue matrix extracellularly. These fragments are subsequently ingested and digested by the macrophages, intracellularly. TGF-β, one of the cytokines secreted by macrophages, enhances type IV collagenase secretion by monocytes.[24]

Connective tissue degradation by collagenase is also a function of fibroblasts induced by factors secreted by macrophages such as interleukin-1.[25] Thus, macrophages play a pivotal role in tissue debridement by secreting proteolytic enzymes, as well as factors that regulate the secretion of collagenase by fibroblasts.

Tissue remodelling

Macrophages play a crucial role in tissue remodelling. They provide the surface membrane receptor for factor Va–factor X interaction and subsequent thrombin formation, which leads to extravascular fibrin deposition.[26] Macrophages also produce fibronectin, which is a chemoattractant for fibroblasts.[27] Fibronectin cross-links with fibrin to form the provisional matrix which facilitates cellular migration. A recent report has also suggested that macrophages produce collagen.[28]

Macrophages secrete polypeptide growth factors and angiogenic factors which influence fibroplasia and neovascularization and which modulate extracellular matrix production by other cells in the wound.[29–32] These include TGF-β,[33] PDGF,[34,35] TGF-α,[31] basic fibroblast growth factor,[36] macrophage-derived growth factor (MDGF)[37] and interleukins. The secretion of these growth factors is a property of macrophages which is amplified by various agents, including endotoxins, lipopolysaccharides and fibronectin. TGF-β is autoinductive and also induces the secretion of other growth factors by activated macrophages.[24,38]

Hence macrophages regulate debridement, cellular infiltration, angiogenesis, extracellular matrix deposition and remodelling during the process of wound healing.

Lymphocytes

Lymphocytes are a group of immunocompetent cells which can be divided into two main subgroups: thymus-dependent lymphocytes (T lymphocytes) and the bone marrow-dependent lymphocytes (B lymphocytes). T lymphocytes appear to regulate the process of wound healing. They migrate into the wound along with the macrophages. Wound lymphocytic infiltration is a dynamic process with maximal infiltration of both T-helper and T-suppressor cells in the superficial part of healing wounds by 7 days postinjury.[39] Mice depleted of T lymphocytes show a significant decrease in the breaking strength and in the collagen content of experimental wounds.[40] Studies suggest that T lymphocytes modulate fibroplasia and collagen deposition in wounds, with the T-suppressor cells having a counterregulatory role in wound healing. Lymphocytes also secrete several soluble peptides such as interferon-γ and the interleukins. Interferon-γ modulates the function of monocytes and macrophages and also inhibits collagen production by fibroblasts, thus having a possible role in regulating collagen deposition in wound repair.[41]

Fibroplasia and neovascularization

The inflammatory response to injury initiates fibroplasia and new blood vessel formation.

Fibroplasia and wound contraction

Fibroblasts entering the wound appear to originate from undifferentiated mesenchymal cells, i.e. lying along the adventitia of blood vessels, in muscle and hair follicles.[42] However, some workers have reported that wound fibroblasts originate from leukocytes.

Around 72 h after injury, fibroblasts migrate into the wound site and commence dividing. This is facilitated by active phagocytosis and degradation of the extracellular matrix by collagenases and plasmin. Collagenases, secreted by neutrophils, macrophages and fibroblasts, degrade collagen into fragments and these collagen fragments are chemotactic to fibroblasts.[43] Plasma fibronectin incorporated in the fibrin clot and cellular fibronectin, released by macrophages and fibroblasts, also promote fibroblast migration into the wound.[44] In addition, cytokines released by platelets, inflammatory cells and fibroblasts such as PDGF, TGF-β and fibroblast growth factor (FGF) also act as fibroblast chemoattractants and mitogens.[18,45,46]

The main function of the fibroblasts is synthesis of the extracellular matrix. Initially, fibroblasts deposit a loose matrix composed of fibronectin, which is important for cell–substrate interaction.[47] With time, fibronectin synthesis diminishes and collagen synthesis increases. Extracellular matrix deposition by fibroblasts is modulated by growth factors.

Some fibroblasts that migrate into the wound undergo phenotypic changes. Their cytoplasm has a well-developed actin microfilamentous system and is packed with cisternae of rough endoplasmic reticulum and their nuclei show indentations similar to that found in smooth-muscle cells.[48] These fibroblasts have been named myofibroblasts and are believed to cause wound contraction *in vivo*. Factors governing this phenotypic conversion into myofibroblasts and wound contraction are currently not well-defined, although recent studies show that TGF-β_1 upregulates α-smooth-muscle actin expression and the differentiation of granulation tissue-derived fibroblasts into myofibroblasts.[49] However, skin autografts are moderate inhibitors of wound contraction. It is the dermal component of the skin which appears to inhibit contraction as epithelial grafts alone do not prevent wound contraction.[50] One study showed that exogenous addition of PDGF or TGF-β_1 to excisional wounds inhibited the differentiation of fibroblasts into myofibroblasts, although both growth factors accelerated wound healing.[51]

Ehrlich[52] opposes the concept of myofibroblasts being responsible for contractile forces during wound contraction and suggests that wound contraction occurs by forces produced by most fibroblasts and this contraction is modulated by the extracellular matrix. In embryonic wounds, a continuous filamentous actin cable acts as a pursestring to close the wound.[53]

Neovascularization

Fibroplasia is accompanied by neovascularization of the wound. Capillary buds sprout from adjacent blood vessels and grow into the wound space. This is a complex process involving degradation of the basement membrane and stimulation, migration and proliferation of endothelial cells and tube formation.

Proximal to the leading edge of migrating and proliferating cells, the endothelial cells begin to form tube-like structures. Lumen formation occurs via intercellular and intracellular mechanisms. The intercellular mechanism appears to involve the development of spaces in the plasma membrane of adjacent cells or the joining of plasma membrane processes of the same and adjacent cells by organized junctional complexes. The intracellular mechanism involves intracellular vacuolization followed by vacuolar fusion and cell–cell plasma membrane fusion resulting in ring cells.[54] Once formed, these tube-like structures are stabilized by the continuous basal lamina that envelope them and the matrix that surrounds these cells. The capillaries then branch and form loops, establish a blood flow and eventually form a plexus.

Many extracellular factors have been shown to regulate angiogenesis. These can be described as stimulators or inhibitors of angiogenesis. Acidic and basic FGF, vascular endothelial cell growth factor (VEGF)/vascular permeability factor (VPF), platelet-derived endothelial cell growth factor (PD-ECGF), epidermal growth factor (EGF), TGF-α, angiogenin, angiotropin, TGF-β, tumour necrosis factor-α (TNF-α) and some low-molecular-weight compounds such as prostaglandins are stimulators of angiogenesis. The mechanism of action of these stimulators is variable. FGF, VEGF/VPF, PD-ECGF and TGF-α directly stimulate endothelial cell migration and proliferation; TGF-β and TNF-α are inhibitors of endothelial cell proliferation, but they can induce three-dimensional tube formation and angiogenesis.[54–59]

Thrombospondin, platelet factor IV and interferon-γ are endothelial cell inhibitors and have been shown to be antiangiogenic *in vivo*. Prolyl hydroxylase inhibitor and hydrocortisone are antiangiogenic, probably due to their interference with the integrity of basement membrane. Metalloproteinase inhibitors have also been shown to be antiangiogenic *in vivo* and *in vitro*.[60]

The repair process continues with the formation of extracellular matrix. When this is accomplished, the abundant newly formed capillaries are no longer required and undergo regression. The endothelial cells at the migrating end undergo mitochondrial swelling, platelets adhere to them and vascular stasis occurs followed by endothelial cell death and phagocytosis by macrophages.[61]

Re-epithelialization

Cutaneous wounding causes a breach in the protective barrier of an organism, exposing the body to detrimental external factors and loss of body fluids. The body attempts to close this breach rapidly even before the deeper tissues are repaired. As already described, injury is followed by clot formation which bridges the gap to form a temporary protective cover; this is soon followed by migration of epithelial cells. In full-thickness wounds the migrating epithelial cells originate from the wound margins. However, if the dermis is retained, as in partial-thickness wounds, the epithelial cells are mainly derived from the dermal appendages.

The process of re-epithelialization has been studied in great detail.[62] Damaged skin signals the transition of keratinocytes from a sedentary to a migratory phenotype. The marginal cells flatten out and form cytoplasmic projections; they lose desmosomal and hemidesmosomal contacts, retract their tonofilaments and form peripheral cytoplasmic filaments. Associated with this change is the modulation of the integrins expressed by these keratinocytes. Activated migrating keratinocytes express β_1, α_5 and vitronectin integrin receptors. These receptors are necessary for adhesion of keratinocytes to fibronectin, the provisional matrix on which the keratinocytes migrate.[63] The epithelial cells move horizontally under the clot to bridge the gap. They move as a sheet rather than as single cells, thus maintaining cell–cell contact away from the wound margins. Cells at the leading edge of the migrating epidermis become phagocytic, ingesting the plasma clot and debris along their path.

At some distance behind the leading edge there is proliferation of epithelial cells. Once the gap is bridged, the epidermal cells reassemble the basement membrane proteins to which they anchor firmly and revert to their original phenotype. The factors that stimulate the migration and proliferation of epithelial cells are unknown, although EGF, epithelial-derived growth factor (EDGF), TGF-β and TGF-α stimulate migration of keratinocytes[64,65] and EGF and EDGF have both been reported to accelerate re-epithelialization of wounds.[66–69] Scatter factor is a protein, isolated from embryo fibroblasts and capable of scattering epithelial cells.[70] The exact role of scatter factor in wound healing is yet to be determined. Recently, keratinocyte growth factor (KGF), a member of the FGF family, was shown to be secreted by fibroblasts and has proliferative effects on epithelial cells. This may represent epithelial–mesenchymal interaction during wound healing.

Extracellular matrix formation and remodelling

With the appearance of fibroblasts in the wound, extracellular matrix begins to be laid down. This is a dynamic process which undergoes continuous change in composition until the final stage of regeneration/mature scar formation is reached. The extracellular matrix is composed of glycoproteins, glycosaminoglycans, collagens and proteoglycans.

Fibronectin

The fibronectins are a group of adhesive glycoproteins that form part of the provisional matrix at the site of tissue injury. Fibronectin is present in the plasma and is also secreted by many cells including macrophages, epithelial cells, endothelial cells, and fibroblasts. Plasma fibronectin is secreted by hepatocytes.

The distribution and role of fibronectin in wound healing have been extensively studied.[71,72] Following injury, plasma fibronectin is cross-linked to fibrin in the presence of factor XIIIa and is incorporated into the blood clot that forms in the wound. This fibrin–fibronectin network not only forms a scaffolding for the various cells to migrate on, but fibronectin fragments are also chemotactic to monocytes,[17] fibroblasts[73] and endothelial cells.[74] Fibronectin enhances phagocytosis of wound debris by monocytes, fibroblasts and epidermal cells and has also been reported to activate monocytes and stimulate TNF-α secretion.[71,75] Fibronectin binds growth factors such as TGF-β in the early phases of wound healing and may protect them from degradation and result in sustained effect of the growth factors.

Thus fibronectin is an important glycoprotein which plays a multifactorial role in wound healing.

Hyaluronan

Hyaluronan is an extremely hydrophilic linear polysaccharide made up of alternating glucuronic acid and *N*-acetylglucosamine residues. It is a non-sulphated glycosaminoglycan which interacts with proteoglycans to provide stability and elasticity to the extracellular matrix of all tissues. By virtue of its hydrophilic properties, hyaluronan can swell to make space between collagen and cells, thus enabling the latter to migrate. In early healing wounds, there is increased deposition of hyaluronan.[76] The presence of hyaluronan at this stage may facilitate the migration and proliferation of the epidermal cells, macrophages and fibroblasts. Growth factors implicated in wound healing have all been reported to stimulate hyaluronan synthesis by cultured human fibroblasts. Fragments of hyaluronan have been reported to be angiogenic.[77]

In the later stages of wound healing, fibroblasts deposit collagens and the hyaluronan content decreases.

Proteoglycans

Proteoglycans are macromolecules composed of core proteins with glycosaminoglycan side chains. The glycosaminoglycans covalently bound to the core protein may be heparin, heparan sulphate, chondroitin sulphate, dermatan sulphate or keratan sulphate. The core proteins are important for targeting the proteoglycans to their anatomical sites and for the stability of their associations with cell membranes and the extracellular matrix. The glycosaminoglycans influence tissue hydration, elasticity, the cationic composition of the tissues and participate in binding to extracellular proteins, growth factors, enzymes and cell surface receptors. Proteoglycans exhibit great diversity in their structure and function[78] and can act as matrix organizers, regulators of cell function and modulators of growth factor functions.

Collagens

Collagens may be defined as extracellular structural proteins whose function depends on the presence of triple helical domains. Connective tissue collagens fall into three main classes: the fibrillar collagens (types I–III, V and XI); the basement membrane collagens (type IV) and the interstitial collagens (types VI–VIII). Type IX, XII and XIV collagens have been found in association with the banded fibrillar collagens, while type X collagen is mainly found in cartilage.[79,80]

The skin contains collagen types I, III–VII, XII and XIV. Collagen types I and III contain three polypeptide chains which form a triple helix and have a short non-helical region at both ends. The collagen molecules associate in a quarter staggered fashion to form banded fibrils. Normal dermis consists mainly of collagen types I and III. Collagen III forms 10–50% of the total collagen content depending on fetal age, while in the mature adult dermis, 85% of the collagen is of type I. Collagen type IV is highly glycosylated, with the helix interrupted by several short non-helical regions and a globular domain near the carboxyl terminal. It apparently aggregates at its ends to form mat-like structures associated with other basement membrane components. Collagen V has a large amino-terminal globule compared to collagen types I and III. Collagen type VI has a dumbbell shape with two globular domains separated by a long triple helical domain. In skin, type VI filaments are concentrated around endothelial basement membranes, forming a loose sheath around blood vessels, nerves and fat cells. Collagen type VI network is also widespread in the rest of the dermis. Type VII collagen forms anchoring fibrils.

Normal oral mucosa is characterized by loose reticular network of collagen types III and VI in the subepithelial region and a deeper stromal region composed mainly of collagen types I and III. Collagen type V is also present as a fibrillar component of the interstitial connective tissue.[81]

Collagen biosynthesis is a complex process which is regulated at various stages during normal collagen metabolism. During wound healing there seem to be many factors which regulate collagen formation. PDGF, released by degranulating platelets, causes chemoattraction and proliferation of fibroblasts. TGF-β, released by platelets, macrophages and fibroblasts, induces increased collagen production by upregulating the collagen messenger RNA and decreasing collagenase production.[82] MDGF with PDGF-like and FGF-like activites increase collagen synthesis by increasing fibroblast proliferation. There is a rapid turnover of collagen and degradation is brought about by several proteinases secreted by macrophages, granulocytes, fibroblasts, endothelial cells and epithelial cells. Plasminogen activator, released into the wound during clot formation, and also secreted by the inflammatory cells, fibroblasts, endothelial cells and keratinocytes, activates procollagenases to form collagenases.

Collagenases are proteinases that can cleave the triple helix of collagen at neutral pH. Matrix metalloproteinases are secreted as zymogens which are activated by physical, chemical or enzymatic agents.[83] Interstitial collagenase degrades collagen types I–III and VII. The molecule then becomes susceptible to various other proteases such as gelatinases and elastases in the extracellular matrix or intracellularly to lysosomal products such as the cathepsins. Collagen IV and the other components of the extracellular matrix such as fibronectin, elastin, proteoglycans and laminin are degraded by stromelysins, gelatinases, plasmin and polymorphonuclear leukocyte elastase.[84] The activity of the collagenases is regulated by several proteinase inhibitors which are present in the blood or in the tissues. The tissue metalloproteinase inhibitors (TIMP) are secreted by fibroblasts, endothelial cells, macrophages and mast cells. The principal collagenase inhibitor in the blood is α_2-macroglobulin.

Collagens have multiple functions in wound healing. Fibrillar collagens are involved in platelet aggregation; collagen fragments are chemotactic for various inflammatory cells and fibroblasts; collagen type V appears to influence epithelial cell migration by preventing cell adhesion to fibronectin;[85] collagen VII helps anchor the epidermis to the dermis; fibroblasts synthesize the extracellular matrix which provides anchoring points and connecting cables for the myofibroblasts to bind and cause wound contraction as well as provide the necessary tensile strength and elasticity to the healing wound.

During the process of wound healing, the composition of the extracellular matrix changes continuously with time. Initially, it is composed of high levels of non-sulphated glycosaminoglycans such as hyaluronan followed by an increasing deposition of sulphated glycosaminoglycan proteoglycans and collagens. In the early stages, collagen type III predominates while later increasing amounts of collagen type I are deposited.[86]

Basement membrane formation

Basement membranes are thin, amorphous sheet-like structures composed of lamina lucida, lamina fibroreticularis and lamina densa. Basement membranes separate epithelium and endothelium from the connective tissue stroma, serving as a boundary between the different tissues. They also serve as an anchoring matrix by virtue of specialized units such as the hemidesmosomes and anchoring fibrils, for the cells to withstand sheer forces. Basement membranes function as selective filters to prevent loss of essential fluid and proteins.

Basement membranes have a complex structure and are made up of collagens IV–VII (type VIII is found in blood vessels and ligamentum nuchae), laminin, entactin and heparan sulphate proteoglycans along with certain antigens such as the bullous pemphigoid antigen (BPA). Collagen IV forms a network and provides tissue support; collagen type VII forms anchoring fibrils which anchor the lamina densa to the underlying dermis;[87] laminin binds cells to the substrate and has also been shown to affect cell motility, proliferation and differentiation; heparan sulphate proteoglycans provide a substrate for cell attachment and also bind growth factors like FGF and protect them from degradation. Tenascin, a glycoprotein, is also found in some basement membranes, including dermal–epidermal junctions, hair follicles and subepidermal capillaries. Recent immunolocalization studies of healing wounds showed that tenascin appeared beneath migrating epithelial cells before laminin and its distribution was spatially and temporally different from that of fibronectin. Tenascin immunolocalized in the dermal–epidermal junctions and homogeneously in the granulation tissues of healing wounds, suggesting that it is important in wound healing.[88,89] However, more recently, Saga *et al.*[90] reported normal wound healing in tenascin null mutant mice.

Regeneration or scar formation

The end-product of the healing process which restores tissue integrity without restoration of the normal architecture and/or function of the tissue is known as scar tissue. Postnatal wounds heal by scar formation. By contrast, cutaneous wounds in early fetal life heal by regeneration and without scar formation.[89,91]

Fetal wound healing

Recent studies on fetal wounds in mice,[89] sheep,[92] rabbits[93,94] and monkeys,[95,96] have demonstrated several differences between adult and fetal wound healing. Fetal wounds heal rapidly, without a scab formation, with reduced inflammatory and angiogenic response, a different growth factor profile and extracellular matrix composition, and with enhanced regeneration of the epithelial and mesenchymal tissues and no scar.[89]

Several investigators[11,89,92,97,98] have reported differences in the inflammatory response during fetal wound healing, consisting of a reduced inflammatory response, mainly a polymorphonuclear cell infiltration, and an absence of immunoglobulins (IgG and IgM) in fetal compared to neonatal and adult wounds.

Another major difference reported between fetal and adult wound healing is the composition of the extracellular matrix. Hyaluronan is deposited in both adult and fetal wound matrix[99,100] but it is short-lived in the adult and sustained in the fetus. Whitby and Ferguson[89] also reported early deposition of fibronectin and tenascin in fetal wounds compared to adult wounds and they proposed that early epithelialization in fetal wounds may be due to early appearance of tenascin.[101,102] The collagens were also deposited earlier in fetal wounds compared to adult wounds and arranged in a reticular pattern resembling that of normal skin, whilst that in adults was abnormally arranged.

Regeneration in adults

It is now becoming apparent that the transition from scarless healing to healing with scar formation occurs gradually *in utero*.[103] Goss[104] has reviewed the regenerative capabilities of mammals in postnatal life. Rabbits can regenerate their ears when a composite disc consisting of both surfaces and cartilage is excised *en masse*. However, if the cartilage is excised prior to excision of the skin, the ear does not regenerate. Deer can regenerate their antlers periodically, but no other part of their body. Another mammalian organ, the liver, is unique in that it can regenerate after partial excision. However, liver forms scar tissue in response to incisional wounds and inflammatory stimuli, often resulting in extensive fibrosis and loss of function. There are reports of very young children regenerating their fingertips following amputation distal to the terminal interphalangeal joints, provided they are not covered by full-thickness skin grafts.[105] Unfortunately, such examples are exceptions as healing in postnatal life is characterized by scar formation.

Scars

Cutaneous scars may be classified into normal and pathological scars, which are further subdivided into keloid and hypertrophic scars. As described earlier, the process of wound healing leads to extracellular matrix deposition which is then remodelled. The new tissue, so-called scar tissue, does not resemble normal skin in its architecture or function.

The macroscopic appearance of a normal scar changes with time. The re-epithelialized wound appears as a depression which fills in and gradually forms a firm, red, often raised area. This gradually blanches, becomes softer and flattens out. Normal scars can be hypopigmented or hyperpigmented and linear scars can stretch with time. Meyers and McGrouther[106] showed that stretching of scars occurred when there was increased uniaxial tension on the scar, whilst hypertrophic scarring was common with multiaxial tension.

Various factors have been described which govern the quality of cutaneous scars. The nature of the injury, its depth and extent, the presence or absence of infection, healing by primary or secondary intention, surgical repair techniques, the site of the wound, vascularity of the tissue and the presence of underlying pathology have all been described as factors affecting the quality of healing and scar formation. Wounds on the face, oral mucosa and scrotum heal with minimal scarring, probably due to high vascularity and possibly due to laxity of the skin in the case of the scrotum.[107] These site-specific differences in scar formation may be due to the site-specific fibroblasts.[108]

There appears to be a series of unidentified 'stop signals' in the process of normal wound healing which control the balance between extracellular matrix synthesis and degradation, terminating the process with a mature 'normal' scar. However, in some individuals, this balance is disturbed and pathological scarring occurs. Hypertrophic scars are raised scars which remain within the confines of the original wound whilst keloids are cutaneous scars which grow beyond the confines of the original wound and both these conditions are due to excessive collagen. Several predisposing factors are recognized.

Hypertrophic scars are common following thermal injury whilst keloids can occur even after trivial injury and occasionally no injury can be recalled in predisposed individuals. Dark-skinned races are more prone to keloid formation and this led to the hypothesis that abnormal scarring was related to an aberration in the metabolism of melanocyte-stimulating hormone.[109] However, abnormal scarring, both hypertrophic and keloid, is not uncommon in white-skinned Caucasians. Whilst no area of the body is immune from abnormal scarring, keloids are more common in the presternal, deltoid and upper back regions of the body. Hypertrophic scarring and keloids tend to occur in areas of increased skin tension such as the presternal region and deltoid region, although the earlobe, which is free of tension is a frequent site for keloids.[109] Younger individuals are more prone to abnormal scarring.[110] Pathological scars differ from normal scars in their extracellular matrix composition,[110–114] immune response[115] and growth factor profile and response.[116–118]

Role of cytokines in wound healing

Cytokines provide the basis for intercellular communication in multicellular organisms. They are multifunctional, regulating migration, proliferation, differentiation and function of the differentiated cell. The effects of a cytokine on a particular cell depend on the presence of other cytokines and on the extracellular matrix surrounding that cell.[119] Cytokines play a major role in wound healing, influencing all phases of the healing process[120,121] and they act by autocrine, paracrine, juxtacrine, intracrine, matricrine and endocrine mechanisms (Fig. 6.1). An autocrine mechanism of action may be defined as one in which the cytokine produced by a cell binds to its own receptors. TGF-β, PDGF and basic FGF are examples of growth factors exhibiting autocrine mechanisms of action. The paracrine mechanism of action is when the growth factor acts on other cells in the vicinity. TGF-β secreted by inflammatory cells induces extracellular matrix production by fibroblasts in a paracrine fashion. Pro-TGF-α, which is membrane-bound via a transmembrane domain and a cytoplasmic domain, can bind to a membrane receptor on an adjacent cell and activate signal transduction in a juxtacrine manner.[122] Acidic and basic FGFs do not have the classical signal peptide sequences and the mechanism of secretion is not well-defined. However, intracellular basic FGF has been shown to be translocated to the nucleolus and may affect the cell by an intracrine mechanism of action.[36] Cytokines such as TGF-β and basic FGF bind to the extracellular matrix. Some of the matrix-bound cytokines such as fibronectin-bound TGF-β and heparan sulphate-bound basic FGF are biologically active and can bind to their respective cell membrane receptors. Binding of the cytokines to the extracellular matrix not only protects them from degradation but also concentrates the growth factors around the responding cells. This mechanism, by which cytokines are delivered to the cells via the extracellular matrix, may be defined as the matricrine mechanism. Cytokines such as insulin-like growth factor are transported to remote sites in an endocrine fashion via plasma. Cytokines have specific cell surface receptors to which they bind and elicit a

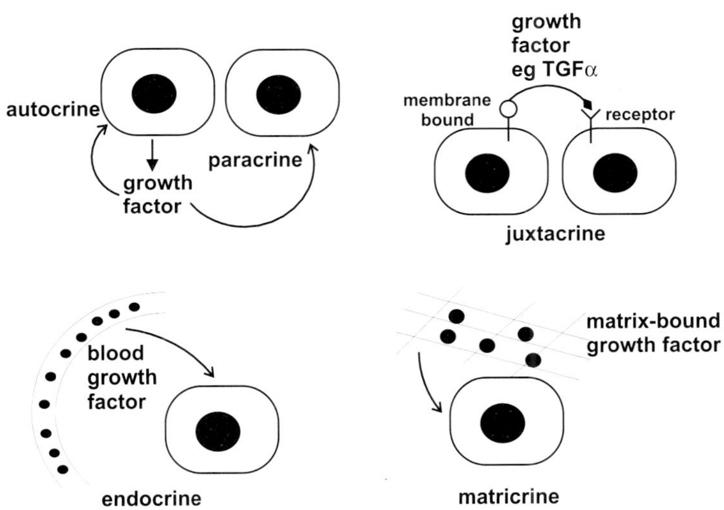

Fig. 6.1 The various mechanisms of actions of growth factors at a cellular level. TGFα = Transforming growth factor α.

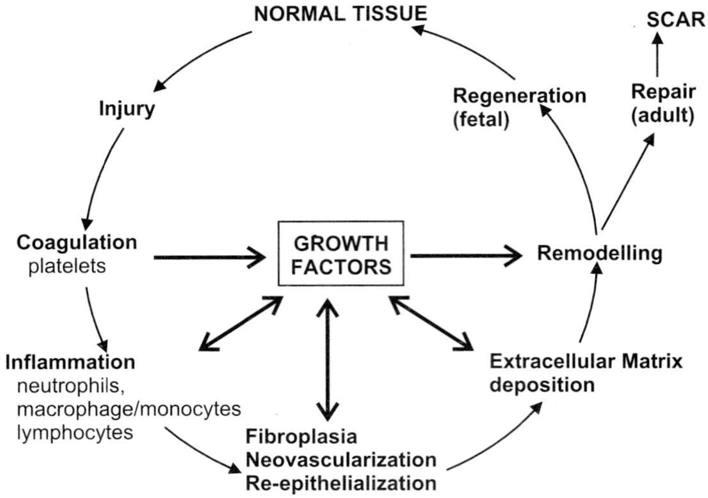

Fig. 6.2 Growth factors play a central role in wound healing. They are released by degranulating platelets soon after injury. Growth factors are chemotactic to the inflammatory cells, chemotactic and mitogenic to fibroblasts, endothelial cells and epithelial cells. All these cells also produce growth factors which influence fibroplasia, neovascularization and re-epithelialization and extracellular matrix deposition and remodelling.

sequence of biochemical events in the target cells (Fig. 6.2).

Numerous studies have demonstrated the effects of exogenous addition of various cytokines to wounds in normal and compromised animals as well as in clinical trials.[123,124] Some of the major cytokines involved in wound healing are described in some detail.

Transforming growth factor-β

TGF-β represents a large family of factors with diverse activities. The structural prototype for this superfamily is TGF-β_1, which is a disulphide-linked dimer of two identical chains of 112 amino acids. TGF-β exists in multiple isoforms which are approximately 64–82% homologous to each other.[125] TGF-βs 1, 2 and 3 are expressed in mammalian cells and tissues and their genes have been localized to chromosomes 19, 1 and 14 respectively in humans.[125]

TGF-β plays a central role in wound healing. Relatively large amounts of TGF-β are present in platelets and these are released by degranulation of the α-granules after injury. TGF-β is a potent chemoattractant of macrophages, neutrophils and fibroblasts and these cells in turn can secrete TGF-β when activated. It induces activation and autocrine release of other growth factors by macrophages, fibroblasts and endothelial cells and induces proliferation of cells and angiogenesis. TGF-β also stimulates extracellular matrix synthesis and prevents its degradation by upregulating the expression of TIMPs and downregulating the expression of proteases.

Exogenous addition of TGF-β has been shown to accelerate wound-healing and increase wound-breaking strengths.[126–128] TGF-β has also been shown to reverse the wound-healing impairment caused by Adriamycin,[129] glucocorticoids[130] and irradiation. Thus TGF-β appears to be an important cytokine influencing and coordinating all the phases of wound healing.

Whilst TGF-β appears to play a key role in tissue repair, excessive or abnormal production of TGF-β can be detrimental, producing fibrosis.

Shah *et al.*[131,132] have reported control of cutaneous scarring by exogenous addition of neutralizing antibodies to TGF-$\beta_{1,2}$ to full thickness wounds on the dorsal skin of adult rats. Early addition of neutralizing antibody to TGF-$\beta_{1,2}$ reduced the inflammatory response, neovascularization and early extracellular matrix deposition in healing wounds without reducing the tensile strength of these wounds. Most importantly, the architecture of the neodermis in wounds treated with neutralizing antibody to TGF-$\beta_{1,2}$ resembled that of normal dermis, i.e. no scar, whilst the control wounds healed with obvious scarring. By manipulating the TGF-β isoform profile of healing wounds, they demonstrated that TGF-β_1 and TGF-β_2 were implicated in 'normal cutaneous scarring' whilst exogenous addition of TGF-β_3 reduced cutaneous scarring.[133] Using the same experimental wound model, they also demonstrated that using excess mannose-6-phosphate, which competitively inhibits binding of latent TGF-β to mannose-6-phosphate receptors required for activation of latent TGF-β, reduced cutaneous scarring.[134]

Platelet-derived growth factor

PDGF is a ubiquitous mitogen principally affecting growth of connective tissue-forming cells such as dermal fibroblasts[135] and arterial smooth-muscle cells.[136] PDGF is stored in the α-granules of platelets but can be formed by various cells such as activated arterial endothelial cells, activated monocytes and macrophages, and activated fibroblasts.[34] PDGF exists as three different isoforms: PDGF-AA, PDGF-BB and PDGF-AB. Each of these isoforms binds to a different spectrum of receptor phenotypes.

Degranulating platelets release their stores of PDGF, along with TGF-β, platelet factor 4, platelet-derived angiogenic factor and PD-EGF. By its mitogenic and chemotactic actions, PDGF and the other factors cause an influx of neutrophils, monocytes, macrophages, fibroblasts, endothelial cells and smooth-muscle cells. These cells are also sources of PDGF, thus maintaining the levels of PDGF at various times during wound healing. PDGF modulates the extracellular matrix by increasing the collagen indirectly by upregulating TGF-β_1 and glycosaminoglycan synthesis, as well as increasing its turnover by increasing the secretion of collagenase.

Fibroblast growth factor

FGFs are a family of seven structurally related peptides which bind to specific receptors. FGFs also have a high affinity for heparin which protects them from proteolysis.

The presence of increased levels of basic FGF at sites of brain injury[137] and in synovial fluid following injury to the joint[138] have suggested an endogenous role for FGF in wound healing. Broadley *et al.*[139] placed slow-release pellets containing a monospecific neutralizing antibody to FGF into polyvinyl sponges implanted subcutaneously in rats. They reported a decrease in the DNA, protein and collagen content of sponges harvested on days 7, 9 and 12 postimplantation compared to control sponges suggesting an intrinsic role for FGF in wound healing.

Buntrock *et al.*[140] noted that the acceleration of wound healing by FGF was associated with an increased migration and proliferation of fibroblasts and an increased collagen synthesis by the fibroblasts. They also reported increased proliferation of endothelial cells and pericytes and new vessel formation.

Recent studies have also implicated a role for KGF (keratinocyte growth factor, a member of the FGF family) in wound healing.[141]

Epidermal growth factor/transforming growth factor-α

EGF and TGF-α are members of the EGF family which share similar biological activities. EGF is a single-chain acidic polypeptide with an isoelectric point of 4.5 containing 53 amino acid residues. TGF-α is a single-chain polypeptide of 50 amino acids that is structurally related to EGF.[142]

Hutson *et al.*[143] and Niall *et al.*[144] showed that wound healing of the skin was enhanced by licking the wounds and this was attributed to the presence of EGF. However, topical application of EGF in aqueous vehicles to partial thickness scalds in rats failed to accelerate healing.[145,146] In contrast, Buckley *et al.*[147] reported increased formation of granulation tissue when exogenous EGF was added to subcutaneously implanted polyvinyl alcohol sponges. These reports and *in vitro* studies suggest that cell proliferation requires a continuous exposure to EGF. It has been proposed that EGF and TGF-α are released at the site of injury by degranulating platelets[148] and wound macrophages.[149] EGF/TGF-α is chemotactic to fibroblasts and endothelial cells and mitogenic to keratinocytes, fibroblasts and endothelial cells and induces angiogenesis. EGF/TGF-α thus appears to play a role in wound healing.

Recently a new member of the EGF family has been identified. It is called heparin-binding (HB) EGF as it has affinity for heparin but binds to EGF receptors. HB-EGF is secreted by macrophages and is mitogenic to fibroblasts, keratinocytes and smooth-muscle cells but not endothelial cells. It may be involved in macrophage-mediated cellular proliferation.[150]

Recent advances in the molecular and cellular mechanisms of wound healing and scarring will undoubtedly influence our management of surgical and traumatic wounds. Acceleration of wound healing and, importantly, prevention and control of scarring will most certainly be feasible in the near future.

References

1. Kaplan KL. Platelet granule proteins: localization and secretion. In: JL Gordon (ed) *Platelets in Biology and Pathology*, vol. 2, pp. 77–90. Amsterdam: Elsevier, 1981.
2. George JN, Nurden AT, Phillips DR. Molecular defects in interactions of platelets with the vessel wall. *N Engl J Med* 1984; **311**: 1084–1098.
3. Knighton DR, Hunt TK, Thakral KK, Goodson WH. Role of platelets and fibrin in the healing sequence. An *in vivo* study of angiogenesis and collagen synthesis. *Ann Surg* 1982; **196**: 379–387.
4. Anderson DC, Schmasteig FC, Arnaout MA *et al.* Abnormalities of polymorphonuclear leukocyte function associated with a heritable deficiency of high molecular weight surface glycoproteins (GP138): common relationship to diminished cell adherence. *J Clin Invest* 1984; **74**: 536–551.
5. Harlan JM, Killen PD, Senecal FM, *et al.* The role of neutrophil membrane glycoprotein GP-150 in neutrophil adherence to endothelium *in vitro*. *Blood* 1985; **66**: 167–178.
6. Anderson DC, Springer, TA. Leukocyte adhesion deficiency: an inherited defect in the Mac-1, LFA-1 and p150,95 glycoproteins. *Annu Rev Med* 1987; **38**: 175–194.
7. Pohlman, TH, Stanness, KA, Beatty, PG, Ochs, HD, Harlan, JM. An endothelial cell surface factor(s) induced *in vitro* by lipopolysaccharide, interleukin-1 and tumor necrosis factor increases neutrophil adherence by a CDW18–dependent mechanism. *J Immunol* 1986; **136**: 4548–4553.
8. Shaw, JO. Leukocytes in chemotactic fragment-induced lung inflammation. *Am J Pathol* 1980; **101**: 283–291.
9. Simpson DM, Ross R. The neutrophilic leukocyte in wound repair. A study with antineutrophil serum. *J Clin Invest* 1972; **51**: 2009–2023.
10. Anderson L, Attstrom R, Fejerskor O. Effect of experimental neutropenia on oral wound healing in guinea pigs. *Scand J Dent Res* 1978; **86**: 237–247.
11. Ferguson MWJ, Howarth G. (1992) Marsupial models of scarless fetal wound healing. In: Adzick NS, Longaker MT (eds) *Fetal Wound Healing*, pp. 95–125, New York: Elsevier, 1992.
12. Alexander JW, Bossert JE, McClellan MA, Altemier WA. Stimulants of cellular proliferation in wounds. *Arch Surg* 1971; **103**: 167–174.
13. Leibovitch SJ, Ross R. The role of the macrophage in wound repair. A study with hydrocortisone and antimacrophage serum. *Am J Pathol* 1975; **78**: 71–91.
14. Bar-Shavit R, Kahn A, Fenton JW, Wilner GD. Chemotactic response of monocytes to thrombin. *J Cell Biol* 1983; **96**: 282–285.
15. Postlethwaite AE, Kang AH. Collagen and collagen peptide-induced chemotaxis of human blood monocytes. *J Exp Med* 1976; **143**: 1299–1307.
16. Senior RM, Griffin GL, Mecham RP, Wrenn DS, Prasad KU, Urry DW. Val-Gly-Val-Ala-Pro-Gly, a repeating peptide in elastin, is chemotactic for fibroblasts and monocytes. *J Cell Biol* 1984; **99**: 870–874.
17. Norris DA, Clark RAF, Swigart LM, Huff JC, Weston WL, Howell SE. Fibronectin fragment(s) are chemotactic for human peripheral blood monocytes. *J Immunol* 1982; **129**: 1612–1619.
18. Wahl SM, Hunt DA, Wakefield LM *et al.* Transforming growth factor type β induces monocyte chemotaxis and growth factor production. *Proc Natl Acad Sci USA* 1987; **84**: 5788–5792.
19. Deuel TF, Senior RM, Huang JS, Griffin GL. Chemotaxis of monocytes and neutrophils to platelet-derived growth factor. *J Clin Invest* 1982; **69**: 1046–1049.
20. Riches DWH. The multiple roles of macrophages in wound healing. In: Clark RAF, Henson PM (eds) *Molecular and Cellular Biology of Wound Repair*, pp. 213–239, New York: Plenum Press, 1988.
21. Danon D, Kowatch MA, Roth GS. Promotion of wound repair in old mice by local injection of macrophages. *Proc Natl Acad Sci USA* 1989; **86**: 2018–2020.
22. Werb Z, Banda MJ, Jones PA. Macrophage proteinases degrade matrix proteins. *J Exp Med* 1980; **152**: 1340–1357.
23. Parakkal PF, Macrophages: The time course and sequence of their distribution in the post-partum uterus. *J Ultrastruc Res* 1972; **40**: 284–291.
24. Wahl SM, Allen JB, Weeks BS, Wong HL, Klotman PE. Transforming growth factor β enhances integrin expression and type IV collagenase secretion in human monocytes. *Proc Natl Acad Sci USA* 1993; **90**: 4577–4581.

25. Postlethwaite AE, Lachman LB, Mainardi CL, Kang AH. Interleukin 1 stimulation of collagenase production by cultured fibroblasts. *J Exp Med* 1983; **157**: 801–806.
26. Tracey PB, Rohrbach MS, Mann KG. Functional prothrombinase complex assembly on isolated monocytes and lymphocytes. *J Biol Chem* 1983; **258**: 7264–7267.
27. Tsukamoto Y, Helsel WE, Wahl SM. Macrophage production of fibronectin, a chemoattractant for fibroblasts. *J Immunol* 1981; **127**: 673–679.
28. Brown LF, Dubin D, Lavigne L, Logan B, Dvorak HF, Van de Water L. Macrophages and fibroblasts express embryonic fibronectins during cutaneous wound healing. *Am J Pathol* 1993; **142**: 793–801.
29. Thakral KK, Goodson WH, Hunt TK. Stimulation of wound blood vessel growth by wound macrophages. *J Surg Res* 1979; **26**: 430–436.
30. Hunt TK, Knighton DR, Thakral KK, Goodson WH, Andrews WS. Studies on inflammation and wound healing: angiogenesis and collagen synthesis stimulated *in vivo* by resident and activated wound macrophages. *Surgery* 1984; **96**: 48–55.
31. Rappolee DA, Mark D, Banda MJ, Werb Z. Wound macrophages express TGF-α and other growth factors *in vivo*: analyses by mRNA phenotyping. *Science* 1988; **241**: 708–712.
32. Sunderkotter C, Goebeler M, Schulze-Osthoff K, Bhardwaj R, Sorg C. Macrophage-derived angiogenesis factors. *Pharm Ther* 19791; **51**: 195–216.
33. Assoian RK, Fleurdelys BE, Stevenson HC *et al.* Expression and secretion of type beta transforming growth factor by activated human macrophages. *Proc Natl Acad Sci USA* 1987; **84**: 6020–6024.
34. Shimokado K, Raines EW, Madtes DK, Barrett TB, Benditt EP, Ross R. A significant part of macrophage-derived growth factor consists of two forms of PDGF. *Cell* 1985; **43**: 277–288.
35. Allam, M, Martinet, N, Gallati, H, Martinet, Y. (1992) Differential expression of PDGF-A and B chain genes and production of AA and AB dimers by activated human blood monocytes. *Biochimie* 1992; **74**: 1097–1101.
36. Baird A, Bohlen P. Fibroblast growth factors. In: Sporn MB, Roberts AB (eds) *Peptide Growth Factors and Their Receptors I*, pp. 369–418. Berlin: Springer Verlag, 1990.
37. Pencev D, Grotendorst GR. Human peripheral blood monocytes secrete a unique form of PDGF. *Oncogene Res* 1988; **3**: 333–342.
38. Van-Obberghen-Schilling E, Roche NS, Flanders KC, Sporn MB, Roberts AB. Transforming growth factor β_1 positively regulates its own expression in normal and transformed cells. *J Biol Chem* 1988; **263**: 7741–7746.
39. Fishel RS, Barbul A, Beschorner WE, Wasserkrug HL, Efron G. Lymphocyte participation in wound healing. *Ann Surg* 1987; **206**: 25–29.
40. Peterson JM, Barbul A, Breslin RJ, Wasserkrug HL, Efron G. Significance of T-lymphocytes in wound healing. *Surgery* 1987; **102**: 300–305.
41. Kovacs EJ. Fibrogenic cytokines: the role of immune mediators in the development of scar tissue. *Immunol Today* 1991; **12**: 17–23.
42. MacDonald RA. Origin of fibroblasts in experimental healing wounds; autoradiographic studies using tritiated thymidine. *Surgery* 1959; **46**: 376.
43. Postlethwaite AE, Seyer JM, Kang AH. Chemotactic attraction of human fibroblasts to type I, II and III collagens and collagen derived peptides. *Proc Nat Acad Sci (USA)* 1978; **75**: 871–875.
44. Grinnell F, Feld M, Minter D. Fibroblast adhesion to fibrinogen and fibrin substrata: requirement for cold-insoluble globulin (plasma fibronectin). *Cell* 1980; **19**: 517–525.
45. Seppa HEJ, Grotendorst GR, Seppa SI, Schiffmann E, Martin GR. Platelet-derived growth factor is chemotactic for fibroblasts. *J Cell Biol* 1982; **92**: 584–588.
46. Postlethwaite AE, Keski-Oja J, Moses HL, Kang AH. Stimulation of the chemotactic migration of human fibroblasts by transforming growth factor-β. *J Exp Med* 1987; **165**: 251–256.
47. Grinnell F, Billingham RE, Burgess L. Distribution of fibronectin during wound healing *in vivo*. *J Invest Dermatol* 1981; **76**: 181–189.
48. Gabbiani G, Ryan GB, Majno G. Presence of modified fibroblasts in granulation tissue and their possible role in wound contraction. *Experientia* 1971; **27**: 549–550.
49. Desmouliere A, Geinoz A, Gabbiani F, Gabbiani G. Transforming growth factor β_1 induces α-smooth muscle actin expression in granulation tissue myofibroblasts and in quiescent and growing cultured fibroblasts. *J Cell Biol* 1993; **122**: 103–111.
50. Rudolph R. Inhibition of myofibroblasts by skin grafts. *Plast Reconstr Surg* 1979; **63**: 473–480.
51. Pierce GF, Berg JV, Rudolph R, Tarpley J, Mustoe TA. Platelet-derived growth factor-BB and transforming growth factor beta 1 selectively modulate glycosaminoglycans, collagen and myofibroblasts in excisional wounds. *Am J Pathol* 1991; **138**: 629–646.
52. Ehrlich HP. Wound closure: evidence of co-operation between fibroblasts and collagen matrix. *Eye* 1988; **2**: 149–157.
53. Martin P, Lewis J. Actin cables and epidermal movement in embryonic wound healing. *Nature* 1992; **360**: 179–182.
54. Madri JA, Pratt, BP. Angiogenesis. In: Clark RAF, Henson PM (eds) *Molecular and Cellular Biology of Wound Repair*, pp. 337–358. New York: Plenum Press, 1988.
55. Banda MJ, Knighton DR, Hunt TK, Werb Z. Isolation of a nonmitogenic angiogenesis factor from wound fluid. *Proc Natl Acad Sci USA* 1982; **79**: 7773–7777.
56. Klagsbrun M, D'Amore PA. Regulators of angiogenesis. *Annu Rev Physiol* 1991; **53**: 217–239.
57. Schreiber AB, Winkler ME, Derynck R, Transforming growth factor alpha: a more potent angiogenic

mediator than epidermal growth factor. *Science* 1986; **232**: 1250–1253.
58. Roberts AB, Sporn MB, Assoian RK *et al.* Transforming growth factor type β: rapid induction of fibrosis and angiogenesis *in vivo* and stimulation of collagen formation *in vitro*. *Proc Natl Acad Sci USA* 1986; **83**: 4167–4171.
59. Folkman J, Klagsbrun M. Angiogenic factors. *Science* 1987; **235**: 442–447.
60. Moses MA, Langer R. A metalloproteinase inhibitor as an inhibitor of neovascularization. *J Cell Biochem* 1991; **47**: 230–235.
61. Ausprunk DH, Falterman K, Folkman J. The sequence of events in the regression of corneal capillaries. *Lab Invest* 1978; **38**: 284–294.
62. Stenn KS, De Palma L. Re-epithelialization. In: Clark RAF, Henson PM (eds) *Molecular and Cellular Biology of Wound Repair*, pp. 321–335. New York: Plenum Press, 1988.
63. Guo M, Kim LT, Akiyama SK, Gralnick HR, Yamada KM, Grinnell F. Altered processing of integrin receptors during keratinocyte activation. *Exp Cell Res* 1991; **195**: 315–322.
64. Hebda PA. Stimulatory effects of transforming growth factor-beta and epidermal growth factor on epidermal cell outgrowth from porcine skin explant cultures. *J Invest Dermatol* 1988; **91**: 440–445.
65. Hebda PA. The acceleration of epidermal wound healing in partial thickness burns by transforming growth factor-beta. *J Invest Dermatol* 1989; **92**: 442.
66. Mansbridge JN, Hanawalt PC. Role of transforming growth factor beta in the maturation of human epidermal keratinocytes. *J Invest Dermatol* 1988; **3**: 336–340.
67. Brown GL, Curtsinger L, Brightwell JR *et al.* Enhancement of epidermal regeneration by biosynthetic epidermal growth factor. *J Exp Med* 1988; **163**: 1319–1324.
68. Brown GL, Curtsinger L, Jurkiewicz MJ, Nahai F, Schultz G. Stimulation of healing chronic wounds by epidermal growth factor. *Plast Reconstr Surg* 1991; **88**: 189–194.
69. Brown GL, Nanney LB, Griffen J *et al.* Enhancement of wound healing by topical treatment with epidermal growth factor. *N Engl J Med* 1989; **321**: 76–79.
70. Stoker M, Gherardi E. Regulation of cell movement: the motogenic cytokines. *Biochem Biophys Acta* 1991; **1072**: 81–102.
71. Clark RAF. Fibronectin matrix deposition and fibronectin receptor expression in healing and normal skin. *J Invest Dermatol* 1990; **94**: 128S–134S.
72. Clark RAF, Lanigan JM, Dellapelle P, Manseau E, Dvorak HF, Colvin RB. Fibronectin and fibrin provide a provisional matrix for epidermal cell migration during wound re-epithelialization. *J Invest Dermatol* 1982; **79**: 264–269.
73. Postlethwaite A, Keski-Oja J, Balian G, Kang AH. Induction of fibroblast chemotaxis by fibronectin. Localization of the chemotactic region to a 140 000 molecular weight non-gelatin binding fragment. *J Exp Med* 1981; **153**: 494–499.
74. Bowersox JC, Sorgente N. Chemotactic response of vascular endothelial cells to fibronectin. *J Cell Biol* 1980; **87**: 64a.
75. Beezhold DH, Personius C. Fibronectin fragments stimulate tumour necrosis factor secretion by human monocytes. *J Leukocyte Biol* 1992; **51**: 59–64.
76. Dunphy JE, Upuda KN. Chemical and histochemical sequences in normal healing wounds. *N Engl J Med* 1955; **253**: 847–851.
77. West DC, Kumar S. Hyaluronan and angiogenesis. In: D Evered and J Whelan (eds) *The Biology of Hyaluronan*, pp. 187–207. Chichester: Wiley, 1989.
78. Gallagher JT. The extended family of proteoglycans: social residents of the pericellular zone. *Curr Opin Cell Biol* 1989; **1**: 1201–1218.
79. Burgeson RE. New collagens, new concepts. *Annu Rev Cell Biol* 1988; **4**: 551–577.
80. Gordon MK, Olsen BR. The contribution of collagenous proteins to tissue-specific matrix assemblies. *Curr Opin Cell Biol* 1990; **2**: 833–838.
81. Schuppan D, Becker J, Boehm H, Hahn EG. Immunofluorescent localization of type-V collagen as a fibrillar component of the interstitial connective tissue of human oral mucosa, artery and liver. *Cell Tissue Res* 1986; **243**:535–543.
82. Ignotz RA, Massague J. Transforming growth factor-β stimulates the expression of fibronectin and collagen and their incorporation into the extracellular matrix. *J Biol Chem* 1986; **261**: 4337–4345.
83. Woessner JF. Matrix metalloproteinases and their inhibitors in connective tissue remodeling. *FASEB J* 1991; **5**: 2145–2154.
84. Werb Z, Alexander CM. Proteinases and matrix degradation. In: Kelly WN, Harris ED, Ruddy S, Sledge CB (eds) *Textbook of Rheumatology*, 4th edn. pp. 248–268. Philadelphia: WB Saunders, 1993.
85. Stenn KS, Madri JA, Roll FJ. Migrating epidermis produces AB2 collagen and requires continual collagen synthesis for movement. *Nature* 1979; **277**: 229–232.
86. Merkel J, Dipaolo BR, Hallock GG, Rice DC. Type I and type III collagen content of healing wounds in fetal and adult rats. *Proc Soc Exp Biol Med* 1988; **187**: 493–497.
87. Sakai LY, Keene DR, Morris NP, Burgeson RE. Type VII collagen is a major structural component of anchoring fibrils. *J Cell Biol* 1986; **103**: 1577–1586.
88. Mackie EJ, Halfter W, Liverani D. Induction of tenascin in healing wounds. *J Cell Biol* 1988; **107**: 2757–2767.
89. Whitby DJ, Ferguson MWJ. The extracellular matrix of lip wounds in fetal, neonatal and adult mice. *Development* 1991; **112**: 651–668.
90. Saga Y, Yagi T, Ikawa Y, Sakakura T, Aizawa S. Mice develop normally without tenascin. *Genes Dev* 1992; **6**: 1821–1831.

91. Rowlatt U. Intrauterine wound healing in a 20 week human fetus. *Virchows Arch A Pathol Anat Histopathol* 1979; **381**: 353–361.
92. Longaker MT, Whitby DJ, Adzick NS. Studies in fetal wound healing: VI. Second and early third trimester fetal wounds demonstrate rapid collagen deposition without scar formation. *J Paediatr Surg* 1990; **25**: 63–69.
93. Adzick NS, Harrison MR, Glick PL *et al.* Comparison of fetal, newborn and adult wound healing by histologic, enzyme-histochemical and hydroxyproline determinations. *J Paediatr Surg* 1985; **20**: 315–319.
94. Krummel TM, Nelson JM, Diegelmann RF, Lindblad RF *et al.* Fetal response to injury in the rabbit. *J Paediatr Surg* 1987; **22**: 640–643.
95. Sopher D. A study of wound healing in the foetal tissues of the cyanomalgus monkey. In: Perkins FT, O'Donoghue, PN (eds) *Breeding Simians for Developmental Biology* pp. 327–335. London: Laboratory Animal Handbooks, 1975.
96. Hallock GG, Rice DC, McClure HM. *In utero* lip repair in the rhesus monkey: an update. *Plast Reconstr Surg* 1987; **80**: 855–858.
97. Whitby DJ, Ferguson MWJ. Immunohistochemical localization of growth factors in fetal wound healing. *Dev Biol* 1991; **147**: 207–215.
98. Dixon JB. Inflammation in the foetal and neonatal rat: the local reactions to skin burns. *J Pathol Bacteriol* 1960; **80**: 73–82.
99. De Palma RL, Krummel TM, Durham LA. Characterization and quantitation of wound matrix in the fetal rabbit. *Matrix* 1989; **9**: 224–231.
100. Mast BA, Flood LC, Haynes JH *et al.* Hyalaluronic acid is a major component of the matrix of fetal rabbit skin and wounds: implications for healing by regeneration. *Matrix* 1991; **11**: 63–68.
101. Longaker MT, Whitby DJ, Ferguson, MWJ. Studies in fetal wound healing: III. Early deposition of fibronectin distinguishes fetal from adult wound healing. *J Paediatr Surg* 1989; **24**: 799–805.
102. Whitby DJ, Longaker MT, Harrison MR, Adzick NS, Ferguson MWJ. Rapid epithelialization of fetal wounds is associated with the early deposition of tenascin. *J Cell Sci* 1991; **99**: 583–586.
103. Lorenz HP, Whitby DJ, Longaker MT, Adzick NS. (1993) Fetal wound healing. The ontogeny of scar formation in the non-human primate. *Ann Surg* 1993; **217**: 391–396.
104. Goss RJ. (1992) Regeneration versus repair. In: JK Cohen, RF Diegelmann, WJ Lindblad (eds) *Wound Healing. Biochemical and Clinical Aspects*, pp. 20–40. Philadelphia: Saunders, 1992.
105. Illingworth CM. Trapped fingers and amputated finger tips in children. *J Paediatr Surg* 1974; **9**: 853–858.
106. Meyer M, McGrouther DA. A study relating wound tension to scar morphology in the presternal scar using Langers technique. *Br J Plast Surg* 1991; **4**: 291–295.
107. Efimov EA, Boukina TV. On the completeness of skin regeneration and reorganization of scars in warm-blooded animals. In: Taban CH, Boilly B (eds), *Keys for Regeneration. Monographs in Developmental Biology*, vol. 23, pp. 165–174. Basel: Karger, 1992.
108. Schor SL, Schor AM. Clonal heterogeneity in fibroblast phenotype: implications for the control of epithelial-mesenchymal interactions. *Bioessays* 1987; **7**: 200–204.
109. Rockwell WB, Cohen IK, Ehrlich HP. Keloids and hypertrophic scars: a comprehensive review. *Plast Reconstr Surg* 1989; **84**(5): 827–837.
110. McCauley RL, Chopra V, Li YY, Henderson DN, Robson MC. Altered cytokine production in black patients with keloids. *J Clin Immunol* 1992; **12**, 300–308.
111. Canniff JP, Harvey W, Harris M. Oral submucous fibrosis; its pathogenesis and management. *Br Dent J* 1986; **160**: 429–434.
112. Canniff JP, Batchelor JR, Dodi K and Harvey W. HLA typing in oral submucous fibrosis. *Tissue Antigens* 1985; **26**: 138–142.
113. Harris M, Haque M and Meghji S. *Oral submucous fibrosis responds to intralesional interferon gamma. Betel quid and tobacco chewing among the Bangladeshi community in the United Kingdom.* Bedi R. and Jones P (eds). London: Centre for Transcultural Oral Health, 1995.
114. Abergel RP, Pizzurro D, Meeker CA *et al.* Biochemical composition of the connective tissue in keloids and analysis of collagen metabolism in keloid fibroblast cultures. *J Invest Dermatol* 1985; **84**: 384–390.
115. Linares HA. Proteoglycan-lymphocyte association in the development of hypertrophic scars. *Burns* 1990; **16**: 21–24.
116. Russell SB, Trupin KM, Rodriguez-Eaton S, Russell JD, Trupin JS. Reduced growth-factor requirement of keloid-derived fibroblasts may account for tumor growth. *Proc Natl Acad Sci USA* 1988; **85**: 587–591.
117. Peltonen J, Hsiao LL, Jaakkola S *et al.* Activation of collagen gene expression in keloids: co-localization of type I and VI collagen and transforming growth factor-β1 mRNA. *J Invest Dermatol* 1991; **97**: 240–248.
118. Babu M, Diegelmann R, Oliver N. Keloid fibroblasts exhibit an altered response to TGF-β. *J Invest Dermatol* 1992; **99**: 650–655.
119. Nathan C, Sporn M. Cytokines in context. *J Cell Biol* 1991; **113**: 981–986.
120. McGrath MH. Peptide growth factors and wound healing. *Clin Plast Surg* 1990; **17**: 421–432.
121. Martin P, Hopkinson-Woolley J, McCluskey J. Growth factors and cutaneous wound repair. *Prog Growth Factor Res* 1992; **4**: 25–44.
122. Wong ST, Winchell LF, McCune BK *et al.* The TGF-α precursor expressed on the cell surface binds to the EGF receptor on adjacent cells, leading to signal transduction. *Cell* 1989; **56**: 495–506.

123. Ksander GA. Exogenous growth factors in dermal wound healing. *Annu Rep Med Chem* 1989; **24**: 223–232.
124. Robson MC, Phillips LG, Thomason A, Robson LE, Pierce GF. Platelet-derived growth factor BB for the treatment of chronic pressure ulcers. *Lancet* 1992; **339**: 23–25.
125. Roberts AB, Sporn MB. The transforming growth factors-β. In: Sporn MB, Roberts AB (eds) *Peptide Growth Factors and their Receptors I*, pp. 419–472. Berlin: Springer Verlag, 1990.
126. Mustoe TA, Pierce GF, Thomason A, Gramates P, Sporn MB, Deuel TF. Accelerated healing of incisional wound in rats induced by transforming growth factor-β. *Science* 1987; **237**: 1333–1336.
127. Mustoe TA, Landes A, Cromack DT *et al.* Differential acceleration of healing of surgical incisions in the rabbit gastrointestinal tract by platelet-derived growth factor and transforming growth factor, type beta. *Surgery* 1990; **108**: 324–330.
128. Ksander GA, Ogawa Y, Chu GH, McMullin H, Rossenblatt JS, McPherson JM. Exogenous transforming growth factor-β_2 enhances connective tissue formation and wound strength in guinea pig dermal wound healing by secondary intent. *Ann Surg* 1990; **211**: 288–294.
129. Salomon GD, Kasid A, Bernstein E, Buresh C, Director E, Norton JA. Gene expression in normal and doxorubicin-impaired wounds: importance of transforming growth factor-beta. *Surgery* 1990; **108**: 318–323.
130. Amento EP, Beck S. TGF-β and wound healing. In: *Clinical Applications of TGF-β*, vol. 157, pp. 115–129. Chichester: Wiley, 1991.
131. Shah M, Foreman DM, Ferguson MWJ. Control of scarring in adult wounds by neutralising antibody to transforming growth factor β. *Lancet* 1992; **339**: 213–214.
132. Shah M, Foreman DM, Ferguson MWJ. Neutralising antibody to TGF-$\beta_{1,2}$ reduces cutaneous scarring in adult rodents. *J Cell Sci* 1994; **107**: 1137–1157.
133. Shah M, Foreman DM, Ferguson MWJ. Neutralization of TGF-β_1 and TGF-β_2 or exogenous addition of TGF-β_3 to cutaneous rat wounds reduces scarring. *J Cell Sci* 1995; **108**: 985–1002.
134. Foreman DM, Shah M, Ferguson MWJ. Reduction of scar tissue formation in adult rodent wound healing by mannose-6–phosphate. *Second annual meeting of ETRS-abstract book.* (ISBN 095 262090 1).
135. Rutherford RB, Ross R. Platelet factors stimulate fibroblasts and smooth muscle cells quiescent in plasma serum to proliferate. *J Cell Biol* 1976; **69**: 196–203.
136. Ross R, Glomset JA, Kariya B, Harker L. A platelet-derived serum factor that stimulates the proliferation of arterial smooth muscle cells *in vitro*. *Proc Natl Acad Sci USA* 1974; **71**: 1207–1210.
137. Logan A, Frautschy SA, Gonzalez AM, Baird A. A time course for the focal elevation of synthesis of basic fibroblast growth factor and one of its high-affinity receptors (flg) following a localized cortical brain injury. *J Neurosci* 1992; **12**: 3828–3837.
138. Hamerman D, Taylor S, Kirschenbaum I *et al.* Growth factors with heparin binding affinity in human synovial fluid. *Proc Soc Exp Biol Med* 1987; **186**: 384–389.
139. Broadley KN, Aquino AM, Woodward SC. Monospecific antibodies implicate basic fibroblast growth factor in normal wound repair. *Lab Invest* 1989; **61**: 571–575.
140. Buntrock P, Buntrock M, Marx I, Kranz D, Jentzsch KD, Heder G. Stimulation of wound healing, using brain extract with fibroblast growth factor activity III. Electron microscopy, autoradiography and ultrastructural autoradiography of granulation tissue. *Exp Pathol* 1984; **26**: 247–254.
141. Werner S, Peters KG, Longaker MT, Fuller-Pace F, Banda MJ, Williams LT. Large induction of keratinocyte growth factor expression in the dermis during wound healing. *Proc Natl Acad Sci USA* 1992; **89**: 6696–6900.
142. Marquardt H, Hunkapiller MW, Hood LE, Todaro GJ. Rat transforming growth factor type I: structure and relation to epidermal growth factor. *Science* 1984; **223**: 1079–1082.
143. Hutson JM, Niall M, Evans D, Fowler R. Effect of salivary glands on wound contraction in mice. *Nature* 1979; **279**: 793–795.
144. Niall M, Ryan GB, O'Brien BM. The effect of epidermal growth factor on wound healing in mice. *J Surg Res* 1982; **33**: 164–169.
145. Thornton JW, Hess CA, Cassingham V, Bartlett RH. Epidermal growth factor in the healing of second degree burns: a controlled animal study. *Burns* 1981; **8**: 156–160.
146. Arturson G. Epidermal growth factor in the healing of corneal wounds, epidermal wounds and partial-thickness scalds. *Scand J Plast Reconstr Surg* 1984; **18**: 33–37.
147. Buckley A, Davidson JM, Kamerath CD, Wolt TB, Woodward SC. Sustained release of epidermal growth factor accelerates wound repair. *Proc Natl Acad Sci USA* 1985; **82**: 7340–7344.
148. Pesonen K, Viinikka L, Myllylae G, Kiuru J, Perheentupa J. Characterization of material with epidermal growth factor immunoreactivity in human serum and platelets. *J Clin Endocrinol Metab* 1989; **68**: 486–491.
149. Higashiyama S, Abraham JA, Miller J, Fiddes JC, Klagsbrun M. A heparin-binding growth factor secreted by macrophage-like cells that is related to EGF. *Science* 1991; **251**: 936–939.
150. Marikovsky M, Breuing K, Liu PY *et al.* Appearance of heparin-binding EGF-like growth factor in wound fluid as a response to injury. *Proc Natl Acad Sci USA* 1993; **90**: 3889–3893.

7

Bone remodelling – cellular and biochemical aspects

Sajeda Meghji, Jonathan R Sandy and Malcolm Harris

Introduction

Bone is a specialized connective tissue that makes up, together with cartilage, the skeleton. These tissues serve three functions: first, mechanical support and site of muscle attachment for locomotion; second, protection for vital organs and bone marrow; and third, a metabolic reserve of ions for the entire organism, especially calcium and phosphate. It is a highly dynamic connective tissue with a capacity for continuous remodelling. Bone is composed of a variety of cell types and an extracellular organic matrix which has become calcified.

The two principal cell types, the osteoblast and the osteoclast, are the major effectors in the turnover of bone matrix. The osteoblast produces the matrix, which in a well-regulated process becomes calcified to form initially the partially calcified osteoid and ultimately fully mineralized bone. This mineral matrix can be dissolved by the activity of the osteoclast when activated. At any given time the processes of bone synthesis and bone breakdown are going on simultaneously and the status of the bone represents the net result of a balance between the two processes. This phenomenon is now widely called coupling of bone resorption and formation.

The extracellular organic matrix of bone consists predominantly of type I collagen (85–95%). The non-collagenous constituents are composed of proteins and proteogylcans which are specific to bone and the dental hard connective tissues (Fig. 7.1). Two-dimensional

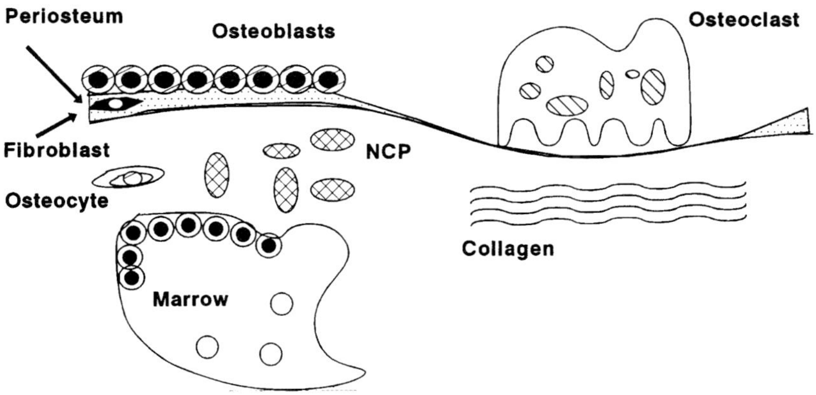

Fig. 7.1 Bone is composed of a variety of cell types and an extracellular organic matrix. The cells include osteoblast, osteocytes, osteoclasts and periosteal fibroblasts. The matrix consists of collagen (85–95%) and non-collagenous proteins (NCP) such as osteonectin, proteoglycan I, proteoglycan II, osteopontin, osteocalcin, sialoprotein II and matrix GLA protein.

electrophoretic analysis of the non-collagen proteins of bone suggests that there may be well over 200 of them.[1] Many of these proteins are identified as originating from plasma or other non-bone sources, for example, α_2-glycoprotein and β_2-microglobulin. The non-collagenous protein products of the bone cells include osteonectin, proteoglycan I, proteoglycan II, osteopontin (sialoprotein I), sialoprotein II, osteocalcin and matrix GLA protein, all of which appear to contribute to the structure and functional qualities of bone.

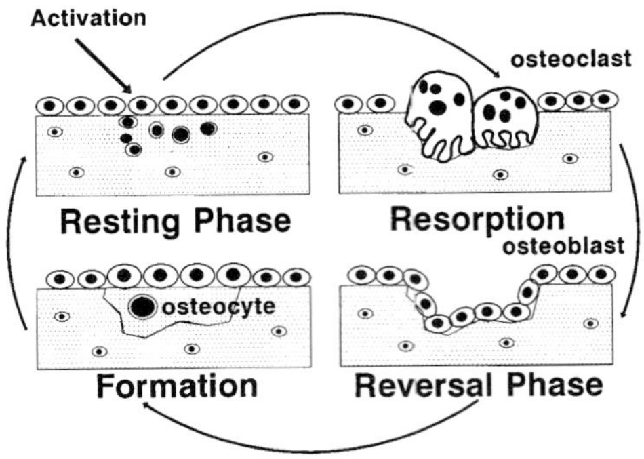

Fig. 7.2 Bone remodelling is a constantly dynamic process. Normal bone breakdown equals new bone formation.

Bone remodelling

Bone remodelling is a finely balanced process regulated by systemic and local humoral factors. The principal effector cells are the bone-forming osteoblast and the osteoclast, the major bone-resorbing cell. Except during growth, a balance between bone resorption and formation is normally maintained. In the normal adult skeleton, bone formation equals resorption, and this is a constant dynamic process throughout life (Fig. 7.2). Any dysfunction of the local or systemic regulatory systems will lead to pathological changes in the rate of bone formation or resorption and a clinical disease of the skeleton.

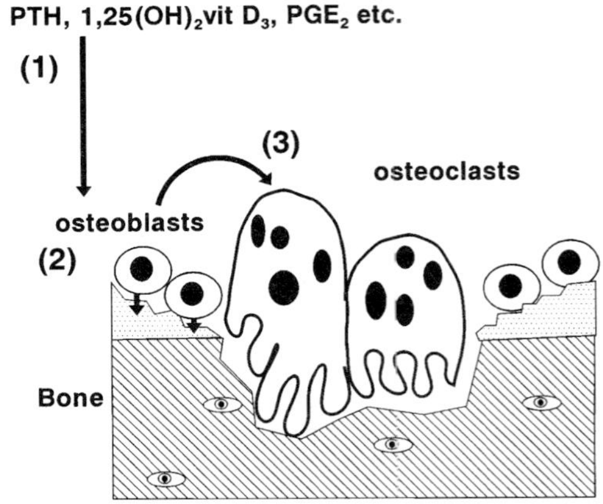

Fig. 7.3 The role of the osteoblast in bone resorption: three steps are probably involved. (1) A bone-resorbing agent such as parathyroid hormone (PTH) or prostaglandin E_2 (PGE_2), stimulates the osteoblasts to synthesize and release collagenase and plasminogen activator which digest the osteoid, exposing the mineralized matrix which may be chemotactic to the osteoclast. (2) The bone-resorbing agent also induces a change of shape of the osteoblast, facilitating the access of the osteoclasts to the bone surface and (3) the osteoblast releases a short-range soluble activator for the osteoclast.

Bone resorption

Resorption is the removal of the mineral and organic components of the extracellular matrix of bone under the action of osteolytic cells, of which the most important is the osteoclast. The osteocyte may function as a local bone resorber, ensuring the natural renewal of bone.

The process involves three steps, each of which may be individually regulated by physiological, pathological or pharmacological mediators. The first involves the formation of osteoclast progenitors in the haematopoietic tissues followed by their vascular dissemination and the generation of resting preosteoclasts and osteoclasts in the bone itself. The second phase consists of osteoclast activation at the surface of the mineralized bone. Here osteoblasts appear to play a major role, not only by retracting to expose the mineral to the osteoclast and preosteoclasts, but also by releasing a soluble factor that activates these cells (Fig. 7.3). The third step involves the activated osteoclast resorbing the bone. During bone resorption, the clasts create for themselves cavities known as Howship's lacunae, which correspond closely in size to the area of bone surface enclosed by the cell. This active surface is described as having a ruffled border which consists of many infoldings of the cell membrane, resulting in finger-like projection of the cytoplasm. Thus an extensive surface is created which is well-suited for an

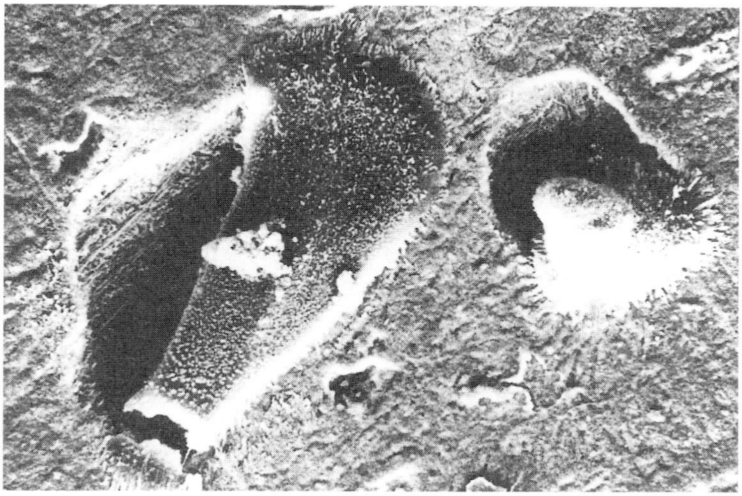

Fig. 7.4 Electron micrograph of two osteoclasts on a surface of a dentine slice, showing resorptive pits.

intensive exchange between the cell and the bone, and is effectively sealed off from the extracellular environment by a tight junction between the bone and the periphery of the osteoclast. Osteoclasts can also move about on the surfaces of bone and dentine slices *in vitro* and leave discontinuous tracks of resorptive activity behind them (Fig. 7.4).[2] In order to carry out bone resorption the osteoclast can secrete organic acids maintaining a sufficiently low pH in the microenvironment at the bone surface, to dissolve the hydroxyapatite crystals. The resorption of the organic matrix is enzymatic principally by lysosomal enzymes. A lysosome is an intracellular membrane-enclosed vacuole containing lytic enzymes.

Biochemical studies have shown that there is a good correlation between lysosomal enzyme release and the progress of bone resorption.[3,4] Those hormones which stimulate bone resorption also appear to increase the synthesis and secretion of various lysosomal enzymes. The osteoclast lysosomes and their lytic enzymes participate in continuous processes of exocytosis and endocytosis at the ruffled border. Enzymes are released into the extracellular bone matrix (exocytosis) and the solubilized matrix components are taken up into the cell within vacuoles termed phagosomes (endocytosis) for further intracellular digestion. The introduction of endocytosed materials to the lysosomal digestive enzymes occurs by the fusion of the phagosome and lysosomes.[5]

Other enzymes involved are metalloproteinases such as collagenase and stromelysins which are dependent on the presence of the metal ion zinc at the active site and serine proteinases such as elastase. All these proteinases would not retain much activity in the low pH of the ruffle border.

The metalloproteinases are secreted into tissues predominantly in the inactive procollagenase form. It is also known that osteoblasts release collagenase especially in response to resorbing agents such as parathyroid hormone (PTH).[6,7] This synthesis of collagenase by osteoblasts suggests that they also contribute to matrix degradation either by digesting the non-mineralized layer of osteoid on the bone surface to facilitate osteoclast activity or by degrading the demineralized matrix when exposed by osteoclastic activity.

Bone formation

Bone formation is an essential process for the maintenance of bone mass and strength. It is also modulated by both systemic hormones and local factors. Bone formation occurs by one of two routes: first, a direct development of bone from mesenchymal cells, as in the calvarium, called intramembranous ossification, and second, an intervening cartilage model precedes the formation – the proliferation of mesenchymal cells is followed by their differentiation into chondrocytes which become hypertrophied and calcified. The calcified cartilage is then replaced by bone which is then remodelled. Formation of bone by this route occurs in long bones and is called endochondral ossification. However, these two modes of ossification do not produce significantly different kinds of bone.[8]

Whatever the means, osteogenesis is a prolonged process which takes several months. The cellular events involved in bone formation include the attraction of osteoblast precursors to the site of resorption by a process of chemotaxis. Their stimulation is followed by differentiation to mature cells which are capable of synthesizing bone proteins. Osteoblasts synthesize and secrete the extracellular organic matrix of bone, including type I collagen, osteocalcin, osteopontin, osteonectin, alkaline phosphatase and proteoglycans as well as the growth-regulatory factors which are stored within the bone matrix. Collagen is initially secreted from the cell surface in an orderly manner, so that the fibrils are oriented parallel to the long axis of the cells.[9] When the osteoblasts become embedded in the matrix which they have produced they become by definition osteocytes, which may continue to produce a limited amount of collagen before becoming completely embedded. However, most of the collagen is produced by the active osteoblasts on the bone-forming surface where they form a pavement-like sheet of closely packed cells.

The mediators of bone remodelling (Table 7.1)

Parathyroid hormone

PTH is an 84-amino-acid single-chain polypeptide secreted by the four parathyroid glands. It has a direct effect on bone turnover, increasing rates of both new bone formation and bone resorption. Physiological concentrations appear to promote bone formation, increase the distal tubular reabsorption of calcium by the kidney, but decrease reabsorption of phosphate. Intermittent administration or low concentration of PTH can stimulate bone formation, probably by increasing the production of local growth factors such as an insulin-like growth factor-1 (IGF-1) and transforming growth factor-1 (TGF-β).[10–12] Increased concentrations promote osteoclastic bone resorption. It stimulates bone resorption both *in vivo* and *in vitro*.[13,14] PTH can also indirectly increase the absorption of calcium by the gut by the stimulation of 1,25-dihydroxy vitamin D_3 synthesis in the kidneys. In high concentrations, PTH inhibits osteoblastic collagen synthesis,[15] this is probably at the level of gene transcription.[16]

Table 7.1 Regulators of bone remodelling

Systemic	*Local*
Polypeptide hormones	
Parathyroid hormone	*Eicosanoids*
Calcitonin	Prostaglandins (PGs)
Insulin	Leukotrienes (LTs)
Growth hormone	
Steroid hormones	
1,25-Dihydroxy vitamin D_3	*Cytokines*
Glucocorticoids	Interleukin-1 (IL-1)
Sex steroids	Interleukin-6
	Tumour necrosis factor (TNF)
Thyroid hormones	
	Growth factors
	Insulin-like growth factor 1 (IGF-1)
	Transforming growth factor β (TGF-β)
	Fibroblast growth factor (FGF)
	Platelet-derived growth factor (PDGF)
	Other
	Parathyroid hormone-related peptide (PTHrp)
	$β_2$-microglobulin

Parathyroid hormone-related peptide (PTHrP)

A number of tumours associated with hypercalcaemia have been found to produce factors that are clearly not PTH, but appear to bind to PTH receptors and so mimic some of the hormone's actions. This factor has now been purified, and the responsible gene has been cloned.[17–20] In each case, there is considerable homology between the PTHrP and PTH within the N-terminal region (8 of the first 13 residues) while the remaining sequence differs substantially. An N-terminal fragment of PTHrP, (PTHrP-1-34) NH_2 has recently been synthesized and its biological properties evaluated.[21,22] When administered *in vivo* this peptide produces hypercalcaemia, reduces serum phosphate, elevates circulating levels of 1,25-dihydroxy vitamin D_3 and increases the excretion of cyclic adenosine monophosphate (cAMP) and phosphate. Similarly, Sato *et al.*[23] showed that PTHrP stimulates bone resorption *in vitro* and increases the serum calcium levels in mice. The biological profile displayed by this peptide suggests that PTH antagonists could inhibit all or most of its actions. In this way the hypercalcaemia produced by malignant tumours with its debilitating anorexia, nausea, diarrhoea, polyuria, polydipsia and depression can be controlled by corticosteroids and bisphosphonates.

Vitamin D metabolites

The vitamin D metabolites are steroid-like compounds which are derived from the plant ergosterol, fish oils and ingested in the diet, or synthesized in the skin by exposure of epidermal cells to ultraviolet light. The cholecalciferol is hydroxylated in the kidney and then further hydroxylated in the liver to produce the active hormone.

Thus the major active metabolite of vitamin D is 1,25-dihydroxy-cholecalciferol. The major physiological role of 1,25-dihydroxy vitamin D_3 (1,25 $(OH)_2D_3$) is to increase calcium and phosphate absorbtion in the intestine. 1,25 $(OH)_2D_3$ can also enhance bone resorption and inhibit bone formation.[24,25] Its effect on bone resorption appears to be by the differentiation of committed progenitor cells into mature cells.[26] Pharmacological doses of vitamin D can prevent bone loss in animal models.[27,28]

Eicosanoids

The products of the lipoxygenase and cyclooxygenase pathways are collectively referred to as eicosanoids since they arise from eicosatetraenoic acid (arachidonic acid; Fig. 7.5).

The prostanoids, which are the prostaglandins (PGE_2, PGI_2, etc.) and their related substances,

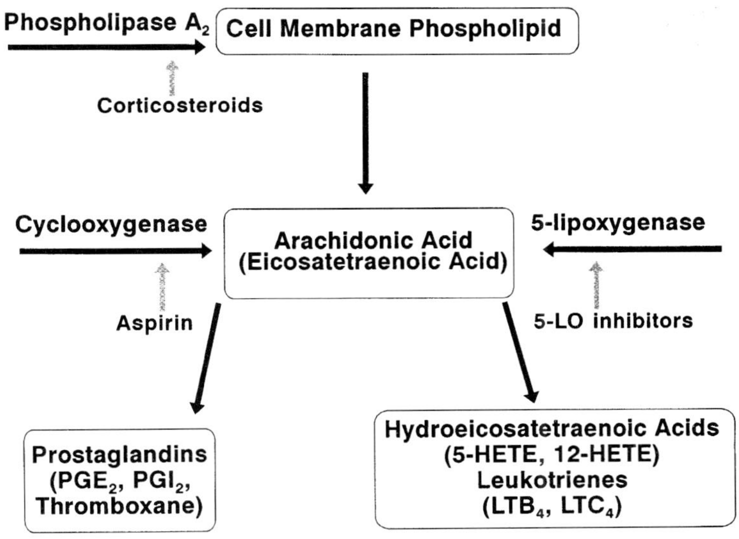

Fig. 7.5 Pathways of arachidonic acid (eicosatetraenoic acid) metabolism showing sites of inhibition by corticosteroids, non-steroidal anti-inflammatory analgesics and 5-lipoxygenase (5-LO) inhibitors.

the thromboxanes, are synthesized from membrane phospholipids by the action of phospholipase A_2 to produce arachidonic acid. This is then metabolized by the cyclooxygenase pathway to give the prostanoids or by the lipoxygenase pathway to give leukotrienes.

Prostanoids (PGs)

Prostaglandins have been shown to have multiple effects on bone cells. The first demonstration that PGs could modify bone metabolism was by Klein and Raisz,[29] who showed that PGE_2 stimulated bone resorption *in vitro* in fetal long bone cultures. This was later confirmed in mouse calvarial organ cultures by Tashjian *et al.*[30] The effects of PGs on osteoclast formation has also been studied. In human bone marrow culture systems, PGE_2 inhibits the formation of osteoclasts,[31] whereas in the mouse culture system PGs stimulate the formation of osteoclasts.[32] PGs also mediate the effects of other bone-resorbing factors, for example, complement-induced bone resorption *in vitro* is inhibited by indomethacin[33] (inhibitor of the cyclooxygenase pathway; Fig. 7.5). Similarly, epidermal growth factor, phorbal esters and platelet-derived growth factor stimulated bone resorption in mouse calvariae by generating PGs.[34,35] PGs were also shown partially to mediate the effect of interleukin-1 (IL-1) on bone resorption *in vivo*.[36]

Until recently it was thought that PGs were only local pathological mediators of bone destruction, in particular where there is inflammation. High concentrations of PGs have been demonstrated in dental cysts,[37] inflamed gingival tissues,[38] synovial fluids from rheumatoid joints[39] and breast carcinoma.[40] However, more recently it has been shown that prostaglandins also an have effect on bone formation. In organ cultures, stimulation of DNA, collagen and non-collagenous protein synthesis is observed with low concentrations of PGE_2 or in presence of glucocorticoids, whereas PGE_2 inhibits collagen synthesis at high concentrations.[41] Administration of PGE_2 *in vivo* may also stimulate bone formation.[42–45]

Lipoxygenase metabolites

Although the involvement of PGs in bone physiology has been studied for almost 20 years, the other major pathway of arachidonate metabolism, the lipoxygenase pathway, has received very little attention. The first evidence that leukotrienes and hydroxyeicosatetraenoic acids (HETEs) stimulate bone resorption was recently shown by Meghji *et al.*[46] demonstrating a potency *in vitro* several orders of magnitude greater than PGs. More recent work has shown that the leukotrienes LTD_4, LTE_4 and 5-HETE act directly on the osteoclast to resorb bone.[47] The possibility of lipoxygenase metabolite involvement in localized bone destruction is strengthened by reports of their synthesis in inflamed and malignant tissues. Sidhagen *et al.*[48] found that lipoxygenase metabolism of ^{14}C-arachidonate in explanted inflamed gingival tissue exceeded cyclooxygenase activity by approximately 10-fold. Similarly, Matejka *et al.*[49] found hydroxy-fatty acids (predominantly 5-HETE) to be a major product of odontogenic cysts. Porteder *et al.*[50] showed that samples from human oral squamous cell carcinoma synthesized approximately equal amounts of cyclooxygenase and lipoxygenase products. As the HETEs and leukotrienes are active at concentrations at least 100-fold lower than PGE_2,[46] it is probable that their production in dental cysts, squamous cell carcinoma and periodontal disease is an important contribution to the bone resorption which characterizes these lesions.

The cytokines

One of the most important breakthroughs in our understanding of bone biology in recent years has been the identification of the role of cytokines in bone remodelling. Several of these cytokines are potent mediators of bone metabolism (Table 7.1). Osteoclast-activating factor (OAF) was the name given to the bone-resorbing factor from human mononuclear leukocytes. This was first described by Horton *et al.*[51] and this activity was found to be IL-1.[52] IL-1 is a potent stimulator of bone resorption, acting both directly and by increasing local prostaglandin synthesis.[53] IL-1 is also an inhibitor of bone formation.[54] IL-1 does not have a direct action on the osteoclast but, like PTH, acts via the osteoblast.[55] IL-1 has been shown to cause hypercalcaemia when infused or injected into normal intact mice. This experimental hypercalcaemia can be inhibited by indomethacin, which suggests that it is mediated by prostaglandin synthesis.[35,56] Furthermore it has a direct promotional effect on osteoclast formation.[57] IL-1 has been associated with bone destruction by pathological lesions such as odontogenic cysts,[58] and solid tumours such as oral squamous cell carcinoma,[59] and an ameloblastoma associated with hypercalcemia.[60]

Tumour necrosis factor-α (TNF-α) and TNF-β in purified forms can also stimulate bone resorption *in vitro*. The bone-resorbing effect is mediated through osteoblasts and is of similar potency to IL-1 and can be inhibited by interferon-γ (IFN-γ).[61–63] Tashjian *et al.*.[64] have reported that the bone-resorbing effect is mediated via prostaglandin production. TNF also inhibits bone collagen and non-collagenous protein synthesis, an effect which can be inhibited by indomethacin and enhanced by IFN-γ.

The physiological role of these cytokines is not clear; they could play a role in the development of the bone marrow cavity. IL-1 and TNF clearly have a role in inflammatory bone loss in arthritis and periodontal disease as well as in the bone loss associated with haematopoietic malignancies.[65] The role of other cytokines such as IL-4, IL-6 and leukaemia-inhibitory factor (LIF) is less clear: both IL-6 and LIF have been implicated as stimulators of bone resorption and formation.[66,67] IL-4 and IFN-γ can also inhibit resorption.[53,68]

Growth factors

The bone matrix is unique because of its abundant mineralized extracellular matrix which absorbs proteins. It contains a number of growth factors with important actions in the regulation of bone remodelling. These growth factors include transforming growth factors (TGFs), fibroblast growth factors (FGFs), IGFs, platelet-derived growth factor (PDGF) and bone morphogenetic proteins. All of these growth factors have profound effects on bone cells, particular those of the osteoblastic lineage. And frequently, these factors are synthesized by osteoblasts, although some growth factors are derived from the cells of the immune or haematological system and are present in the bone microenvironment.

Transforming growth factors

TGFs are polypeptides that were initially defined by their ability to induce surface-adherent cells to form anchorage-independent colonies in soft agar suspension cultures. This process was considered to be linked to neoplastic transformation because tumour-derived cells can form colonies spontaneously.

Transformation growth factor-β family

TGF-β is a polypeptide with a molecular weight of 25 000 and is synthesized by many cells types, including osteoblasts. Three forms of TGF-β which seem to have similar biological activities are present in bone: TGF-β1, TGF-β2, and TGF-β3. TGF-β stimulates the replication of precursor cells of the osteoblast lineage and it also has a direct stimulatory effect on bone collagen synthesis.[69] TGF-β also decreases bone resorption. Hormones capable of inducing bone resorption, such as PTH, increase the release of active TGF-β from bone, which could then suppress further bone resorption, thus initiating the bone-forming phase of remodelling.[70]

Bone morphogenetic proteins (BMPs)

The BMPs are members of the extended TGF-β family. The concept of BMPs is derived from the early work of Urist,[71] which showed that implantation of demineralized bone matrix subcutaneously or in muscle would induce cartilage and bone formation in rodents. The first BMPs identified chemically were TGF-β1 and TGF-β2. Subsequently, six distinct BMPs have been identified with sequence homology to TGF-β.

Fibroblast growth factors

The mineralized bone matrix also contains heparin-binding FGFs.[72] Acid and basic FGFs are polypeptides with an approximate molecular weight of 17 000 synthesized by a variety of cell types. FGF stimulates osteoblast replication, which results in an increased cell population capable of synthesizing bone collagen.[73]

Insulin-like growth factors

IGFs are growth hormone-dependent polypeptides with a molecular weight of 7600. Two forms have been characterized: IGF-I and IGF-II: they are synthesized by a variety of cell types, including osteoblasts. IGF stimulates osteoblast mitogenesis as well as collagen synthesis.[74] It has also been shown to stimulate bone formation *in vivo*.[75] Bone cells are also capable of producing IGF-binding proteins.[76] These can either block or enhance the effect of locally produced IGFs.[77–79]

Platelet-derived growth factor

PDGF is a polypeptide with a molecular weight of 30 000. It was initially isolated from platelets and was considered important in the early phases of wound healing.[80] PDGF, like the other growth factors, can be synthesized by osteoblast-like cells.[81] It is a potent bone cell mitogen, and can enhance bone collagen synthesis.[82] PDGF has also been shown to enhance periodontal regeneration in conjunction with IGF-I.[83] PDGF may also be a regulator of osteoclastic bone resorption. It can stimulate bone resorption in neonatal mouse calvariae.[35]

Bacterial products

Bacterial products, such as lipopolysaccharide,[84] capsular material,[85] lipoteichoic acids,[86] muramyl dipeptide[87] and peptidoglycans,[88] have been shown to stimulate bone resorption *in vitro*. The implication of bone resorption induced by the bacterial products is particularly important for the pathology of periodontal diseases and osteomyelitis. These bacterial products may also act as foreign antigens and induce monocyte macrophages and then bone cells to produce prostaglandins and cytokines such as IL-1 leading to bone resorption.

Mechanical stress

The relationship between mechanical forces and bone remodelling has been known for over a century.[89] This is particularly apparent in cancellous bone, where immobilization increases bone resorption and decreases formation.[90,91] This shows that mechanical stress is necessary for the normal coupling of bone remodelling. Mechanical bone remodelling is also utilized by orthodontists where forces exerted on tooth roots enable teeth to move through alveolar bone (this will be discussed in more detail in the next chapter).

The osteoblast–osteoclast relationship (Table 7.2)

Although the osteoclast is the principal bone-resorbing cell, it is the osteoblast that contains the receptors for the major bone-resorbing agents such as PTH, the eicosanoids (PGE_2, PGI_2, LTB_4, etc.), 1,25-dihydroxy vitamin D_3 and cytokines such as IL-1 and TNF. The osteoblasts, having recognized the resorptive signal, somehow transmit it to the osteoclast. Rodan and Martin[92] hypothesized that bone-resorbing agents, such as PTH, may induce a change of shape in the osteoblast which would facilitate the access of osteoclasts to the bone surface. Thus, at low concentrations PTH promotes bone formation, but at high concentrations it will facilitate bone destruction.

An additional theory is that, in response to certain levels of PTH, osteoblasts secrete short-range soluble activators for osteoclasts.[93] As yet, these osteoblast–osteoclast factors have not been characterized and reports have suggested substances with diverse molecular weights. McSheehy and Chambers[94,95] showed that the OAF produced by osteoblasts had a relative molecular weight (Mr) of 500–1000 Da and was inhibited by lipoxygenase inhibitors, implying that the factor is a lipoxygenase metabolite of arachidonic acid (Fig. 7.5). This is possible since lipoxygenase metabolites of arachidonic acid also stimulate bone resorption *in vitro*.[46] However, Perry *et al.*[96] reported that the OAF is bigger than 25 kDa. Meghji *et al.*[97]

Table 7.2 Bone-resorbing factors that act via the osteoblast

Agent	*Source*
Parathyroid hormone	Parathyroid
Vitamin D_3	Liver via kidney from skin
Interleukin-1	Monocytes (major source) Many other cell types, including keratinocytes, fibroblasts and tumour cells
Tumour necrosis factor	Monocytes

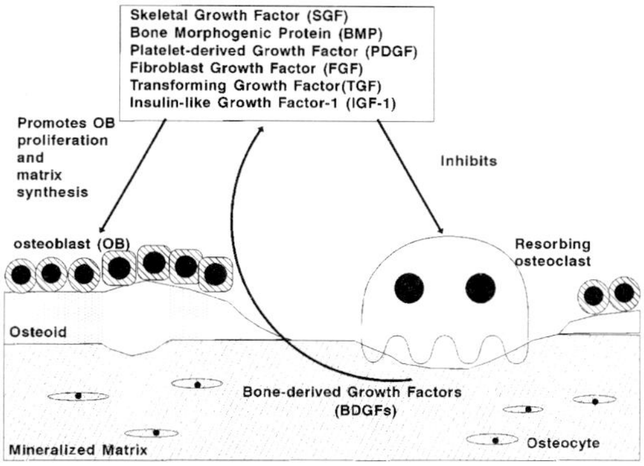

Fig. 7.6 During resorption the osteoclasts release polypeptide growth factors which stimulate osteoblasts to proliferate and synthesize matrix proteins and inhibit the action of the osteoclast.

confirmed that the activity is heterogeneous, and not a single factor, and that osteoblasts spontaneously produce four major peaks of bone-resorbing activity when fractionated by gel permeation on high-performance liquid chromatography. Osteoblasts, therefore appear to play a pivotal role in the regulation of bone resorption. The osteoclast, apart from its osteolytic function, also plays an important role in the development and growth of bone by releasing polypeptide growth factors from the extracellular mineralized matrix (Fig. 7.6).

Inhibitors of bone remodelling (Table 7.3)

These include calcitonin, cortisol, IFN-γ, bisphosphonates, plicamysin and actinomycin D. Calcitonin is synthesized by the C cells in the thyroid gland. It has a molecular weight of 3500 Da and is composed of 32 amino acids. The precise biological role of calcitonin remains unclear. It was first recognized in 1962 by Copp *et al.*[98] as a serum calcium-lowering agent. It inhibits osteoclastic bone resorption rapidly and effectively.[99] It acts directly on the osteoclasts to cause an increase in cAMP generation and contraction of the osteoclast cell membrane.[100,101] It probably also causes the dissolution of osteoclasts into mononuclear cells.[102] However, this effect is only transient. Wener *et al.*[103] showed that calcitonin inhibited PTH-mediated bone resorption only for the first 3 days of culture. When they included cortisol, however, this escape from inhibition of bone resorption is prevented. Similar observations are seen *in vivo* when patients with hypercalcaemia are treated with calcitonin.[104]

It remains unclear why osteoclasts escape from the effects of calcitonin. It could be due to a downregulation of calcitonin binding or receptor numbers in the continued presence of calcitonin. Alternatively, it may result from the emergence of a population of osteoclasts which are not sensitive to calcitonin.

It has been proposed that calcitonin is necessary during growth to protect the body against postprandial hypercalcaemia following a calcium-containing meal. This may explain why infants have much higher levels of calcitonin.[105] Calcitonin has no major effects on bone formation, vitamin D metabolism or absorption of calcium from the gut. It causes regression of central giant cell granulomas and aneurysmal bone cysts of the jaws when 0.5 mg (100 IU) is administered daily subcutaneously for a year.[106]

Table 7.3 Factors that inhibit bone resorption

Agent	*Function/use*
Calcitonin	Acts directly on osteoclasts
Glucocorticoids	Inhibits eicosanoid synthesis
Bisphosphonates	Inhibits osteoclastic bone resorption, probably by making the mineralized surface inaccessible to the cell by binding to the hydroxyapatate crystals
Indomethacin and asprin	Inhibits prostaglandin synthesis
Interferon-γ	Inhibits both proliferation and differentiation of osteoclast progenitors
Tranforming growth factor-β	Inhibits osteoclast formation and differentiation
Interleukin-1 receptor antagonist (IL-1ra)	Binds to IL-1 receptors. Also effective against tumour necrosis factor

Other factors inhibiting bone resorption include the corticosteroids, IFN-γ and various pharmacological inhibitors such as the bisphosphonates and cytotoxic drugs such as plicamycin and actinomycin D. The bisphosphonates and calcitonin are used to retard bone turnover in Paget's disease. The bisphosphonate sodium etidronate is invaluable in preventing reankylosis of the temporomandibular joint following surgery for ankylosis. IFN-γ has attracted a significant research effort. It is a multifunctional cytokine which is produced by immune cells and inhibits both proliferation and differentiation of osteoclast progenitors. Gowen *et al.*[53] demonstrated *in vitro* that IFN-γ specifically inhibits bone resorption induced by TNF and IL-1.

Another cytokine which inhibits osteoclastic bone resorption is IL-1 receptor antagonist.[107] IL-1 receptor antagonist is a cytokine produced by monocytes and monocytoid cell lines. It is a very effective inhibitor of osteoclastic bone resorption stimulated by IL-1 and TNF. IL-4 also inhibits bone resorption *in vitro*.[108]

In summary, bone, despite its apparently solid and inert form, is probably the most dynamic and complex of body tissues. We are only just beginning to discover the many factors which influence the interactions of its formation and destruction.

References

1. Delmas PD, Tracy RP, Riggs BL, Mann KG. Identification of non-collagenous proteins of bovine bone by two dimensional electrophorosis. *Calcif Tissue Int* 1984; **36**: 308–316.
2. Boyde A, Ali NN, Jones SJ. Resorption of dentine by isolated osteoclasts *in vitro. Br Dent J* 1984; **156**: 216–220.
3. Eilon G, Raisz LG. Comparison of the effects of stimulators and inhibitors of resorption on the release of lysosomal enzymes and radioactive calcium from fetal bone in organ culture. *Endocrinology* 1978; **103**: 1969–1975.
4. Vaes G. Collagenase, lysosomes and osteolytic bone resorption. In: Wooley DE, Evanson JM (eds) *Collagenase in Normal and Pathological Connective Tissue*, pp. 185–207. Chichester: John Wiley, 1980.
5. De Duve C. An integrated view of lysosome function. In: Berlin RD, Herrman H, Lepow IH, Tanzer JM (eds) *Molecular Basis of Biological Degradative Processes*, pp. 25–38. New York: Academic Press, 1978.
6. Sakamoto S, Sakamoto M. Biochemical and immunohistochemical studies on collagenase in resorbing bone in tissue culture. *J Periodont Res* 1982; **17**: 523–526.
7. Heath JK, Atkinson SJ, Meikle MC, Reynolds JJ. Mouse osteoblasts synthesize collagenase in response to bone resorbing agents. *Biochim Biophys Acta* 1984; **802**: 151–154.
8. Ham AW, Cormack DW. In: *Histology*, pp. 377–462. (Conference proceedings) Philadelphia: Lippincott, 1979.
9. Jones SJ, Boyde A, Pawley JB. Osteoblasts and collagen orientation. *Cell Tissue Res* 1975; **159**: 73–80.
10. Canalis E, Centrella M, Burch W, McCarthy T. Insulin-like growth factor-1 meditates selective anabolic effects of parathyroid production in bone culture. *J Clin Invest* 1989; **83**: 60–65.
11. Hock JM, Gera I. Effects of continuous and intermittent administration and inhibition of resorption on the anabolic response of bone to parathyroid hormone. *J Bone Mineral Res* 1992; **7**: 65–72.
12. Pfeilschifter J, Mundy GR. Modulation of type β transforming growth factor activity in bone cultures by osteotropic hormones. *Proc Natl Acad Sci USA* 1987; **84**: 2024–2028.
13. Barnicot NA. The local action of parathyroid and other tissue on the bone in intracerebral grafts. *J Anat* 1948; **83**: 233–248.
14. Raisz LG. Bone resorption in tissue culture. Factors influencing the response to parathyroid hormone. *J Clin Invest* 1965; **44**: 103–116.
15. Raisz LG, Kream BE. Regulation of bone formation. *N Engl J Med* 1983; **309**: 29–35.
16. Kream BE, Peterson DN, Raisz LG. Parathyroid hormone blocks the stimulatory effect of insulin-like growth factor on collagen synthesis in cultured 21-day fetal rat calvariae. *Bone* 1990; **11**: 411–415.
17. Moseley JM, Kubota M, Diefenbach-Jagger H. Parathyroid hormone related protein purified from a human lung cancer cell line. *Proc Natl Acad Sci USA* 1987; **84**: 5048–5052.
18. Stewart AF, Wu T, Goumas D, Burtis WJ, Broadus AE. N-terminal amino acid sequence of two novel tumour-derived adenylate cyclase-stimulating proteins: identification of parathyroid hormone-like and parathyroid hormone-unlike domains. *Biochem Biophys Res Commun.* 1987; **146**: 672–678.
19. Strewler GJ, Stern PH, Jacobs JW *et al.* Parathyroid hormone-like protein from human renal carcinoma cells: structural and functional homology with parathyroid hormone. *J Clin Invest* 1987; **80**: 1083–1811.
20. Suva LJ, Winslow GA, Wettenhall REH *et al.* A parathyroid hormone-related protein implicated in malignant hypercalcaemia: cloning and expression. *Science* 1987; **237**: 893–896.
21. Horiuchi N, Caufield MP, Fisher JE *et al.* Similarity of synthetic peptide form human tumour to parathyroid hormone *in vivo* and *in vitro*. Science 1987; **238**: 1566–1569.

22. Kemp BE, Moseley JM, Rodda CP *et al.* Parathyroid hormone-related protein of malignancy: active synthetic fragments. *Science* 1987; **238**: 1568–1570.
23. Sato K, Fujii Y, Kasono K. Parathyroid hormone-related protein and interleukin-1 alpha synergistically stimulated bone resorption *in vitro* and increase serum calcium concentration in mice *in vivo*. *Endocrinology* 1989; **124**: 2172–2178.
24. Raisz LG, Trummel L, Wener JA. Effect of glucocorticoids on bone resorption in tissue culture. *Endocrinology* 1972; **90**: 961–967.
25. Raisz LG. Recent advances in bone cell biology: interactions of vitamin D with other local and systemic factors. *Bone Mineral* 1992; **9**: 191–197.
26. Roodman GD, Ibbotson KJ, MacDonald BR. 1,25-dihydroxyvitamin D3 causes formation of multinucleated cells with several osteoclast characteristics in cultures of primate marrow. *Proc Natl Acad Sci USA* 1985; **82**: 8213–8217.
27. Erben RG, Weiser H, Sinowatz F, Rambeck WA, Zucker H. Vitamin D metabolites prevent vertebral osteopenia in ovariectomised rats. *Calcif Tissue Int.* 1992; **50**: 228–236.
28. Nakamura T, Nagai Y, Yamato H, Suziki K, Orimo H. Regulation of bone turnover and prevention of bone atrophy in ovariectomized beagle dogs by the administration of $24,25(OH)_2D_3$. *Calcif Tissue Int* 1992; **50**: 221–227.
29. Klein DC, Raisz LG. Prostaglandins: stimulation of bone resorption in tissue culture. *Endocrinology* **86**: 1970; 1436–1440.
30. Tashjian AH, Voelkel EF, Levine L *et al.* Evidence that the bone-stimulation factor produced by mouse fibrosarcoma cells is prostaglandin E_2: a new model for the hypercalcaemia of cancer. *J Exp Med* 1972; **136**: 1329–1343.
31. Chenu CC, Kurihara T, Mundy GR, Roodman GD. Prostaglandin E_2 inhibits formation of osteoclast-like cells in long-term human marrow cultures but is not a mediator of the inhibitory effects of transforming growth factor β. *J Bone Mineral Res* 1990; **5**: 677–681.
32. Akatsu T, Takahashi N, Debari K *et al.* Prostaglandins promote osteoclast line cell formation by a mechanism involving cyclic adenosine 3'5'-monophosphate in mouse bone marrow cell cultures. *J Bone Mineral Res* 1989; **4**: 29–35.
33. Raisz LG, Sandberg AL, Goodson JM, Simmons HA, Mergenhagen SE. Complement-dependent stimulation of prostaglandin synthesis and bone resorption. *Science* 1974; **185**: 789–791.
34. Tashjian AH, Wright DR, Ivey JL, Pont A. Calcitonin binding sites in bone: relationships to biological response and 'excape'. *Rec Prog Horm Res* 1978; **34**: 285–334.
35. Tashjian AH, Hohmann EL, Antoniades HN, Levine Ll. Platelet-derived growth factor stimulates bone resorption via a prostaglandin mediated mechanism. *Endocrinology* 1982; **111**: 118–124.
36. Boyce BF, Aufdemorte TB, Garrett IR, Yates AJP, Mundy GR. Effects of interleukin-1 on bone turnover in normal mice. *Endocrinology* 1989; **123**: 1142–1150.
37. Harris M, Jenkins MV, Bennett A, Wills MR. Prostaglandin production and bone resorption by dental cysts. *Nature* 1973; **245**: 213–215.
38. Goodson JM, Dewhirst F, Brunetti A. Prostaglandin E_2 levels in human gingival tissue. *J Dent Res* 1973; **52**: 182.
39. Robinson HJJr, Granda JL. Prostaglandins in synovial inflammatory disease. *Surg Forum* 1974; **25**: 476–477.
40. Bennett A, McDonald AM, Simpson JS, Stampford IF. Breast cancer. Prostaglandins and bone metatases. *Lancet* 1975; **i**: 1218–1220.
41. Raisz LG, Fall PM. Biphasic effects of prostaglandin E_2 on bone formation and cultured neonatal mouse calvariae: interactions with cortisol. *Endocrinology* 1990; **126**: 1076–1079.
42. Akamine T, Jee WSS, Ke HZ, Li ZJ, Lin BY. Prostaglandin E_2 prevents bone loss and adds extra bone to immobilized distal femoral metaphysis in female rates. *Bone* 1992; **13**: 11–22.
43. Jee WSS, Akamine T, Ke HZ, Li XJ, Tang LY, Zeng QQ. Prostaglandin E_2 prevents disuse-induced cortical bone loss. *Bone* 1992; **13**: 153–160.
44. Ke HZ, Jee WSS, Mori S, Li XJ, Kimmel DB. Effects of long-term daily administration of prostaglandin E_2 on maintaining elevated proximal tibial metaphyseal cancellous bone mass in male rats. *Calcif Tissue Int* 1992; **50**: 245–252.
45. Mori S, Jee WSS, Li XJ. Production of new trabecular bone in osteopenic ovariectomized rats by prostaglandin E_2. *Calcif Tissue Int* 1992; **50**: 80–87.
46. Meghji S, Sandy JR Scutt AM, Harvey W, Harris M. Stimulation of bone resorption by lipoxygenase metabolites of arachidonic acid. *Prostaglandins* 1988; **36** 139–149.
47. Gallwitz WE, Mundy GR, Lee CH *et al.* 5-Lipoxygenase metabolite of arachidonic acid stimulates osteoclasts to resorb calcified matrices. *J Biol Chem* 1993; **268**: 10087–10094.
48. Sidhagen B, Hamberg M, Fredholm BB. Formation of 12L-hydroxyyeicosatetraenoic acid (12-HETE) by gingival tissue. *J Dent Res* 1982; **61**: 761–763.
49. Matejka M, Porteder H, Ulrich W, Watzek G, Sinzinger H. Prostaglandin synthesis in dental cysts. *Br J Oral Maxillofac Surg* 1985; **23**: 190–194.
50. Porteder H, Matejka M, Ulrich W, Sinzinger H. The cyclo-oxygenase and lipoxygenase pathways in human oral cancer tissue. *J Maxillofac Surg* 1984; **12**: 145–147.
51. Horton JE, Raisz LG, Simmons HA, Oppenheim JJ, Mergenhagen, E. Bone resorbing activity in supernatant fluid from cultured human peripheral blood leukocytes. *Science* 1972; **177**: 793–795.
52. Dewhirst FE, Stashenko, PP, Mole JE, Tsurumachi T. Purification and partial sequence of human osteoclast activating factor: identity with interleukin 1 beta. *J Immunol* 1985; **135**: 2562–2568.

53. Gowen M, Mundy GR. Actions of recombinant interleukin-1, interleukin-2 and interferon gamma on bone resorption *in vitro*. *J Immunol* 1986; **136**: 2478–2482.
54. Marusic A, Raisz LG. Cortisol modulates the actions of interleukin-1a on bone formation, resorption and prostaglandin production in cultured mouse parietal bones. *Endocrinology* 1991; **129**: 2699–2706.
55. Thomson BM, Saklatvala J, Chambers TJ. Osteoblasts mediate interleukin-1 stimulation of bone resorption by rat osteoclasts. *J Exp Med* 1986; **164**: 104–112.
56. Boyce BR, Yates AJP, Mundy GR. Bolus injections of recombinant human interleukin-1 causes transient hypocalcemia in normal mice. *Endocrinology* 1989; **125**: 2780–2783.
57. Pfeilschifter J, Mundy GR, Roodman GD. Interleukin-1 and tumour necrosis factor stimulate the formation of human osteoclast-like cells *in vitro*. *J Bone Miner Res* 1989; **4**: 113–118.
58. Meghji A, Harvey, W, Harris M. Interleukin-1-like activity in cystic lesions of the jaw. *Br J Oral Maxillofac Surg* 1989; **27**: 1–11.
59. Meghji S, Sandy JR, Scutt A, Harvey W, Harris M. Macromolecular osteolytic factor released by squamous cell carcinoma is interleukin-1. *Br J Cancer* 1988; **58**: 139–149.
60. Macperhson DW, Hopper C, Meghji S. Hypercalcaemia and the synthesis of interleukin-1 by an ameloblastoma. *Br J Oral Maxillofac Surg* 1991; **29**: 29–33.
61. Thomson BM, Mundy GR, Chambers TJ. Tumour necrosis factors alpha and beta induce osteoblastic cells to stimulate osteoclastic bone resorption. *J Immunol* 1987; **138**: 775–779.
62. Bertolini DR, Nedwin GE, Bringman TS, Smith DD, Mundy GR. Stimulation of bone resorption and inhibition of bone formation *in vitro* by human tumour necrosis factors. *Nature* 1986; **319**: 516–518.
63. Gowen M, Nedwin G, Mundy GR. Preferential inhibition of cytokine-stimulated bone resorption by recombinant interferon gamma. *J Bone Mineral Res* 1986; **1**: 469–474.
64. Tashjian AH Jr, Voelkel EF, Levine L. Tumour necrosis factor stimulates prostaglandin production and bone resorption in cultured mouse calvaria. In: Cohn DV, Martin TJ, Meunier PJ (eds) *Calcium Regulation and Bone Metabolism*; vol. 9, pp. 320–324. Amsterdam: Elsevier. 1987
65. Kawano M, Yamamoto I, Iwato K *et al*. Interleukin 1 beta rather than lymphotoxin as the major bone resorbing activity in human multiple myeloma. *Blood* 1989; **73**: 1646–1649.
66. Lowe C, Cornish J, Martin TJ , Reid IR. Effects of leukemia inhibitory factor on bone resorption and DNA synthesis in neonatal mouse calvarial. *Calcif Tissue Int* 1991; **49**: 394–397.
67. Roodman GD. Perspectives – interleukin-6: an osteotropic factor? *J Bone Mineral Res* 1992; **7**: 475–478.
68. Shioi A, Teitelbaum SL, Ross FP *et al*. Interleukin-4 inhibits murine osteoclast formation *in vitro*. *Cell Biochem* 1991; **47**: 272–277.
69. Centrella M, McCarthy T, Canalis E. Transforming growth factor beta is bifunctional regulation of replication and collagen synthesis in osteoblast-enriched cell cultures from fetal rat bone. *J Biol Chem* 1987; **262**: 2869–2874.
70. Pfeilichifter J, Seyedin SM, Mundy GR. Transformation growth factor beta inhibits bone resorption in fetal rat long bone cultures. *J Clin Invest* 1988; **82**: 680–685.
71. Urist MR. Bone: formation by autoinduction. *Science* 1965; **150**: 150.
72. Hauschka PV, Mavrakos AE, Iafrati MD, Doleman SE, Klagsbrun M. Growth factors in bone matrix. *J Biol Chem* 1986; **261**: 12665–12674.
73. Canalis E, Centrella M, McCarthy TL. Effects of basic fibroblasts growth factor on bone formation *in vitro*. *J Clin Invest* 1988; **81**: 1572–1577.
74. Canalis E. Effect of insulin-like growth factor I on DNA and protein synthesis in cultured rat calvaria. *J Clin Invest* 1980; **66**: 709–719.
75. Spencer EM, Liu CC, Si ECC, Howard GA. *In vivo* actions of insulin-like growth factor-I (IGF-I) on bone formation and resorption in rates. *Bone* 1991; **12**: 21–26.
76. McCarthy TL, Centrella M, Canalis E. Regulation of insulin factor binding protein (IGF0BP) expression in primary osteoblast enriched cultures. *J Bone Mineral Res* **6**: 1991; 209–480.
77. Ernst M, Rodan GA. Increased activity of insulin-like growth factor (IGF) in osteoblastic cells in the presence of growth hormone (GH). Positive correlation with the presence of the GH-induced IGF-binding protein BP-3. *Endocrinology* 1990; **127**: 807–814.
78. Feyen JHM, Evans DB, Bickert C, Heinrich GF, Geisse S, Kocher HP. Recombinant human (cys^{281}) insulin-like growth factor-binding protein-2 inhibits both basal and insulin-like factor-1-stimulated proliferation and collagen synthesis in fetal rat calvariae. *J Biol Chem* 1991; **266**: 19469–19474.
79. Schmid C, Rutishauser J, Schlapfer I, Froesch ER, Zapf J. Intact but not truncated insulin-like growth factor binding protein-3 (IGFBP-3) blocks IGF-1 induced stimulation of osteoblasts. Control of IGF signalling to bone cells by IGFBP-3-specific proteolysis. *Biochem Biophys Res Commun* 1991; **179**: 579–585.
80. Burgess WH, Wehlman T, Firesel R, Johnson WV, Maciag T. Multiple forms of endothelial cell growth factor. *J Biol Chem* 1985; **260**: 11389–11392.
81. Graves DT, Owen AJ, Barth RK *et al*. Detection of c-*sis* transcripts and synthesis of PDGF-like proteins by human osteosarcoma cells. *Science* 1984; **226**: 972–974.
82. Canalis E. Platelet derived growth factor stimulates DNA and proteins synthesis in cultured fetal rat calvaria. *Metabolism* 1980; **30**: 970–975.

83. Lynch SE, Williams RC, Polson AM *et al*, A combination of platelet-derived and insulin-like growth factors enhances periodontal regeneration. *J Clin Periodont* 1989; **16**: 545–548.
84. Hausmann E, Raisz LG, Miller WA. Endotoxin: stimulation of bone resorption in tissue culture. *Science* 1989; **168**: 862–864.
85. Wilson M, Kamin S, Harvey W. Bone-resorbing activity of purified capsular material from *Actinobacillus actinomycetemcomitans. J Perio Res* 1985; **20**: 484–491.
86. Hausmann E, Luderitz O, Knox, K Weinfeld N. Structural requirements for bone resorption by endotoxin and lipoteichoic acid. *J Dent Res* 1975; **54**: B94–B99.
87. Dewhirst FE. N-acetyl muralmyl dipeptide stimulation of bone resorption in tissue culture. *Infect Immun* 1982; **35**: 133–137.
88. Lensgraf EJ, Greenblatt, JJ, Bawden JW. Effect of group A streptococcal peptidoglycan and group A strepococcal cell wall on bone in tissue culture. *Arch Oral Biol* 1979; **24**: 495–498.
89. Wolff J. (1892) Das gesetz der transformation der knochen. Berlin: Hirschwald.
90. Weinreb M, Rodan GA, Thompson DD. Osteopenia in the immobilised rat hind limb is associated with increased bone resorption and decreased bone formation. *Bone* 1989; **10**: 187–194.
91. Jee SS, Li XJ. Adaptation of cancellous bone to over-loading in the adult rat: a single photon absorptiometry and histomorphometry study. *Anat Rec* 1990; **227**: 418–426.
92. Rodan GA, Martin TJ. Role of osteoblasts in hormonal control of bone resorption – a hypothesis. *Calcif Tissue Int* 1981; **33**: 349–351.
93. Wong GL. Paracrine interactions in bone-secreted products of osteoblasts permit osteoclasts to respond to parathyroid hormone. *J Chem* 1984; **259**: 4019–4022.
94. McSheehy PMJ, Chambers TJ. Osteoblastic cells mediate osteoclastic responsiveness to parathyroid hormone. *Endocrinology* 1986; **118**: 824–828.
95. McSheehy PM, Chambers TJ. Osteoblast-like cells in the presence of parathyroid hormone release soluble factor that stimulates osteoclastic bone resorption. *Endocrinology* 1986; **119**: 1654–1659.
96. Perry HM, Skogen W, Chappel JC, Wilner GD, Kahn AJ, Teitelbaum SL. Conditioned medium from osteoblast-like cells mediate parathyroid hormone induced bone resorption. *Calcif Tissue Int* 1987; **40**: 298–300.
97. Meghji S, Sandy JR. Scutt AM, Harvey W, Harris M. Heterogeneity of bone resorbing factors produced by murine osteoblasts *in vitro*: modulation by parathyroid hormone and mononuclear cell products. *Arch Oral Biol* 1988; **33**: 773–778.
98. Copp DH, Cameron EC, Cheney EC *et al*. Evidence for calcitonin – a new hormone from the parathyroid that lowers blood calcium. *Endocrinology* 1962; **70**: 638–649.
99. Friedman J, Au WYW, Rais LG. Responses of fetal rat bone to thyrocalcitonin in tissue culture. *Endocrinology* 1968; **82**: 149–156
100. Heersche JNM, Marcus R, Aurbach GD, Calcitonin and the formation of 3'5'-AMP in bone and kidney. *Endocrinology* 1974; **94**: 241–247
101. Chambers TJ, Magnus CJ. Calcitonin alters behaviour of isolated osteoclasts. *J Pathol* 1982; **136**: 27–39.
102. Baron R, Vignery A. Changes in the osteoclastic pools and the osteoclast nuclei balance after a single injection of salmon calcitonin in the adult rat. In: Meunier PJ. (ed) *Bone Histomorphometry*, pp. 147–156. Paris: Laboratoires Armour Montagu, 1976.
103. Wener JA, Gorton SJ, Raisz LG, Escape from inhibition of resorption in cultures of fetal bone treated with calcitonin and parathyroid hormone. *Endocrinology* 1972; **90**: 752–759.
104. Binstock ML, Mundy GR. Effect of calcitonin and gluccocorticoids in combination in malignant hypercalcaemia. *Ann Intern Med* 1980; **93**: 269–272.
105. Sunday ME, Wolfe HJ, Roos BA, Chin WW, Spindel ER. Gastrin-releasing peptide gene expression in developing hyperplastic and neoplastic human thyroid C-cells. *Endocrinology* 1988; **122**: 1551–1558.
106. Harris M. Calcitonin cures central giant cell granulomas of the jaws. *Br J Maxillofac Surg* 1991; **29**: 136.
107. Seckinger P, Klein-Nulend J, Alander C, Thompson RC, Dayer J-M, Raisz LG. Natural and recombinant human IL-1 receptor antagonist block the effects of IL-1 on bone resorption and prostaglandin production. *J Immunol* 1990; **145**: 4181–4184.
108. Watanabe K, Tanaka Y, Morimoto I *et al*. Interleukin-4 as a potent inhibitor of bone resorption. *Biochem Biophys Res Commun* 1990; **172**: 1035–1041.

8

Bone remodelling in the jaws – clinical considerations

Jonathan R. Sandy, Sajeda Meghji and Malcolm Harris

Introduction

The mandible and maxilla provide an ideal site for the study of pathological bone changes because of their accessibility and the unique interface between the dentition and its skeletal support.

The following conditions will be discussed:

1. Tooth eruption.
2. Periodontal disease.
3. Odontogenic cysts.
4. Squamous cell carcinoma.
5. Hypercalcaemia of malignancy.
6. Hyperparathyroidism.
7. Giant cell granuloma.
8. Paget's disease.
9. Osteoporosis.
10. Osteopetrosis.
11. Iatrogenic bone remodelling in orthodontic movement.

Regardless of the individual process, these changes share common cellular and biochemical processes.

Tooth eruption

Most tooth eruption studies have used one of two model systems which provide very different bases for the process. The continuously erupting incisor model, found in rodents, features tooth movement which continues throughout the life of the animal. This model provides animals of controlled genetic stock at low cost and, not surprisingly, the literature on continuously erupting teeth is extensive. Animals such as dogs, cats and primates have succedaneous dentitions, enabling the development of the dental follicle and enamel organ, resorption of the exfoliating precursor and root growth of the erupting tooth to be examined. These models are expensive and not easily controlled genetically. There are numerous theories of tooth eruption which reflect our incomplete understanding. All these theories have contributed and provoked research to support or refute hypotheses which are now briefly reviewed.

Pulp theory

This theory suggests that a propulsive force is generated by the pulp through three mechanisms. First, growth of dentine, second interstitial pulp growth and third, a hydraulic effect generated by the pulp vasculature. Perhaps the strongest evidence against this theory is the work of Herzberg and Schour[1] who removed the pulp of rodent incisors and found that its eruption rates were unaffected.

Vascular theory

The mechanism behind this theory to some extent overlaps the pulp theory. The force of eruption comes from the pressure in the blood vessels within or below the tooth. This theory has been discounted by some for the same reasons as the pulp theory. In addition, use of hypotensive drugs appears to have no effect on eruption rates.[2] However, Moxham[3] critically appraises previous work and suggests that at least part of the eruptive force is generated by a non-functional force.

Root elongation theory

This theory attributes tooth eruption to elongation of the roots. It suggests that the tooth erupts by the root pushing against an immovable base. A series of case observations and experiments where roots of the teeth have erupted into functional occlusion would seem to disprove this hypothesis. Furthermore, Marks and Cahill,[4] using young dogs, took teeth at the beginning of eruption, removed their pulps and killed the periodontal ligament cells by freeze-thawing. These inert, rootless teeth with no periodontal ligaments were reimplanted and still managed to erupt by compensatory bone growth.

Alveolar bone growth

The importance of bone growth in tooth eruption was demonstrated with a series of classical experiments by Brash[5] using madder-fed pigs. Madder is a dye which binds to newly formed bone and Brash noticed large amounts of bone laid down beneath the crypts of erupting teeth. These observations have been confirmed,[6] but although bone formation is clearly involved in tooth eruption, the cause-and-effect relation is still unclear.

Periodontal ligament theory

This theory suggests that the impetus for tooth eruption is derived from the periodontal ligament. Evidence for this came from some key observations by Moxham and Berkovitz[7] where root transection failed to prevent the incisor segment superficial to the transection from erupting. This strongly implicates the periodontal ligament in the eruption process, and questions the contribution from alveolar bone, root growth, or indeed pulpal pressure. Evidence against this theory includes studies with lathyritic agents such as β-aminoproprionitrile. Lathyritic compounds inhibit the intermolecular cross-linking of the polypeptide chains in the collagen molecule and should therefore inhibit teeth from erupting. Despite administration of these drugs, rat incisors continue to erupt normally.[8]

The periodontal ligament theory has also gained some support from tissue culture experiments. If a fibroblast is cultured on a substrate on which it can move, it vibrates using contractile mechanisms generated by its cytoskeleton. The actin molecule has a particularly prominent role. As the fibroblast moves, it elongates on a leading edge, and leaves the trailing end of the cell adherent to the substrate. Eventually, the latter edge will detach.[9] If these cells are cultured on thin silicon sheets then as they move the contractile element is sufficiently strong to cause the rubber to wrinkle. This effect can also be seen when these cells are embedded in three-dimensional gels[10] and this is true for fibroblasts derived from the periodontal ligament.[11] This model has been adapted to show that periodontal ligament fibroblasts are capable of generating sufficient contractile force to lift a piece of root, against gravity towards the top of a tissue culture well.[12] Direct evidence for this tractional effect has still not been presented, but these models have at least added weight to the argument that the periodontal ligament has some role in the process of eruption.

Follicular theory

This theory attributes a critical role to the dental follicle for the eruption of teeth. It seems probable that the loose connective tissue of the dental follicle is a rich source of factors which are responsible for both bone formation and resorption. Indeed, the follicle is certainly capable of producing eicosanoids, cytokines and growth factors which could not only resorb the overlying deciduous roots and alveolar bone but also induce bone formation at the base of the follicle. The role of these has been outlined in the section on bone remodelling. It seems surprising, perhaps, that so little has been done to determine the interplay of these factors with tooth eruption, rather than some of the mechanistic approaches described previously. It is over 30 years since epidermal growth factor (EGF) was isolated from mouse submandibular glands.[13] When the original bioassay was used for the purification of EGF incisor eruption was accelerated in newborn mice. As our understanding of the role of these factors in bone remodelling increases, we are more likely to be able to explain tooth eruption in terms of cellular and molecular interactions.

Genetic input

If tooth eruption is to be explained at the cellular and molecular level, a degree of genetic control is highly likely. In normal development of the occlusion, incisors erupt before premolars and this process of eruption is often disturbed in a number of genetic disorders. A classification of these relationships has been presented by Sauk.[14] These comprise:

1. Inherited defects, primarily involving enamel – amelogenesis imperfecta.
2. Syndromes with enamel involvement.
3. Disorders associated with supernumerary teeth and/or crowding of teeth.
4. Growth retardation syndromes.
5. Conditions associated with tissue overgrowth of the gingivae and the presence of hyperplastic frenula.
6. Miscellaneous disorders. These include: premature exfoliation, such as hypophosphatasia, juvenile periodontosis and Papillon–Lefèvre syndrome.

In summary, there is no simple explanation of tooth eruption, which is clearly a multifactorial event.

Periodontal disease

Periodontal disease is one of the commonest inflammatory diseases of bone. Chronic inflammation of the gingiva is associated with the loss of the alveolar bone and periodontal ligament leading to the loss of the dentition. The role of bacteria in the initiation of periodontitis and the destruction of alveolar bone is well-recognized, although the detailed causal relationship remains uncertain. Bone-resorbing agents derived from bacteria include lipopolysaccharides (LPS), lipoteichoic acids, peptidoglycans, muramyl dipeptides and bacterial capsular material, also called surface-associated material (SAM). This is the solubilized outer material of the bacteria, commonly known as slime layers.

In studying the role of bacteria in connective tissue destruction, much attention has focused on the biological activity of the LPS of the outer membrane of the cell wall of Gram-negative bacteria (Fig. 8.1). However, the osteolytic activity and cytotoxic effect on fibroblasts are substantially less than the SAM derived from periodontopathic bacteria such as *Actinobacillus*

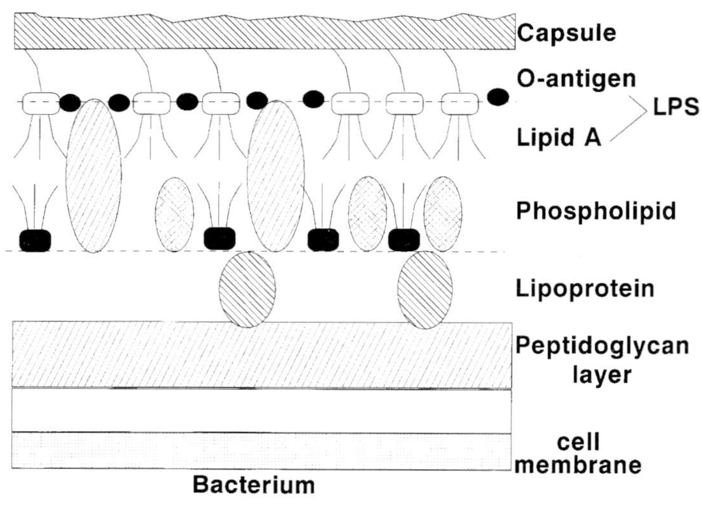

Fig. 8.1 Cross-section of a Gram-negative bacterium showing the active outer layers. Capsule = surface-associated material; LPS = lipopolysaccharide.

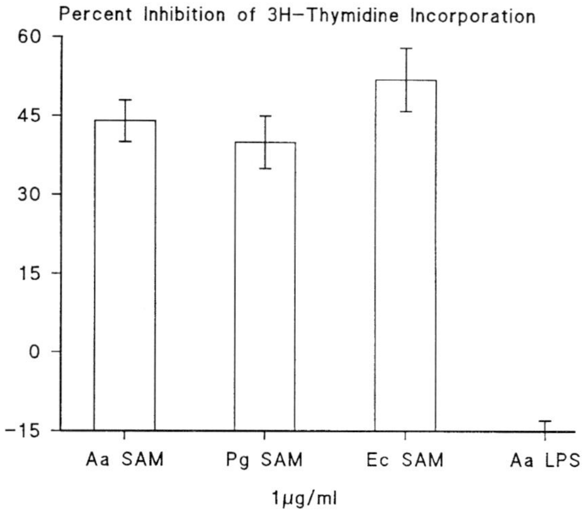

Fig. 8.2 The inhibitory effect of surface-associated material (SAM; 1 μg/ml) from *Actinobacillus actinomycetemcomitans* (Aa), *Porphyromonas gingivalis* (Pg), *Eikenella corrodens* (Ec) and lipopolysaccharide (LPS) from Aa on fibroblast DNA synthesis. This was measured as incorporation of tritiated thymidine into DNA by human gingival fibroblasts. The results are shown as percentage inhibition of tritiated thymidine incorporation.

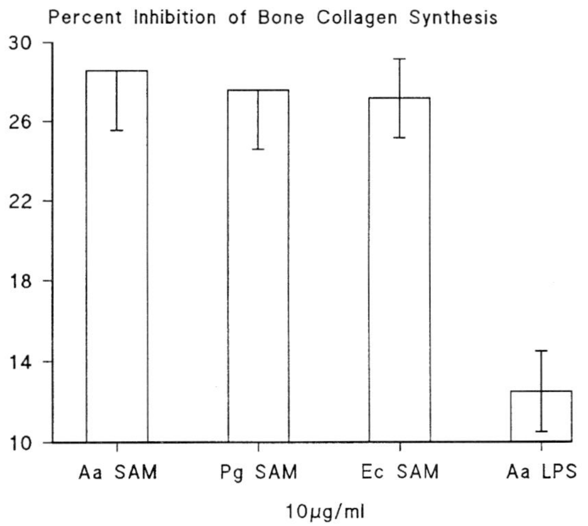

Fig. 8.3 The inhibitory effect of surface-associated material (SAM; 10 μg/ml) from *Actinobacillus actinomycetemcomitans* (Aa), *Porphyromonas gingivalis* (Pg) and *Eikenella corrodens* (Ec) on bone collagen synthesis by cultured murine calvaria compared with Aa lipopolysaccharide (LPS). Results are shown as per cent inhibition of collagen synthesis.

actinomycetemcomitans, Porphyromonas gingivalis and *Eikenella corrodens*[15] (Fig. 8.2).

The effect of SAM on bone was investigated on osteoblast proliferation, collagen synthesis

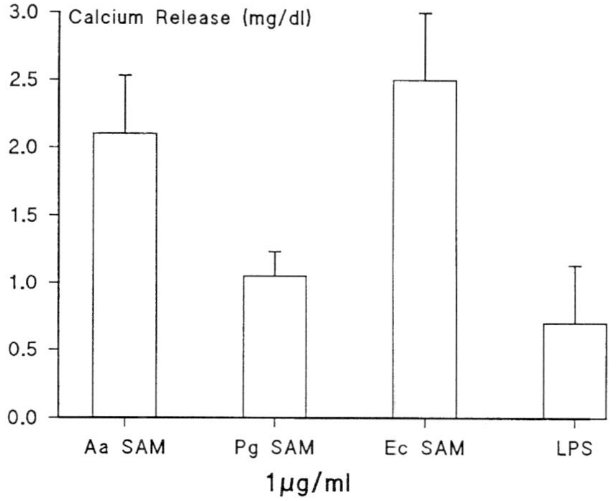

Fig. 8.4 The bone resorbing activity (measured as calcium release in mg/dl) of capsular material, surface-associated material (SAM; 1 μg/ml) from *Actinobacillus actinomycetemcomitans* (Aa), *Porphyromonas gingivalis* (Pg) or *Eikenella corrodens* (Ec) and LPS from Pg. Each point represents the mean and standard deviation from five cultures.

and bone resorption. SAM from all three pathogens significantly inhibited DNA and collagen synthesis by murine calvaria and isolated osteoblasts (Fig. 8.3).[16] This SAM inhibitory effect on DNA and collagen synthesis was blocked by 1 μmol/l indomethacin, which suggested that the effect was prostanoid-mediated. The SAM from all three oral pathogens was found to be the most potent bacterial bone-resorbing agent yet isolated, at the same concentration that inhibited osteoblast proliferation (Fig. 8.4).[17,18] Selective inhibitors were used to define the mechanisms by which these materials stimulate bone resorption. These were indomethacin to inhibit prostanoid synthesis, interleukin-1 (IL-1) receptor antagonist to antagonize locally produced IL-1 and neutralizing antibodies to murine tumour necrosis factor (TNF) and IL-6.

The results showed that the bone resorption induced by SAM from *P. gingivalis* appeared to be mediated by a mixture of prostaglandins, IL-1 and TNF (Fig. 8.5). The activity of *E. corrodens* SAM was principally TNF and some prostaglandins, which contrasted with the bone resorption induced by SAM from *A. actinomycetemcomitans*, which was not significantly inhibited by any of these inhibitors. However, all SAM has potent bone-resorbing activity[18]

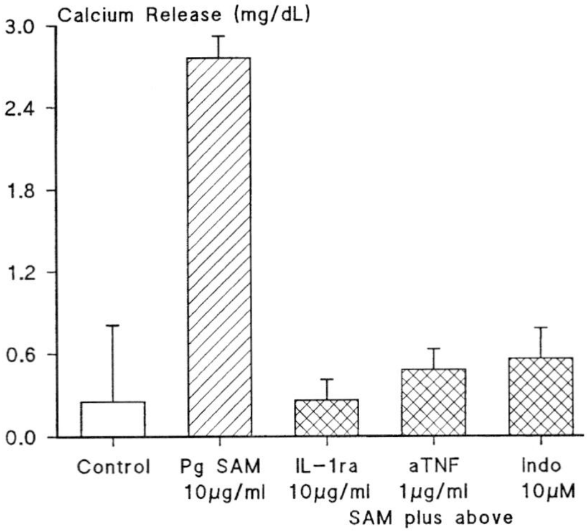

Fig. 8.5 The inhibition of the bone resorption induced by surface-associated material (SAM) from *Porphyromonas gingivalis* (Pg) by interleukin-1 receptor antibody (IL-1ra; 10 μg/ml) neutralizing anti-tumour necrosis factor (a-TNF) antibody (1 μg/ml) and indomethacin (10^{-6} mol/l). The control represents the release of calcium in unstimulated cultures. Each bar represents the mean and standard deviation of five cultures.

and antibodies to its constituents are also found in patients with periodontal disease.[19]

Serum from patients with severe generalized periodontitis (SGP) contained high titres of antibodies to *P. gingivalis* which completely inhibited the bone resorption induced by SAM from this organism. Conversely, serum from patients with low titres of antibodies to *P. gingivalis* failed to inhibit resorption. Similarly, sera from patients with localized juvenile periodontitis containing high titres of antibody to SAM from *A. actinomycetemcomitans*[20] also inhibited bone resorption. This suggests that the antibody response to SAM may have a protective effect in patients with periodontal disease. SAM from periodontopathogens also stimulate cytokine synthesis by human gingival fibroblasts, and human peripheral blood mononuclear cells.[21]

Odontogenic cysts

The odontogenic cyst is an ideal structure to explore the cellular origin of bone-resorbing factors, especially the eicosanoids and cytokines. It consists of an outer connective tissue capsule and the inner epithelial lining. Within the capsule of the periapical cyst, aggregates of

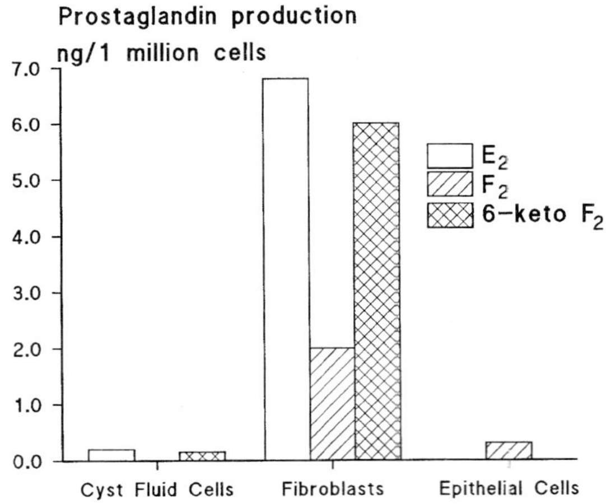

Fig. 8.6 Prostaglandin synthesis by cyst fluid cells, cyst capsule fibroblasts and cyst epithelial lining cells cultured for 48 h. Results are shown as ng/10^6 cells. The fibroblast is the principal source. This fibroblast production of prostaglandins is enhanced by the addition of the cytokine mixture. MCF = Monocyte cell factor (not shown here).

inflammatory cell are also found. If its component parts, that is the epithelial cells, the fibroblasts of the capsule, and mixed cells of both constituents, are cultured in parallel with cyst fluid cells (Fig. 8.6), the prostaglandin production of each can be measured and compared.[22] It can be seen that there is very little prostaglandin synthesis by cells of the cyst fluid and the epithelial cells, whereas fibroblasts derived from the cyst capsule produce substantial amounts of prostaglandin E_2 and 6-keto prostaglandin $F_2\alpha$. Furthermore, when culture

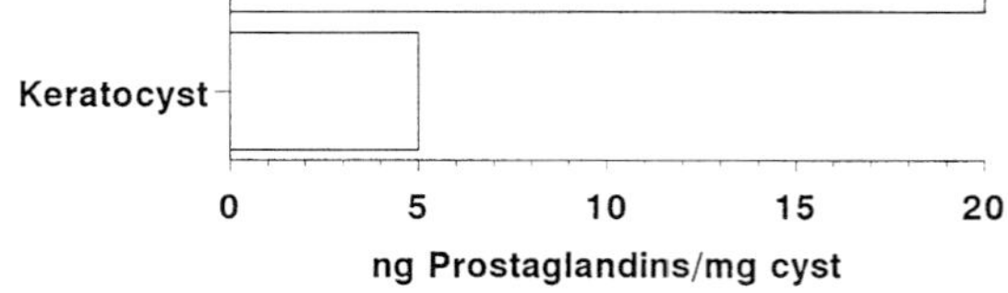

Fig. 8.7 Prostaglandin synthesis by the odontogenic cysts. Results are shown as ng/prostaglandin per mg cyst tissue. The thin-walled keratocyst, when corrected for prostaglandin release per unit area, produces the least.

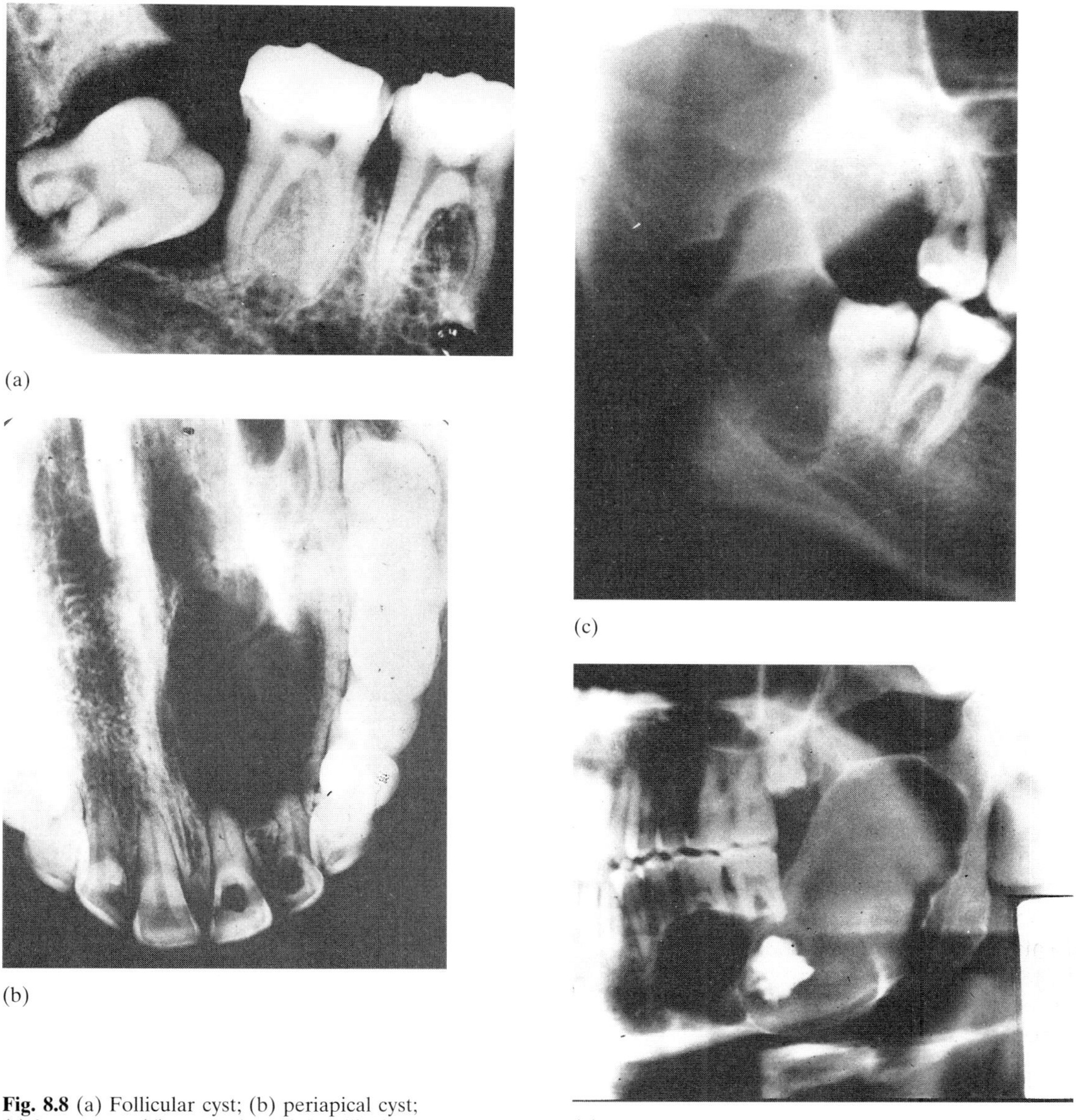

Fig. 8.8 (a) Follicular cyst; (b) periapical cyst; (c) keratocyst; (d) aggressive adult follicular cyst.

medium from stimulated monocytes–monocyte cell factor (MCF), now known to be a cytokine mixture,[23] was added to the fibroblasts, the prostaglandin production was substantially increased.[22] More recent work has shown the odontogenic cyst also synthesizes the cytokines IL-1 and IL-6.[24–26] Thus, this important cytokine interaction takes place within the tissue.

Cysts expand within the alveolus and adjacent basal bone by virtue of their ability to release these osteolytic factors. This can be shown *in vitro* by placing fragments of cyst in culture and transferring the culture medium after 24 h to an adjacent bone culture where resorption is seen to take place. Arising out of this observation was the finding that cyst-derived prostaglandins were involved in this bone resorption. Similarly, collagenase[27] and leukotrienes[28] were found to be released as osteolytic agents by cyst fragments. Quantitative studies showed that there appeared to be a hierarchy of cyst-resorbing capacity (Fig. 8.7).[29] The common small adolescent follicular cyst (Fig. 8.8a) was the least potent bone resorber, especially when compared

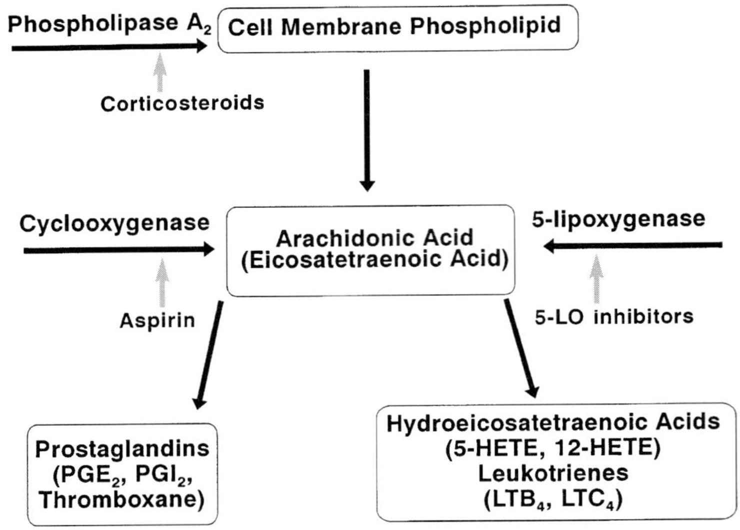

Fig. 8.9 Pathways of arachidonic acid (eicosatetraenoic acid) metabolism showing sites of inhibition by corticosteroids, non-steroidal anti-inflammatory analgesics and 5-lipoxygenase (5-Lo) inhibitors.

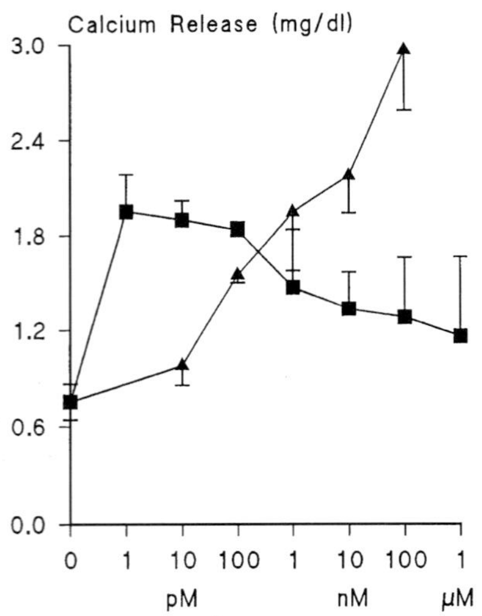

Fig. 8.10 The effect of leukotriene B_4 (■) and prostaglandin E_2 (▲) on bone, showing that the leukotriene is 1000 times more active a resorbing agent in the range of concentration expected *in vivo*. The results are shown as means of net calcium release (mg/dl, ± s.d.) of each concentration (n = 5).

to the periapical cyst (Fig. 8.8b). When prostaglandin production (μg/g) of the thin-walled keratocyst (Fig. 8.8c) is adjusted for mass per unit area, it is also found to be a relatively poor bone resorber (Fig. 8.7). These estimates tend to match the clinical presentation of the cyst. Thus, most follicular cysts appear to have limited growth potential and remain less than twice the diameter of the crown of the tooth enclosed, whereas keratocysts, although spread insidiously through the mandible, rarely resorb the cortical plates and expand the body of the mandible. An exception, which is not well-recognized, is the follicular cyst arising in an adult (Fig. 8.8d), which can grow to a considerable size, resorb tooth roots and mimic an ameloblastoma.

For some time the lipoxygenase products of the arachidonic acid cascade – the leukotrienes (Fig. 8.9) – were not examined for their ability to be released by odontogenic cysts or resorb bone. However, when a leukotriene such as leukotriene B_4 or 12-hydroxyeicosatetraenoic acid (12-HETE) is compared to prostaglandin E_2,[30] it can be seen (Fig. 8.10) that the leukotriene and the HETE are 10–100 times more potent bone resorbers than the prostaglandins. Furthermore, when cysts are cultured in the presence of ^{14}C-labelled arachidonic acid, although all produce substantial amounts of prostaglandins, only the radicular and the dentigerous (follicular) cysts synthesize comparable amounts of HETEs. The keratocyst by contrast produces very little HETE. Thus odontogenic cysts are capable of synthesizing leukotrienes, HETEs, as well as prostanoids, and this varying profile may also reflect their clinical behaviour. The benign odontogenic tumour, the ameloblastoma, also releases osteolytic eicosanoids.[31]

Oral squamous cell carcinoma

Oral squamous cell carcinomas often invade the jaws (Fig. 8.11) and produce extensive resorption of bone by osteoclast activation. This may be demonstrated when the media of squamous cell carcinoma cultured *in vitro* is transferred to bone in culture (Fig. 8.12). The resorption is only partially inhibited by indomethacin[25] suggesting both a prostaglandin and non-prostaglandin resorptive agent. This carcinoma osteolytic agent was found to stimulate fibroblasts to release PGE_2 which accounts for the component inhibited by non-steroidal anti-inflammatory analgesics. The non-prostanoid agent was demonstrated to be the cytokine IL-1 by Meghji *et al.*[32] and was inhibited by the addition of anti-interleukin-1 (Fig. 8.12). This macromolecular cytokine, together with IL-6 and TNF-α, plays an important role in much bone destruction. IL-1α and IL-6 have also been shown to be synthesized by ameloblastoma, carcinoma, some multiple myelomas and lymphomas, all of which also release eicosanoids and metalloproteinases in response to these cytokines.

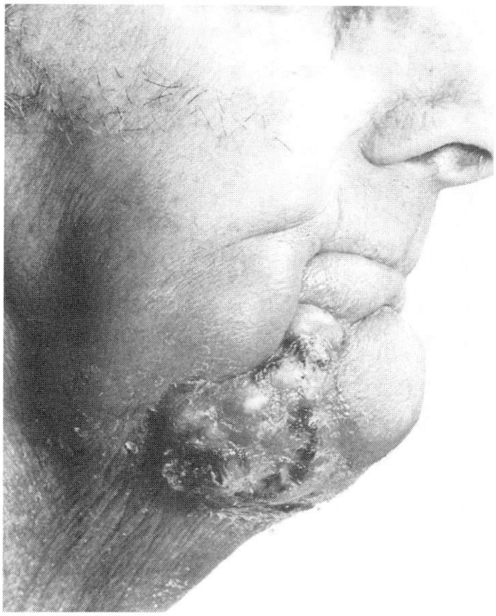

(a)

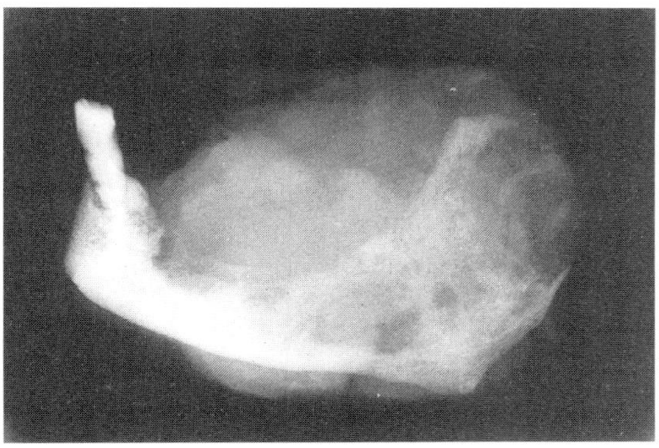

(b)

Fig. 8.11 (a, b) An aggressive mandibular squamous cell carcinoma showing extensive bone and soft-tissue destruction. The bone invasion appears to be facilitated by cytokine and eicosanoid production (see also Fig. 8.10).

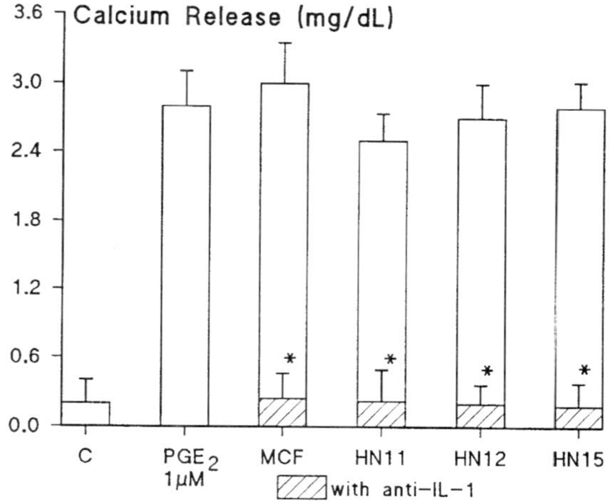

Fig. 8.12 The osteolytic effects of three dialysed squamous cell carcinoma culture media (HN11, HN12, HN15; diluted 1:10; open bars) and the effect of the same media in the presence of antihuman interleukin-1 (closed bars) on bone resorption. The amount of calcium released into the culture media during a 48-h incubation of mouse calvaria with the test media is the measure of bone resorption. Blank medium alone (C), mononuclear cell factor (MCF; diluted 1:10) and prostaglandin E_2 (PGE_2 1 μmol) were used as controls.

Hypercalcaemia of malignancy (oncogenic hypercalcaemia)

This condition is not often recognized in relation to malignant lesions of the jaws. The

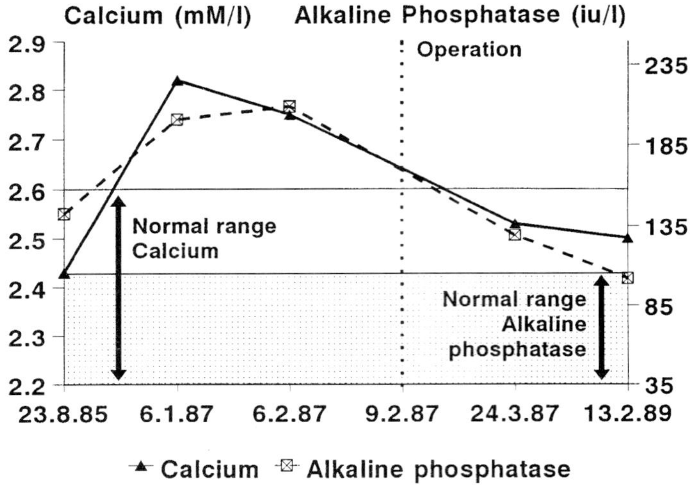

Fig. 8.13 Biochemistry results showing the preoperative raised serum calcium and alkaline phosphatase with its subsequent postoperative fall.

anorexia, nausea, polyuria, polydipsia, lethargy, constipation, depression and muscle wasting which are characteristic of chronic hypercalcaemia may be mistaken for the effects of the tumour or therapy rather than high levels of circulating calcium. Accelerated bone resorption by osteoclasts is the primary pathogenic mechanism in most instances of hypercalcaemia.[33] This is seen with metastatic squamous cell carcinoma, where the hypercalcaemia is considered to be due to circulating IL-1, TNF, parathyroid hormone-related peptide (PTHrp), and transforming growth factor-α (TGF-α).[34] Control is achieved by the adminstration of corticosteroids, indomethacin and bisphosphonates, which block eicosanoid release[35] and osteoclast action on bone respectively.

An important observation was that a benign tumour, an ameloblastoma, may also produce hypercalcaemia. Macpherson *et al.*[36] showed that a large ameloblastoma confined to the mandible without any evidence of malignancy or metastases was associated with hypercalcaemia and a raised alkaline phosphatase, both of which fell to normal levels after removal of the tumour (Fig. 8.13). Subsequent follow-up over a period of 4 years confirmed the lack of malignancy or metastatic spread and the patient maintained a normal calcium chemistry. The hypercalcaemia was shown to be due to the release of PTHrp. This observation would suggest that all osteolytic tumours may be capable of causing hypercalcaemia and this condition should be renamed oncogenic hypercalcaemia.

Hyperparathyroidism

Primary hyperthyroidism as a cause of hypercalcaemia ranks equally in incidence with hypercalcaemia associated with malignant disease. The characteristics of primary hyperthyroidism are hypercalcaemia occurring in association with elevated levels of parathyroid hormone. This disease is caused by a benign, solitary adenoma 80% of the time when the remaining three parathyroid glands are normal. Primary hypercalcaemia may also be due to a hyperplasia of all four parathyroid glands in response to hypocalcaemia caused by chronic renal disease.

A very rare presentation of primary hyperparathyroidism is parathyroid carcinoma. The pathophysiology of primary hyperparathyroidism is essentially the loss of the nomal feedback control of parathyroid hormone secretion by extracellular calcium. In addition to the symptoms of hypercalcaemia and hypercalciuria there is a reduction of overall bone density, seen as a radiographic loss of the lamina dura around the teeth, 'tufting' of the terminal phalanges of the fingers and 'pepper pot' radiolucencies of the skull. In addition the 'giant cell' (osteoclast) granulomas of the gingiva or within bone may develop. The patients may present with renal colic due to calculus formation. Plasma calcium, parathyroid hormone and alkaline phosphatase are raised and phosphate is reduced. Urinary calcium is also raised.

The giant cell granuloma

The giant cell granuloma of the jaws occurs as a peripheral lesion, that is, an epulis and an intraosseous central lesion. They are indistinguishable from similar lesions occurring in hyperparathyroidism and therefore all cases must be investigated biochemically to exclude raised serum calcium, alkaline phosphatase and immunoreactive parathyroid hormone levels. Where there is any doubt, a bone scan and 24-h urinary calcium and hydroxyproline are also invaluable.

The central giant cell granuloma appears to occur more commonly in females than males, but principally at the onset of adolescence. The peripheral giant cell granuloma occurs in females and males in the order of 6:4 and the peak instance is 40–60 years. Flanagan *et al.*[37] have shown that the multinucleated giant cells resorb bone *in vitro*, are inhibited by calcitonin and bind to osteoclast-specific monoclonal antibodies. This supports the concept that these lesions are really osteoclast granulomas, recruited by promoting factors which seem likely to be released by the fibroblastic spindle cells found in abundance within the lesion. However, the cause of this focal transient disturbance, which appears to be in response to a surge of pubertal growth and sex hormones, remains a mystery, but their occurrence in the tooth-bearing areas of the jaws suggests an odontogenic cellular source of PTHrp or a disturbance in the tooth eruption process.

The standard therapy of the central giant cell granuloma has been curettage to eliminate the lesion, but not infrequently there is a recurrence and excision leaves a gross deformity. In order to avoid ablative surgery for a benign lesion in children, human calcitonin (0.5 mg; 100 IU) was injected daily deep subcutaneously in a series of 4 patients.[38] After 12 months of this therapy the lesions remitted, although in 1 case, small local recurrences took place requiring further calcitonin, which was delivered by nasal inhaler over a period of 2 years (Fig. 8.14).

This therapy, despite the dramatic effect that it has in eliminating the granuloma, does not interfere with skeletal development. In the adult a course of bisphosphonate would also be appropriate,[39] but would cause rickets in children.

Paget's disease

Paget's disease of bone is an idiopathic disorder of bone remodelling. The process is initiated by increases in osteoclast-mediated bone resorption, with subsequent compensatory increases in new bone formation, resulting in a disorganized mass of woven and lamellar bone at affected skeletal sites. The structural change produces bone that is expanded in size, less compact, more vascular, and more suscepitible to deformity or fracture than normal bone. The skull calvarium shows a 'cotton wool'-like thickening which may also affect the maxilla and the cementum of the tooth roots. For some reason the mandible is rarely affected. There is also an increased tendency for osteosarcoma formation.

An ethnic and geographic distribution of Paget's disease has been noted. It is common in the UK, Australasia and North America, but rare in Scandinavia, Spain, Italy and Asia.[40] The aetiology of Paget's disease remains unknown, however, there is some evidence that there may be a genetic element in this disease as a number of familial cases have been reported.[41,42] An autosomal dominant pattern of inheritance[43] has demonstrated an association with human leukocyte D, A9 and B15 loci. In addition, there is also support for a viral aetiology for this disease. Rebel *et al.*[44] were the first to describe ultrastructural abnormalities in the osteoclasts of affected patients; this has since been demonstrated by numerous other workers.[45] These nuclear and cytoplasmic inclusions resemble the nucleocapsids of the paramyxovirus family, which includes canine distemper virus.[46] More recently, Frausto *et al.*[47] have shown that abnormal virus-infected osteoclasts could be generated *in vitro* from the bone marrow of patients with Paget's disease of bone and that they may play a role in regulating the behaviour of the osteoclasts in this disease[48] The

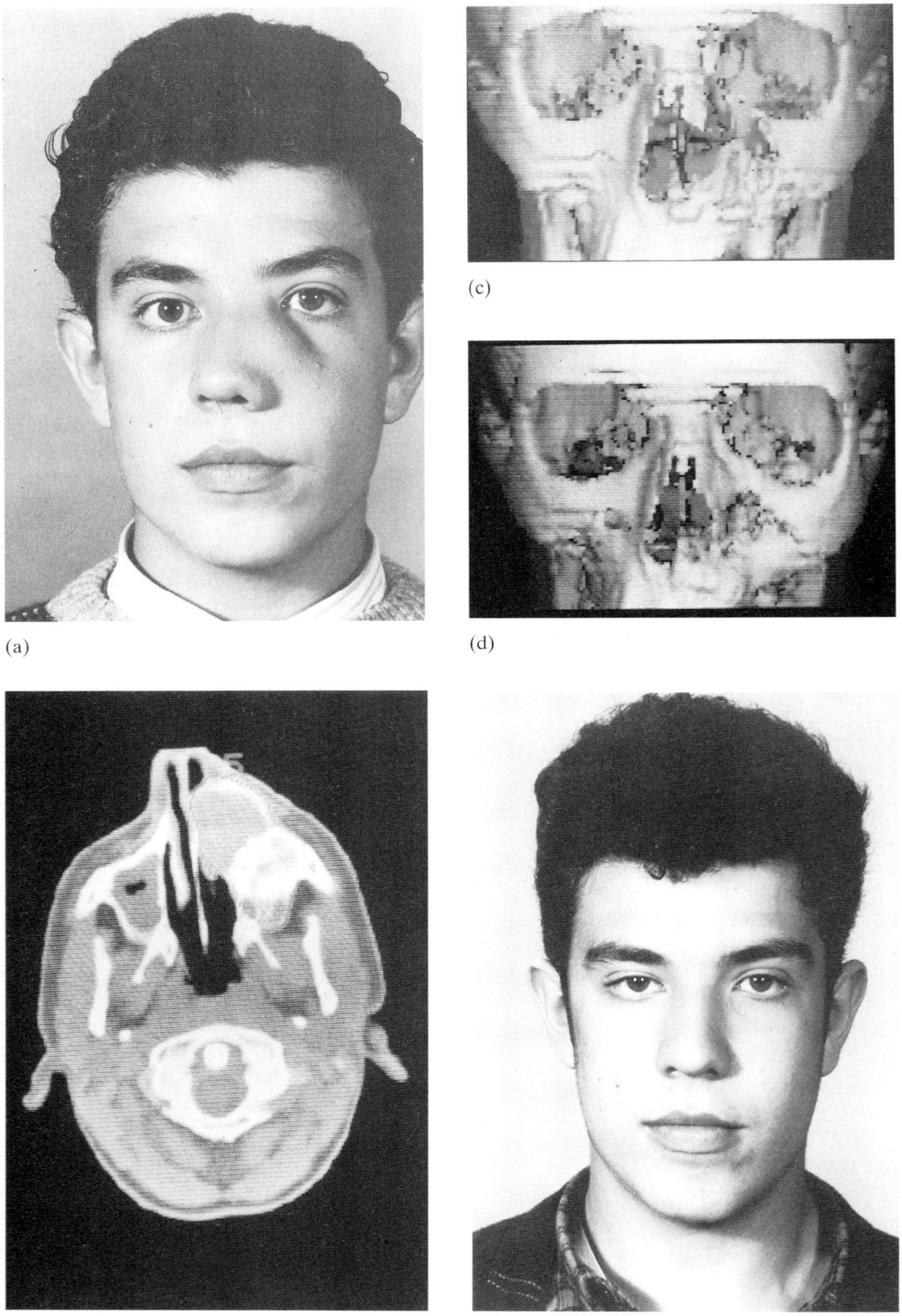

(a) (b) (c) (d) (e)

Fig. 8.14 (a, b) Giant cell granuloma of the maxilla invading the orbit and ethmoidal cells regressing with calcitonin therapy. (c) Three-dimensional reconstruction showing loss of orbital floor and medial wall. (d) Bone formation 2 years later. (e) Three years after calcitonin therapy.

current thoughts are that the large, functionally hyperactive osteoclasts are a product of a virus-mediated increase in cell fusion between osteoclasts and osteoclast progenitor cells. Despite the lack of definitive proof of a viral aetiology, many investigators believe that a common viral infection, perhaps in early life, in a genetically susceptible host predisposes to an osteoclast lesion that is manifested in adulthood as the abnormality that produces Paget's disease.

Osteoporosis

Osteoporosis is characterized by low bone mass, as a result of an imbalance between the activities of osteoclasts and osteoblasts. Postmenopausal osteoporosis may be triggered by the depletion in sex hormones and by a prior deficiency in calcium. Initially the pattern of bone loss is consistent with an increase in bone resorption[49,50] However, during the latter stages of development of osteoporosis, the pattern and rate of bone loss are consistent with a decrease in bone formation due to a reduction in the number of osteoblasts.[50–53] Why this reduction in osteoblast numbers occurs is currently unknown. It may be due to either reduction of the size of the stromal cell population or an impairment in the process of the osteogenic commitment of the stromal stem cells.

There is also evidence that there may be an imbalance between the differentiation of osteoblasts and the marrow adipocytes which could be a contributory factor in the elderly. In osteoporotic patients the volume of marrow adipose tissue is increased at sites of marked bone atrophy and decreased bone formation[54,55]

As far as treatment is concerned, oestrogen therapy is useful in the prevention of osteoporosis; however, the treatment of established osteoporosis is still a major problem. During the last decade, much attention has focused on the bisphosphonate compounds. Bisphosphonates are synthetic analogues of pyrophosphates developed as inhibitors of plaque formation on teeth. Russell *et al.*[56] showed that they also inhibited osteoclastic bone resorption by binding to bone mineral and thereby preventing the osteoclast from resorbing bone. Osteoclasts are also thought be metabolically impaired because they ingest the bisphosphonates bound to the bone surface.[57] This mode of action was supported by the finding that osteoclasts acquire a degenerative morphological appearance and change in function not only *in vivo*[58] but also *in vitro*.[59] It is also thought that bisphosphonate acts on the osteoclasts via the osteoblast.[60]

Osteopetrosis (Albers–Schönberg disease)

Osteopetrosis is a bone disease characterized by an increased bone mass that obliterates the marrow spaces and impairs haematopoiesis. It is caused by impaired osteoclastic bone resorption. This could be due to decreased osteoclast formation or decreased capacity of preformed osteoclasts to resorb bone. Not only are the bones dense and fragile, but they are also susceptible to chronic infection with impaired healing. Studies in animal models of osteopetrosis have shown that there is a defect in the coding region of the colony-stimulating factor-1 (CSF-1) gene, with subsequent impaired production of biological active CSF-1.[61] The result is a decrease in osteoclast formation, particularly during the neonatal period. The disease can be cured by treating animals with CSF-1.[61] Autosomal recessive infantile osteopetrosis has recently been treated with bone marrow transplantation,[62,63] which resulted in good responses, restoring normal osteoclastic bone resorption. Recombinant interferon-γ treatment in a study with 8 young patients has also shown good response.[64]

Orthodontic tooth movement

Bone also remodels in response to function and conversely shows a marked loss in its density and growth potential without mechanical stress, as seen in long bones in patients with poliomyelitis or in the mandible after ankylosis of the temporomandibular joint in early childhood. For this reason the study of orthodontic tooth movement helps to integrate both physical and biochemical concepts of bone remodelling.

Mechanical forces exerted on tooth roots and transmitted to the surrounding tissues of the periodontium initiate the remodelling activity, which facilitates the movement of teeth through bone. Bone is resorbed in areas perceived to be subjected to pressure and deposited at sites of tensile mechanical stress. Orthodontic models have provided much information, for instance Gianelly[65] noted that when excessive forces compressed the roots against the scoket wall, localized resorption ceased but so-called undermining resorption was seen in the adjacent alveolar bone, suggesting that ischaemia was associated with the former and venous congestion with the reactive undermining resorption.

The role of the periodontal vessels is also suggested by the differential resistance of cementum to resorption. It is postulated that the peripheral disposition of the periodontal vessels and the insulation of the cementum by the dense insertion of periodontal fibres are protective factors. Cementum may also possess an anti-invasive factor, again protecting its surface from mechanical resorptive factors. How tissues respond to physical stress at a cellular level has come from models for studying mechanical strain within bone. The technique of externally loading bones *in vivo* over various time periods was first used in a classic series of studies in rabbits by Hert *et al.*[66,67] They, and later Lanyon and co-workers,[68,69] showed that continuous loading of bone was unable to stimulate bone remodelling whereas intermittent forces applied over several weeks produced an increase in bone deposition on both the endosteal and periosteal surfaces of the cortex, irrespective of the type of force, i.e. compressive or tensile. The magnitude of the reaction was greater in younger animals.

The role of tension and compression in orthodontic tooth movement was based on histological studies of the periodontium, in which collagen fibre bundles are the predominant morphological feature. Despite this it seems unlikely that the periodontal ligament is able to generate differential pressures. Bien[70] suggested that the periodontal ligament acts as a continuous hydrostatic system through the socket with three distinct fluid compartments: the cells of the periodontal ligament, the vascular and lymph vessels, and the interstitial fluids. He proposed that any force would therefore be distributed evenly throughout the system. Hence it seems doubtful that the principal fibres of the periodontal ligament are capable of transferring forces directly to the adjacent bone. In crucial experiments, Heller and Nanda[71] disrupted collagen metabolism and function in rats by the systemic administration of lathyritic agents. In spite of this, the histological response of the alveolar bone to orthodontic forces was normal. Similarily, studies with radioactive isotopes to examine rates of cell proliferation and collagen metabolism showed no striking differences between tension and pressure sites, which suggests that metabolic activity was similar whichever side was examined.

When teeth are moved, the crowns of teeth are displaced 10 times more than the reduction in periodontal ligament width, suggesting that bone also deforms quite readily. Bone bending can produce associated physical phenomena such as piezoelectric currents, but it is not clear how these and other physical forces such as magnetic and electric fields produce cellular effects. Electric stimuli have a similar effect to mechanical stress.[72–74] Electric fields and piezoelectric effects have also been an area of interest, especially in promoting healing of bony defects.[75] Piezoelectric forces are generated when crystalline structures, such as bone are deformed. These currents have been suggested as the prime mechanism by which tooth movement and Wolff's law is modulated.[76] It is not clear how mechanical stress, the effects of electric currents or piezoelectric stimuli exert a specific cellular effect, especially as many of the experiments designed to measure their generation have been performed using dry tissue. Furthermore, the action potential in adjacent nerves is of considerably greater magnitude than the piezoelectric phenomenon. In the face of this evidence it seems unreasonable to equate cellular activation with these potentials.

Animal models have clearly demonstrated many important changes associated with mechanical stress. However, the major drawback of experiments carried out *in vivo* is the difficulty of determining the individual responses of different cell types. For this reason the development of tissue culture models has proved useful in determining the responses tissues make when exposed to mechanical forces. The *in vivo* evidence described earlier suggests that bone is unable to discriminate between tension and compression. *In vitro* models have provided some indication as to how this differential response may occur.

Change in cell shape: as a mechanism for the transduction of mechanical forces

The development of techniques to isolate and culture monolayers of single cell types, together with methods for deforming cell layers or altering cell shape, have suggested that a relationship exists between cell shape and metabolic activity. Folkman and Moscona[77] showed that flattened cells synthesize more DNA than rounded cells. Other workers have produced evidence that catabolic rather than anabolic events are associated with rounded cells.[78] Agents such as phorbol esters cause a rounding-up of synovial fibroblasts with an alteration in gene expression. This results in an increase of collagenase and plasminogen activator production, but a reduction in the synthesis of extracellular matrix proteins such as collagen and fibronectin.

Similar findings have been made in epithelial cells where shape change was induced by non-chemical means.[79,80] Prostaglandins and parathyroid hormone induce shape change in bone cell cultures which are associated with changes in the microfilament system rather than microtubules.[81] To date, there is little published work regarding changes in the cytoskeleton with mechanical forces, but Banes *et al.* found a decrease in tubulin and suggested that this may have a role in the mediation of mechanical stress.[82] It is conceivable then that in pressure sites cells are rounded and have catabolic effects and in tension sites cells are flattened and are therefore in a synthetic mode. It is important to realize that shape change by cultured cells *in vitro* in response to various hormones and growth factors may not neccessarily occur *in vivo*.

Prostaglandins and tooth movement

One of the clearest examples of how *in vivo* and *in vitro* investigative means have been used to improve clinical practice in orthodontics comes from the role of prostaglandins in orthodontic tooth movement.

Prostaglandins were first discovered by Von Euler in 1934.[83] The compound was isolated from human semen and it was believed at the time that the prostate gland was the major source. It is now known that prostaglandins are produced by nearly all tissues, but the name has been retained. Similarly leukotrienes, which are also metabolites of arachidonic acid, were originally demonstrated in leukocytes and were called leukotrienes. Both prostaglandins and leukotrienes have a common parent substrate – arachidonic acid. The major metabolites of this pathway are shown in Figure 8.9.

Much of the information which first implicated prostaglandins in the transduction of mechanical stimuli was derived from experiments using tissue culture models. Essentially cells are grown on a substrate and the culture surface distorted; this then stimulates the cells. It is possible using bioassays and biochemical techniques to detect what substances cells produce in response to this perturbation. One of the first models which was developed using this approach was described by Harell *et al.*[84] These workers have suggested that mechanical distortion evokes the following sequence of events. First, activation of the enzyme phospholipase A_2 with subsequent release of arachidonic acid results in increased prostaglandin E_2 production, which in turn elevates cyclic adenosine monophosphate (cAMP) production. Second, there is also an increase in intracellular Ca^{2+} and stimulation of DNA synthesis. The ability to mimic or inhibit these changes by addition of exogenous prostaglandin E_2 or indomethacin respectively suggests that mechanical forces are mediated by prostaglandin production.[85] The increase in DNA synthesis has been confirmed by other workers.[86,87] It is of interest that the *in vivo* and *in vitro* data are mutually supportive in that intermittent forces have a greater effect on stimulating activity compared to continuous forces.

Based largely on this *in vitro* work, Yamasaki and coworkers,[88] using a rat model of tooth movement, demonstrated that injection of prostaglandins increased osteoclast numbers. Indomethacin, which inhibits prostaglandin synthesis, inhibited the appearance of osteoclasts. Further work showed that local prostaglandin injection could also increase the rate of orthodontic tooth movement in primates.[89] This culminated in the clinical use of prostaglandin E_1 to increase the efficiency of orthodontic appliances.[90] It must be noted that the frequency of injections (approximately weekly) would deter many patients, although their use in adult patients is routine in some dental schools (Yamasaki, personal communication).

An alternative approach to demonstrate the role of prostaglandins in bone remodelling is the use of cyclooxygenase inhibitors (non-steroidal anti-inflammatory drugs or NSAIDs). Experiments using NSAIDs have shown that bone remodelling in fractured femurs can be reduced if prostaglandin synthesis is blocked[91] and inhibition of tooth movement by indomethacin has been reported in experimental animals.[92] However, an earlier report in a rabbit model found only a significant decrease in osteoclast numbers and not in the degree of tooth movement, suggesting that prostaglandins alone do not account for bone remodelling associated with tooth movement.[93] Leukotrienes and HETEs produced from the same substrate (arachidonic acid) could account for this discrepancy. A rat orthodontic model has been used to demonstrate that inhibition of leukotriene synthesis can significantly reduce orthodontic tooth movement.[94]

Second messenger systems activated by mechanical forces

Some indication that second messengers are involved in the transduction of mechanical forces was made in the previous section.

All cells have internal signalling systems, which convert external stimuli such as hormones or mechanical forces into internal signals known as second messengers. The second messenger classically associated with mechanical force transduction is cAMP. A schematic diagram of the control of this system is shown in Fig. 8.15. A further second messenger system was also starting to be unravelled in the 1950s by Hokin and Hokin[95] who showed an increase in phosphate incorporation into cell membrane phospholipids in response to many stimuli.

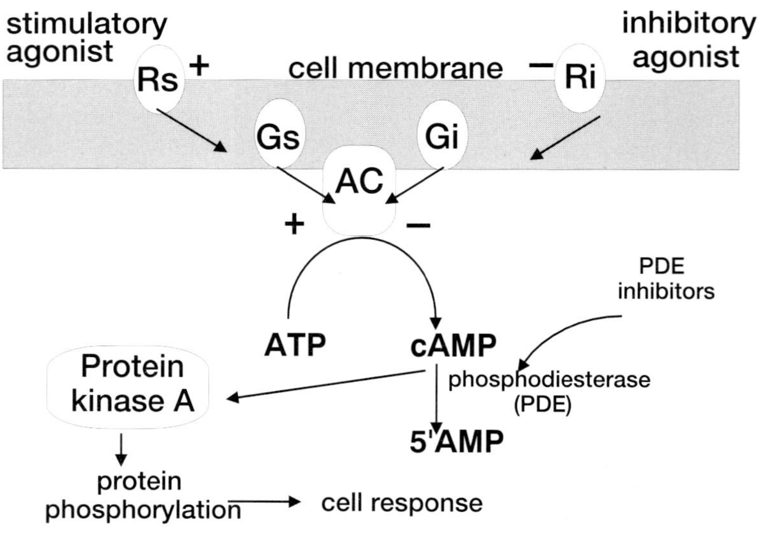

Fig. 8.15 Schematic diagram of the cellular events which regulate cyclic adenosine monophosphate (cAMP) production. The production of this second messenger pathway is regulated by stimulatory (Rs) and inhibitory (Ri) receptors. These interact with their respective G proteins (Gs and Gi) to stimulate or inhibit production of adenylate cyclase. This enzyme results in the formation of cAMP from adenosine triphosphate (ATP). The inactivation of cAMP is effected by phosphodiesterase. cAMP is known to activate protein kinase A, an enzyme responsible for protein phosphorylation. (AC = Adenyl Cyclase).

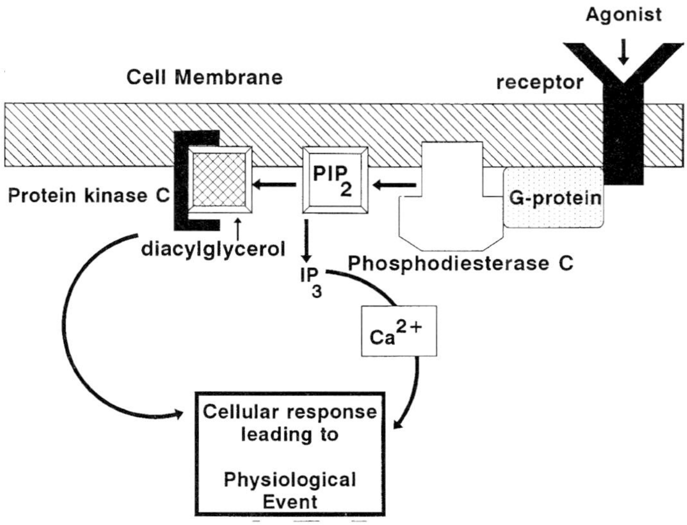

Fig. 8.16 The membrane events which result in the production of inositol phosphates are similar to those for generation of cyclic adenosine monophosphate, i.e. an agonist binds to a receptor followed by a receptor–G protein interaction. The phosphodiesterase (a phospholipase C) cleaves phosphatidylinositol bisphosphate into diacylglycerol and inositol trisphosphate (IP_3). Intracellular calcium $[Ca^{2+}]_i$ is mobilized from the endoplasmic reticulum by IP_3.
Diacylglycerol remains within the plane of the cell membrane and activates protein kinase C. The continued action of these two second messenger pathways accounts for early and sustained cell responses.

The real importance of the phospholipids as messenger systems was not fully appreciated until the 1980s. The first demonstration that products of the inositol lipids could cause release of intracellular stores of calcium brought together a number of observations and hypotheses.[96] The phosphoinositide pathway has been reviewed extensively by Berridge[97] and is illustrated in Figure 8.16.

The basic scheme suggests that breakdown of phosphatidylinositol 4,5-bisphosphate in response to activation of cell surface receptors leads to inositol trisphosphate (IP_3) formation with the subsequent release of Ca^{2+} from intracellular stores. IP_3 is a mediator of mitogenesis in a variety of cell types. In addition to the production of inositol phosphates, diacylglycerol is formed and this remains within the plane of the cell membrane and activates protein kinase C. The production of these two pathways results in the activation of a large number of intracellular processes such as protein phosphorylation. With these developments, the importance of second messengers other than cAMP in mediating the effects of mechanical deformation has been realized. Although it seems likely that the Ca^{2+} changes previously reported by Harell and co-workers[84] might have occurred as the result of a cAMP-dependent Ca^{2+} flux through cell membranes, the effects of hormones or mechanical stress cannot be explained by cAMP elevation alone.

The phosphoinositide pathway could certainly account for many of the changes seen in mechanically deformed tissues. This includes an elevation of intracellular Ca^{2+} and an increase in DNA synthesis. Furthermore, osteoblasts elevate inositol phosphates as well as cAMP in response to PGE_2 and parathyroid hormone.[98] Recent work with second messenger production in mechanically deformed osteoblasts has also shown that there is dual elevation of at least two second messenger pathways, cAMP and the inositol phosphates.[99] Binderman *et al.*[85] have also presented indirect evidence that diacylglycerol, the other arm of the phosphatidylinositol pathway, may be involved in transduction of mechanical stress.

Cytokines as possible mediators of mechanically induced bone remodelling

Cytokines can be defined as small proteins with either paracrine or endocrine functions involved in local inflammation or immunoregulation. Within this definition are the interleukins, TNF-α and -β, the interferons (IFN-α, IFN-β and IFN-γ), CSF and growth factors. Cytokines are produced by a wide variety of cell types, often in response to stimulation by other members of the cytokine network. IL-1 has a central role; it has many actions on different target cells and can induce high levels of expression of many other cytokines. The isolation and purification of these factors continue at great pace. An excellent series of articles in the *Lancet*[100–105] has reviewed these factors together with their relevance in health and disease.

Cytokines can influence connective tissue remodelling and these include the interleukins, tumour necrosis factors, interferons, polypeptide growth factors and CSF. IL-1α and IL-1β have recently been immunolocalized in the periodontal tissues of cat canine teeth following the application of a tipping force.[106] This work has provided the first experimental evidence to support the suggestion that cytokines regulate some remodelling processes during orthodontic tooth movement Some *in vitro* data also exist. Mechanically deformed osteoblasts produce a wide range of molecules some of which are capable of causing bone resorption.[107] These include four osteolytic factors with molecular weights of 40–50, 14–15, 5–6 and less than 1 kDa (Fig. 8.17).[107]

Further studies revealed that secretion of the osteolytic activity from stressed osteoblasts was dependent on 5-lipoxygenase activity but not cyclooxygenase activity. This osteolytic activity was not blocked by neutralizing

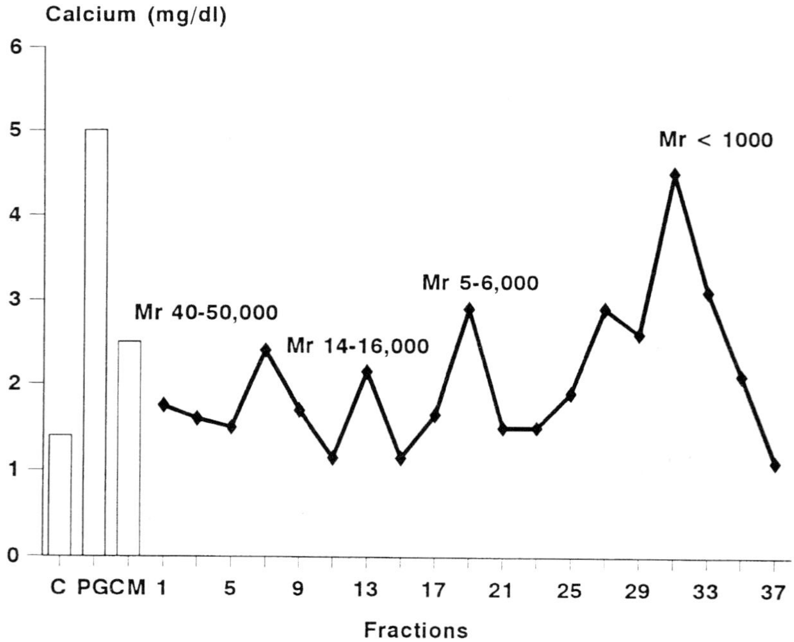

Fig. 8.17 Mechanically stressed osteoblasts release four major peaks of bone-resorbing activity. Control cultures (C) show the level of endogenous bone resorption. Prostaglandin E_2 (PG) was included as a positive control. Culture medium (CM) from the osteoblasts was tested to show the bone resorbing activity before fractionation. High-perfomance liquid chromatograpy fractionation of the osteoblast culture media shows four peaks, suggesting four distinct factors. The results are expressed as mean calcium release (mg/dl). The relative molecular weights (M_r) of the major peaks are indicated.

antibodies to the major osteolytic cytokines, namely, IL-1α and β, IL-6 or TNF-α. Fractionation of the media from the mechanically stimulated osteoblasts isolated at least three separate protein fractions and one lipid fraction. One of these proteins with a molecular mass of 15 kDa may represent a novel mediator of bone resorption.[108]

Collagen turnover and mechanical stimuli

Collagen represents 50% of protein in vertebrates. In bone this proportion increases to 90% and this is even higher in the periodontal ligament. Clearly then, the interaction between applied forces and collagen turnover is an important part of tooth movement. Much of the evidence for the changes in collagen turnover have been derived from *in vitro* studies using organ culture techniques. These comprise culturing various cranial bones together with their sutures, which are mechanically deformed by wires or coil springs.[109–111] Alternatively, blocks of mouse alveolar bone containing three molars have been successfully cultured and mechanical forces were applied to the teeth using multistranded orthodontic wires.[112]

With these techniques, it has been demonstrated that mechanical forces induce an initial increase in DNA synthesis, alkaline phosphatase activity and an increase in collagen synthesis. More detailed investigation showed that the relationship between mechanical stress and collagen synthesis was discriminating. Normally fibroblasts synthesize type I collagen, but in response to tensile mechanical stress the cells synthesized significant quantities of type III collagen.[112] Type III collagen is found in fetal tissues, uterus wall, blood vessel walls and periodontal ligament. Such tissues are characterized either by high turnover or functional loading, which suggests that the biomechanical environment of a connective tissue cell is an important determinant of the type of collagen synthesized. Mechanical stress has also been shown to stimulate not only the synthesis of structural macromolecules such as collagen, but also the enzymes responsible for their specific hydrolysis. Meikle *et al.*[113] reported an increase in the production of the metalloproteinases collagenase, gelatinase (type IV collagenase) and stromelysin by mechanically deformed sutures, with a concomitant increase in their specific inhibitor – tissue inhibitor of metalloproteinase (TIMP). Subsequent experiments using sensitive immunocytochemical methods demonstrated the presence of active collagenase bound to collagen within the suture together with a local decrease in TIMP, suggesting collagen breakdown. This collagenase activity was found to correspond to the site of increased cell proliferation in the cranial suture and other animal models of tooth movement.

Conclusion

Osteoclast activity has proved to be substantially more complex than Howship ever anticipated. Despite this, common biochemical mechanisms appear to account for a diversity of pathological bone conditions, which are readily studied in the jaws.

References

1. Herzberg F, Schour I. Effects of the removal of pulp and Hertwig's sheath on the eruption of incisors in the albino rat. *J Dent Res* 1941; **20**: 264.
2. Main JHP, Adams D. Experiments on the rat incisor into the cellular proliferation and blood-pressure theories of tooth eruption. *Arch Oral Biol* 1966; **11**: 163–178.
3. Moxham BJ. The role of the periodontal vasculature in tooth eruption. In: *The Biological Mechanisms of Tooth Eruption and Root Resorption*, pp. 207–223. Alabama: EBSCO Media, 1988.
4. Marks SC, Cahill DR. Experimental study in the dog of the non-active role of the tooth in the eruptive process. *Arch Oral Biol* 1984; **29**: 311–322.
5. Brash JC. Growth of the alveolar bone and its relation to the movements of teeth, including eruption. *Int J Orthodont* 1928; **14**: 196–223.
6. Cahill DR, Marks SC. Tooth eruption: evidence for the central role of the dental follicle. *J Oral Pathol* 1980; **9**: 189–200.
7. Moxham BJ, Berkovitz BKB. The effects of root transection on the unimpeded eruption rate of the rabbit mandibular incisor. *Arch Oral Biol* 1974; **19**: 903–909.
8. Berkovitz BKB, Migdalski A, Solomon M. The effect of the lathyritic agent amino-acetnitrile on the unimpeded eruption rate in normal and root-resected rat lower incisors. *Arch Oral Biol* 1972; **17**: 1755–1763.
9. Abercrombie M. The crawling movement of metazoan cells. In: *Cell Behaviour*, pp. 19–48. Cambridge: Cambridge University Press, 1982.

10. Bell E, Ivarsson B, Merrill C. Production of a tissue-like structure by contraction of collagen lattices by human fibroblasts of different proliferative potential *in vitro*. *Proc Natl Acad Sci* 1979; **76**: 1274–1278.
11. Bellows CG, Melcher AH, Aubin JE. Contraction and organization of collagen gels by cells cultured from periodontal ligament, gingiva and bone suggest functional differences between cell types. *J Cell Sci* 1981; **50**: 299–314.
12. Bellows CG, Melcher AH, Aubin JE. An *in vitro* model for tooth eruption utilizing periodontal ligament fibroblasts and collagen lattices. *Arch Oral Biol* 1983; **28**: 715–722.
13. Cohen S. Isolation of a mouse submaxillary gland protein accelerating incisor eruption and eyelid opening in the newborn animal. *J Biol Chem* 1962; **237**: 1555–1562.
14. Sauk JJ. Genetic disorders involving tooth eruption anomalies. In: *The Biological Mechanisms of Tooth Eruption and Root Resorption*, pp. 171–179. Alabama: EBSCO Media, 1988.
15. Meghji S, Wilson M, Henderson B, Kinnane D. Anti-proliferative and cytotoxic activity of surface-associated material from periodontopathogenic bacteria. *Arch Oral Biol* 1992; **37**: 637–644.
16. Meghji S, Henderson B, Nair S, Wilson M. Inhibition of bone DNA and collagen production by surface associated material from bacteria implicated in the pathology of periodontal disease. *J Periodontol* 1992; **63**: 736–742.
17. Wilson M, Meghji S, Barber P, Henderson B. Biological activities of surface associated material from *Porphyromonas gingivalis. FEMS Immunol Med Microbiol* 1993; **6**: 147–156.
18. Meghji S, Wilson M, Barber P, Henderson B. Bone resorbing activity of surface associated material from *Actinobacillus actinomycetemcomitans* and *Eikenella corrodens*. *J Med Micro* 1994; **41**: 197–203.
19. Meghji S, Henderson B, Kirby A, Newman HN, Wilson M. Serum antibody response to surface-associated material from periodontopathogenic bacteria. *FEMS Immunol Med Microbiol* 1995; **10**: 101–108.
20. Meghji S, Henderson B, Wilson M. High titre anti-sera from patients with periodontal disease inhibits bacterial capsule-induced bone breakdown. *J Periodont Res* 1993; **281**: 115–121.
21. Reddi K, Wilson M, Poole S, Meghji S, Henderson B. Relative cytokine-stimulating activities of surface components of the oral periodontapathic bacterium *Actinobacillus actinomycetemcomitans*. *Cytokine* 1995; **7**: 534–541.
22. Harvey W, Foo GC, Gordon D, Meghji S, Evans A, Harris M. Evidence for fibroblasts as the major source of prostacyclin and prostaglandin synthesis in dental cysts in man. *Arch Oral Biol* 1984; **29**: 223–229.
23. Dewhirst FE, Stashenko PP, Mole JE, Tsuramachi T. Purification and partial sequence of human osteoclast-activating factor, identity with interleukin 1β. *J Immunol* 1985; **135**: 2562–2568.
24. Bando Y, Henderson B, Meghji S, Harris M. Immunocytochemical localization of cytokines and adhesion receptor in radicular cysts. *J Oral Pathol Med* 1993; **22**: 221–227.
25. Meghji S., Henderson B, Bando Y, Harris M. Interleukin-1 is the principal osteolytic cytokine produced by keratocysts. *Arch Oral Biol* 1992; **36**: 935–943.
26. Meghji S, Harvey W, Harris M. Interleukin 1–like activity in cystic lesions of the jaw. *Br J Oral Maxillo Fac Surg* 1989; **27**: 1–11.
27. Donoff RB, Harper E, Guralnick WC. Collagenolytic activity in keratocysts. *J Oral Surg* 1972; **30**: 879–884.
28. Matejka M, Porteder H, Kleinert W, Ulrich W, Watzek G, Sinzinger H. Evidence that PGI_2–generation in human dental cysts is stimulated by leukotrienes C_4 and D_4. Br *J Oral Maxillofac Surg* 1985; **23**: 190–194.
29. Harris M, Jenkins MV, Bennett A, Wills MR. Prostaglandin production and bone resorption by dental cysts. *Nature* 1973; **245**: 213–215.
30. Meghji S, Sandy JR, Scutt A, Harvey W, Harris M. Stimulation of bone resorption by lipoxygenase metabolites of arachidonic acid. *Prostaglandins* 1988; **36**: 139–149.
31. Meghji S, Sandy JR, Harvey W, Harris M. Ameloblastoma, characterisation and identification of bone resorbing factors *in vitro*. *Calcif Tissue Int* 1988; **42**: A44.
32. Meghji S, Sandy JR, Scutt A, Harvey W, Harris M. Macromolecular osteolytic factor released by squamous cell carcinoma is interleukin 1. *Br J Cancer* 1988; **58**: 17–21.
33. Attie MF. Treatment of hypercalcaemia. *Endocrinol Metab Clin North Am* 1989; **18**: 807–828.
34. Mundy GR, Martin TJ. Hypercalcaemia of malignancy – pathogenesis and treatment. *Metabolism* 1982; **31**: 1247–1277.
35. Gibbs J, Dillon MJ, Lang S, Meghji S, Pritchard J. Indomethacin responsive hypercalcaemia associated with a renal sarcoma. *Arch Dis Child* 1990; **65**: 1168–1169
36. Macpherson DW, Hopper C, Meghji S. Hypercalcaemia and the synthesis of interleukin 1 by an ameloblastoma. *Br J Maxillofac Surg* 1991; **29**: 29–33.
37. Flanagan AM, Tinkler SMB, Horton MA, Williams DM, Chambers TJ. The multinucelate cells in giant cell granulomas of the jaws are osteoclasts. *Cancer* 1989; **62**: 1139–1144.
38. Harris M. Central giant cell granulomas of the jaws regress with calcitonin therapy. *Br J Oral Maxfac Surg* 1992; **30**: 313–318.
39. Davis JP, Archer DJ, Fisher C, Wimalawansa SJ, Baldwin D. Multiple recurrent lesions associated with high circulating levels of parathyroid hormone-related peptide in a young adult. *Br J Maxillofac Surg* 1991; **29**: 102–105.

40. Smith R. Disorders of the skeleton: Paget's disease. In: Weatherall DJ, Ledingham JGG, Worell DA (eds) *Oxford Text of Medicine*, pp. 17.19–17.22. Oxford: Oxford Medical Publications, 1989.
41. Irvine RE. Familial Paget's disease with early onset. *J Bone Joint Surg* 1953; **4**: 104–110.
42. Wu RKI, Trumble TE, Ruwe PA. Familial incidence of Paget's disease and secondary osteogenic sarcoma. *Clin Orthop* 1991; **265**: 306–309.
43. Siris ES, Ottman R, Flaster E, Kelsey JL. Familial aggregation of Paget's disease of bone. *J Bone Miner Res* 1991; **6**: 495–500
44. Rebel A, Basle MF, Pouplard A, Malkani K, Filmon R, Le Patezpur A. Bone tissue in Paget's disease of bone. *Arth Rheum* 1974; **23**: 1104–1114.
45. Kahn AJ. The viral aetiology of Paget's disease of bone: a new perspective. *Calcif Tissue Int* 1990; **47**: 127–129.
46. Gherarardi G, Iocascio U, Bonnuci E. Fine structrue of nucleii and cytoplasm of osteoclasts in Paget's disease of bone. *Histopathology* 1980; **4**: 63–65.
47. Frausto A, Mills B, Singer F, Roodman GD. Multinucleated cells fromed in long-term marrow cultures from Paget's pateints express viral antigens. *J Bone Miner Res* 1990; **5** (suppl 2): 791.
48. Roodman GD, Kurihara N, Osaki Y, Signer FS. Il-6 is an autocrine/paracrine factor for pagetic osteoclasts. *J Bone Miner Res* 1990; **5** (suppl 2): 793.
49. Parfitt AM. The three organizational levels of bone remodelling: implications for the interpretation of biochemical markers and the mechanisms of bone loss. In: Christiansen C, Overgaard K (eds) *Osteoporosis 1990. Third International Symposium on Osteoporosis*, pp. 329–434. Copenhagen: Osteopress ApS, 1990.
50. Parfit AM. The cellular basis of bone remodelling. The quantum concept reexamined in the light of recent advances in cell biology. *Calcif Tissue Int* 1984; **36**: s37–s45.
51. Compston JE, Croucher PI. Histomorphmetric assessment of trabecular bone remodelling in osteoporosis. *Bone Mineral* 1991; **14**: 91–102.
52. Compston JE, Vedi S, Mellish RWE, Croucher PE, O'Sullivan MM. Reduced bone formation in non-steroid treated patients with rheumatoid arthritis. *Ann Rheum Dis* 1989; **48**: 483–487.
53. Cohen-Solal ME, Shih M-S, Lundy MW, Parfitt AM. A new method of measuring cancellous bone erosion depth: application to the cellular mechanisms of bone loss in postmenopausal osteoporosis. *J Bone Miner Res* 1991; **12**: 1331–1337.
54. Novotny JR, Duehrsen U, Welch K, Layton JE, Cebon JS, Boyd AW. Cloned stromal cell lines derived from human Whitlock/Witte-type long-term bone marrow cultures. *Exp Hematol* 1990; **18**: 775–784.
55. Burkhardt R, Kettner G, Bohm W. Changes in trabecular bone, haematopoiesis and bone marrow vessels in aplastic anaemia, primary osteoporosis and old age. A comparative and histomorphometric study. *Bone* 1987; **8**: 157–164.
56. Russell RGG, Muhlbauer RC, Bisaz S *et al.* The influence of pyrophosphate, condensed phosphates, phosphonates, and other phosphate compounds on dissolution of hydroxapatite *in vitro* and on bone resorption indices by parathyroid hormone and in thyroparathyroidectomised rats. *Calcif Tissue Res* 1970; **6**: 183–196.
57. Fleisch H. Bisphosphonates: pharmacology and use in the treatment of tumor-induced hypercalcemic and metastatic bone disease. *Drugs* 1991; **42**: 919–944.
58. Schenk RWA, Merz R, Muehbauer R, Russel RGG, Fleeisch H. Effect of ethane-1,1–diphosphonate (EHDP) and dichoromethylene diphosphonate (Cl2MDP) on tibial epiphysis and metaphysis of rats. *Calcif Tissue Res* 1976; **11**: 196–214
59. Flanagan AM, Chamber TJ. Dichloromethylenebisphosphonate (Cl_2MDP) inhibits bone resorption through injury to osteoclasts that resorb the Cl_2MDP-coated bone. *Bone Mineral* 1989; **6**: 33–43.
60. Sahni M, Guenther H, Fleisch H, Collin P, Martin TJ. Bisphosphonates act on rat bone resorption through the mediation of osteoblasts. *J Clin Invest* 1993; **91**: 2004–2011.
61. Kodoma H, Yamasaki A, Nose M *et al.* Congenital osteoclast defieciency in osteopetrotic (op/op) mice is cured by injections of macrophage colony stimulating factor. *J Exp Med* 1991; **173**: 269–272.
62. Coccia PF, Krivit W, Cervenka J *et al.* Successful bone marrow transplantation for infantile malignant osteopetrosis. *N Engl J Med* 1980; **302**: 701–708
63. Kaplan FS, August CS, Fallon MD *et al.* Successful treatment of infantile malignant osteopetrosis by bone marrow transplantation: a case report. *J Bone Joint Surg* 1988; **70**: 617–623.
64. Key LL, Ries WL, Rodriguez RM *et al.* Recombinant interferon-gamma therapy for osteopetrosis. *J Pediatr* 1992; **121**: 119–124.
65. Gianelly AA. Force induced changes in the vascularity of periodontal ligament. *Am J Orthodont* 1969; **55**: 5–15.
66. Hert J, Liskova M, Landrgot B. Influence of the long-term, continuous bending on the bone. An experimental study on the tibia of the rabbit. *Folia Morphol* 1969; **XVII**: 389–399.
67. Hert J, Liskova M, Landa J. Reaction of bone to mechanical stimuli. Part 1. Continuous and intermittent loading of tibia in rabbit. *Folia Morphol* 1971; **XIX**: 290–300.
68. Lanyon LE, Rubin CT. Static vs dynamic loads as an influence on bone remodelling. *J Biomechanics* 1984; **17**: 897–905.
69. Rubin CT, Lanyon LE. Regulation of bone mass by mechanical strain magnitude. *Calcif Tissue Int* 1985; **37**: 411–417.
70. Bien SM. Haemodynamic damping of tooth movement. *J Dent Res* 1966; **45**: 907–914.

71. Heller IJ, Nanda R. Effect of metabolic alteration of periodontal fibres on orthodontic tooth movement. *Am J Orthodont* 1979; **75**: 239–257.
72. Davidovitch Z, Steigman S, Finkelson MD *et al.* Immunohistochemical evidence that electric currents increase periosteal cell cyclic nucleotide levels in feline alveolar bone *in vivo*. *Arch Oral Biol* 1980; **25**: 321–327.
73. Davidovitch Z, Finkelson MD, Steigman S, Shanfeld JL, Montgomery PC, Korostoff E. Electric currents, bone remodelling and orthodontic tooth movement. I. The effect of electric currents on periodontal cyclic nucleotides. *Am J Orthod* 1980; **77**: 14–32.
74. Davidovitch Z, Finkelson MD, Steigman S, Shanfeld JL, Montgomery PC, Korostoff E. Electric currents, bone remodelling and orthodontic tooth movement. II Increase in rate of tooth movement and periodontal cyclic nucleotide levels by combined force and electric current. *Am J Orthod* 1980; **77**: 33–47.
75. Friedenberg ZB, Brighton CT. Bioelectric potentials in bone. *J Bone Joint Surg* 1966; **48–A**: 915–923.
76. Bassett CAL, Becker RO. Generation of electrical potentials by bone in response to mechanical stress. *Science* 1962; **137**: 1063–1064.
77. Folkman J, Moscona A. Role of cell shape in growth control. *Nature* 1978; **273**: 345–349.
78. Aggeler J, Frisch SM, Werb Z. Changes in cell shape correlate with collagenase gene expression in rabbit synovial fibroblasts. *J Cell Biol* 1984; **98**: 1662–1671.
79. Hong HL, Brunette DM. Effect of cell shape on proteinase secretion by epithelial cells. *J Cell Sci* 1987; **87**: 259–267.
80. Unemori EN, Werb Z. Reorganization of polymerized actin: a possible trigger for induction of procollagenase in fibroblasts cultured in and on collagen gels. *J Cell Biol* 1986; **103**: 1021–1031.
81. Beertsen W, Heersche JNM, Aubin JE. Free and polymerized tubulin in cultured bone cells and Chinese hamster ovary cells: the influence of cold and hormones. *J Cell Biol* 1982; **95**: 387–393.
82. Banes AJ, Gilbert J, Taylor D, Monbureau O. A new vacuum-operated stress-providing instrument that applies static or variable duration cyclic tension or compression to cells *in vitro*. *J Cell Sci* 1985; **75**: 35–42.
83. Von Euler US. Contributions to the understanding of the pharmacologic effect of secretions and extracts from secondary male sex glands. *Naunyn-Schmeideberg's Arch Exp Pathol Pharmakol* 1934; **175**: 78–84.
84. Harell A, Dekel S, Binderman I. Biochemical effect of mechanical stress on cultured bone cells. *Calcif Tissue Res* 1977; **22** (suppl): 202–207.
85. Binderman I, Zor U, Kaye AM, Shimshoni Z, Harell, A, Somjen D. The transduction of mechanical force into biochemical events in bone cells may involve activation of phospholipase A_2. *Calcif Tissue Int* 1988; **42**: 261–266.
86. Hasegawa S, Sato S, Saito S, Suzuki Y, Brunette DM. Mechanical stretching increases the number of cultured bone cells synthesising DNA and alters their pattern of protein synthesis. *Calcif Tissue Int* 1985; **37**: 431–436.
87. Buckley MJ, Banes AJ, Levin LG *et al.* Osteoblasts increase their rate of division and align in response to cyclic, mechanical tension *in vitro*. *Bone Miner* 1988; **4**: 225–236.
88. Yamasaki K, Miura F, Suda T. Prostaglandin as a mediator of bone resorption induced by experimental tooth movement in rats. *J Dent Res* 1980; **59**: 1635–1642.
89. Yamasaki K, Shibata Y, Fukuhara T. The effect of prostaglandins on experimental tooth movement in monkeys (*Macaca fuscata*). *J Dent Res* 1982; **61**: 1444–1446.
90. Yamasaki K, Shibata Y, Imai S, Tani Y, Shibasaki Y, Fukuhara T. Clinical application of prostaglandin $E_1(PGE_1)$ upon orthodontic tooth movement. *Am J Orthod* 1984; **85**: 508–518.
91. Sudman E, Bang G. Indomethacin-induced inhibition of Haversian remodelling in rabbits. *Acta Orthopaed Scand* 1979; **50**: 621–627.
92. Chumbley AB, Tuncay OC. The effect of indomethacin (an aspirin-like drug) on the rate of orthodontic tooth movement. *Am J Orthod* 1986; **89**: 312–314.
93. Sandy JR, Harris M. Prostaglandins and tooth movement. *Eur J Orthodont* 1984; **6**: 175–182.
94. Mohammed AH, Tatakis DN, Dziak R. Leukotrienes in orthodontic tooth movement. *Am J Orthod Dentofac Orthop* 1989; **95**: 231–237.
95. Hokin MR, Hokin LE. Enzyme secretion and the incorporation of 32P into phospholipids of pancreas slices. *J Biol Chem* 1953; **203**: 967–977.
96. Streb H, Irvine RF, Berridge MJ, Schulz I. Release of Ca^{2+} from a nonmitochondrial intracellular store in pancreatic acinar cells by inositol-1,4,5–trisphosphate. *Nature* 1983; **306**: 67–69.
97. Berridge MJ. Inositol trisphosphate and diacylgycerol: two interacting second messengers. *Annu Rev Biochem* 1987; **56**: 159–193.
98. Farndale RW, Sandy JR, Atkinson SJ, Pennington SR, Meghji S, Meikle MC. Parathyroid hormone and prostaglandin E_2 stimulate both inositol phosphates and cyclic AMP accumulation in mouse osteoblast cultures. *Biochem J* 1988; **252**: 263–268.
99. Sandy JR, Meghji S, Farndale RW, Meikle MC. Dual elevation of cyclic AMP and inositol phosphates in response to mechanical deformation of murine osteoblasts. *Biochim Biophys Acta* 1989; **1010**: 265–269.
100. Metcalf D. Haemopoietic growth factors 1. *Lancet* 1989; **1**: 825–827.
101. Metcalf D. Haemopoietic growth factors 2. *Lancet* 1989; **1**: 885–886.
102. O'Gara A. Interleukins and the immune system. *Lancet* 1989; **1**: 943–946.
103. Balkwill FR. Interferons. *Lancet* 1989; **1**: 1060–1063.
104. Tracey KJ, Vlassara H, Cerami A. Cachectin/tumour necrosis factor. *Lancet* 1989; **1**: 1122–1125.

105. Ross R. Platelet-derived growth factor. *Lancet* 1989; **1**: 1179–1182.
106. Davidovitch Z, Nicolay OF, Ngan PW, Shanfeld JL. Neurotransmitters, cytokines and the control of alveolar bone remodelling in orthodontics. *Dent Clin North Am* 1988; **32**: 411–435.
107. Sandy JR, Meghji S, Scutt AM, Harvey W, Harris M, Meikle MC. Murine osteoblasts release bone-resorbing factors of high and low molecular weights: stimulation by mechanical deformation. *Bone Miner* 1989; **5**: 155–168.
108. Nair SP, Meghji S, Henderson B. Osteolytic factors released by rat osteoblast-like cells in response to mechanical deformation. *Bone* 1994; **15**: 133.
109. Meikle MC, Reynolds JJ, Sellers A, Dingle JT. Rabbit cranial sutures *in vitro*: a new experimental model for studying the response of fibrous joints to mechanical stress. *Calcif Tissue Int* 1979; **28**: 137–144.
110. Hickory WB, Nanda R. Effect of tensile force magnitude on release of cranial suture cells into S phase. *Am J Dentofac Orthop Orthodont* 1987; **91**: 328–334.
111. Meikle MC, Heath JK, Hembry RM, Reynolds JJ. Rabbit cranial suture fibroblasts under tension express a different collagen phenotype. *Arch Oral Biol* 1982; **27**: 609–613.
112. Duncan GW, Yen EHK, Pritchard ET, Suga DM. Collagen and prostaglandin synthesis in force-stressed periodontal ligament *in vitro*. *J Dent Res* 1984; **63**: 665–669.
113. Meikle MC, Sellers A, Reynolds JJ. Effect of tensile mechanical stress on the synthesis of metalloproteinases by rabbit coronal sutures *in vitro*. *Calcif Tissue Int* 1980; **30**: 77–82.

9

Muscle function and the control of facial form

Nigel Hunt

Introduction

The genetic basis of facial form is covered in Chapter 1, but for many years, scientific opinion has varied as to the relative contribution of genetic and environmental factors in the control of facial form and craniofacial development. Sicher,[1] for example, was of the opinion that growth of the craniofacial region was almost totally under genetic control. This view was supported to a large extent by Scott,[2] although he recognized that growth at the cranial sutures was secondary to the expansion of the developing brain. However, with regard to the maxilla and mandible, Scott considered the inherent growth of the cartilagenous nasal septum and condylar cartilage as the primary factors which pushed the bones away from the cranial base. It is now recognized that the condylar cartilage has a limited influence on total mandibular growth and probably contributes no more than 20% of the ascending ramus height and very little to the growth of the mandibular body.[3] Therefore, unilateral enlargement of the mandible is no longer considered to be the sole result of condylar cartilage overgrowth. Of the two recognizable presentations, in hemimandibular elongation (Fig. 9.1), where the affected side deviates across the midline to give a contralateral cross-bite, the asymmetry may originate in the condyle. By comparison, in cases of hemimandibular hyperplasia, not only are the condyle and ascending ramus enlarged but there is also downward bowing of the body of the mandible, suggesting that there is intrinsic overgrowth throughout the mandible to the midline. Figure 9.2 shows such a case. Note that the excess growth is in the vertical plane and there is no deviation of the lower dental midline or the chin point. These disorders appear to be genetically determined and may occur individually or even together on complementary sides of the mandible.[4]

Such examples are uncommon and ignore the importance of the neuromuscular influence on skeletal growth. This concept was probably first noted by Wolff who related bone density and skeletal structure to function.[5] Subsequently, Moss[6]. proposed that growth of the craniofacial complex was due to the effect of function on its components, each component being termed a functional matrix. Functional matrices are defined as not only the tissues and their structures but also the craniofacial cavities that serve to perform functions, for example respiration, speech or sight. Therefore, once bone formation has been initiated, subsequent craniofacial growth is dependent on localized functional activity that is in turn directed by both genomic and non-genetic information. This is probably exemplified in children with ankylosis of the temporomandibular joints where the loss of function gives rise to reduced growth of the body of the ipsilateral mandible (Fig. 9.3), or the early loss of an eye in infancy will give rise to a small orbit and facial asymmetry.

Therefore, most now agree that the ultimate size and shape of the human face arise through the effects of a predetermined genetic blueprint, the so-called homeobox or H*ox*

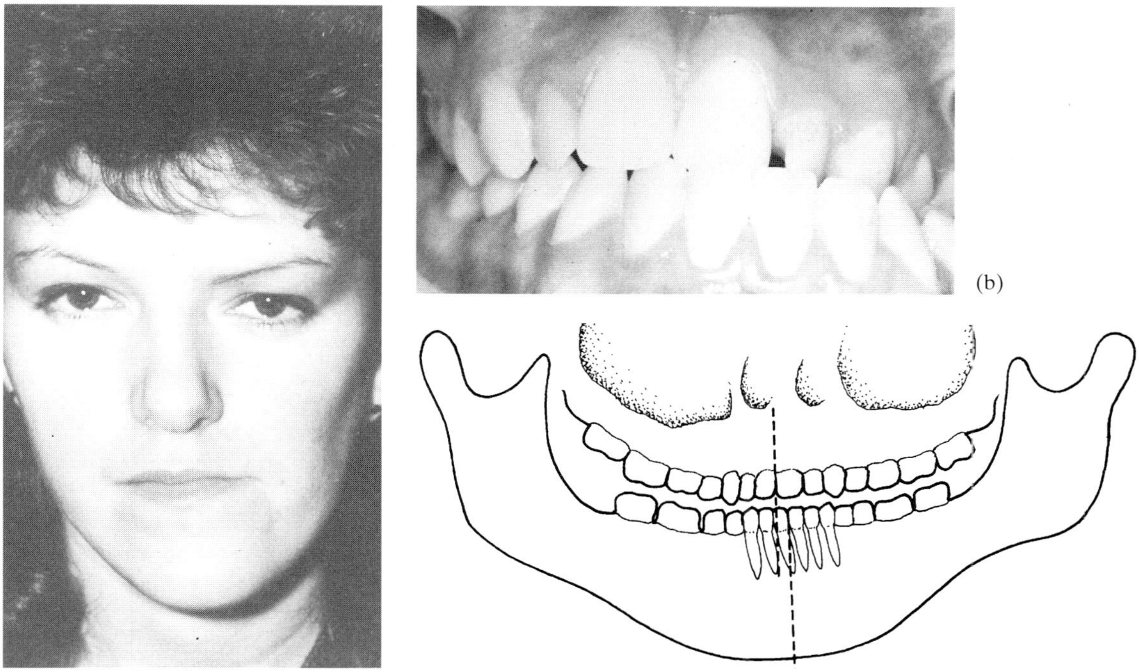

(a) (b) (c)

Fig. 9.1 Right-sided hemimandibular elongation showing (a) deviation of the chin point and (b) the dental midline to the contralateral side, with a marked cross-bite. (c) The affected ascending ramus is longer than the left side.

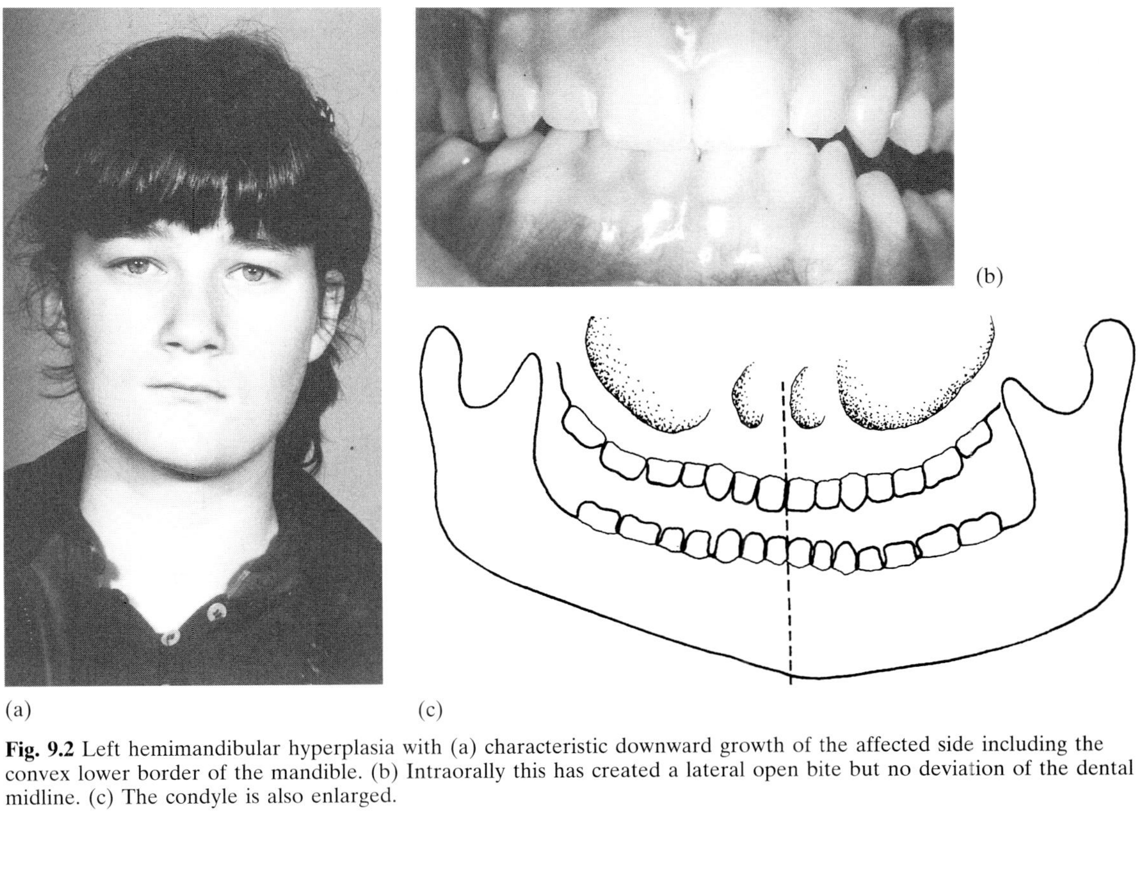

(a) (b) (c)

Fig. 9.2 Left hemimandibular hyperplasia with (a) characteristic downward growth of the affected side including the convex lower border of the mandible. (b) Intraorally this has created a lateral open bite but no deviation of the dental midline. (c) The condyle is also enlarged.

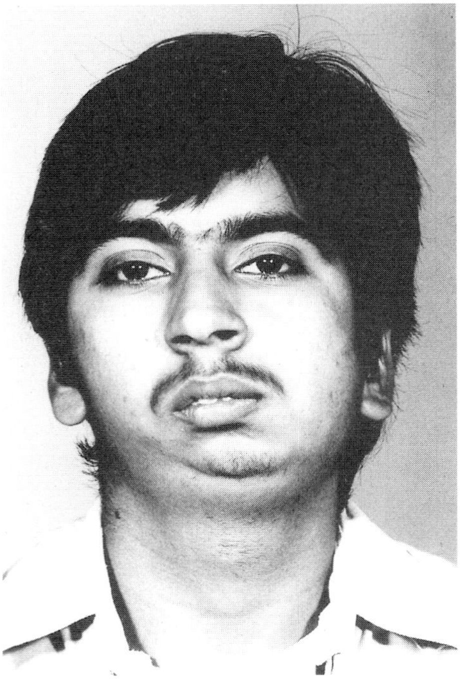

(a)

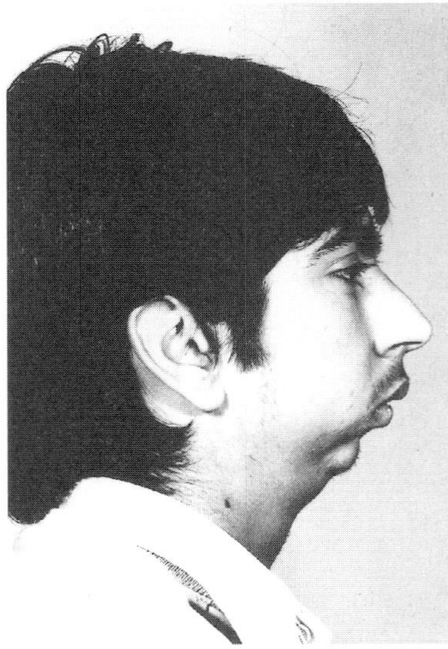

(b)

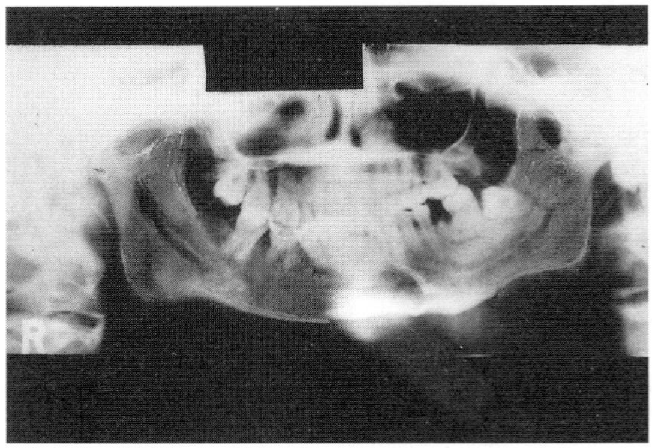

(c)

Fig. 9.3 Ankylosis of the left temporomandibular joint with asymmetrical growth of the mandible. The ankylosed side shows limited growth due to loss of the condylar growth cartilage and limitation of function. Contralateral growth of the condyle and body continues within the limits of restricted function, creating relative elongation and deviation to the ankylosed side.

genes, which will create the family resemblance but which may be modified by environmental influences. Some of these environmental influences may themselves be genetically controlled (epigenetic factors). Examples of environmental factors which influence facial growth may include nasopharyngeal function, in particular the mode of respiration[7] such as mouth or nose breathing, and head posture. Congenital nasal obstruction such as choanal atresia, or acquired due to turbinate enlargement, gives rise to the characteristic adenoidal facies consisting of a narrow upper dental arch, an obtuse gonial angle with increased lower facial height and a short posterior facial height.

With head posture, the degree of extension of the head on the cervical spine may be related to abnormal variations in facial morphological features.[8] The most obvious is a reduced middle and lower facial height due to persistent flexion of the cervical spine. More recently, attention has focused on the possible environmental role of the muscles of mastication which, through their origins and insertions, may directly influence the ultimate form and relationships of the mandible and maxilla, especially in the vertical dimension.

The effect of muscle function on bone growth

The effect of altered muscle function and impaired mechanical forces on skeletal growth in general is well-appreciated. Reduced muscle activity, for example, following poliomyelitis, is associated with a marked reduction in bone growth in the affected limb of a growing child.

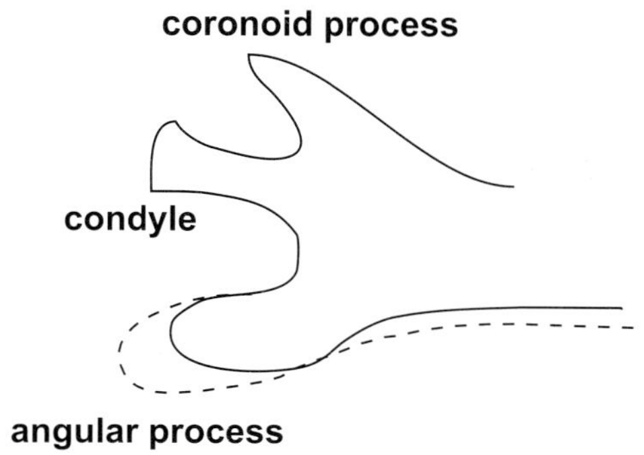

Fig. 9.4 The effect of surgically repositioning the masseter muscle at a reduced length in dogs. Note the underdevelopment of the angular process, the reduced condyle to angular process distance and the absence of the sigmoid notch following surgery (solid outline) compared to normal growth (dashed outline).

Similarly, muscle wasting following splint immobilization is associated with a diminished rate of bone growth in an arm or leg.

With regard to facial development, the relationship between muscle function and both the size and shape of the jaws has been studied extensively in animal models. Measurable changes in skeletal morphology have been observed following a variety of procedures including alteration in the physical consistency of the diet. Animals fed a soft diet demonstrated a reduced rate of appositional growth at the mandibular angle compared to those fed a normal hard diet.[9] Surgical intervention, for example, detachment of the origin of the temporalis muscle or removal of all or part of the muscle, resulted in a shortened or absent coronoid process.[10] Similarly, removal or surgical repositioning of the masseter muscle at a reduced length results in a smaller gonial angle[11,12] (Fig. 9.4).

The clinical case studies of patients with pathological muscular disorders[13–15] indicate how progressive weakness of the mandibular elevator muscles can lead to a downward and backward rotation of the mandible away from the maxilla with a resultant long face deformity and anterior open bite (Fig. 9.5). Muscular dystrophy may be associated with degenerative or inflammatory muscle damage, nerve malfunction or connective tissue changes, and so both disturbed muscular contractile and connective tissue factors may influence facial morphogenesis.

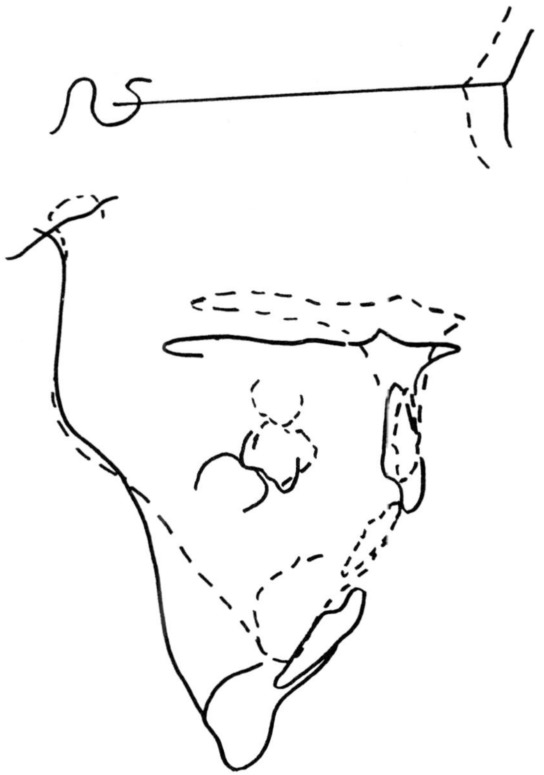

Fig. 9.5 Cephalometric tracings of the facial changes seen in progressive muscular dystrophy. Note the downward and backward growth rotation of the mandible between 4 years (dashed outline) and 8 years (solid outline).

Evidence of a correlation between muscle function and facial morphology comes from a series of experiments using electromyographic (EMG) and gnathodynamic techniques. These investigations show that in adults a significant correlation exists between a large bite force and/or high EMG activity when swallowing, biting or chewing and the facial features of a large mandible and a reduced gonial angle. Furthermore, these individuals have a rectangular-shaped profile characterized by a large posterior face height, a small anterior face height and a tendency towards a short face. Conversely, individuals with high maxillary–mandibular plane angles, a long face and skeletal open bite have markedly reduced EMG activity in the mandibular elevator muscles and a reduced or weak bite force (Fig. 9.6). Whether this variation in bite force is a cause or an effect of the skeletal morphology remains unclear.

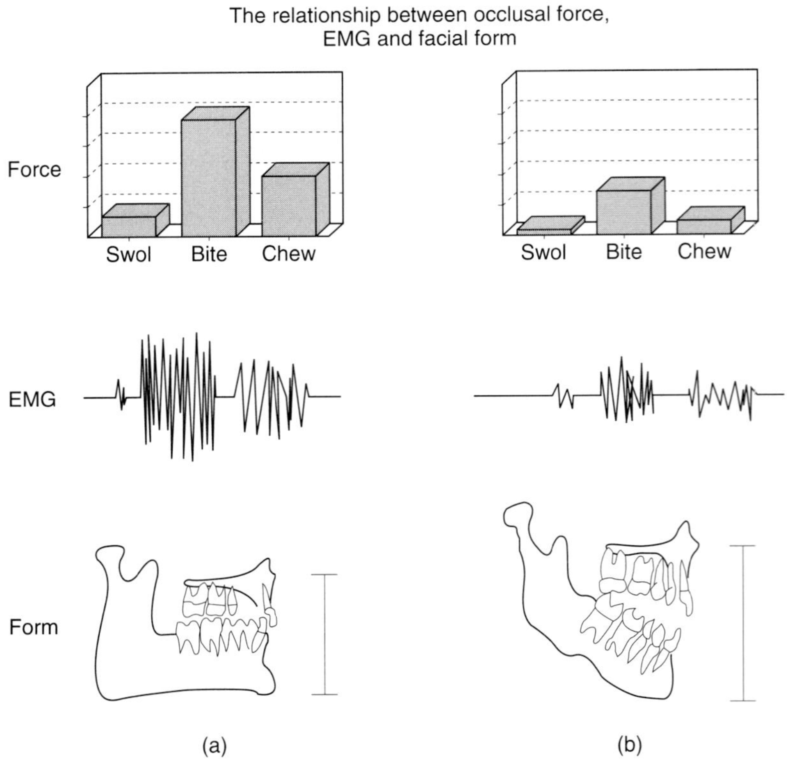

Fig. 9.6 The relationship between facial form, electromyogram (EMG) activity of the masticatory muscles and maximum occlusal force. (a) Reduced gonial angle and anterior face height are associated with large occlusal forces; conversely, (b) reduced bite forces relate to an obtuse gonial angle, an increased face height and an anterior open bite.

The hypothesis that masticatory muscle strength partly determines facial form is supported by a study where children with developing features of long face deformity were given daily chewing exercises, with the result that there was a significant increase in maximum bite force and the corresponding muscle activity after 1 year.[16] Morphologically, the majority of these children exhibited an upward and forward growth rotation of the mandible over the review period. It was concluded that exercises aimed at strengthening the muscles of mastication could have a beneficial influence on controlling the long face pattern of development. Whether or not this constitutes a permanent change has yet to be established.

Whilst it is appreciated that variations in muscle structure and function can be related to variations in craniofacial morphology, it is at present impossible to determine in some cases whether the abnormalities in muscle structure and function affect facial form, or whether the abnormalities of form have led to variation in muscle structure and function. The question as to which abnormality came first remains controversial. Support for the hypothesis that variations in muscle strength are an effect rather than a cause of the variation in morphology has arisen through investigations of occlusal force during swallowing, chewing and maximal biting in both long-face and normal children and adults. A comparison of the occlusal force in abnormal and normal children prior to the pubertal growth spurt has shown that there was no statistical difference between the two groups.[17] However, a similar comparison in normal and long-face adults demonstrated significantly reduced force levels in the long-face group which were equivalent to those seen in children[18] (Fig. 9.7). It would appear, therefore, that those children with a developing long face failed to increase their

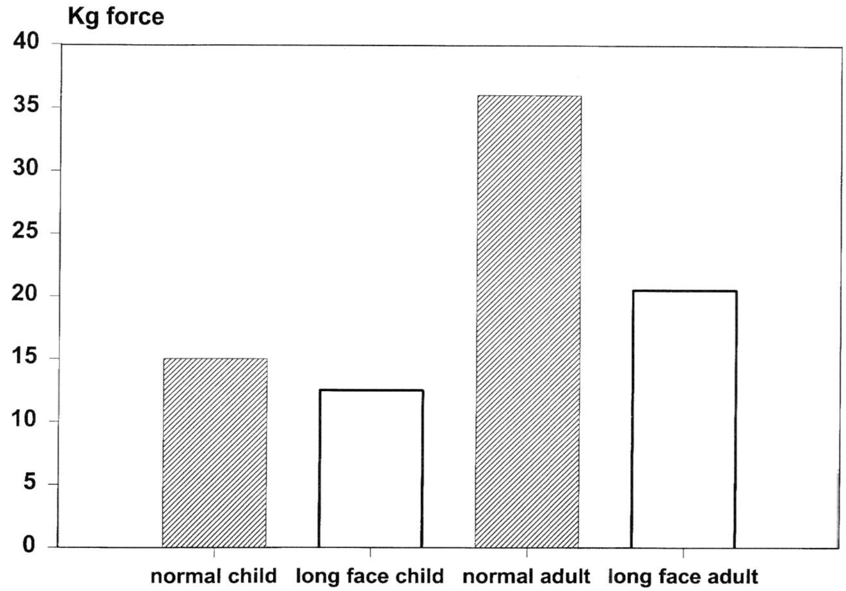

Fig. 9.7 The maximum occlusal force recorded in normal and long-face children and adults.

muscle strength during the adolescent period. This suggests that the clinically identifiable abnormal growth pattern precedes the occlusal force disturbance, and therefore the reduced bite force seen in the adult group is more likely to be the result of rather than a direct cause of the facial abnormality.

A further explanation of the variation in bite force levels observed in individuals with abnormal morphology has been based upon the geometric arrangement of the muscles as part of the jaw lever system.[19] If one assumed that the contractile force of the temporalis (*T*: newtons) and the masseter (*M*: newtons) muscles were constant for all facial morphologies, which is improbable, the total elevator force is proportional to the length of their moment arms, i.e. the perpendicular distances of the line of muscle action from the condyle. The bite force (BF) they exert together is also proportional to the moment arm of the biting teeth. This is represented by the following equation:

$$(T \times \text{ma.t}) + (M \times ma.m) = (\text{BF} \times ma.i)$$

Therefore:

$$\text{BF} = \frac{(T \times ma.t) + (M \times ma.m)}{ma.i}$$

where *ma* is the moment arm of the muscles (*ma.m* and *ma.t*) or incisor (*ma.i*) teeth.

As can be seen from Figure 9.8, where the temporalis and masseter muscle moment arms are short and the bite force moment arm is long, the ratio produces a significantly smaller bite force than with the short-face moment arms. This probably applies more appropriately when considering the greater bite force of the molars with a shorter moment arm.

The greater bite force reported for patients with features of the short-face syndrome, which is characterized by reduced maxillary height and gonial angle, may be partly due to the greater mechanical advantage of the temporalis and masseter muscles. However, it must be stressed that two-dimensional models and single lines of action of muscle vectors do not necessarily correspond to those of complex muscles which exhibit differential fibre activity and differences in muscle bulk.

The maximal isometric strength of a muscle is usually proportional to the total cross-sectional area of its fibres[20] and so it would be reasonable to expect the cross-sectional dimensions of the masticatory muscles to correlate with skeletal morphological features. Modern imaging techniques, including computed tomography (CT), ultrasonography

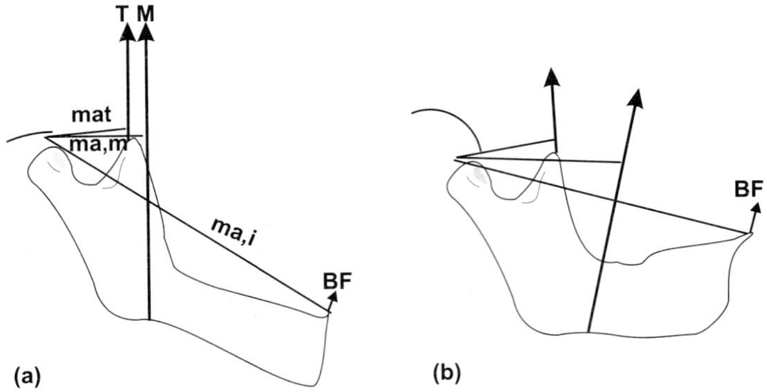

Fig. 9.8 The mechanical advantage of the long face (a) is less than the short face (b) as the temporalis (T) and masseter (M) muscle moment arms (ma,t and ma,m) are short and the incisor moment arm (ma,i) is long compared to the short face. The formula for bite force (BF) in the text confirms this.

and magnetic resonance imaging (MRI) scans enable clinicians accurately to assess the three-dimensional structure and dimensions of muscles. The results of such studies have shown relationships between the width, length, depth, cross-sectional area and muscle volume and the shape of the mandible and the mandibular/maxillary structural relationship. Using CT, it has been shown that large masseter and medial pterygoid cross-sectional areas are associated with brachycephalic (short) skulls, with a long mandible having a small gonial angle. Also large masseter and temporalis cross-sectional areas correlated with increased facial width.[21] Furthermore, CT muscle volume assessment has demonstrated an inverse correlation between masseter and medial pterygoid volumes and the size of the mandibular plane and gonial angles. Similarly, there was a positive correlation of muscle volume with other cephalometric variables, for example, posterior face height.[22] More recently, ultrasound studies have also demonstrated relationships between both the thickness of masseter muscle[23] and its volume,[24] with vertical cephalometric measures of facial form.

Muscle structure in relation to form

The recognition that muscle function may play a role in craniofacial morphogenesis has led to research into the histochemical properties of the contractile components of the muscles of mastication in both laboratory animals and human subjects. Skeletal muscles are composed of fibres which are long multinucleated cells specialized to generate force and movement. The muscle fibres are arranged in bundles or fasiculi surrounded by a loose collagenous connective tissue sheath termed the perimysium (Fig. 9.9), and each muscle fibre is encased in a delicate connective tissue envelope, composed mainly of reticulin fibres, termed the endomysium. The nuclei of muscle fibres are flattened and lie peripherally in the zone within the cell membrane or sarcolemma. The cytoplasm of each fibre (the sarcoplasm) is striated due to the parallel arrangement of contractile proteins into cylindrical structures termed myofibrils. The myofibrils are, in turn, composed of numerous myofilaments of the contractile proteins actin, myosin, troponin and tropomyosin B, only visible under the electron microscope. Two distinct types of myofilament can be identified: thick myofilaments consisting of the fibrous protein myosin and the thin myofilaments composed of the globular proteins actin and troponin.

The actin filaments consist of two chains of globular units in the form of a long double helix with the smaller troponin molecules

Fig. 9.9 Structural levels within a skeletal muscle. The enzyme adenosine triphosphatase is located in the heads of the myosin myofilaments.

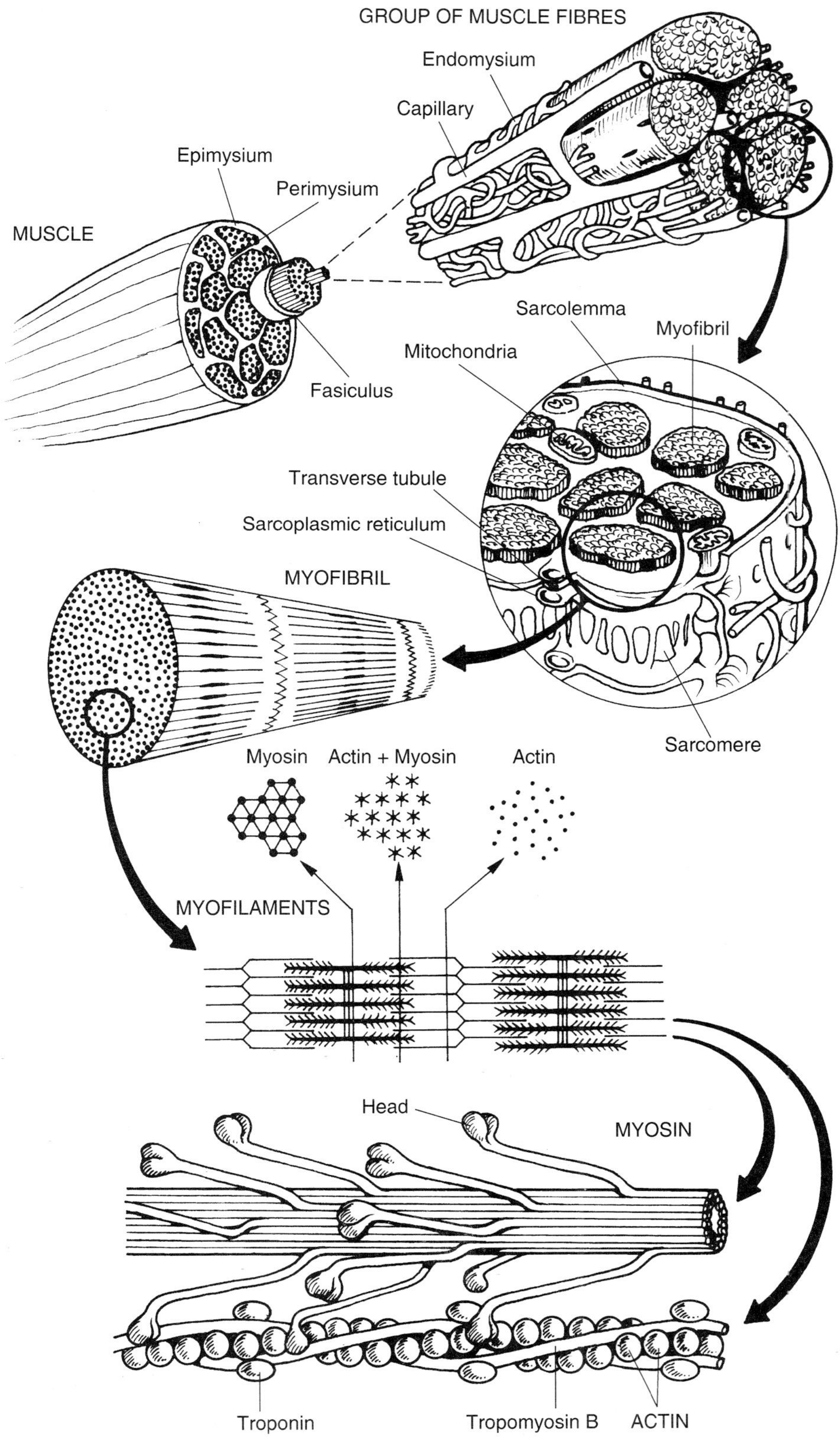
GROUP OF MUSCLE FIBRES
Endomysium
Capillary
Epimysium
Perimysium
MUSCLE
Fasiculus
Sarcolemma
Myofibril
Mitochondria
Transverse tubule
Sarcoplasmic reticulum
MYOFIBRIL
Sarcomere
Myosin
Actin + Myosin
Actin
MYOFILAMENTS
Head
MYOSIN
Troponin
Tropomyosin B
ACTIN

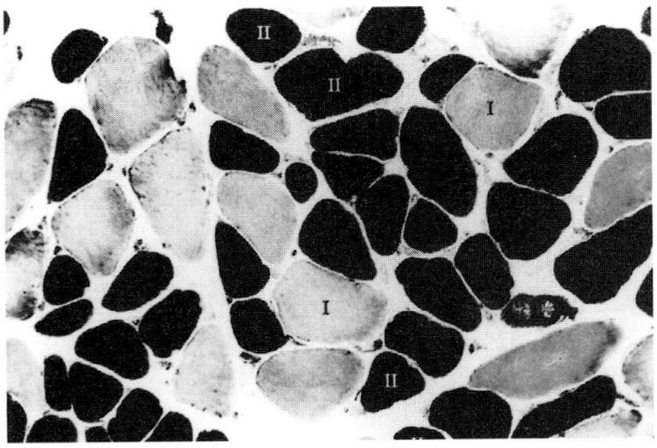

Fig. 9.10 Adenosine triphosphatase staining of human masseter muscle fibres. Note that under alkaline conditions, the slow-acting type I fibres are pale-staining, whereas the fast-type II fibres are darkly staining.

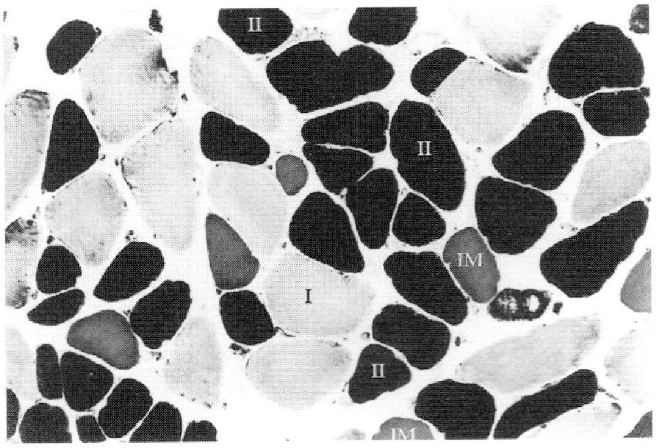

Fig. 9.11 Adenosine triphosphatase staining of human masseter muscle fibres at pH 9.4. Note the pale-staining type I fibres, the darkly staining type II fibres and fibres with an intermediate intensity (type IM).

attached at intervals along its length by means of tropomyosin B molecules present in the groove between the two actin chains. In transverse section, each myosin filament is surrounded by six actin filaments in a regular hexagonal pattern. Each myosin molecule consists of two heavy-molecular-weight and four light-molecular-weight polypeptide chains. The two myosin heavy chains (MHCs) intertwine to form a double-alpha helix termed the rod. At the end of the rod the MHCs split and form two globular heads containing adenosine triphosphatase (mATPase). Contraction of muscle fibres occurs through the interaction of the heads of the myosin filament, with the actin–troponin myofilament complex activated by the mATPase. Although the precise role of the myosin light chains is not known, light-chain–heavy-chain interactions are considered to play an important part in the conversion of chemical energy into movement.[25]

The intensity of the staining reaction for mATPase and its stability at varying pH have formed the basis for the histochemical classification of muscle fibre types (Fig. 9.10). When combined with other histochemical stains, for example succinate dehydrogenase activity to identify oxidative potential and fatigue, the human mandibular elevator muscles have been noted to possess several fibre types which are broadly divided into either slow or fast fibres with subgroups of each type. Slow-twitch or type I fibres have a low (weak-staining) intensity for myofibrillar ATPase under alkaline conditions. These fibres have a high oxidative capacity and, whilst only capable of producing low force levels, are resistant to fatigue. The fast-twitch or type II fibres are generally divided into two subtypes: type IIA and IIB fibres. Whilst the IIB fibres have properties which are in direct contrast to type I fibres, i.e. a low oxidative capacity, a high force capability and a rapid fatigue rate, type IIA fibres possess intermediate features with a fast contraction rate but a slow rate of fatigue.

On the basis of these metabolic profiles, type I fibres are primarily responsible for the maintenance of posture or slow repetitive movements, type IIA fibres for fast repetitive movements and type IIB fibres for explosive movement or for the development of maximum tension over a limited period of time. The presence of these fibre types in masticatory muscles is similar to other skeletal muscles. However, unlike other skeletal muscles, two other fibres with unusual ATPase activity have been noted in healthy human masticatory muscle. These have been designated the IIC and intermediate (IM) fibres,[26,27] which are distinct from the type I and II fibres in that they provide a variable staining intensity under alkaline conditions (Fig. 9.11). The precise role of these fibres is uncertain, although they are often associated with damaged muscle which is undergoing repair and it has been suggested that they may represent regenerating, immature muscle fibres or precursors of other muscle fibre types.

Immunocytochemistry, using antibodies raised against the MHC, as well as electrophoretic techniques have improved our understanding of these myosin types

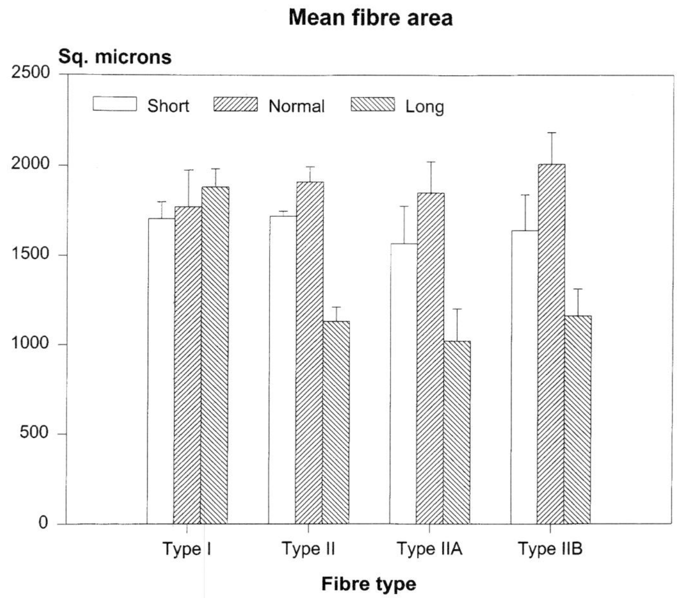

(a)

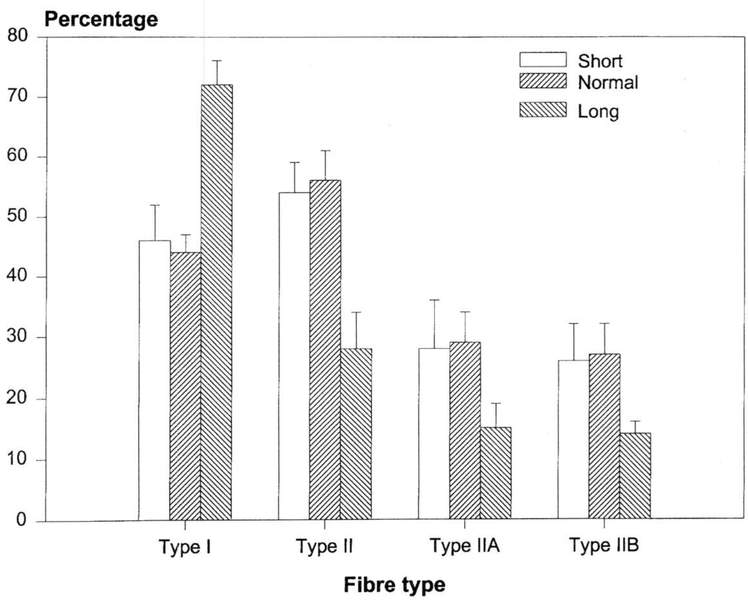

(b)

Fig. 9.12 Variation in muscle fibre structural characteristics for different facial groups. (a) Long-face patients appear to have a significant reduction in type IIA and IIB mean fibre areas. (b) There is a significant increase in total cross-sectional area of type I fibres in the long-face group but a reduction in all other types.

(isoforms).[28,29] In addition to confirming the presence of predominantly slow and fast myosins in the type I and II fibres respectively, it has been confirmed that the type IIC and IM fibres contain a neonatal MHC which is characteristic of developing muscle and never found in normal adult limb muscle. The presence of this isoform may provide the means by which the masseter muscle can adapt to its varying functional demands.[30] Most studies undertaken to correlate muscle fibre type to craniofacial morphology are based upon muscle biopsy samples from patients with vertical dysplasias undergoing surgery. Unfortunately, these studies have been based upon small sample numbers and present contradictory results.[31–33] Recently, the muscle fibre characteristics of long, short and normal vertical facial proportion groups have been compared[34] (Fig. 9.12). Having established that

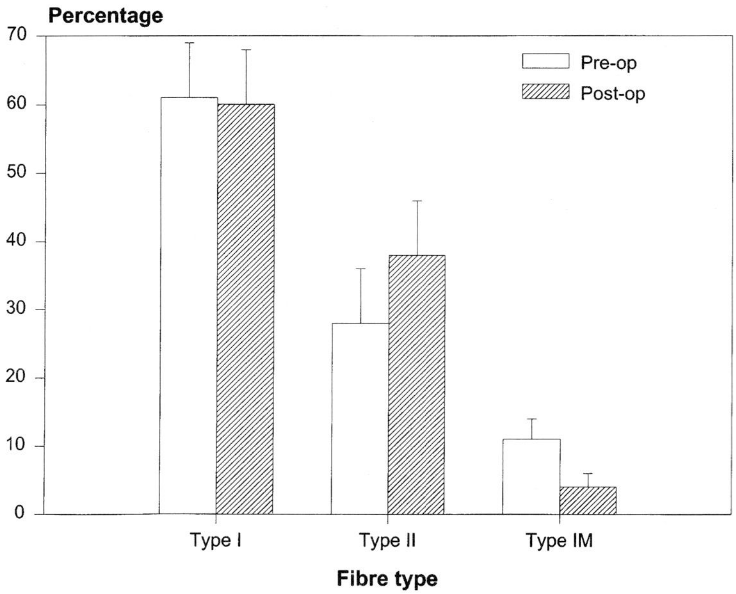

Fig. 9.13 Changes in fibre profile in response to orthognathic surgery. The principal changes are an increase in the contribution of type II fibres coupled with a reduction in intermediate fibres.

a single muscle biopsy could be considered as representative of the muscle architecture providing anatomical location was standardized, it was noted that the relative size of the type I fibres was comparable between the facial groups. However, both the size and the proportion of the type II fibres in the long-face subjects were significantly reduced compared to the other groups. This reduction in type II fibres correlated well with the reduced occlusal bite force seen within this group.

As mentioned previously, type II fibres are capable of fast action but are easily fatigued, whereas type I fibres are responsible for more sustained activity. If muscle composition and activity influence facial form to a significant extent, it is more likely to be effected through the type I fibres rather than the less frequently recruited type II fibres. As there was no significant difference between the abnormal and control groups with regard to type I fibre size, the fibre cross-sectional area of type I fibres may not be important in influencing vertical skeletal relationships. However the *relative* contribution of the type I and II fibres to the total percentage cross-sectional area of muscle fibres or the ratio of the fibres to the quantity of extracellular matrix may be worthy of further consideration.

Muscle and bone homeostasis

The obvious cause-and-effect relationship between muscle structure and function and skeletal morphology must be in physiological balance prior to orthodontic or surgical treatment. Any procedure which interferes with this relationship, for example orthognathic surgery, will upset that balance. If relapse is not to occur, then adaptation must take place. The possible mechanisms by which adaptation can occur in the musculoskeletal system have been excellently reviewed by McNamara *et al.*[35] These include adaptation within the central nervous system, within the muscle fibres, at the muscle–tendon or muscle–bone interface and within the bone itself.

A change in muscle structure and function following orthognathic surgery has been clearly demonstrated. For example, correction of the long-face deformity results in a gradual increase in bite force to more normal levels. This change is seen in conjunction with an alteration in the muscle fibre profile to that of a more normal picture, as seen in individuals with balanced facial features (Fig. 9.13).[36] Typically, in the case of long-face patients, this involves an increase in the contribution of the type II fibres to the overall fibre cross-sectional area, and a reduction in the prevalence of intermediate fibres. The precise mechanism by which this change in fibre type occurs is unclear, although it is interesting to note that those patients who exhibit a relatively large proportion of intermediate fibres prior to surgery appear to adapt well to the new environment following operation. On the other hand, those patients who demonstrate a relatively low prevalence of intermediate fibres appear to have a greater likelihood of surgical relapse.[37]

Further work is required to clarify this issue, but if the concept is valid then a whole range of therapeutic opportunities are feasible. Human masseter muscle can be grown in tissue culture from explants and tissue disaggregations and modification of the relative prevalence of myosin isoforms can be achieved by the addition of growth factors and hormones, especially 3,5,3-triiodothyronine. The possibility of permanently altering the myosin expression of cloned myogenic stem cells (satellite cells) by the manipulation of the culture conditions or gene transfection is being investigated. The unique ability of satellite cells to fuse with existing fibres means that if this work is successful then cell transplantation techniques may alter masticatory muscle structure, and therefore function, as has been proposed for the management of Duchenne muscular dystrophy.[38,39] Duchenne muscular dystrophy results from the failure to express the cytoskeletal protein dystrophin. Cell therapy, therefore, aims to replace dystrophin by seeding muscle with autologous satellite cells which have been engineered *in vitro* to express the protein.

The response of muscle to increased length

During growth, the increase in length of a bone is associated with an increase in length of the muscles, mainly through the addition of sarcomeres at the ends of existing myofibrils. Little is known about the factors involved in the control of sarcomere number; however, it is appreciated that the adjustment of both sarcomere number and muscle length can occur rapidly. An illustration of this can be seen by the rapid attainment of the correct number of sarcomeres following the release of plaster cast immobilization of a limb.[40]

The ability of mature muscles to adapt to a change in functional length has also been demonstrated. These experiments have usually involved the fixation of limbs either in a flexed or extended position, both with and without denervation. The adjustment of sarcomere number to the functional length does not seem to be dependent upon direct neural control, but rather a myogenic response to the amount of passive tension to which the muscle becomes subjected.[41] This mechanism of the addition or removal of sarcomeres in order for a muscle to adapt to a change in functional length maintains maximal functional overlap of the myosin cross-bridges and the actin filaments.[42]

One example of a clinical situation where muscles need to adapt to an increased functioning length is that arising through surgery to increase the length of a limb. The concept of bone lengthening was first described by Codivilla in 1905, when an increase in femur length was achieved through repeated distraction of the callus formed following an oblique osteotomy.[43] The technique of stretching a callus was further popularized by Ilizarov *et al.* who described the transosseous osteosynthesis technique following corticotomy in tubular bones.[44] Whilst the histological changes associated with the increase in bone length at differing rates of distraction have been reported on numerous occasions, the response of muscle to leg lengthening has received relatively little attention. Recently, it has been shown in rabbits that although new contractile tissue forms during lengthening, damage to muscle through the proliferation of fibrous tissue between the muscle fibres can be seen at distraction rates of greater than 1 mm per day. Overall, it has been shown that muscle responds only favourably at rates of distraction slower than those known to lead to the most prolific bone formation.[45]

The adaptation of bone distraction techniques for the correction of both developmental and traumatic abnormalities of the face and jaws has been reported.[46] Whilst the majority of studies have been undertaken in animals, the technique has now been applied to mandibular lengthening in children.[47,48] However, before clinicians can be confident of the long-term stability of this application of the technique, as well as others such as the possibility of inferior positioning of the maxilla, further clarification of the adaptive response of the muscles and the other soft-tissue investments is required.

References

1. Sicher H. *Oral Anatomy*. St Louis: CV Mosby, 1952.
2. Scott JH. The growth of the craniofacial skeleton. *Int J Med Sci* 1962; **438**: 276–286.
3. Sprinz R. Surgery on the condyle and its effect on the growing mandible in rats. *J Dent Res* 1976; **55**: 112.
4. Obwegeser HL, Makek MS. Hemimandibular hyperplasia – hemimandibular elongation. *J Max-fac Surg* 1986; **14**: 183–208.
5. Wolff J. *Das Gesetz der Transformation der Knochen*. Berlin: Hirschwald, 1892.
6. Moss ML. The functional matrix. In: Kraus BL, Riedel RA (eds) *Vistas in Orthodontics*. Philadelphia: Lea & Febiger, 1962.
7. Linder-Aronson S. Respiratory function in relation to facial morphology and the dentition. *Br J Orthod* 1979; **6**: 59–71.
8. Solow B, Kreiborg S. Soft-tissue stretching: a possible control factor in craniofacial morphogenesis. *Scand J Dent Res* 1977; **85**: 505–507.
9. Kiliaridis S. Masticatory muscle function and craniofacial morphology – An experimental study in the growing rat fed a soft diet. *Swed Dent J* 1986; suppl 36.
10. Boyd TG, Castelli WA, Huelka DF. Removal of the temporalis muscle from its origin: effects on the size and shape of the coronoid process. *J Dent Res* 1967; **46**: 997–1001.
11. Horowitz SL, Shapiro HH. Modification of skull and jaw architecture following removal of the masseter muscle in the rat. *Am J Phys Anthropol* 1955; **13**: 301–308.
12. Nanda SK, Merow WW, Sassouni V. Repositioning of the masseter muscle and its effect on skeletal form and structure. *Angle Orthod* 1967; **37**: 304–308.
13. Proffit WR, Gamble JW, Christianssen RL. Generalized muscle weakness with severe anterior open bite. A case report. *Am J Orthod* 1968; **54**: 104–110.
14. Kreiborg S, Jensen BL, Møller E, Björk A. Craniofacial growth in a case of congenital muscular dystrophy. *Am J Orthod* 1978; **74**: 207–215.
15. Kiliaridis S, Mejersjö C, Thilander B. Muscle function and craniofacial morphology: a clinical study in patients with myotonic dystrophy. *Eur J Orthod* 1989; **11**: 131–138.
16. Ingervall B, Bitsanis E. A pilot study of the effect of masticatory muscle training on facial growth in long-face children. *Eur J Orthod* 1987; **9**: 15–23.
17. Proffit WR, Fields HW, Nixon WL. Occlusal forces in normal and long face adults. *J Dent Res* 1983; **62**: 566–571.
18. Proffit WR, Fields HW. Occlusal forces in normal and long face children. *J Dent Res* 1983; **62**: 571–574.
19. Throckmorton GS, Finn R, Bell WH. Biomechanics of differences in lower facial height. *Am J Orthod* 1980; **77**: 410–420.
20. Weijs WA, Hillen B. The relationship between the physiological cross-section of the human jaw muscles and their cross-sectional area in computer tomograms. *Acta Anat* 1984; **118**: 129–138.
21. Weijs WA, Hillen B. Correlation between the cross-sectional area of jaw muscles and craniofacial size and shape. *Am J Phys Anthrop* 1986; **70**: 423–431.
22. Gionhaku N, Lowe AA. Relationship between jaw muscle volume and craniofacial form. *J Dent Res* 1989; **68**: 805–809.
23. Bakke M, Tuxen A, Vilmann P, Jensen BR, Vilmann A, Toft M. Ultrasound image of human masseter muscle related to bite force, electromyography, facial morphology and occlusal factors. *Scand J Dent Res* 1992; **100**: 165–171.
24. Benington PCM, Hunt NP. Masseter muscle volume and facial form. *J Dent Res* 1994; **73**: 795.
25. Lowey S, Waller GS, Trybus KM. Skeletal muscle myosin light chains are essential for physiological speeds of shortening. *Nature* 1993; **365**: 454–456.
26. Ringqvist M. Histochemical enzyme profiles of fibres in human masseter muscles with special regard to fibres with intermediate myofibrillar ATPase reaction. *J Neurol Sci* 1973; **18**: 133–141.
27. Eriksson P-O. Muscle fibre composition of the human mandibular locomotor system. *Swed Dent J* 1982; **12** (suppl): 1–44.
28. Billiter R, Weber H, Lutz H, Howald H, Eppenberger HM, Jenny E. Myosin types in human skeletal muscle fibres. *Histochemistry* 1980; **65**: 249–259.
29. Sciote JJ, Rowlerson AM, Hopper C, Hunt NP. Fibre type classification and myosin isoforms in the human masseter muscle. *J Neurol Sci* 1994; **126**: 15–24.
30. Butler-Browne GS, Eriksson P-O, Laurent C, Thornell L-E. Adult human masseter muscle fibres express myosin isozymes characteristic of development. *Muscle Nerve* 1988; **11**: 610–120.
31. Finn RA, Gonyea WJ, Bell WH. Histochemical characteristics of masseter muscle in patients with vertical maxillary dysplasias. *J Dent Res* 1980; **59**: 458.
32. Boyd S, Gonyea WJ, Finn RA, Woodward CE, Bell WH. Histochemical study of the masseter muscle in patients with vertical maxillary excess. *J Oral Maxillofac Surg* 1984; **42**: 75–83.
33. Shaughnessy T, Fields H, Westbury J. Association between craniofacial morphology and fibre-type distributions in human masseter and medial pterygoid muscles. *Int J Adult Orthod Orthog Surg* 1989; **4**: 145–155.
34. Hunt NP. A comparison of the masseter muscle fibre profile in subjects with normal and diverse vertical facial morphology. Submitted for publication to *Br J Orthod* 1997 (in press).

35. McNamara JA, Carlson DS, Yellich GM, Hendricksen RP. Musculo-skeletal adaptation following orthognathic surgery. In: Carlson DS, McNamara JA (eds) *Muscle Adaptation in the Cranio-facial Region*. Michigan: University of Michigan, Ann Arbor, 1978.
36. Hunt NP. The effect of orthognathic surgery on the fibre profile of masseter muscle. Submitted for publication to *Br J Orthod* 1997 (in press).
37. Hunt NP. Musculo-skeletal adaptation to disturbances of the cranio-facial complex. *PhD* thesis. 1992, University of London.
38. Watt DJ, Lambert K, Morgan JE, Partridge TA, Sloper JC. Incorporation of donor muscle precursor cells into an area of muscle regeration in the host mouse. *J Neurol Sci* 1982; **57**: 319 –331.
39. Partridge TA. Myoblast transfer: a possible therapy for inherited myopathies? *Muscle Nerve* 1991; **14**: 197–212.
40. Williams PE, Goldspink G. Longitudinal growth of striated muscle fibres. *J Cell Sci* 1971; **9**: 751–767.
41. Goldspink G, Tabary C, Tabary JC, Tardieu C, Tardieu G. Effect of denervation on sarcomere number and muscle extensibility to the functional length of the muscle. *J Physiol (Lond)* 1974; **236**: 733–742.
42. Goldspink G. The adaptation of muscle to a new functional length. In: Anderson DJ, Matthews B (eds) *Mastication*, pp. 90–99. Bristol: J. Wright, 1976.
43. Codivilla A. On the means of lengthening in the lower limbs, muscles and tissues which are shortened through deformity. *Am J Orthopaed Surg* 1905; **2**: 353.
44. Ilizarov GA, Devyatov AA, Karnerim VK. Plastic reconstruction of longitudinal bone defects by means of compression and subsequent distraction. *Acta Chir Plast* 1980; **22**: 32–41.
45. Simpson AHRW, Williams PE, Kyberd P, Goldspink G, Kenright J. The response of muscle to leg lengthening. *J Bone Joint Surg* 1995; **77B**: 630–636.
46. Rachmiel A, Potparic Z, Jackson IT *et al.* Midface advancement by gradual distraction. *Br J Plast Surg* 1993; **46**: 201–207.
47. Michieli S, Miotti B. Lengthening of the mandibular body by gradual surgical-orthodontic distraction. *J Oral Surg* 1977; **35**: 187–192.
48. McCarthy JG, Schreiber J, Karp N, Thorne CH, Grayson BH. Lengthening the human mandible by gradual distraction. *Plast Reconst Surg* 1992; **89**: 1–10.

10

The structure and functions of the dentogingival junction and periodontal ligament

Douglas Luke

The dentogingival junction and periodontal ligament perform unique functions. The former makes a seal where a tooth punctures the integument; the latter, nominally a ligament, cushions the tooth during mastication while sheltering the cells which remodel the bony socket. A special feature of both tissues is the rapid turnover of their major components.

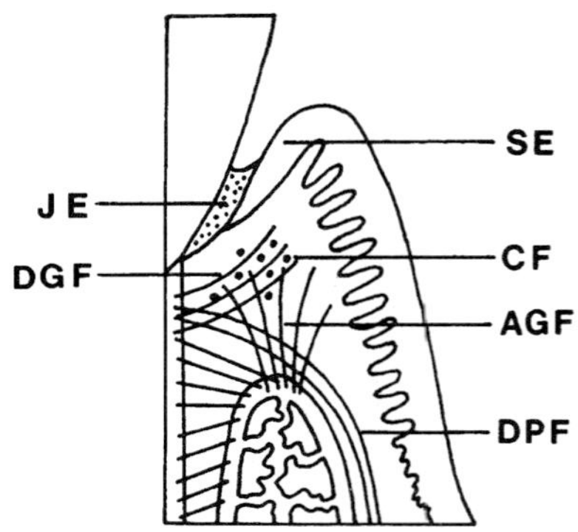

Fig. 10.1 Diagrammatic vertical section through gingiva and neck of tooth, showing junctional epithelium (JE), sulcular epithelium (SE), dentogingival fibres (DGF), circular fibres (CF), alveologingival fibres (AGF) and dentoperiosteal fibres (DPF). From Luke[10] with permission.

Dentogingival junction

The integrity of this potential site of weakness is maintained by local adaptations of both epithelium and connective tissue and it is protected by the contours of teeth, including marginal ridges, which deflect away food.

Junctional epithelium

A vertical section through the gingiva and neck of a tooth (Fig. 10.1) passes through three types of epithelium. The oral surface of the gingiva is typically keratinized and is continuous over the gingival crest with the lining of the gingival sulcus. In primates, sulcular epithelium does not usually form keratin, although it can be persuaded to do so, at least partially, if the sulcus is clean and sterile.[1]

Junctional epithelium (JE) is a unique type of oral epithelium: cells born in the basal layer remain immature as they migrate coronally, parallel to the tooth surface. The JE, therefore, does not exhibit the stratification typical of oral epithelia and the bulk of its cells are relatively undifferentiated. For example, their tonofilaments are sparse and consist of cytokeratins which resemble those of basal cells from other regions of oral mucosa. In health, JE lacks rete pegs and is quite thin, tapering at its apical extremity to a layer only a few cells in depth; intercellular desmosomal connections are few and the intercellular spaces are large.

Cells are surrounded by a coat or glycocalyx which consists of the projecting carbohydrate portions of glycoproteins and glycolipids, the major parts of which are embedded in the plasma membrane. The precise composition of the glycocalyx varies with cell type and the carbohydrates in the coat of JE cells are characteristic of basal rather than mature cells. Membrane-coating granules (MCGs), which are usually discharged from cells in the middle layers of oral epithelium, have not been definitely identified in the JE. The material in these granules, probably a lipid or glycolipid, augments the glycocalyx and is important in limiting the permeability via the intercellular route.

The above features explain why JE is very permeable, a fact confirmed by studies tracing the passage of large molecules, for example horseradish peroxidase, into and out of the sulcus. Through it flows gingival fluid which contains protective factors such as serum antibodies and polymorphs. The amount and composition of this fluid vary with the degree of inflammation in the subjacent tissue and it may be useful as an indicator of disease; for example, the content of sulphated glycosaminoglycan (GAG) seems to be related to the rate of alveolar bone destruction. Cells also migrate through the JE; indeed, in mild gingivitis more than half its volume may be contributed by polymorphs, monocytes and lymphocytes. One estimate suggests that 3000 neutrophils enter the mouth via this route every minute. Occasional Langerhans cells, the most peripheral component of the immune system, also occur in the JE.[2]

Although gingival fluid has defensive properties, it is unlikely that JE is primarily designed to be permeable. More significantly, the immature nature of its cells allows them to form an attachment at the tooth surface in addition to the normal basement membrane between the JE and the underlying connective tissue of the gingiva. Such an attachment system could not form if the cells of the JE followed the usual differentiation pathway of stratified epithelium. It is also probable that the thinness of the JE allows the cells at the tooth surface to be more metabolically active than would be the case if they were at a greater distance from their nutritional source via blood vessels in the lamina propria of the connective tissue.

Basement membrane consists of two components: a basal lamina about 80 nm wide adjacent to the basal epithelial cell membrane, and a deeper, thicker and more diffuse reticular lamina. The basal lamina, which contains collagen type IV as well as glycoproteins such as laminin, is produced by epithelial cells, whereas the reticular lamina contains collagens type I and III of fibroblastic origin.

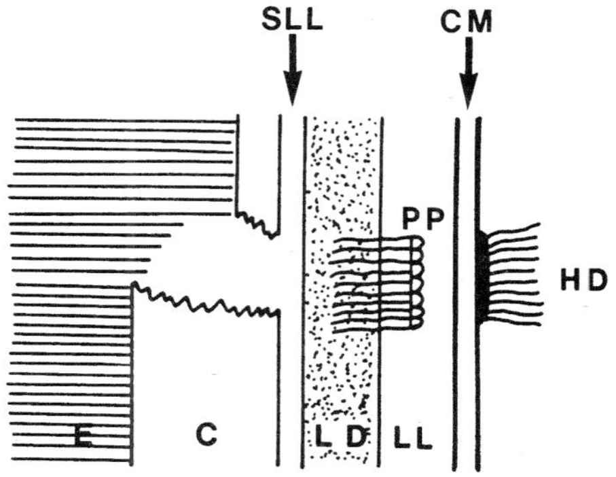

Fig. 10.2 Ultrastructure of epithelium–tooth interface. CM = Cell membrane; HD = hemidesmosome; LL = lamina lucida; LD = lamina densa; PP = pyramidal particles; SLL = sublamina lucida; C = cuticle; E = enamel. After Kobayashi *et al.*[3]

Ultrastructural investigations have revealed a basal lamina between the JE and the tooth surface (Fig. 10.2) which is often regarded as evidence of an organic union between epithelium and tooth. However, this is only partly correct: obviously a complete basement membrane cannot be formed where there are no fibroblasts to provide its reticular layer. A problem therefore remains: what sticks the basal lamina to the tooth? In the critical zone, Kobayashi *et al.*[3] have identified a structureless layer, about 5 nm thick, which they term the sublamina lucida (SLL).

The nature of the attractive forces in the SLL is a matter for speculation. Perhaps the negatively charged enamel surface and basal lamina are united by an electrostatic coupling, mediated by divalent calcium ions. Alternatively, weak forces of the van der Waals type, due to mutual distortion of the electron clouds of molecules, may be involved. Whatever the nature of the attractive forces, cells of the JE seem to be more adherent to the tooth surface than to one another, because if the marginal gingiva is pulled away from the tooth, the tear occurs within the JE and some cells remain attached to the enamel.

A further obstacle to understanding the attachment mechanism is that the enamel surface in this region is often covered by a cuticle (probably unmineralized enamel matrix), or even afibrillar cementum. If dentogingival collagen fibres are damaged, the JE can of course migrate apically and adhere to the cementum of the root. An attachment with ultrastructural features typical of JE has also been observed where an implant emerges through the mucosa.[4]

What controls the peculiar phenotype of JE? It is true that JE originates from reduced enamel epithelium, but its characteristic features reappear after surgical excision, suggesting that its phenotype is locally controlled. One possibility is that its cells are stimulated to divide by the almost invariable inflammatory infiltrate in the subjacent connective tissue or by bacterial mitogens seeping from the gingival sulcus. JE certainly has a fast turnover rate, being replaced in a matter of days, compared to the 3 or 4 weeks needed for renewal of the more complex epithelium of the hard palate. This rapid turnover allows insufficient time for its cells to produce the materials needed for a permeability barrier (MCGs, intercellular junctions). In other words, a vicious circle may exist, with bacterial products evoking an inflammatory response beneath the JE which increases its rate of cell proliferation, thereby producing an immature, leaky epithelium.

However, there is some experimental evidence that the special features of the JE are controlled by an inductive stimulus from the connective tissue. Inductive mechanisms of this nature are responsible for maintaining the individual characteristics of integumental epithelium and are referred to as epithelium–mesenchymal interactions. When basal epithelial cells are cultivated on deep rather than superficial mucosal connective tissue, they remain immature. The JE is close to the coronal aspect of the periodontal ligament, which can be considered to be a deep connective tissue, and may be influenced by it rather than by the gingival lamina propria.

The JE is obviously a friable tissue; in estimating sulcus depth, a probe tip will almost certainly pass into it. According to one study, the tip penetrated more than halfway between its coronal and apical extremities.[5] Other studies suggest that the probe tip may only be arrested by the dentogingival collagen fibres. Nevertheless, such measurements, perhaps made with a probe which minimizes the applied force, are useful especially for evaluating changes with time or following treatment.

Connective tissue

Collagen bundles in the gingiva are organized in such a way that they maintain the tissue in close contact with the tooth (Fig. 10.1). The named groups include circular fibres, but these actually run in semicircles around the buccal and lingual aspects of a tooth, being anchored to the cement at the approximal aspects of the neck. Transseptal fibres connect teeth around the arch and together with their associated fibroblasts have been implicated as causative factors in approximal drift. Gingival collagen, including that of the transseptal fibre system, has a slower turnover rate than that of the periodontal ligament and following orthodontic tooth movement the retention time must be sufficient to allow these fibres to remodel. Pericision, or cutting the gingival fibres around a tooth, has been used to expedite renewal of this collagen following orthodontic treatment.

Near to the JE and the sulcular epithelium, blood vessels form loops and coils, probably with complex arteriovenous communications resembling glomeruli; the blood flow through this intricate system will contribute to the turgor of the tissue. Connective tissue resilience is further enhanced by proteoglycans. The monomeric unit of these polymers consists of GAGs linked to a protein. Monomers are attached to a back bone of hyaluronic acid, forming large proteoglycan molecules. They are very hydrophilic but can lose water and alter their degree of aggregation under load, thereby dissipating stress applied to a tissue. The contour of the tooth, its contact areas and marginal ridges, also protects the vulnerable dentogingival junction from mechanical injury during mastication.

Periodontal ligament

The periodontal ligament (PDL) is appropriately named in that it anchors the tooth in its socket, but it differs in several important respects from other ligaments.

Structure

The PDL normally varies in width from 0.15 to 0.38 mm and is thinnest at mid-root level.

Being a dense connective tissue, the predominant cell type in the PDL is the fibroblast, although osteoblasts and cementoblasts, associated respectively with bone and cementum, are also recognized constituents, as are osteoclasts. Fibroblasts of the PDL have numerous intercellular connections including adhesive contacts and communicating (gap) junctions. In the latter, the gap of about 3 nm between the cells is bridged by protein channels which allow ions and very small molecules to pass from cell to cell. Fibroblasts are involved in the production and breakdown of collagen and ground substance and can modulate into overtly mobile and contractile cells, sometimes called myofibroblasts. In this state they contain numerous actin filaments, united by sliding cross-links of myosin. Fibroblast contraction and migration have been implicated as causative factors in eruption. A fluctuating population of defensive cells is found in the PDL, including macrophages, lymphocytes and neutrophil polymorphs. Mast cells have also been described, but are probably few in number.

Surprisingly for a ligament, the PDL contains epithelial cells, the rests of Malassez, which are the remnants of Hertwig's root sheath. In thin sections, these are seen as small clumps located on the cemental side of the ligament (Fig. 10.3) but in reality they constitute a cylindrical network around the root, somewhat like a fishnet stocking. They occasionally proliferate, perhaps stimulated by infection, especially endotoxins, and form the lining of a cyst. Their proliferation determines the expansion of the cyst and may also stimulate adjacent fibroblasts to organize a capsule and secrete bone-resorbing factors. It is possible that they have a related normal function and discourage mineralization of the PDL, thereby preventing ankylosis.

Most of the collagen is type I, although about 20% is type III. The individual fibrils have diameters of about 55 nm, rather smaller than those of most ligaments. The type I fibrils are mostly grouped into the well-known principal fibre bundles which become the Sharpey fibres where they are embedded and mineralized in cementum and bundle bone. When relaxed, the type I fibres are crimped or wavy, the waves having a periodicity of about 16 μm. The bundles vary in diameter across the PDL, being about 7 μm at the cemental side and 15 μm at their insertion into bone. In the central zone they are 1–4 μm thick. These facts suggest that bundles split and reform in an intermediate plexus, although this structure, visible in thin histological sections, may be due to a more subtle rearrangement, the bundles at the edge of the PDL combining to form sheets in the centre. The more numerous but finer bundles entering cementum compared with bone have been suggested as one reason why cementum resorbs less readily than bone; the fibres obscure the cementum surface and physically discourage attack by large osteoclasts.

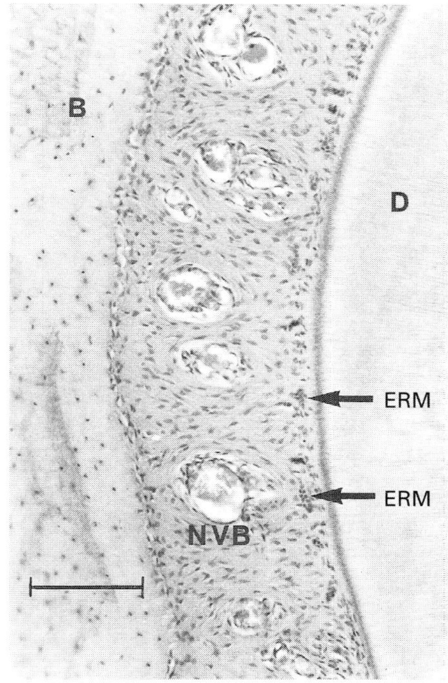

Fig. 10.3 Transverse section of periodontal ligament. Note epithelial rests of Malassez (arrowed ERM), dentine (D), bone (B) and neurovascular bundles (NVB). Stained with haematoxylin and eosin. Bar indicates 0.1 mm.

There are several other ways in which cementum might deter resorption. Cementocytes near the surface may produce an anti-invasion factor which repels osteoclasts. The PDL capillary network, which could be a source of bone-resorbing factors and precursors of osteoclasts, is nearer the bone surface than the cementum. It is also very likely that cementoblasts, which generally line the surface of the cementum, differ metabolically from osteoblasts. For example, cementoblasts do not possess receptors for parathyroid hormone; perhaps cementoblasts are also less responsive to pressure than are osteoblasts and are unable to communicate with, and attract, osteoclasts. Despite these protective mechanisms, cementum does of course resorb during the shedding of deciduous teeth and, not infrequently, during orthodontic treatment.

One remarkable characteristic of PDL collagen is its rapid turnover, with a half-life of only 10–15 days. This is about five times faster than gingival collagen, which in turn is renewed more rapidly than dermal collagen. The rapid renewal of collagen does not seem to be related to functional activity; it does not vary with the eruption rate and may even increase around unopposed teeth. The glycoprotein fibronectin is also found in the PDL. It is important in attaching cells and collagen to each other and also linking them to adjacent substrates, creating an attachment system called a fibronexus. Fibroblasts of the PDL are particularly well-endowed with fibronexi. Fibronectin has been used therapeutically to aid reattachment of collagen to cementum, although this has not been uniformly successful.

Although true elastin does not exist in the PDL, apart from that in the walls of blood vessels, a related substance, oxytalan, is present. This material is revealed by elastic tissue stains provided that the section has been oxidized. Its fine fibres, 1–2 μm thick, are composed of cylindrical microfibrils. Unlike the principal collagen bundles, oxytalan fibres run parallel to the root, often embedded in cementum and terminating as loops around neurovascular bundles. The function of these fibres is unclear; they may play a role in tooth support by keeping blood vessels open when the PDL is compressed. Alternatively, they may aid the neural mechanoreceptors in detecting loads applied to teeth. Eluanin is another immature form of elastin which has recently been revealed in the PDL. Like oxytalan, it forms a meshwork surrounding the collagen fibre bundles.

The cells and fibres are embedded in a highly hydrated ground substance, the major constituents of which are proteoglycans. The predominant GAGs in PDL are dermatan sulphate and chondroitin-4-sulphate. The degree of polymerization and hydration of these proteoglycans varies with the functional state of the tissue.

Compared with other ligaments, the PDL is unusually vascular. Branches of intraosteal vessels traverse the socket wall; others pass into the PDL from the apical vessels and some from gingival vessels. The penetrating vessels which pass through the cribriform plate are more numerous in posterior than anterior teeth; they are also found most frequently in the gingival third and are least common in the middle third of the ligament. The vessels are generally thin-walled and mainly run vertically in the PDL. A system of capillaries exists, nearer the bone surface than the tooth. The PDL is well-supplied with arteriovenous anastomoses and veins drain to a network around the root apex. It is unlikely that this high vascularity is merely associated with the rapid metabolic turnover of the PDL. More plausible reasons are first, that the blood flow dissipates as heat energy generated in the PDL during mastication and second that it provides a hydrodynamic damping mechanism to absorb masticatory forces.

There is little doubt that lymphatic vessels exist in the PDL, although they have not been thoroughly studied. They are less numerous than blood vessels and the main route of drainage follows the veins towards the tooth apex and thence alongside the dental vessels.

Like its blood supply, the PDL is innervated from several sources. Branches of dental nerves run coronally from the apical region and these are supplemented by fibres which enter via the cribriform plate. A vast array of differently shaped nerve endings has been described in the ligament and a force applied to a tooth could additionally be detected by endings in the gingiva or periosteum. Most numerous are free endings which ramify in tree-like arrangements around the connective tissue elements and are thought to be mechanoreceptors and perhaps nociceptors. Specialized nerve endings have been classified into four morphological types.[6] Ruffini corpuscles occur around the root apex, often in close association with collagen fibres, suggesting a role as mechanoreceptors. Coiled endings are located at the mid-root region and two less common types, spindle-like and expanded endings, are occasionally found around the apex. It is not known if each structural type of ending has a unique purpose.

Functionally, PDL mechanoreceptor endings are often separated into two groups. Slowly adapting units respond to small (2–10 μm) displacements of a tooth and can be activated by very small forces (1–2 g). Rapidly adapting units have higher thresholds (20 g) and can signal rates of change of a stimulus, but they are poor indicators of its duration. Linden[7] has attempted to locate and map the distribution of PDL mechanoreceptors in the cat. All the receptors he identified showed directional sensitivity and responded maximally when the ligament in that area was stretched by a horizontal force on the crown. When a point force is applied to a crown, the least displacement occurs at a fulcrum about halfway down the root. Mechanoreceptors were mapped between the fulcrum and the apex and the threshold of activation and speed of adaptation depended on their position relative to the fulcrum. Thus, at the apex, furthest from the fulcrum, the receptors are subjected to the greatest displacement and behave as slowly adapting units with a low threshold of activation. On the other hand, those nearest the fulcrum are distorted least and act as rapidly adapting, high-threshold units. It is possible, therefore, that the different functional characteristics of PDL mechanoreceptors depend not on their morphological type but on their position in the ligament relative to a fulcrum of movement. Some of the cell bodies of these receptors are located in the trigeminal ganglion and others in the mesencephalic nucleus of the fifth cranial nerve.

Whatever their precise structure, the significance of these PDL receptors is that the speed, amplitude and duration of tooth displacement are encoded and transmitted to the brain. It is probable that the major role of all these receptors, including the nociceptors, is in the control of the biting force.

Supporting functions

The PDL has several functions, some of which have been alluded to above. Envisaged as separating rather than joining tooth and bone, it provides space for cellular remodelling and hence continued eruption and approximal drift. Its sensory potential plays an important part in the control of mastication. Additional to these functions, which are considered elsewhere in this volume, the PDL must support the tooth during mastication.

It used to be thought that masticatory forces, averaging around 10 kg on a molar tooth, were transmitted to the alveolar bone as tension, mainly by stretching of the obliquely arranged principal collagen bundles. There are, however, several problems with this simple idea. The fibres may be too long and wavy to straighten out, at least under relatively small loads which nevertheless displace the tooth in the socket. Also, intrusive loads dilate the margins of a socket, quite the reverse of what would be expected if force is transmitted to the bone as tension. On the other hand, horizontally applied forces may be resisted by stretching of collagen fibres.

Much can be learned about the supporting mechanism by considering the rate of tooth movement when an axial load is applied and removed (Fig. 10.4). Intrusion is biphasic; an initial rapid displacement is followed by a slower movement. Recovery displays the reverse conformation. Rapidly repeated loadings produce a progressively greater intrusion of the tooth. These characteristics correspond to a well-known biomechanical property of soft connective tissues, known as viscoelasticity. The loaded tooth support system exhibits elasticity in recovering its original position, but it also shows viscosity during the slow phases of the movement.

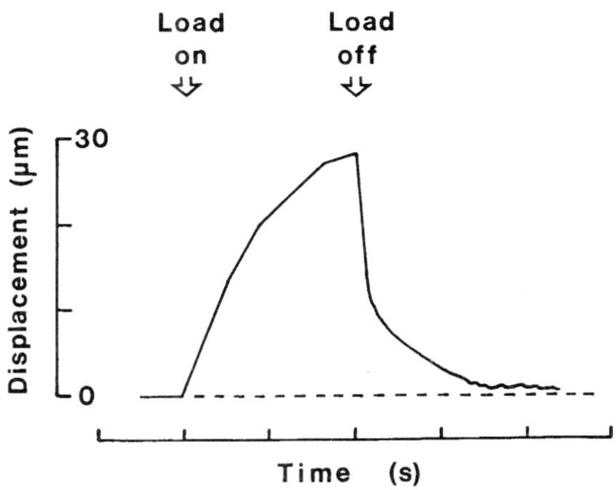

Fig. 10.4 Time sequence of displacement of a tooth following application and removal of an axial load of 5 N (approximately 500 g). Modified after Picton and Wills.[8]

Precisely which structural features of the PDL and alveolar bone are responsible for the various rates of movement under load is a matter for speculation. During the early intrusive phase, blood may be squeezed out of the PDL via the cribriform plate. This function of the extensive blood supply has been called hydrodynamic damping and its importance is confirmed by the reduction in intrusive displacement following the infiltration of a vasoconstrictor into the ligament. Rapidly repeated loadings will tend to expel progressively more blood from the ligament and retard its re-entry. The slow phase of the intrusive movement may be due to the loss of water from proteoglycans and the partial disaggregation of these large polymers. Probably the alveolar bone's resistance to distortion finally limits tooth movement. The abundant collagen fibres must also be important in all these events, but they are unlikely to act as a simple suspensory ligament.

When the load is removed, the initial fast recovery phase may be due to the elastic recoil of the alveolar bone and the subsequent slower phase is associated with the reconstitution of the hydrated proteoglycans and refilling of the PDL blood vessels. The importance of the overall support mechanism is that the load applied to a tooth is dissipated relatively slowly, rather than being suddenly resisted by the bone of the socket.

The slow recovery phase may take several seconds, so that during mastication the tooth becomes progressively more intruded into the socket. If a tooth is not in regular contact with others in the opposite jaw, the factors responsible for extrusion will continue to act, producing an eruptive force estimated to be 1 g for an incisor. In particular, the aggregation of proteoglycans into larger molecules will allow them to attract a greater volume of water. Within a matter of hours, the rapid turnover of collagen in the PDL will have stabilized the tooth and in the succeeding days changes in the bony socket will have further consolidated its new, extruded position. Thus, as Picton[9] has persuasively argued, tooth eruption can be explained as a continuation of the mechanisms responsible for extrusion following the removal of an axial load, supplemented by the rapid reconstitution of collagen.

References

1. Kristoffersen EK, Caffesse RG, Nasjleti CE, Kristoffersen TØ. Ultrastructural study of induced keratinization in sulcular gingival epithelium in rhesus monkeys. *Acta Odontol Scand* 1983; **41**: 227–240.
2. Juhl M, Stoltze K, Reibel J. Distribution of Langerhans cells in clinically healthy human gingival epithelium with special emphasis on junctional epithelium. *Scand J Dent Res* 1988; **96**: 199–208.
3. Kobayashi K, Rose GG, Mahan CJ. Ultrastructure of the dento-epithelial junction. *J Periodont Res* 1976; **11**: 313–330.
4. McKinney RV, Stefflick DE, Koth DL. Evidence for a junctional epithelial attachment to ceramic dental implants. *J Periodontol* 1985; **56**: 579–591.
5. Polson AM, Caton JG, Yeaple RN, Zander HA. Histologic determination of probe tip penetration into the gingival sulcus of humans using an electronic pressure-sensitive probe. *J Clin Periodontol* 1980; **7**: 479–488.
6. Maeda T, Kannari K, Sato O, Iwanaga T. Nerve terminals in human periodontal ligament as demonstrated by immunohistochemistry for neurofilament protein (NFP) and S-100 protein. *Arch Histol Cytol* 1990; **53**: 259–265.
7. Linden RWA. An update on the innervation of the periodontal ligament. *Eur J Orthod* 1990; **12**: 91–100.
8. Picton DCA, Wills DJ. Viscoelastic properties of the periodontal ligament and mucous membrane. *J Prosthet Dent* 1978; **40**: 263–272.
9. Picton DCA. The periodontal enigma: eruption versus tooth support. *Eur J Orthod* 1989; **11**: 430–439.
10. Luke DA. The structure and functions of the dentogingival junction and periodontal ligament. *Br Dent J* 1992; **172**: 187–200.

Further reading

Berkovitz BKB, Moxham BJ, Newman HN. *The Periodontal Ligament in Health and Disease*, 2nd edn. London: Mosby-Wolfe, 1995.

Mackenzie IC. Nature and mechanisms of regeneration of the junctional epithelial phenotype. *J Periodont Res* 1987; **22**: 243–245.

Picton DCA. Tooth mobility – an update. *Eur J Orthod* 1990; **12**: 109–115.

Squier CA. Keratinization of the sulcular epithelium – a pointless pursuit? *J Periodontol* 1981; **52**: 426–429.

Squier CA. The permeability of oral mucosa. *Crit Rev Oral Biol Med* 1991; **2**: 13–32.

Stern IB. Current concepts of the dentogingival junction: the epithelial and connective tissue attachments to the tooth. *J Periodontol* 1981; **52**: 465–476.

11

The structure and function of the temporomandibular joint

Gavin McKay and Robert Yemm

Introduction

The mammalian craniomandibular articulation is a comparatively modern evolutionary feature, being as recent as 70×10^6 years old. Prior to this vertebrates had various types of jaw articulations, at their simplest with Meckel's cartilage articulating indirectly with the otic capsule, These articulations are now in the middle ear. The modern jaw joint develops anterolateral to the otic capsule, from the first branchial arch mesenchyme, and is therefore innervated by the fifth (trigeminal) cranial nerve.

The evolution of the mammalian temporomandibular joint (TMJ) was associated with the acquisition of socketed teeth, primary and secondary dentitions; somatic growth ceases at maturity and a complex functional dentition features precision occlusion. The teeth had ceased to constitute a simple food-trapping mechanism and had come to be part of a more evolved, more sensitive and better integrated feeding system, as well as having other roles, including being used for communication.

In humans, the TMJ, like all other movable joints, is characterized by having a synovial membrane lining the non-articulating surfaces within a joint capsule. However, in other ways it is an atypical joint, as will be highlighted in the description below.

General description

The human TMJ is said to be almost unique in that it is a freely movable union between two membrane bones: temporal above and mandible below. This, however, is not strictly true because, although the basic mandible has been defined in membrane bone by the 10th week *in utero*, cartilage growth centres begin to appear from the 12th week. The condylar is the first and most important of these to develop. The condylar cartilage is not a typical articular cartilage; it is defined as a secondary cartilage because it develops on (and is therefore secondary to) a pre-existing piece of membrane bone. This contrasts with the normal situation in which joints are usually found between endochondral bones. Another unique feature is that this is the only movable joint to play a significant role in bone growth of the mandible, through the activity of a growth centre contained within the joint capsule.

The TMJ (Fig. 11.1) is principally between the articular part of the inferior surface of the squamous temporal bone – comprising a cranially convex glenoid fossa and an articular eminence more anteriorly – and the mandibular condyle. The glenoid fossa is formed by not only the articular part of temporal bone but also by part of the tympanic plate of temporal posteriorly, from which it is separated by the squamotympanic fissure; more medially tegmen tympani protrudes between the squamous and the petrous part of the temporal. The posterior margin of the glenoid fossa is defined by a lateral postglenoid process (squamous temporal) and this continues medially as a postglenoid ridge in the tympanic plate. The medial and anteromedial boundary of the articular area are

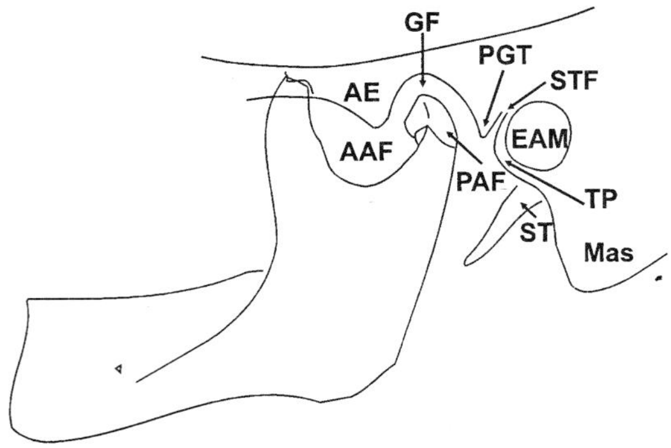

Fig. 11.1 The spatial relationship of the mandibular condyle to the membranous temporal bone. The gap between the posterior aspect of the neck of condyle and the tympanic plate and mastoid process is exaggerated in this and subsequent figures, for clarity. AE = Articular eminence; GF = glenoid fossa; PGT = postglenoid tubercle (lateral end of postglenoid ridge); STF = squamotympanic fissure; EAM = external auditory meatus; TP = tympanic plate; ST = styloid process; Mas = mastoid process; AAF = anterior articular facet; PAF = posterior articular facet.

defined by the median glenoid plane. In those cases where the postglenoid ridge is continued into the medial boundary, it is known as the entoglenoid process. Between the zygomatic root and the median glenoid plane (which are not articular areas) there is an extension of the articular surface – anterior to the crest of the articular slope – called the preglenoid plane. The boundary of this part of the joint is often not well-demarcated. The condylar process comprises a thin neck and an expanded condylar head which is somewhat flattened anteroposteriorly (ventrodorsally) and elongated lateromedially, so that it has lateral and medial poles. The lateral pole is the more pointed and does not extend far beyond the lateral surface of the ramus. The medial pole projects further medially, is thicker, smoother and more rounded. The condylar head does not sit upright on its neck but is inclined forwards. This forward inclination, combined commonly with a more or less well-defined transverse crest between the poles, results in a smaller, principal articular surface (or facet) anteriorly and a larger, less functional, posterior articular facet. The long axis of the condylar head (the hinging axis – see below) is not perfectly transverse but, in the plane of the cranial base, is rotated so that the lateromedial line points some 8–15° posteriorly.

Disc

Each human TMJ is essentially a double joint due to the presence of an intra-articular disc (Fig. 11.2). The articular surfaces are of fibrous tissue (not the normal articular cartilage): condylar perichondrium and temporal periosteum. It is technically classified as a ginglymoarthrodial articulation which, by definition, is capable of hinge-type movements (*ginglymos*: a hinge) and gliding movements (*arthrodia*: a sliding joint). The intra-articular disc acts not only to separate two joint cavities but also to adapt for the changing contours of the rotating condylar head as it glides across the different parts of the temporal bone. To enable this there are two specializations: the interjoint disc is not uniformly thick but is modified in different regions, and the periosteal covering of the temporal bone is padded as required.

The disc is a collagenous fibrous tissue sheet of variable thickness (derived from three

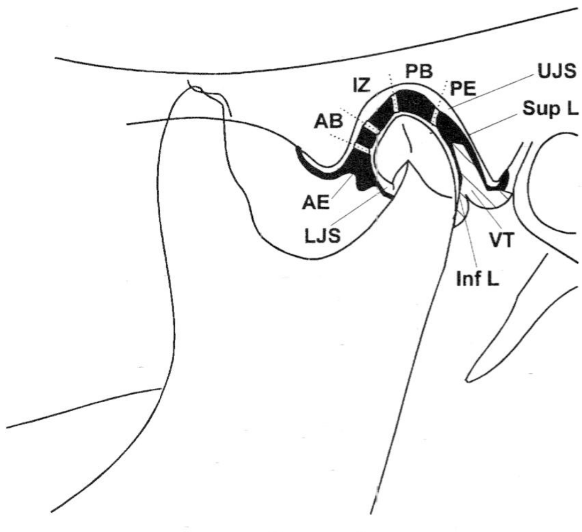

Fig. 11.2 The lateral view of the disc is shown with the five zones highlighted. Note the vascular tissue posteriorly. The upper surface of the disc is pear-shaped when viewed from above, has a larger surface area than the lower and is concavoconvex from anterior to posterior in a vertical plane. It is somewhat like a baseball cap: the convex part covers the head and the anterior concave part (the tapering element of the pear shape) is the projecting rim that extends over the articular crest on to the preglenoid plane. LJS = Lower joint space; AE = anterior extension; AB = anterior band; IZ = intermediate zone; PB = posterior band; PE = posterior extension; UJS = upper joint space; Sup L = superior lamina; VT vascular tissue; Inf L = inferior lamina.

developmental strata) that completely divides the jaw into upper and lower compartments. The underside of the disc is concave and fits closely over the condylar head like a cap, but one which is bound to the lateral and medial poles of the head. This ensures that the condylar head can be rotated (about the axis through its poles) within the lower joint cavity and that the disc plus condyle must move together across the temporal bone surface. At its margins, the disc blends with the fibrous joint capsule and in front is continuous with the tendon of the lateral pterygoid muscle.

The presence of cartilage cells within the disc is believed to be a degenerative change related to non-physiological function stresses. The classical description of the disc recognizes five zones from anterior to posterior (Fig. 11.2). In front, there is the anterior extension that is continuous with the tendon of the lateral pterygoid muscle and is vascular on its inferior surface. Posteriorly, the disc is bilaminar: the upper lamina contains well-developed elastic elements together with much vascular tissue. It also contains discomalleolar fibres. There is currently some controversy concerning whether or not there are elastic elements in the lower lamina; the remaining three zones of the disc comprise thickened anterior and posterior bands, which are in fact continuous with each other at the condylar poles forming an ellipsoidal 'doughnut' and a thinner intermediate zone (within the 'doughnut'). There is no doubt that the ellipsoidal doughnut functions to stabilize the condylar head in the glenoid fossa with the jaws at rest. The posterior band is the broader of the two and occupies the depth of glenoid fossa when the jaw is at rest; it is located over the posterior condylar facet. The anterior condylar facet relates to the thinner intermediate zone of the disc, which in turn relates to the articular slope of the temporal bone, from the glenoid fossa to the articular crest, which, by way of compensation for the thinner disc, has a fibrously padded periosteum. The narrow anterior band of the disc overlies the lower margin of the anterior condylar facet and interposes between it and the articular crest. It is conventional to consider the disc to be a flexible, viscoelastic adaptor which helps the moving joint surfaces achieve more effective articular surface congruity than would otherwise be possible. There is some controversy as to whether the anterior and posterior thickened bands are entirely due to the collagen fibres, or whether some thickness is contributed by pooling of a cartilage-like interfibrillar matrix which has flowed to this equilibrium distribution under the resting pressures within the joint.

Capsule

The capsule forms a thin, fibrous connective tissue sleeve about the joint which tapers from above down to the condyle neck. It is attached just peripheral to the margins of the articular surfaces. The collagenous capsular fibres are mainly vertically oriented and are of such a length as to enable the normal range of joint movements. Within the capsule, all the non-articular surfaces form synovial membranes, the surface area of which is usually increased by the development of folds and villi. The synovial fluid is a dialysate of plasma with added mucins and proteins; it contains a variety of cells, mainly lymphoid/macrophage in type.

Ligaments

The capsule itself is too delicate a structure to support the joint unaided and so joint stability is achieved with intrinsic and extrinsic ligaments (Fig. 11.3).

Intrinsic

The main ligament is the temporomandibular, which is located lateral to the capsule, cannot easily be separated from it by dissection, but is easily distinguished by the orientation of its fibres, which pass obliquely posteroinferiorly from a wide (long) origin, lateral to the articular tubercle to a narrower insertion in the neck of condyle, below and behind the lateral pole of the condyle.

So-called collateral ligaments are also found. These are rather narrow bands of collagen fibres that run horizontally backwards on the inner aspect of the capsule, from the lateral and medial aspects of the articular eminence to the respective condylar poles. They obviously restrict distal displacement of the

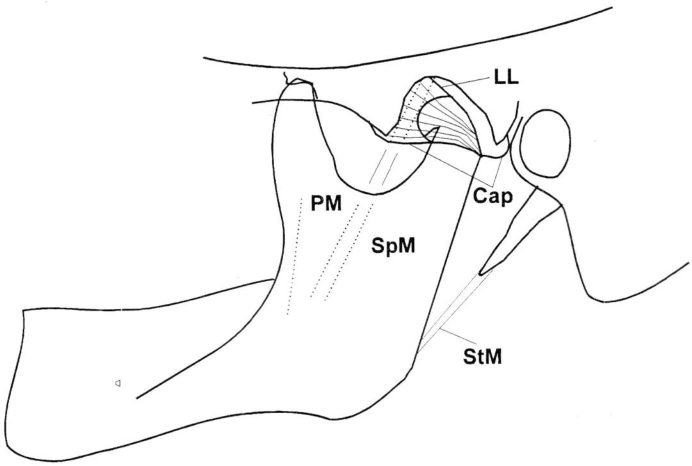

Fig. 11.3 Joint ligaments. The joint capsule is outlined with a heavy line but the capsular fibres are omitted for clarity – they would run more or less vertically. Note that the lateral ligament is somewhat fan-shaped with the fibres running downwards and back to converge on the posterior and lateral aspects of the condylar neck. LL = Lateral ligament; Cap = capsule; StM = stylomandibular ligament; SpM sphenomandibular ligament; PM = pterygomandibular ligament.

condylar head. With the teeth in maximal intercuspal position the collateral ligaments are not fully taut. When tight, these structures, together with the temporomandibular ligaments, help define the clinical ligamentous position.

Extrinsic

There are a number of fibrous connective tissue bands, attached to the mandible which, although not directly involved with the joint, modify the range of movements that are possible. These are also known as accessory ligaments and include the sphenomandibular ligament, the stylomandibular ligament, the pterygomandibular raphe and the temporomandibular ligament of the opposite side which acts as an extrinsic medial ligament.

Innervation

The afferent (sensory) nerve supply to the TMJ is derived from branches of the mandibular division of the trigeminal nerve – most importantly, the auriculotemporal branch but also the masseteric and deep temporal branches. The fibres supplying the joint cover almost the entire range of nerve diameters from large myelinated (A-α and A-β) through small myelinated (A-δ) to small unmyelinated (C) fibres. Contrary to previous suggestions that the cell bodies of these fibres might be located – like those from jaw muscle spindles and some periodontal ligament receptors – in the trigeminal mesencephalic nucleus, it now seems that, like those of most trigeminal fibres, they are located in the trigeminal ganglion. The receptors associated with these fibres are found in the joint capsule and ligament – more so laterally than medially, although there is some dispute as to whether the antero- or posterolateral area is the most heavily innervated. There are few, if any, receptors in the disc or on the articular surfaces.

Morphologically, the receptors are mainly free nerve endings which are associated with the small myelinated and unmyelinated fibres, but there are also three more complex endings, all associated with larger myelinated fibres, viz. Ruffini endings, Golgi tendon organs and paciniform corpuscles. Functionally, the receptors are either nociceptive (detectors of tissue damage or threat of damage) or mechanoreceptive (detectors of mechanical events such as stretch or pressure). Unfortunately, there is little evidence from studies of the TMJ to link the structures and function of these nerves and receptors. However, from what is known of such receptors elsewhere in the body, including in other joints, it seems likely that all the nociceptive fibres will have free nerve endings while the mechanoreceptive fibres will mainly have the more complex receptors. It is also likely that activity from the paciniform endings will be rapidly adapting and thus be able to give information only about transient events such as joint movement while those from the other mechanoreceptors will be more slowly adapting and possibly capable of signalling joint position.

Little is known about the synaptic connections of TMJ afferents within the brainstem, although there is some evidence that these may occur in both the trigeminal main sensory nucleus and the trigeminal spinal nuclei. It is likely that the nerves will subserve both reflex and sensory functions but for technical reasons these have proved difficult to study. There is evidence that activation of TMJ afferents can produce reflexes in the musculature of the tongue but, to the best of our knowledge, there is no evidence at present of such activity triggering reflexes in the more obviously related muscles of the jaws; nevertheless, one would anticipate that it would do so, with one possible function being to limit movement in directions which are inadequately protected by the ligaments. In terms of sensory abilities, it seems that TMJ afferents contribute to our awareness of mandibular position as far as can be ascertained by experiments in which subjects have to move their jaw to a position which they have memorized. Curiously, the loss of afferent input from one TMJ (by local anaesthesia) has as bad an effect on this ability as has the loss of inputs from both joints. More controversial is the question of whether TMJ afferents contribute to our ability to detect or judge the size of objects placed between the teeth; on balance it seems that their role in these abilities, if any, is less than that of afferents from the jaw muscle spindles.

In addition to its afferent innervation the TMJ also receives an efferent–autonomic–supply which is carried in the auriculotemporal nerve as well as in the plexus on the superficial temporal artery. This may be made up largely or entirely of sympathetic fibres supplying the blood vessels of the joint. It may account for the reported innervation of the posterior part of the disc which is said to be almost devoid of sensory receptors.

Blood supply

The superficial temporal branches of the external carotid artery and vein are the principal vascular channels for the TMJ. In addition it is said that any named artery that runs within 2.5 cm of the joint gives one or two branches to it. It is, however, worth highlighting the fact that arteries within bone (temporal, mandible) send multiple branches to the joint capsule. The vascular anteroinferior part of the disc extension is connected via lateral vessels to the vascularized lamina in the posterior part of the disc.

The TMJ and musculature at rest

When not functionally active, the mandible adopts the so-called rest position. The condyles occupy a central, unstrained position in the glenoid fossae, and the upper and lower teeth are separated by the 'freeway space' (interocclusal clearance). The natural teeth are in a position of equilibrium between, on the one hand, eruptive forces and on the other, some of the forces of function (as demonstrated by the tendency of unopposed teeth to overerupt). The presence of the freeway space demonstrates that functional forces exceed those of eruptive potential.

The role of the jaw musculature in determining resting posture is controversial. One possibility is that a state of tonic activity exists which stabilizes jaw position, even at rest. Such a state of activity could be dependent upon muscle spindle activity in jaw-closing muscles. However, mandibular posture at rest is not an exact position, and is subject to change with head and body posture, intraoral contents and air pressure, and lip muscle activity. This variability argues against a precise neuromuscular control mechanism. Unfortunately, it is technically difficult to ascertain the existence of a state of complete muscle inactivity, but it is clear that external circumstances, such as psychological stress, can induce an increase in jaw-closing muscle activity. An alternative explanation of the relative stability of the mandibular rest position is that it depends principally upon the inactive properties of the tissues, particularly on muscle elasticity. External forces exert an influence upon the mandible (e.g. gravity), as do variable but largely uncontrolled degrees of activity in related muscles. This hypothesis can explain much of the variability observed in the resting posture and is consistent with known mechanisms of resting posture control in other parts of the body.

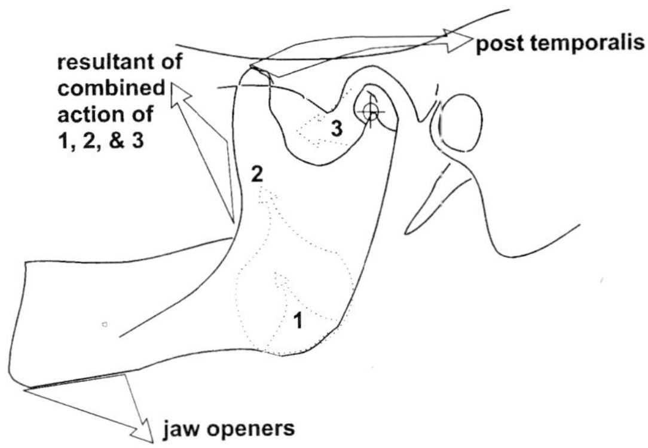

Fig. 11.4 One of the explanations for the relatively low functional loads transmitted to the temporal bone by the condylar head is that it is positively supported by a muscle sling formed from the mechanical couple shown here. A second purpose of this figure is to emphasize that the rest position probably owes its stability to the inactive properties of the tissues acting on the jaw, particularly on muscle elasticity. The vector for the jaw openers is shown to emphasize that these muscles are part of this equation.

Joint movements

In the past some authorities have stated that the TMJ is a non-weight-bearing joint: this cannot be the case, but it is certainly true that only a proportion of the forces generated by mastication are transmitted via the joints. This is because, first, the head of the condyle is supported in space by a sling of jaw muscles, and second, because the forces of mastication are to some extent transmitted via the teeth and periodontal membranes to the maxilla and mandible. In the case of the maxilla these forces are dispersed through the facial buttresses and pterygoid plates to the vault of the skull and cranial base. At its simplest (Fig. 11.4) the muscle sling is seen as a mechanical couple, made up of posterior fibres of temporalis being counteracted by the pterygomasseteric complex, which have the effect of locating the head of the condyle in a low stress-bearing relationship with the glenoid fossa.

The human TMJ is capable of both rotation (hinge) and gliding (translation) movement. Most functional movements involve a combination of the two. Such jaw movements can occur symmetrically in both joints, as when the mandible is raised (closed), lowered (opened), protruded or retruded. Movements also occur in asymmetrical manner, when translation occurs on one side only (or to a greater extent on one side) to produce lateral jaw positions. Such lateral deviation is a normal feature of masticatory function, discussed later in this book.

The total movement capability is limited and imposes a restriction on the extent of mandibular movement relative to the maxilla. For this reason, there exists a maximum range of movement in the normal subject. This has led to the concept of border movements – those performed at the extremes. Assessed in each of the classical anatomical planes (sagittal, coronal, horizontal), the extreme movements are seen as envelopes of movement. These are mainly useful in assessing disturbances of joint or muscle function, where limitation of movement may restrict the size of envelope or introduce asymmetry.

The position of widest opening, or of maximum mandibular protrusion, is associated with the head of the condyle moving forward to the crest of the glenoid eminence. In doing this it is considered that some subjects voluntarily subluxate the joint, in which case the posterior facet of the condyle relates to the preglenoid plane. In closing, the fenestrated elastic sheet in the posterior part of the upper lamina aids in the recoil and helps to ensure that the disc is retracted in synchrony with the condylar head.

The ability of the condyle to move backwards (retrude) within the glenoid fossa is limited. It may be achieved voluntarily (with practice) by combined activity of digastric and some jaw-closing muscles, but is restricted to a distance of about 1 mm. The significance of this is clinical: symmetrical retrusion is regarded as providing a reproducible horizontal relationship between maxilla and mandible (the ligamentous position).

During mandibular movements the space that was occupied by the resting condyle becomes filled by surrounding loose tissue and in particular by the vascular tissue in the posterior part of the disc. In addition the anterior attachment of the disc has to be sufficiently loose to enable all the rotation of the condylar head to take place in the lower joint cavity. As the slack tissue here is put under tension during opening movements, the blood in the anteroinferior part of the disc extension is squeezed along lateral connecting vessels to be displaced to the posterior vasculature, and vice versa on closing. The posterior plexus is no longer regarded as a form of hydraulic buffer against a too rapid posterior displacement of the condyle during closing.

Effectors of TMJ movements

Although some movements of the TMJ are achieved by the action of the lateral pterygoid muscle, which has a direct insertion into the joint (see above), the majority of movements result from the action of muscles attached elsewhere on the mandible. There are several ways of categorizing these muscles but perhaps the simplest way is to classify them as either jaw openers or jaw closers (since all except, perhaps, the lateral pterygoid fit easily into one of these categories) and then note what additional movements can be achieved by each muscle.

The conceptually simplest jaw-opening muscles are those which are responsible for depressing the mandible by producing a rotation of the condylar head – these are the diagastric (anterior belly), mylohyoid and geniohyoid muscles. This action by these muscles can be achieved only if other muscles – particularly the infrahyoid group – act to stabilize the hyoid bone during the mandibular movement; if this does not happen, then elevation of the hyoid rather than depression of the mandible is achieved as in swallowing. Furthermore, there is evidence that these jaw-opening muscles may also contribute to retrusive movements. The other movement of the TMJ during jaw opening – translation of the condylar head on to the articular eminence – is achieved principally by the action of the lateral pterygoid muscle. However, the actions of this muscle are complex since its inferior head is active during jaw opening and its upper head during jaw closing: the role of this latter action is difficult to envisage and is sometimes stated as being to stabilize the TMJ. In addition, the lateral pterygoid acts to protrude the jaw and, if acting unilaterally, to move the mandible to the other side. In this action it will tend to move the condylar head not only forwards but also, to a small extent, medially, while the opposite condyle will rotate within its fossa and may move very slightly laterally.

The jaw-closing muscles, whose actions are responsible for returning the condylar head to its rest position in the glenoid fossa after its displacement, are the masseter, temporalis and medial pterygoid. The masseter, or at least its superficial fibres, can also cause protrusion of the jaw and in so doing move the condylar head towards the articular eminence. The posterior and intermediate parts of the temporalis muscle can retrude the jaw, moving the condylar head to its posterior limit in the fossa. The medial pterygoid, like its lateral counterpart, can also protrude the jaw and, if acting unilaterally, cause movement of the mandible to the opposite side with resultant movements of the condylar heads as described above for the lateral pterygoid.

Control of TMJ movements

The muscles which move the TMJ, like those elsewhere on the body, are subject to both reflex controls and controls arising from within the central nervous system. We will confine our consideration to reflex controls. There are three principal reflexes which control the vertical relationship between the mandible and maxilla and hence TMJ movements – the jaw jerk, jaw-opening and jaw-unloading reflexes.

Jaw jerk reflex

The jaw jerk reflex is sometimes also called the jaw-closing reflex, but the latter term is best avoided to prevent confusion with another reflex which was described in classical work early this century but which has been found only in decerebrate animals and not in

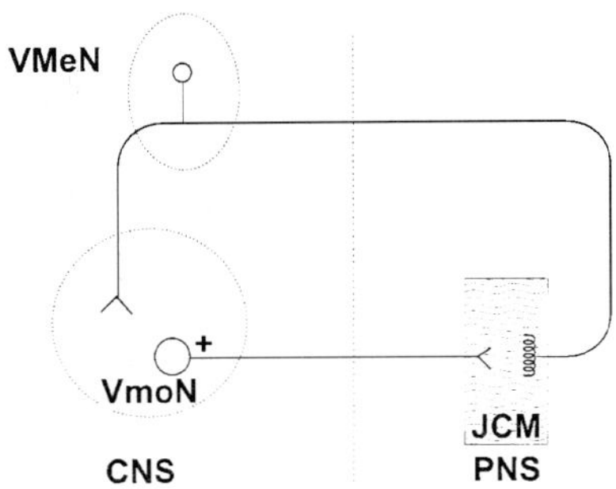

Fig. 11.5 Schematic representation of the pathway for the jaw jerk reflex. Note the monosynaptic connections between the afferent nerves from the spindles in the jaw-closing muscles and the motor neurons for these same muscles. CNS = Central nervous system; PNS = peripheral nervous system; JCM = jaw-closing muscle; VMeN = trigeminal mesencephalic nucleus; VMoN = trigeminal motor nucleus; + excitatory synapse.

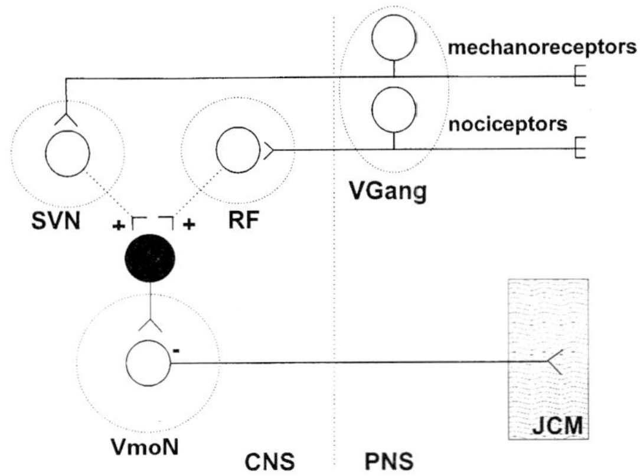

Fig. 11.6 Schematic representation of the pathway for the jaw-opening reflex in humans. Note the polysynaptic connections between mechanoreceptive and nociceptive afferent nerves from the mouth and face and the motor neurons for the jaw-closing muscles and that these connections result in an inhibition of the motor neurons. Abbreviations as in Figure 11.5, plus VGang = trigeminal ganglion; SVN = supratrigeminal nucleus; RF = reticular formation; – = inhibitory synapse. Broken 'axons' represent uncertainty about the number of synapses involved.

humans. The jaw jerk is analogous to the knee jerk and is a stretch reflex whereby stretching the jaw-closing muscles – usually by applying a downwards tap on the chin – produces a reflex contraction of these muscles. The importance of this reflex lies not in it happening as such in everyday life (one rarely receives downward blows on the chin!) but in that it demonstrates the existence of a feedback mechanism from jaw-closing muscles to their own motor neurons in the central nervous system; it is known that this feedback loop comes from muscle spindles within the muscles which, via their primary afferent nerves, make direct (monosynaptic) connections with the motor neurons in the trigeminal motor nucleus (Fig. 11.5). Presumably this feedback mechanism helps with the fine control of jaw/TMJ movements throughout normal function, for example, to take account of different consistencies of food. It should be noted that no such mechanism exists for the jaw-opening muscles since these have few, if any, muscle spindles.

Jaw-opening reflex

The term jaw-opening reflex refers to several reflexes, all of which result in either jaw opening or a cessation of jaw closing. In primates, including humans, these are effected by an inhibition of activity in jaw-closing muscles but do not usually show any activation of jaw-opening muscles as is found in non-primate mammals. Jaw-opening reflexes can be triggered by stimulating mechanoreceptive nerves from most structures within the mouth or nociceptive nerves from the mouth or face; it has also been found that similar jaw reflexes can be evolved from other parts of the body such as the limbs. There is no evidence that these reflexes can be evoked from the TMJ itself but that also seems possible (see above). The pathway for jaw-opening reflexes is polysynaptic, with the first synapse in either the trigeminal sensory nuclei or the adjacent reticular formation and the final one in the trigeminal motor nucleus (Fig. 11.6). The importance of these reflexes probably lies in their ability to prevent injury when biting or chewing objects liable to produce damage, although it is more difficult to speculate as to the function of jaw-opening reflexes triggered from nerves outside the mouth.

Jaw-unloading reflex

The jaw-unloading reflex also involves a cessation of activity in jaw-closing muscles, together with an activation of jaw-opening muscles, but in this case the trigger is rather different. The reflex is evoked when a hard object which is being bitten breaks suddenly, thus 'unloading' the jaw-closing muscles of the resistance against which they were working. The result of the reflex is that the opposing teeth do not then forcefully hit into one another in a fashion which could cause damage. The mechanisms for the reflex are not well-understood, largely because many different receptors in the orofacial region (for example, muscle spindles, periodontal and TMJ mechanoreceptors) will change their levels of activity when the object breaks. The most likely explanation, for which there is some evidence, is as follows. When biting on an object which one knows or suspects might be brittle, one sends excitatory signals not only to the jaw-closing motor neurons but also, as a precaution, to those of the jaw-opening muscles. The jaw-closing motor neurons also receive positive feedback from their own muscle spindles (i.e. via jaw jerk pathway) and there may be negative feedback to the jaw-opener motor neurons from this same source (the phenomenon known as reciprocal inhibition). When the object breaks, the sudden shortening of the muscle would result in a decrease in spindle activity and hence in the overall excitatory drive to the jaw-closing muscles, as well as in a disinhibition of the jaw-opening motor neurons. Thus the decreases and increases in activity in the jaw-closing and opening muscles respectively would be produced.

Horizontal jaw reflexes

In addition to the vertical jaw reflexes just described, there are also horizontal jaw reflexes which involve lateral, protrusive and, maybe, retrusive movements of the jaw in response to stimulation of mechanoreceptors in the periodontium, oral mucosa and again, possibly, the TMJ. Although far less is known about these reflexes than about the vertical ones, they may be of great significance in the function and dysfunction of the TMJ due to their being superimposed upon the normal chewing pattern.

Pain and dysfunction of the TMJ are discussed in Chapter 23.

Further reading

Dubner R, Sessle BJ, Storey AT. *The Neural Basis of Oral and Facial Function*. New York: Plenum, 1978.

Matthews B. Mastication. In: Lavelle CLB (ed.) *Applied Physiology of the Mouth*, pp. 199–244. Bristol: Wright, 1975.

McDevitt WE. *Functional Anatomy of the Masticatory System*. London: Wright, 1989.

Morimoto T. Perception of intraoral stimulation. In: Taylor A (ed.) *Neurophysiology of the Jaws and Teeth*, pp. 369–390. London: Macmillan, 1990.

Sperber GH. *Craniofacial Embryology*. London: Wright, 1989.

Walker A. Functional anatomy of oral tissues: mastication and deglutition. In: Shaw JH, Sweeney EA, Cappuccino CC, Mellor SM (eds) *Textbook of Oral Biology*, pp. 277–296. Philadelphia: Saunders, 1978.

12

Some aspects of mastication and swallowing

Alan J. Thexton

General comments

The processes of chewing and swallowing, taken together, are often considered to represent the totality of the feeding process. However, this overlooks the mechanisms subserving the essential requirement of simply moving food through the oral cavity. The fact that the process of feeding is primarily one of transport is obvious in the neonate and it is only during maturation that the act of chewing is introduced to deal with solid food. This process of mechanical reduction can be regarded simply as an interruption in the transport of food through the oral cavity until the food is mechanically reduced to meet some internal criterion of consistency; only then is the food transported more posteriorly for swallowing.[1] Chewing consequently divides intraoral transport into two stages: stage I represents transport of food from the front of the mouth to the level of the molars/premolars and stage II represents transport from that level to the back of the tongue (Fig. 12.1). In contrast, if the ingested food already meets the internal criteria for swallowing, there will be no true mastication and the food will be moved towards the pharynx for swallowing, without significant interruption between the two stages of transport. It should be noted that the two stages of transport may utilize different mechanisms to move the food items (see next section).

The mechanisms for intraoral transport in normal feeding are now well-described in a number of animals[1–5] but the processes have

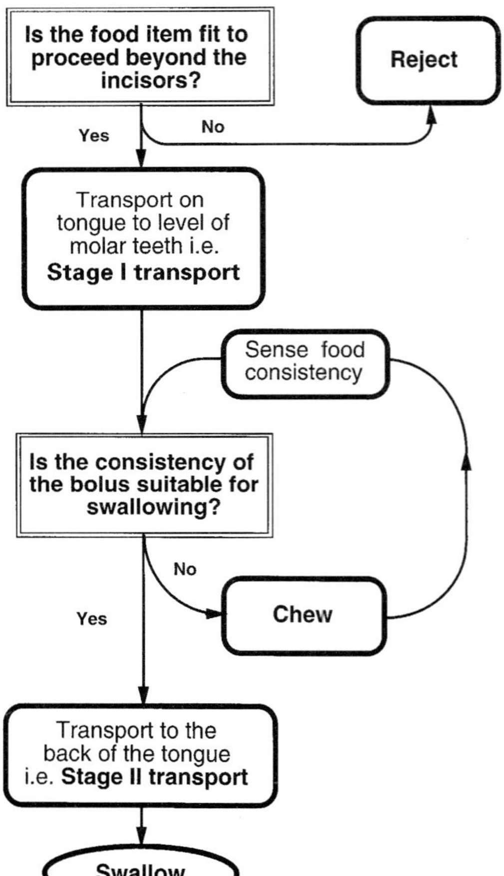

Fig. 12.1 Flow diagram of the choices and actions that, it is suggested, occur as food is taken into the mouth. The reasons for differentiating between transport of food to the back of the tongue and swallowing are discussed in the text.

been little studied during normal feeding in the human, except in relation to swallowing. The mechanisms used by the tongue to select food particles and place them between the occluding teeth is also an area which has been little investigated. However, some general understanding of the criteria on which the tongue selects particles is arising out of studies of chewing efficiency. In such experiments labelled food particles of specified sizes are given and the masticated food is collected after a given number of chewing cycles; the particle size distribution of the processed food may then be assessed. These experiments[6–8] have succeeded in isolating the breakage function of the dentition (a measure of the reduction in size of food particles fractured between occluding teeth) from a selection function (the chance of particular-sized particles being placed between the occluding teeth in the first place).

The chance of selecting a particle for breakage increases disproportionately with increase in particle size, but the efficiency of breakage of the selected particles by the teeth probably peaks at a size that is directly related to the occlusal area of the occluding teeth. Particles that are larger than this optimum remain partly unprocessed after a single chewing stroke, whereas particles that are very much smaller may simply be deformed against the sides of cuspal inclines.[8] In chewing, the process is iterative, so that what is found is a change in the distribution of particle sizes as the number of cycles used to process the food is increased. Furthermore, the median particle size of test foods soon decreases below the optimum for efficient breakage, so that further chewing continues at ever-decreasing levels of efficiency. The Victorian admonition to chew everything 30 times may therefore have been rather excessive.

Until recently the tendency has been to treat the process of selection as a mechanicostatistical function rather than a specific motor response driven by sensory input; this view is perhaps not surprising because the underlying theory of these experiments was based upon the performance of industrial crushing machines. However, it has been shown,[9] on a quantitative basis, that local anaesthesia impairs chewing efficiency. While the most obvious aspects of this finding may not surprise anyone who has had an inferior dental block, it does underline the fact that the most elegantly restored occlusion can be rendered virtually useless if the tongue cannot carry out the functions of transport, food particle selection and positioning.

One of the problems with investigating feeding mechanisms in humans is that there are severe limitations on the experimental techniques that can be used. Consequently, most of the information on the basic mechanisms of feeding has been gathered from animal experiments and a digression into the nature of animal mastication is therefore necessary. The different functional classes of jaw cycle (those producing the intraoral transport of liquids, which may combine the functions of both stage I and stage II transport, those separately producing either stage I or stage II transport for solids and those producing food breakdown and finally the cycles associated with swallowing) all have different profiles of movement, particularly in subprimate omnivores and carnivores. The profile of movement is defined in this context as the angle of jaw opening (gape), measured in the sagittal plane, plotted against time. As food passes through the oral cavity these different cycles arise and change from one to another with no break in the general underlying rhythm of movement, although characteristic cycles of each type are clearly identifiable. In humans and macaques, the jaw movement cycles in an ingestive sequence are, however, less obviously different from each other than is the case in subprimates. Nevertheless, the mechanisms, operating in the obviously different cycle types of subprimates, are now being found to be present in human and macaque jaw cycles subserving the same functions.[10]

The demonstration that the jaw cycles change from one type to another, as the food is processed in normal feeding, raises the question of whether there is a preset pattern for each cycle type that can be selected or switched in by appropriate sensory input or whether there is continuous modulation of a basic pattern by sensory input. The first possibility cannot be totally dismissed on present evidence[11] but, for simplicity, this overview will proceed on the assumption first, that all cycle variation is due to a continuous modulation of a basic pattern and second, that simple reflex responses are capable of integration into the cyclical pattern of movement and, in so doing, will produce changes in those cycles.

In order to present a condensed account of the mechanisms of feeding, three aspects only will be considered:

1. The nature of jaw and tongue movement in mastication and swallowing (in animal models but with a consideration of how these findings shed light on human function).
2. How the masticatory rhythm is generated.
3. The mechanisms by which the jaw cycle profiles may change in response to the ingestion of different-consistency foods (or in response to the progressive breakdown of solid food).

Oral movement

In both the primate and the subprimate animals studied, the general characteristics of the jaw movement cycles depend upon the range of the physical characteristics of the food ingested (Fig. 12.2). This is exemplified on the one hand by the ingestion of liquid, which is associated with a series of stereotyped cycles interspersed with cycles containing a swallow and, on the other hand, the ingestion of a solid which may require an incisor bite, a first stage of transport carrying the food fragments to the cheek teeth (molars and premolars), a variable number of chewing cycles and then a second stage of further transport, followed by a swallow. In cycles with these different functions, the jaw movement differs, depending to a large extent on the associated tongue function. During postnatal maturation, the consistency of food that is ingested shows a progressive change from liquid through pulped food to solids. At the same time the nature of the ingestive sequence changes, so that, in animals, it ceases to consist of a series of relatively homogeneous cycle types and comes to consist of the differing cycle types described previously.

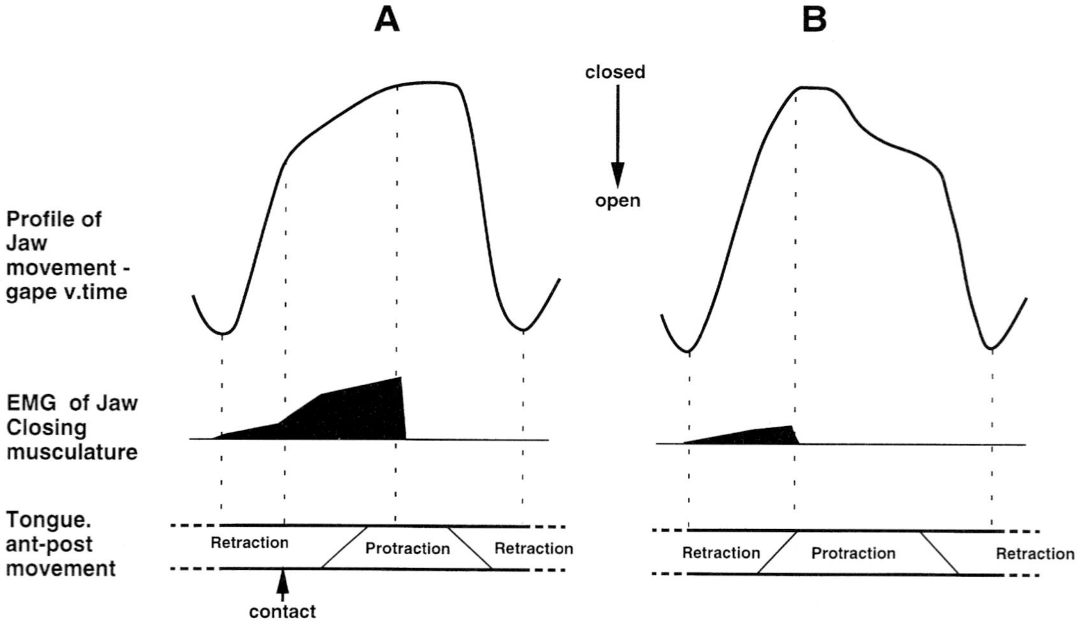

Fig. 12.2 A diagrammatic representation of two cycle types that have been observed in both macaques and humans eating. (A) Hard brittle food; (B) soft food. The profile of jaw movement is that occurring in the sagittal plane. The highly diagrammatic representation of the electromyogram (EMG) activity is intended only to indicate general trends in the amplitude of the signal. Note that the increase in EMG amplitude corresponds with deceleration in jaw-closing; this is clearly evident in A (see arrow marking tooth–food–tooth contact) but unclear in B. The duration of the cycles would be of the order of 0.5–0.8 s. The data summarized in this diagram are based on a human cineradiographic and electromyographic study[10] and two unpublished studies, one carried out at Harvard on the macaque using cineradiography and electromyography and the other carried out at the Royal London Hospital on humans using the Sirognathograph and electromyography.[47,48]

The first stage of transport, in animals, is mainly a function of the tongue working against a rugae-covered hard palate that is flat anteroposteriorly. The mechanism requires that there are extensive anteroposterior movements of the working (dorsal) surface of the tongue against the palate (because the hyoid is positioned relatively posteriorly to the working surface of the tongue in animals, rather than directly underneath the oral surface of the tongue as in humans, the antero-posterior movements of the hyoid make a significant contribution to such tongue movements relative to the palate). The preparatory forward movement of the tongue takes its working surface under the food item which, at that time, is either being held by the teeth or trapped by the rugae. This forward movement is followed by retraction of the tongue; since the simultaneous jaw opening releases the hold on the food, this is then carried back on the surface of the retracting tongue. As a general rule, during transport, tongue protraction takes place at low gapes, mainly during early jaw opening; conversely, tongue retraction takes place mainly when the jaw is wider open (Fig. 12.2). This coordination is not absolute and variation occurs within the limits necessary for effective stage I transport of solids. This really only requires two conditions to be met; first, that time is allowed in the cycle for the tongue to come forward sufficiently and, second, that tongue retraction is timed to occur at a sufficient gape such that the food item can be transported back without being hindered by contact with teeth or mucosal contact.[5,12]

In direct contrast to the subprimates, adult humans have a palate that is free of functionally useful rugae, a roof to the mouth that is effectively curved anteroposteriorly when dentate and a hyoid that is deeply placed underneath the working surface of the tongue; none of these anatomical features are appropriate to efficient stage I transport. Moreover humans can use hands, forks or chopsticks to place food within the mouth. Stage I transport is not therefore an obvious feature of mastication in humans.

Although it seems to be reduced to one or perhaps two cycles at the beginning of the ingestive sequence, stage I transport is nevertheless essential to the movement of a piece of hard food, just broken off by the incisors, to the posterior teeth for processing. The mechanism seems to be the same as that described above – the protracted tongue is positioned underneath the food item and is then retracted while the jaw is still open. In subsequent (chewing) cycles on hard food, tongue excursion is not only considerably reduced but retraction corresponds less to the time when food on the tongue dorsum can be carried backwards unhindered and more to jaw closure, i.e. the potential for food transport is substantially reduced. The reader can test the effectiveness of human stage I transport, by taking small bites from a biscuit or, more obviously, by eating long bits of spaghetti.

The jaw and tongue movements of stage II transport differ from those of stage I (depending upon the species) and usually involve one or more cycles in which the posterior tongue depresses and advances (creating a space posteriorly) whilst the anterior tongue elevates (reducing space anteriorly). This produces a pressure gradient in the food on the tongue, causing it to flow. Transport is consequently produced during tongue protraction rather then during retraction. Such cycles normally occur immediately preceding swallowing in subprimates. Although they would seem to be intrinsically more appropriate to the transport of foods that are soft or liquid, i.e. foods that are capable of flowing, these cycles seem to be the main transport mechanism in anthropoids.[2,3] However, the movements may also produce a limited amount of mechanical processing of some soft foods.

In the case of the ingestion of liquids, transport is the sole function of the jaw/tongue cycle. In animals, e.g. cat,[4] the tongue movements in each cycle preceding a swallow combine the functions of both stage I and stage II transport (but without the increased gape associated with the ingestion of solids) and produce accumulation of the ingestate in the vallecula. This accumulation occurs prior to a swallow and is dependent upon an anatomy that is very different from that of an adult (but not from that of an infant) human (Fig. 12.3).

In general, the anteroposterior movement of the working surface of the tongue is produced by anteroposterior movements of the tongue base (hyoid) together with elongation and shortening of the tongue body itself. These length changes within the body of the tongue

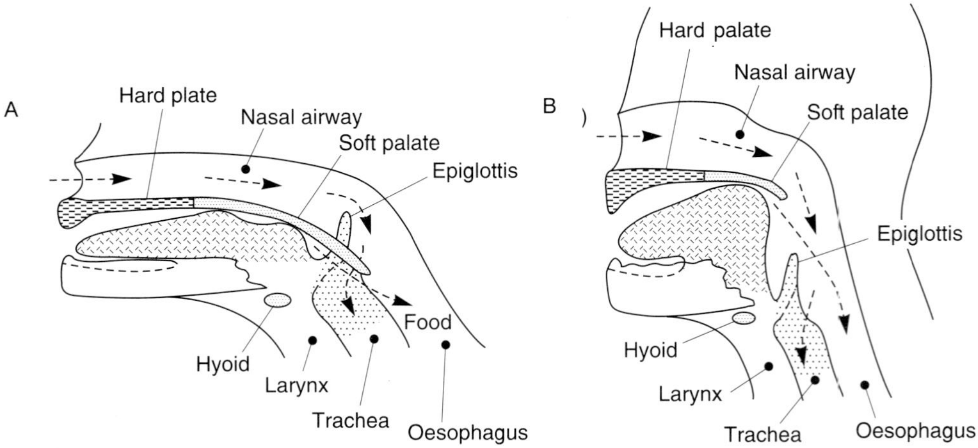

Fig. 12.3 A highly diagrammatic summary of the relative positions, in the parasagittal plane, of tongue, soft palate, epiglottis, larynx and pharynx in (A) a generalized mammal or an infant human and (B) an adult human. The specific differences that should be noted are:

1. In A the tongue is entirely oral, whereas in B it is not, the posterior part having descended to form the upper anterior wall of the pharynx.
2. In A the epiglottis makes contact with the posterior edge of the soft palate and extends above it, whereas in B there is no such contact. The difference reflects primarily a higher position of the larynx in A. The soft palate is shown extending a long way around the edge of the epiglottis and larynx but the extent of this varies with the species.
3. There is a clear supralaryngeal or oral part of the pharynx through which food passes in B but not in A. The space in B forms a resonator for sounds generated by the larynx and is crucial for modifying laryngeal sounds into the articulated speech of humans.
4. There is a single channel through the fauces in B but a division into two lateral food channels in A. Liquids pass in the lateral channels. Depending very much upon which species is considered (and probably depending upon age in the case of the human infant), swallowing of some solids may cause disengagement of the epiglottis from the soft palate; the epiglottis is then presumed to function much as in adult humans.
5. In A, a space exists immediately in front of the epiglottis, bounded above by the soft palate and below by the tongue. During feeding this space is occupied by the accumulating bolus which eventually induces a swallow. In B a bolus cannot accumulate in the same way although there is evidence that leakage of food into this region is the stimulus that elicits a swallow.

may be synchronous in all parts of the tongue or they may be differential, one part elongating whilst another shortens. The movements may subserve transport or may be concerned with food localization, in which case transport may be minimized. The varying coordination of these tongue movements with jaw movements can, in different cases, produce transport in a number of ways, either alone or in combination:

1. By squeezing (in which one component of the force is derived from the tongue acting vertically against the hard palate, so producing a pressure). Note that this may also be used to process some soft foods.
2. By sweeping (dorsum of tongue rolls back in contact with the hard palate and progresses posteriorly).
3. By negative pressure (anterior tongue advances, maintaining a seal against the hard palate while the posterior tongue is depressed).
4. By bodily retraction of the tongue.

It should be noted that the first three mechanisms only operate at low gapes and are more suited to the transport of liquid or soft food (note the long period spent at low gape in Fig. 12.2B). The fourth mechanism can act at any gape, the only requirement being that there is physical clearance between tongue and palate for the substance being transported. In contrast, during chewing, no net transport may be produced; in such cycles the tongue may be raised posteriorly to contact the palate while at the same time reducing its anteroposterior excursion. In addition, as found in humans and cats,[5,13] the tongue may twist around its long axis; this enables food on the dorsum of the tongue to be presented to the occluding surface of the teeth on one side. Such a movement is particularly associated with reduced anteroposterior excursions of the tongue.

If, in chewing cycles, the path of closure of the jaw is going to approximate to any standard path of movement, there are logical consequences. When the jaw opens, the gape between the cheek teeth is greater than is required to disengage from the bolus[14,15] and the subsequent closure of the jaw initially takes place only against gravity. Closure is therefore relatively rapid up to the point at which tooth–food–tooth contact is made; at this point there is a reduction in velocity as closure now has to continue against the resistance of the food.[16] Jaw closure, producing fracture of hard food, clearly requires more power than either jaw closure on soft food or jaw closure in cycles in which transport is the main function. The electromyogram (EMG) activity in the jaw-closing muscles is known to increase considerably at this time. Depending upon the size of the ingested lump of food, over 50% of the time for jaw-closing may consist of a loaded, slow closure (Fig. 12.2A). Conversely, closure on soft food has a high velocity throughout and it may be difficult to demonstrate any deceleration at tooth–food–tooth contact (Fig. 12.2B).

Swallow

The classical description of swallowing divides it into three stages. The first stage of the human adult swallow has been described as a conscious or voluntary movement which takes a prepared bolus to the level of the fauces. At this point a second or pharyngeal stage is said to be reflexly elicited and this is followed, after further passage of the bolus, by the third oesophageal stage.[17]

On the basis of cinefluorographic studies,[17–19] the generally accepted pattern of movement associated with the first two stages of a human command swallow starts with collection of the bolus in a spoon-shaped depression on the anterior tongue. The tongue is sealed anteriorly and laterally against palatal mucosa and posteriorly against the soft palate. The posterior tongue then depresses and the soft palate elevates while the original depression in the tongue proceeds to empty from front to back by sequential elevation of the midline of the anterior tongue. As the bolus is propelled through the pillars of the fauces (the start of the classical second stage), the posterior pharyngeal wall contracts, moving forward to meet the elevating soft palate. At this stage the hyoid elevates and the posterior tongue moves upwards and backwards, sweeping the bolus into the pharynx. The pharynx contracts, elevating the whole structure and it then exhibits a peristaltic wave. The bolus passes down through a relaxed pharyngo-oesophageal sphincter and so into the classical third or oesophageal stage. Because the upper pharynx also serves as a respiratory passage, respiration is inhibited while food is passing through it in the pharyngeal stage of the swallow; during this time the larynx tips forward into the back of the tongue and the epiglottis tips backwards over the entrance to the larynx; these actions protect the airway in adult humans.

At this stage it is worthwhile considering whether the general term swallow is always used by the various workers to mean exactly the same thing. Human swallows have been traditionally studied as they are carried out on command – in this particular situation they are initiated to deal with a single bolus, consciously held in the mouth, using a mechanism that depends very much upon the function of the motor cortex and the premotor cortex to produce another volitional action. This situation should be compared with the multiple unconscious swallows that occur during the normal course of a family meal. In contrast, in most non-human experimental studies, the swallows have been elicited either by direct electrical stimulation of the superior laryngeal nerve in anaesthetized animals or, as in the classical work of Miller and Sherrington,[20] by liquid placed on the posterior part of the tongue in decerebrate animals. In this last-mentioned case the placement of the liquid by cannula precludes the occurrence of any classical first stage. It is also known that superior laryngeal nerve stimulation elicits movements that correspond to the second or pharyngeal stage of swallowing. The fact that the 'swallow' may start with a pharyngeal stage also seems to be true for the mechanism, suggested by Storey,[21] in which the swallow is considered to be elicited reflexly by traces of saliva or food moving posteriorly and entering the vallecula (despite the supposed efficacy of the tongue/soft palate seal).

The general pattern of movement associated with swallowing in normally feeding conscious animals is different from that described from adult humans. After food has been mechanically reduced by chewing, it is transported further posteriorly (stage II transport) in one or more cycles in which the posterior part of the tongue is depressed and moved forwards while the anterior and mid-regions of the tongue are elevated. This leads to movement of softened food posteriorly and its accumulation as a bolus at the back of the tongue in the vallecula, the space between the posterior surface of the tongue and the anterior surface of the epiglottis (Fig 12.3). This ability to accumulate a significant bolus of comminuted, softened or liquid food in the vallecula, prior to a swallow, is associated with two important anatomical features that are not present in the human adult but are present in the human neonate:[22] first, a high larynx positioned intranarially, i.e. the epiglottis and laryngeal opening is at or above the level of the soft palate, and second, a seal between the soft palate and the epiglottis/larynx which extends on either side to a variable extent. There is also an intermediate seal between the tongue dorsum and the palate at about the level of the soft–hard palate junction.[2] These conditions produce a potential space for the temporary storage of a soft/liquid bolus between the posterior tongue, the epiglottis and the palate. The swallow (starting with a pharyngeal stage) only occurs when, following one or more stage II transport cycles, the stored volume in the vallecula reaches some predetermined level. This is very different from the classical description of the human adult swallow. However, within the first year of life of the human infant, the larynx descends (losing its seal with the soft palate) and a single soft palate–tongue seal is produced more anteriorly, on the posterior surface of the tongue.

When, in the decerebrate cat, swallowing is induced experimentally by placing liquid posteriorly on the tongue,[20] the path of movement of points on the posterior tongue and hyoid is found to be triangular in the sagittal plane when recorded cineradiographically. The posterior tongue firstly moves upwards/backwards and then moves forwards, followed by a return to its original position. This movement must characterize the pharyngeal stage because no first stage was permitted. If, on the other hand, the path of movement of points on the posterior tongue and the hyoid is recorded cineradiographically in the intact cat during normal lapping, it is seen to be characterized by a series of regular ellipses except, every few cycles, when the swallows occur.[4] In these swallow cycles, an extra movement of the tongue and hyoid is added to the normal cyclical forward movement of the tongue in an otherwise normal lapping cycle. The added movement consists of the upwards/backwards and then forwards movement that is seen in the decerebrate and which characterizes the pharyngeal stage. This implies that, in a swallow associated with normal rhythmic function, the part of the classical first stage of swallowing is taken by the normal cyclical jaw and tongue movement of ingestive activity. Recently, a cineradiographic study of the human swallow occurring in the context of normal feeding (i.e. *not* swallowing on command) has found that normal rhythmic cyclical behaviour immediately precedes and succeeds the classical pharyngeal stage of swallowing[10] so that the act of swallowing is embedded into a normal cycle, as in animals. Furthermore, evidence was found of food and/or saliva leakage into the valleculae prior to swallowing in a substantial proportion of swallows, despite the supposed tongue–palate seal. It was the entry of material into the valleculae that was usually associated with the onset of swallowing as previously suggested by Storey,[21] in this respect, humans behaved in much the same way as the animal model except that the latter allowed accumulation of a far more significant bolus in the vallecular region before swallowing.

The argument as to whether or not a swallow is a series of voluntary and reflex actions is of limited importance in view of the evidence for a central pattern generator for swallowing[17,23] although the evidence does seem to indicate that the first stage of swallowing is not included in the pattern generated. This central pattern generator, like the one for mastication (see below), can be activated by excitation converging from different sources. Such excitation may arrive from a number of sources; the two most obvious sources are the motor cortex (in response to drive for voluntary action) or a sensory nucleus (receiving sensory input from neurons innervating the posterior tongue or larynx). Activation of the pattern generator may therefore arise from either source or, more importantly, from both working in combination. This implies that, if the central pattern generator for swallowing is only weakly activated, the generation of sensory input by food in the region of the fauces or of the posterior tongue could raise the excitation of the generator sufficiently to trigger the production of swallowing movements, so appearing to elicit a reflex swallow. The ability of centrally and peripherally generated inputs to combine in various ways to generate a swallow has been referred to as divided control. Once activated, the pattern generator will drive the motor neurons involved in a particular temporal sequence, without the need for further sensory input.

Patterns of EMG activity

Even when swallowing is excluded, the movements of feeding involve far more muscles than those that have been narrowly defined as muscles of mastication simply because of their innervation by the trigeminal nerve; the movement of muscles innervated by the facial and by the hypoglossal nerves are equally important. A consideration of the overall pattern of EMG activity in all the circumstances outlined in the previous sections cannot be contained in this brief overview. However, the changes in the activity of the jaw-closing muscles in response to different foods will be considered. The EMG activity recorded from a group of muscle fibres reflects the number and the frequency of muscle action potentials which will determine the mechanical performance of those fibres (for given conditions of muscle length or shortening velocity). Depending upon the conditions under which the electrical signals are recorded, the amplitude of the EMG activity in the jaw-closing muscles can reflect the force of bite.[24]

The rhythmic EMG activity in the jaw-closing muscles starts with a low amplitude at about the time of maximum gape in each cycle and this activity continues as the jaw closes against gravity. However, when tooth–food–tooth contact is made (or shortly after), the amplitude of the EMG activity increases; the increase is large when hard food is contacted but is small when only soft food is contacted (Fig. 12.2). During the ingestion and mastication of a piece of hard food, the cyclical EMG activity in the jaw-closing muscles generally decreases with the progressive comminution and softening of a single small piece of food. The data therefore indicate that the force generated by the jaw muscles in some way responds to the food consistency. It is also known that sudden contact with hard material, hidden in otherwise soft food, causes an abrupt reduction in the EMG and a collapse of biting force. Again the force generated is matched to the food consistency. The mechanisms producing these effects can often be demonstrated as simple reflex actions.

Oral reflexes

The best known reflexes (that have at one time or another been reputed to be involved in mastication) are the jaw jerk, the jaw-opening reflex, the jaw-closing reflex and the unloading reflex. Besides being the essential sensory receptor for the jaw jerk, the muscle spindle is also considered to be involved in the unloading reflex and in producing load compensation, i.e. an automatic adjustment to a requirement for increased force of bite. If in any doubt as to the working of the muscle spindle, the reader should consult a modern physiology textbook. As will become apparent, the experimental evidence for the existence of a specific reflex, elicited by a particular sensory input, is rather less important than how that sensory input interacts with the masticatory rhythm generated by the central nervous system. As in the limbs, the main motor neurons exciting the jaw muscles will be referred to as α motor neurons, but the motor neurons controlling the intrafusal fibres of the muscle spindles will be designated fusimotor neurons (rather than γ motor neurons).[25]

The jaw jerk is a reflex upward movement of the jaw that can be elicited by a sudden downwards deflection of the jaw, e.g. produced by tapping the chin downwards. The reflex should not be confused with the jaw-closing reflex either, as described by Sherrington[26] or by Thexton.[27] The receptors detecting the externally imposed muscle stretch that elicits the jaw jerk are the muscle spindles in the jaw-closing muscles. Activation of these spindles causes a burst of impulses that travel to the central nervous system and produce excitation of the motor neurons of the jaw-closing muscles. Muscle spindles are complex receptors that can have their sensitivity to change of length and to rate of change of length independently altered by the action of the central nervous system, i.e. by fusimotor activity. These receptors are muscle length detectors and, as such, are involved in the maintenance of posture, including that of the mandible, quite apart from any function in mastication (see below). Some general explanation of the more important functions of the muscle spindle (in relation to mastication) will be given later but it is not possible to deal with the functions of the muscle spindle in any detail in this chapter.

The jaw-opening reflex, as classically described in animals, can be elicited by brief mechanical stimuli applied to teeth or mucosa or by electrical stimuli applied to any of the sensory nerve fibres of the second and third divisions of the trigeminal nerve.[26,28] The classically described response consists of activation of the digastric muscle with a simultaneous inhibition of the activity of the elevator muscles of the jaw,[26] in accordance with the concept of reciprocal innervation. However, more recently, evidence has been obtained indicating that the two classical elements of the reflex can be elicited separately by appropriate stimuli.[27,29,30] This is consistent either with the digastric and jaw-closing motor neurons having different thresholds (for their activation and inhibition respectively) by sensory input arriving at the central nervous system by a single common route, or with two quite separate reflex pathways, one for digastric activation and one for jaw-closing inhibition.

In the light of this finding, it is less surprising that the so-called jaw-opening reflex in humans normally only consists of inhibition of the jaw-closing muscles.[31] It is this inhibition, elicited by periodontal loading, that is probably the basis of many of the so-called silent periods that appear in the EMG of the jaw-closing muscles (see Linden[32] for a review of periodontal mechanisms in general). These short periods of electrical silence, each lasting 10–20 ms, occur when the teeth come into sudden contact with each other or with hard food. Silent periods are particularly evident when chewing brittle foods, such as hard biscuit. It should however be noted that a silent period is simply a brief lack of activity and this can arise in a whole variety of ways. First, it can be caused by activation of any receptor that drives an inhibitory reflex arc acting on the elevator motor neurons. Second, a silent period can arise if a sensory input causes a sudden brief excitation of the motor neurons and results in their synchronization; this synchronization of activity is then followed by a very brief period without activity because the refractory periods, that follow each generation of an action potential, will also be synchronized.[31] Subsequently the motor neurons return to their normal asynchronous pattern of firing and produce the normal EMG interference pattern. It is therefore dangerous to ascribe the existence of a silent period to a specific mechanism unless additional information is available.

There are multiple sources of excitation that may act upon the elevator motor neurons but two have received particular attention. First there are a number of reports indicating that brief mechanical stimuli applied to the periodontal membrane or to oral mucosa can produce signs of apparent excitation (in addition to the inhibition described above) in the EMG activity of the jaw-closing muscles.[29,33,34] Knowledge of such an excitatory mechanism, representing a jaw-closing reflex, would be important because it could represent a mechanism whereby bite force could be reflexly increased upon tooth–food–tooth contact. Objections to a simple interpretation of these experiments can however be raised on the following bases:

1. A brief mechanical stimulus applied to a tooth inevitably spreads and may involve distant receptors, such as the jaw-closing muscle spindles, which also cause excitation of the jaw-closing muscles.[31]
2. Any input that simply causes synchronization of motor neurons, even without increasing the total activation, can result in an apparent temporary increase of the peak-to-peak amplitude of the EMG and be mistaken for increased excitation.[35]

However a number of authors have reported that electrical stimulation of mucocutaneous or dental afferent nerve fibres (not spreading to excite other structures) can, under certain experimental conditions, produce signs of elevator motor neuron or EMG excitation.[27,36,37] This indicates that an excitatory pathway to the jaw-closing motor neurons does exist for oral sensory input but this does not necessarily mean that the pathway is actually functional in normal feeding. The matter is far from settled and requires further investigation.

There is no dispute that the α motor neurons of the jaw-closing muscles are excited by the afferents from their muscle spindles and it has been suggested that these sensory receptors are capable of supplying the sensory input that increases the force of bite upon making tooth–food–tooth contact and slowing jaw closure – a load compensation mechanism. An extension of this proposition is that the sensory input from the spindles enables comparison of the executed movement to be made with the intended movement (the motor template) so that corrective action can be taken if any discrepancy arises; this proposition is currently difficult to test because it appears that the motor template itself may vary, depending upon mucosal sensory inputs (see below). The hypothesized mechanism of load compensation is complex and only a simplified description is given here (see Taylor[25] for a more extensive account).

It is necessary to bear in mind that if the spindle were composed purely of sensory elements and the main muscle mass contracted/shortened, the sensory elements in the spindle would be less stretched and would therefore reduce their firing rate. Because the afferents from the spindle form excitatory synapses on the motor neurons, the reduced firing of the spindle would reduce the excitation of the motor neurons as soon as the latter caused muscle contraction. This would mean that excitation arising from a command signal, e.g. from the motor cortex, could be offset by reduction in excitation from the spindles – the command might not be carried out effectively. There is however a fusimotor supply to the spindle which is capable of contracting special muscle fibres (intrafusal muscles) in the spindle; this intrafusal contraction maintains the stretch of the sensory elements and compensates for external muscle shortening. The suggestion is that, in the case of unhindered jaw-closing, the pattern of fusimotor drive to the intrafusal muscles parallels the activation of the α motor neurons so that the two types of muscle shorten to the same extent. As a consequence the sensory endings in the spindle would not be subject to any length change and would not change their firing rate despite the fact that the muscle mass was shortening. Any command signal to the motor neurons would then be carried out faithfully. On the other hand, if tooth contact is made with a hard piece of food, the shortening of the main muscle mass will initially be reduced or stopped because insufficient force will be available to continue closure against the resistance. However, the shortening of the intrafusal muscles continues because the only work being done by the intrafusal muscles is that of stretching the region of the muscle spindle containing the sensory elements. The intrafusal contraction therefore stretches the sensory endings of the spindle which generate action potentials at an increased frequency. These have excitatory effects on the motor neurons of the jaw closing muscles and so increase the force of closure. The crucial requirement of this mechanism is an increase in fusimotor drive during loaded jaw closure; such an increase has been found in some cycles in the cat.[38]

Although much attention has been directed to the excitation produced by stretching muscle spindle afferents, the converse (reduced excitation upon passive shortening) is also important because, when there is a sudden shortening of the muscles, a period of electrical silence occurs in the EMGs of the jaw-closing muscles. Such a shortening can occur in the jaw-closing muscles when a piece of brittle food suddenly yields during biting. Because the muscle spindle afferents normally supply part of the excitation of the jaw-closing motor neurons, the effect of sudden uncompensated shortening of the muscle is a brief failure on the part of the muscle spindles to generate afferent impulses. The resultant fall in the excitation of the motor neurons leads to a period of silence in the EMG; this is known as the unloading reflex. Its effect is to decelerate jaw closure following food fracture.

The effects of some of the oral sensory inputs upon the jaw-closing muscles in particular are summarized in Table 12.1.

Table 12.1 Some oral receptors, their afferent pathways and the effects they exert on jaw-closing muscles

		Cell bodies in ganglion or in mesencephalic nucleus		*Trigeminal nuclei to which central processes project*	*Reflex action on jaw-closing motor neurons*
Periodontal membrane					
Mechanoreceptors	→	Ganglion	→	Main sensory, spinal	Inhibition–disynaptic
Mechanoreceptors	→	Mesencephalic	→	Uncertain	Uncertain but possibly excitation
Nociceptors	→	Ganglion		Spinal	Inhibition–disynaptic
Mucosa and mucoperiosteum					
Mechanoreceptors	→	Ganglion		Main sensory, spinal	Inhibition–disynaptic
Mechanoreceptors	→	Mesencephalic		Uncertain	Uncertain but possibly excitation
Nociceptors	→	Ganglion		Spinal	Inhibition–disynaptic
Muscle					
Spindles	→	Mesencephalic		Motor	Excitation–monosynaptic
Golgi tendon ganglion	→	Ganglion		Probably main sensory and/or Spinal	Inhibition–disynaptic (by analogy with limbs)
Joint capsule					
Mechanoreceptors	→	Ganglion		Probably main sensory and/or Spinal	Inhibition
Nociceptors	→	Ganglion		Spinal	Inhibition (by analogy with limbs)

Notes
1. The above effects are described where possible on the basis of direct evidence but otherwise on the basis of best guess or by analogy with findings in the limbs.
2. The effects upon muscle groups other than the jaw closers may be very different, e.g. temporomandibular joint receptors stimulated during passive jaw opening will reflexly activate the genioglossus and so produce tongue protraction.
3. When the masticatory pattern generator is active, reflex effects (such as those in the table) can be modulated rhythmically in time with masticatory activity. On the other hand, when certain hypothalamic centres are activated, the threshold for the reflexes may be tonically increased or decreased.

Generation of rhythmic movement of the jaws

It has been known for over 150 years that rhythmic jaw movements can be present in anencephalic human infants; in passing, it should be noted that it has also been known from time immemorial that headless chickens can run but it was, for a long time, fashionable to ignore the ability of the lower centres to generate organized movement. The evidence, therefore, indicates that rhythmic movement can be generated by the nervous system in the absence of the cerebral hemispheres. The earliest well-known attempts at explaining the origin of the motor rhythms were all broadly based on the idea of a series of interacting reflexes. The proposition was that each reflex produced a motor response that caused a new sensory input that in turn elicited the next reflex – the reflex chain theory.

One of the earliest attempts at explaining masticatory rhythm[26] proposed that the presence of food in the mouth elicited a jaw-opening reflex and that the jaw opening was followed automatically by a central rebound phenomenon; the latter was considered to cause jaw closure and so lead to force being exerted on the food item by the teeth. The idea was that the jaw-opening reflex was then re-elicited by the periodontal stimulation so that the cycle repeated itself *ad infinitum*. Subsequently Jerge[39] modified the concept by suggesting that the jaw-opening movement itself directly induced a reflex closing which was caused by the reflex response to stretch of muscle spindles in the temporal and masseter muscles during jaw opening. In other words, closure was considered to be due to a jaw jerk. Although at first glance, these concepts did seem to indicate how rhythmic jaw movements might be produced in decerebrate animals or anencephalic infants, when the time course of a simple reflex and the time course of the jaw movement in, say, a cow chewing the cud are considered, one has to conclude that the hypothesis had its faults.

Over roughly the same time period, a quite different set of propositions were advanced by others who had observed that stimulation of the motor cortex and other subcortical structures of animal and humans could produce movements of different parts of the body (see for example Rioch[40] or Penfield and Boldrey[41]). This led to propositions that masticatory movements were voluntary or were, perhaps, in some way learnt but became unconscious (by analogy with the process of learning to ride a bicycle). However this approach failed to explain how rhythmic jaw movements could exist in the anencephalic infant or decerebrate adult animal.

Despite their contradictory nature, both hypotheses seemed to exist side by side for over half a century. Meanwhile, Bremer[42] had published a paper that was fundamental to the basis of present-day thinking on the generation of masticatory rhythm. Unfortunately, perhaps because it was published in French, his paper remained largely ignored by the English-language literature for about 50 years. Bremer was able to show experimentally that masticatory behaviour could be produced either by stimulation of the cerebral hemispheres or by stimulation of the oral cavity. The basic Bremer proposition was that there was a brainstem *centre de corrélation* capable of producing the coordinated rhythmic movements of feeding and that this was capable of being switched on or driven by neuronal activity arriving from different sources, i.e. either by action potentials descending from the cortex in a corticobulbar pathway or arriving from the periphery as trigeminal sensory input. This model therefore avoided some of the contradictions inherent in a narrow interpretation of the reflex chain and the cortically originating theories. The original ideas of Bremer have been extensively refined and extended by Dellow and Lund[43] and subsequently by Lund and coworkers in a series of papers (see, for example, Lund[44]). The existence of a rhythm/pattern generator in the brainstem, reponsible for driving cranial motor neurons to produce the various oral movements of feeding, is now generally accepted.

One interesting aspect of the rhythm generator is that it can cause the fusimotor activity (acting on intrafusal muscle) to fluctuate in a cyclic manner without causing activation of the α motor neurons and muscular activity;[24] this is an example of the separation of rhythm generation from executive action, as indicated in Figure 12.4.

Interaction between oral sensory input and rhythm generator

A matter of some importance is, however, how sensory information from the mouth might interact with the rhythm generator to produce the changes in cyclic oral behaviour that occur with food consistency change. The most obvious mechanism is that the sensory input simply sums with the other sources of excitatory or inhibitory input in the rhythm generator and/or it sums with the rhythmic excitatory output from the rhythm generator at the level of the motor neuron (Fig. 12.4). On theoretical grounds the two destinations would be expected to produce different effects; increased excitation of the rhythm generator would be expected primarily to change the period of its oscillation whereas increased excitation of the motor neurons would be expected to increase the amplitude of the activity with no change in periodicity.

The central nervous system has the general ability to control its own sensory input and there is good evidence that the brainstem rhythm generator has a specific ability to inhibit the digastric reflex (elicited from dental tissues) at certain stages during the jaw cycle, e.g. during jaw closure.[45] The relevance of some of the experimental evidence to normal mastication is however disputed,[30] the critical test being the proof of the ability of the rhythm generator to inhibit, during jaw-closing, the afferents that would normally cause jaw-closing motor neuron inhibition (Fig. 12.5). If proven, it could perhaps explain why brief inhibition of the jaw-closing muscles may be produced experimentally in humans, by a 50 g tap applied to a tooth, whereas forces that are 100–1000 times larger can be applied to the same tooth during mastication. It should also be noted that, during the various forms of cyclic behaviour of the jaws, the modulation of the digastric reflex elicited from the tongue[11] is

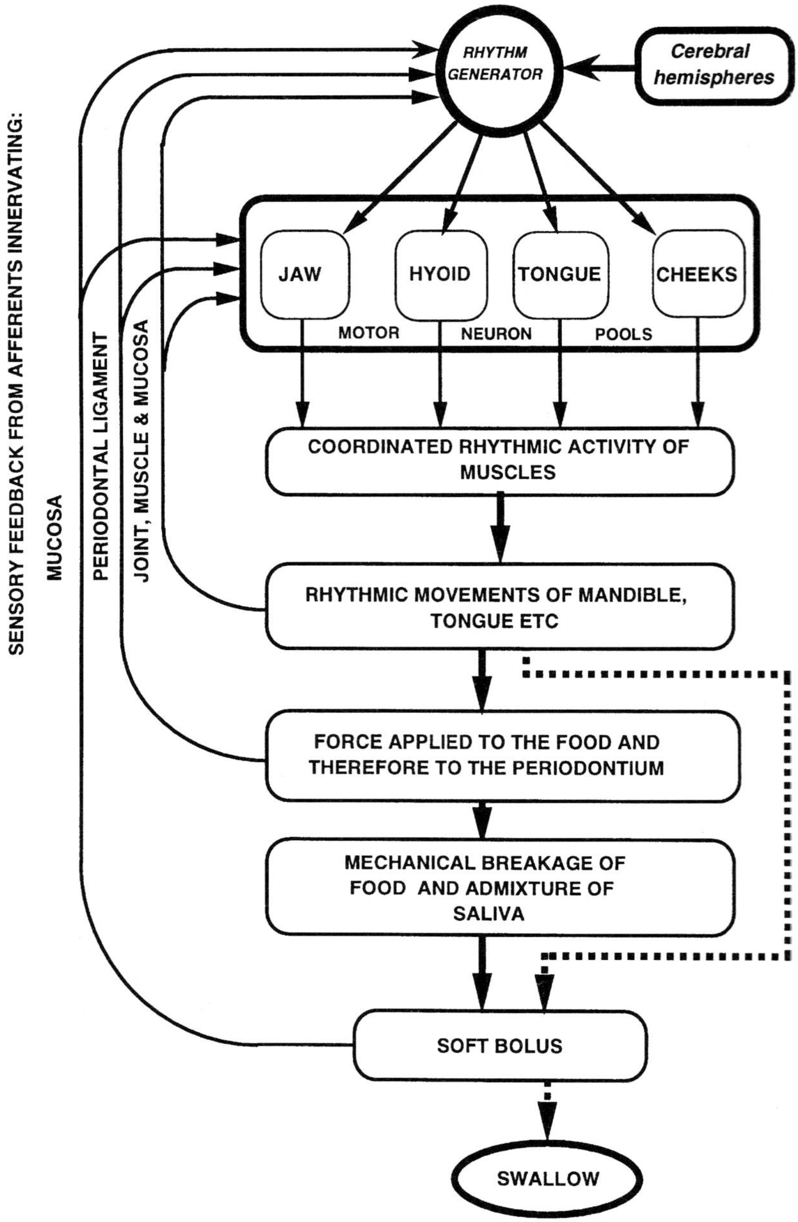

Fig. 12.4 An outline of the probable organization of the systems controlling mastication. The rhythm generator supplies correctly patterned drive to each of the motor neuron pools controlling the jaw-closing/opening muscles, the hyoid-linked muscles, the tongue muscles and cheek/facial muscles. This activation produces rhythmic jaw movements which will cause a variety of sensory inputs to be generated, partly by mucosal contact with the food and partly because of changes of muscle length and joint rotation. At some stage force will be exerted on teeth and stimulate the periodontal receptors. The sensory input that is generated may influence either the rhythm generator itself or the motor neurons driven by it. If hard food is present in the mouth, the mechanical contact with mucosa is likely to be made at points or very localized areas, whereas if the food is soft and flows easily, a broad area of contact with the mucosa is likely to arise. It seems that the latter can change the nature of the masticatory cycle. It is proposed that, in this case, chewing does not occur and transport mechanisms are enhanced, leading eventually to a swallow (see dotted line).

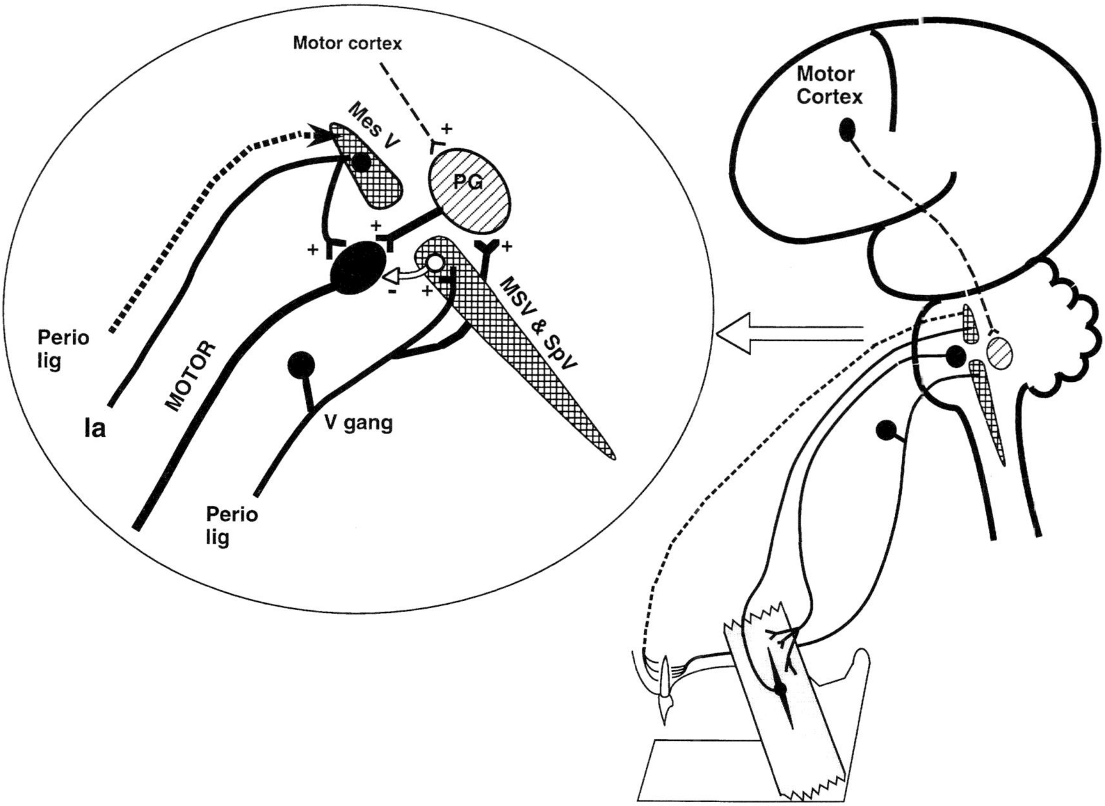

Fig. 12.5 A simplified schematic representation of some afferent and some descending pathways that influence the jaw-closing muscles.

Note that there are two afferent pathways shown originating from mechanoreceptors in the periodontal membrane. In one case the cell bodies are located in the trigeminal ganglion (V gang) and the central processes pass to the main sensory (MSV) and to the spinal nuclei (SpV) of the trigeminal nerve; some of these afferents are known to form a disynaptic inhibitory pathway acting on the motor neurons of the jaw-closing muscles (it should be noted that some mucosal afferents will follow the same path). The cell bodies of neurons forming the other afferent pathway from the periodontal membrane are located in the mesencephalic nucleus (Mes V); the direct reflex action of these neurons is unclear although, if any analogy can be made with the action of the muscle spindle projections to the same nucleus, there is a possibility that they could be involved in some as yet unproven excitatory drive to the jaw-closing motor neurons. Unfortunately, the only case where there is currently good evidence for this action is in the shark.

The muscle spindle afferents are shown with a traditional monosynaptic connection to the jaw-closing motor neurons. Unlike the reciprocal inhibitory system of the limbs, the muscle spindle afferents do not exert a disynaptic inhibition on the motor neurons of muscles that are presumed to be antagonists.

Note that two descending pathways probably exist, arising from the motor area of the cerebral cortex. One pathway, which may make a monosynaptic contact with the motor neuron pool, represents a path to motor neurons carrying instructions for precise voluntary movement; note however that evidence also exists for such a pathway being disynaptic. It is also known that jaw-closing motor neurons may receive their input indirectly from the cerebral cortex, i.e. via interneurons shared with other inputs; this pathway (dashed line) is shown in the figure as contacting interneurons which are associated with a pattern generator (PG). These interneurons associated with the PG also receive input from other peripheral sensory receptors (see also Fig. 12.4). The proposition is that activation of the pathway from cortex to PG would produce rhythmic activity while the other cortically originating pathway (not shown) would be employed in precision non-rhythmic movements.

not necessarily the same as that described by Lund *et al.*[45] for the reflex elicited from purely dental structures.

Occasionally it has been possible to change the natural intraoral sensory input during an established rhythmic activity in a normally feeding animal; this has been accomplished by the simple expedient of hiding solids on the false floor of a container filled with milk and raising the floor during established lapping. In such experiments it has been found that tongue (and possibly palate) contact with particles of solid food suspended in a liquid can be sufficient to change the cycle type from one that is characteristic of liquid transport to one that is characteristic of solid food transport, i.e. by increasing jaw opening so that it coincides with tongue retraction and converts the cycle to one that is appropriate to stage I transport for solids.[12] It is also known that the mucosal stimulation caused by a liquid bolus placed on the back of the tongue will induce a change of cycle type by producing a swallow. It therefore seems possible that mucosal sensory inputs may be generally capable of changing the type of feeding cycle. The possible involvement of periodontal receptors in this process cannot be ignored, if only because some primary afferents innervate not just periodontal membrane but mucosa as well.[47]

Summary

The cycles of jaw and tongue movement during feeding subserve not only the breakage of food but also the transport of food through the oral cavity. In cycles subserving mainly a transport function, e.g. when eating very soft foods, the anteroposterior movements of the tongue (or parts of the tongue) are greater than in chewing cycles. Tongue protraction occurs at a low gape and an increase in protraction is usually associated with a prolongation of the time spent by the jaw at low or moderate gapes. Closure on hard food is associated with a reduction in closing velocity as tooth–food–tooth contact is made and a period of slow jaw closure associated with a big increase in the EMG activity in the jaw-closing muscles; closure on soft food may not show any such change. The profile of jaw movement (gape versus time) consequently varies with food consistency, some of the variation being due to the nature of the tongue movements. The predictable variation in cycle type, with variation in food consistency, strongly suggests that sensory input controls the form of the cyclical tongue and jaw movements.

A basic pattern of movement is probably produced by the activity of a brainstem rhythm/pattern generator which in turn drives the relevant motor neuron pools. The rhythm generator can be driven by nerve impulses descending from higher centres or by nerve impulses arriving as sensory input from the periphery.

It is arguable that sensory input from mucosal receptors (e.g. of palate and tongue) is responsible for controlling cycle type. It is rather more certain that, because of patterned fusimotor drive, the sensory input from muscle spindles ensures some adherence to a motor template – jaw-closing activity is increased when solid food is encountered so that divergence of the path of closure from some norm or template is reduced. It is also reasonably certain that the periodontal afferents exert some form of corrective action in relation to excessive or sudden bite forces on the teeth.

The non-command swallow, i.e. that occurring in normal feeding, appears to consist of the equivalent of the classical second stage of swallowing inserted into the occlusal or initial jaw-opening phase of an otherwise standard cycle. Swallowing is produced by a pattern generator in the brainstem which receives inputs from both cortical and peripheral sources. Leakage of traces of food or saliva into the vallecula appears to be a peripheral sensory input of major importance in inducing a swallow.

References

1. Hiiemae KM, Thexton AJ, Crompton AW. Intra-oral food transport: the fundamental mechanism of feeding. In: Carlson DS, McNamara JA. (eds) *Muscle Adaptation in the Craniofacial Region. Monograph no. 8*, pp. 181–208. Craniofacial Growth Series. Center for Human Growth and Development, University of Michigan, Michigan: Ann Arbor, 1978.
2. Hiiemae KM, Crompton AW. Mastication, food transport and swallowing. In: Hildebrand M, Bramble D, Liem K, Wake D (eds) *Functional Vertebrate Morphology*, pp. 262–290. Cambridge, Massachusetts USA: Belknap Press of Harvard University Press, 1985.
3. Franks HA, Crompton AW, German RZ. Mechanism of intra-oral transport in Macaques. *Am J Phys Anthrop* 1984; **65**: 275–282.
4. Thexton AJ, McGarrick JD. Tongue movement of the cat during lapping. *Arch Oral Biol* 1988; **33**: 331–339.
5. Thexton AJ, McGarrick, JD. Tongue movement in the cat during the intake of solid food. *Arch Oral Biol* 1989; **34**: 239–248.
6. Lucas PW, Luke DA. Methods for analysing the breakdown of food in human mastication. *Arch Oral Biol* 1983; **28**: 813–819.

7. van der Glas HW, van der Bilt A, Olthoff LW, Bosman F. Measurement of selection chances and breakage functions during chewing in man. *J Dent Res* 1987; **66**: 1547–1550
8. van der Bilt A, Olthoff HW, van der Glas LW *et al.* A mathematical description of the comminution of food during mastication in man. *Arch Oral Biol* 1987; **32**: 579–586.
9. Kapur KK, Garrett NR, Fischer E. Effects of anaesthesia of human oral structures on masticatory performance and food particle size distribution. *Arch Oral Biol* 1990; **35**: 397–403.
10. Palmer JB, Rudin NJ, Lara G *et al.* Coordination of mastication swallowing. *Dysphagia* 1992; **7**: 187–200.
11. Thexton AJ, McGarrick JD. Effect of experimentally elicited rhythmic oral activity on the linguodigastric reflex in the lightly anaesthetised rabbit. *Exp Neurol* 1987; **96**: 104–117.
12. Thexton AJ, Crompton AW. Effect of sensory input from the tongue on jaw movement in normal feeding in the opossum. *J Exp Zool* 1989; **250**: 233–243.
13. Abd-el-Malek S. The part played by the tongue in mastication and deglutition. *J Anat* 1955; **89**: 250–254.
14. Thexton AJ, Hiiemae KM, Crompton AW. Food consistency and bite size as regulators of jaw movement during feeding in the cat. *J Neurophysiol* 1980; **44**: 456–474.
15. Lucas PW, Ow RKK, Ritchie GM. *et al.* Relationship between jaw movement and food breakdown in human mastication. *J Dent Res* 1986; **65**: 400–404.
16. Hiiemae KM. Mammalian mastication: a review of the activity of the jaw muscles and the movement they produce in chewing. In: Butler PM, Joysey KA (eds) *Studies on the Development, Structure and Function of the Teeth*, pp. 360–398. London: Academic Press, 1978.
17. Miller AJ. Deglutition. *Physiol Rev* 1982; **62**: 129–184.
18. Ardran GM, Kemp FH. Biting and masticatiom: a cine-radiographic study. *Dent Practitioner* 1960; **9**: 23–36.
19. Ardran GM, Kemp FH. The tongue. In: Lodge T, Steiner RE (eds) *Recent Advances in Radiology*, pp. 77–87. London: Churchill Livingstone, 1975.
20. Miller FR, Sherrington CS. Some observations on the buccopharyngeal stage of reflex deglutition in the cat. *Q J Exp Physiol* 1915; **9**: 147–186.
21. Storey AT. Interactions of alimentary and upper respiratory tract reflexes. In: Sessle BJ, Hannam AJ (eds) *Mastication and Swallowing: Biological and Clinical Correlates*, pp. 22–36. Toronto: University of Toronto Press, 1976.
22. Laitmann JT. The ontogenetic and phylogenetic development of the upper respiratory system and basicranium in man. Yale University Ph.D. Ann Arbor, Michigan: Xerox University Microfilms, 1977.
23. Jean A. Brainstem control of swallowing: localization and organization of the central pattern generator. In: Taylor A. (ed) *Neurophysiology of the Teeth and Jaws*, pp. 294–321. Basingstoke: Macmillan Press, 1990.
24. Hylander WL, Johnson KR. The relationship between masseter force and masseter electromyogram during mastication in the monkey *Macaca fascicularis. Arch Oral Biol* 1989; **34**: 713–722.
25. Taylor A. Proprioceptive control of jaw movement. In: Taylor A (ed) *Neurophysiology of the Teeth and Jaws*, pp. 237–263. Basingstoke: Macmillan Press, 1990.
26. Sherrington CS. Reflexes elicitable from pinna, vibrissae and jaws. *J Physiol* 1917; **51**: 404–451.
27. Thexton AJ. Jaw opening and jaw closing reflexes in the cat. *Brain Res* 1974; **66**: 425–433.
28. Blais M, Genest R, Robillard E. Elements anatomiques du reflexe linguo-maxillaire. *Rev Can Biol* 1943; **2**: 128–113.
29. Thexton AJ. Oral reflexes elicited by mechanical stimulation of palatal mucosa in the cat. *Arch Oral Biol* 1973; **18**: 971–980.
30. Dessem D, Iyadurai OD, Taylor A. The role of periodontal receptors in the jaw-opening reflex in the cat. *J Physiol* 1988; **406**: 315–330.
31. Matthews B. Mastication. In: Lavelle CLB. (ed) *Applied Physiology of the Mouth*, pp. 199–242. Bristol: John Wright, 1975.
32. Linden RWA. Periodontal mechanoreceptors and their functions. In: Taylor A (ed) *Neurophysiology of the Teeth and Jaws*, pp. 52–88. Basingstoke: Macmillan Press, 1990.
33. Goldberg LJ. Masseter muscle excitation induced by stimulation of periodontal and gingival receptors in man. *Brain Res* 1971; **32**: 369–380.
34. Sessle BJ, Schmidt A. Effects of controlled tooth stimulation on jaw activity in man. *Arch Oral Biol* 1972; **17**: 1597–1607.
35. Widmer CG, Lund JP. Evidence that peaks in EMG averages can sometimes be caused by inhibition of motoneurons. *J Neurophysiol* 1989; **62**: 212–219.
36. Kidokoro Y, Kubota K, Shuto S *et al.* Reflex organization of cat masticatory muscles. *J Neurophysiol* 1968; **31**: 695–708.
37. Achari NK, Thexton AJ. Diencephalic influences on the jaw opening reflex in the cat. *Arch Oral Biol* 1972; **17**: 1073–1080.
38. Taylor A, Appenteng K, Morimoto T. Proprioceptive input from the jaw muscles and its influence on lapping, chewing and posture. *Can J Physiol Pharmacol* 1981; **59**: 636–644.
39. Jerge CR. The neurologic mechanism underlying cyclic jaw movements. *J Prosth Dent* 1964; **14**: 667–681.
40. Rioch J. Neural mechanisms of mastication. *Am J Physiol* 1934; **108**: 168–176.
41. Penfield W, Boldrey E. Somatic motor and sensory representation in central cortex of man as studied by electrical stimulation. *Brain* 1937; **60**: 389–443.
42. Bremer F. Physiologie nerveuse de la mastication chez le chat et le lapin. *Arch Int Physiol* 1923; **21**: 309–352.
43. Dellow PG, Lund JP. Evidence for central timing of rhythmical mastication. *J Physiol* 1971; **215**: 1–13.

44. Lund JP. Evidence for a central neural pattern generator regulating the chewing cycle. In: Anderson DJ, Matthews B (eds) *Mastication*, pp. 204–212. Bristol: Wright, 1976.
45. Lund JP, Enomoto S, Hayashi H *et al.* Phase linked variations in the amplitude of the digastric nerve jaw opening reflex response during fictive mastication in the rabbit. *Can J Physiol Pharmacol* 1983; **61**: 1122–1128.
46. Olson KA, Lund JP, Valiquette C, Veilleux D. Activity during mastication of periodontal mechanosensitive neurons of the trigeminal subnucleus oralis of the rabbit. *J Neurophysiol* 1988; **59**: 341–357.
47. Hiiemae KM, Heath MR, Heath G, Kazazoglu E, Murray J, Hamblett K. Natural bites, food consistency and feeding behavior in man. *Arch Oral Biol* 1996; **41**: 175–189.
48. Hiiemae KM, Reese A, Hayenga SM. Patterns of tongue and jaw movement: a cinefluorographic study of feeding in the macaque. *Arch Oral Biol* 1995; **40**: 222–246.

13

Taste

Roger W. A. Linden

Summary

When we eat or drink we perceive a sensation that is often described as taste. A better term for it would be flavour, because the experience is made up of different modalities of sensation. Amongst these modalities are those of smell, touch (texture), temperature and, of course, the chemical sense of taste. In this chapter only the sensations of oral chemoreception will be described. The distribution and the morphology of the chemoreceptors within the oral cavity, the mechanisms involved in the transduction of the signal and the central connections of the nerve fibres innervating the receptors will be discussed.

Introduction

Although this chapter is confined to the sense of taste, one of the special senses of the animal kingdom, it is also important to mention the special sense of smell. Many patients will not realize the role smell plays in what they commonly call taste. For example, we all know that a foul-tasting medicine has little taste if the nose is held during swallowing and that we lose our sense of taste when we have a common cold which blocks our nose. It has been reported that astronauts have complained that they lose their sense of taste while in zero gravity. The cause of this is thought to be congestion in the nose due to the increased capillary pressure in the head, as the heart no longer has to work against gravity and there is a considerable reduction in hydrostatic pressures.

Taste and smell are both forms of chemically induced sensation. They have not been studied as extensively as the other special senses; however, they are important in humans particularly when eating. Patients who have lost their sense of taste or smell report that much of the pleasure of eating is also lost. In addition these patients are also deprived of the natural warning system that alerts one of the presence of toxic substances in the food.

It is important to define carefully the term taste when it is used biologically. The word taste is commonly used to describe the sensation produced by placing food in the mouth. Yet flavour and gustation also describe this sensation. For the purposes of this chapter taste will refer to the sensation experienced during stimulation of oral chemoreceptors and will include stimulation of specialized receptor cells in the taste buds and free nerve endings in the oral cavity. Gustation will be used to describe chemoreception mediated by receptor cells in taste buds, and the common chemical sense will be used to describe chemoreception mediated by free nerve endings. Taste buds are in effect gustatory end-organs.

The popular view of the interplay between taste and olfaction is that the two are closely linked. The perceived intensity of a mixture of odorant and tastant presented into the oral cavity is very close to the sum of the perceived intensities of the unmixed components. This near-perfect additive effect supports the view that there is no true sensory interaction between olfaction and taste. When the nostrils are open so that the odour from the air in the oral cavity can reach the nasal cavity, subjects rate the taste as higher or stronger and when the nostrils are closed, the rating is lower. However, it must be emphasized that this so-called taste sensation is probably a mixture of different modalities of stimuli, not just gustatory and olfactory, but also includes stimulation of common chemical receptors, thermoreceptors and mechanoreceptors signalling textures. All of these could interact in an additive, synergistic or even inhibitory effect to produce the complex sensation of flavour.

Although these definitions apply well to all vertebrates, they do not apply so well to invertebrates which have no receptors that look like taste buds yet still have chemoreceptors, in their mouth parts, that are used in feeding.

In vertebrates, the sense of taste is used not only to detect food but also to determine its suitability for eating. It is said that children grow normally and remain in good health when left alone to select their own diet from a wide variety of natural unprocessed foods. Rats also select food according to their dietary requirements when given a large choice of purified food. Taste appears to play an important role in this selection. There appears to be a relationship between the palatability and nutritive value of eating different foods. The gustatory system has receptors that are tuned to bitter-tasting compounds which are often potentially harmful (e.g. alkaloids). The rejection response to bitter tastes and the acceptance of sweet foods appear to be inborn and not learned responses. It has been demonstrated that newborn infants show preferences to sugar, aversions to acids and bitter stimuli and are relatively indifferent to salt solutions. This suggests that the sense of taste is to some degree functional at birth. However, these preferences and aversions change after birth, with the major changes occurring with salt solutions. The indifference to 0.1–0.2 mol/l salt solutions changes to a preference at 4–24 months, but between the ages of 31 and 60 months children reject these solutions.

The aversion to bitter tastes can be, and often is, overcome in humans by what is called an acquired taste. The bitter taste of hops in beer would be rejected by a baby but savoured by an adult. Salt preference is also seen in many mammals that are salt-depleted. One of the best examples of this is when steel mill workers would add considerable amounts of salt to their beer after their work shift. The beer would be unpalatable at any time other than when they had finished their hard working shift in high temperatures. The evidence, in humans and animals, is that taste plays an important role in this preference for high sodium salt solutions.

In animal studies it has been shown that the initiation and satiation of this need for salt are not dependent on the plasma concentration of Na^+, but are more likely to depend on taste. The salt-depleted animals will lose interest in a high-salt solution after 2–3 min drinking yet their plasma sodium ion concentration takes between 15 and 30 min to reach normal values. Arterial infusion of sodium chloride for 15 min, which produces a rapid rise in plasma sodium ion concentrations, does not appear to affect sodium appetite in the short term in these animals.

From these experiments it would appear that taste is important in satisfying a salt appetite. Similarly, animals made hypoglycaemic by insulin have been shown markedly to increase their intake of sweet-tasting solutions whether they are nutritive or not. This suggests that their appetite for sweet is related to the taste rather than the nutritional value of the solution.

The common chemical sense from free nerve endings in the oral cavity also plays a role in feeding. Chili peppers (*Capsicum* sp.) and pepper (*Piper nigrum*) contain chemicals such as capsaicin and piperine that stimulate chemical nociceptors, particularly those in the oral and anal mucous membranes. These chemicals would be expected to prevent animals from eating the fruits and seeds of these plants. However, humans have acquired a taste for food that strongly stimulates trigeminal chemoreceptors.

For these reasons taste has been described as the chemical gate-keeper to the body. It not only attends to the physiological welfare of the organism by signalling the intensity and quality of the chemicals but it is also very sensitive to the internal state of the organism. The sensitivity of taste to both its internal and external environment means that the organism is usually attracted to nutrients and repulsed by toxins.

The distribution of gustatory taste buds

The specialized end-organs involved in gustation are the taste buds, which are embedded in the stratified epithelium of the tongue, soft palate, pharynx, larynx and epiglottis in humans. The arrangement of taste buds in these regions is uneven in number and discontinuous in spatial distribution. In mammals the majority of taste buds are to be found on the tongue and in humans the distribution of taste buds in the extralingual areas appears to be less extensive in the adult than in newborn infants and children. There appear to be more extralingual taste buds in laboratory animals. The taste buds in fish are situated in areas outside the mouth, in the epidermis of the head and body.

Lingual taste buds are associated exclusively with characteristic papillae, whilst those associated with the soft palate, epiglottis, pharynx and larynx are to be found on smooth epithelial surfaces. In humans the number of taste buds varies considerably from individual to individual, with between 2000 and 5000 taste buds on average distributed on the tongue, palate and epiglottis. However, these numbers can be as low as 500 and as high as 20 000 in some individuals.

Taste buds and gustatory papillae

On the tongue there are three types of gustatory papilla-containing taste buds. The fungiform papillae carry 18%, the foliate papillae 34% and the circumvallate papillae 48% of the taste buds. The fourth type of papilla, the filiform papillae, do not have taste buds associated with them. The dorsum of the tongue is subdivided into an anterior oral two-thirds and a posterior pharyngeal third by a V-shaped groove called the sulcus terminalis.

The fungiform papillae are located on the anterior two-thirds of the tongue (Fig. 13.1) and number about 200 and contain an average of three taste buds each (range 0–21). There is no common agreement on the number of human fungiform papillae without taste buds: reports range from 0 to 85% of the total number. This may be due to individual variation or difficulties in defining the structures to call fungiform papillae. The papillae are shaped like mushrooms with the taste buds

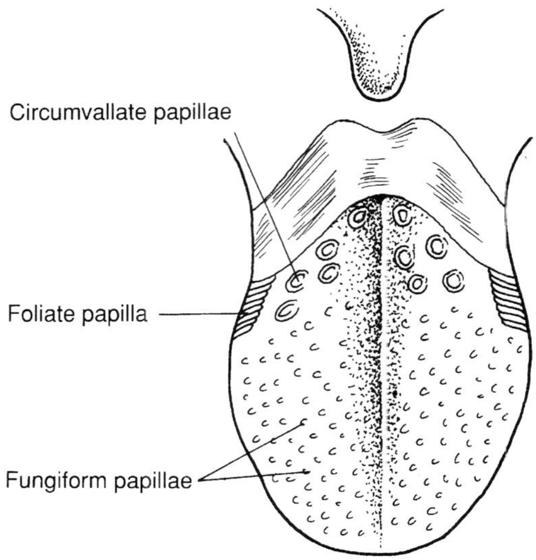

Fig. 13.1 The dorsal surface of the tongue showing the relative distributions of the three types of gustatory papillae.

found in the dorsal surface epithelium of the papillae (Fig. 13.2). The taste buds are innervated by the chorda tympani branch of the facial nerve and the papillae themselves are innervated by the lingual branch of the trigeminal nerve.

The foliate papillae are located on the posterolateral sides of the tongue (Fig. 13.1). There is one foliate papilla on each side of the tongue but each papilla is a large structure arranged in a series of many vertical folds. Up to 20 parallel ridges and furrows have been described, the most rostral of which contain no secretory ducts or taste buds and have been termed lateral rugae. The foliate papillae folds are more caudal to the lateral rugae and are composed of thinner epithelial linings (Fig 13.2). The taste buds lie in these epithelial linings facing a cleft and secretions from lingual salivary glands (von Ebner glands) are released from ducts located between the folds. In the rhesus monkey these folds contain the majority of lingual taste buds, yet many textbooks in the past have reported that in humans the foliate papillae are either regressive or rudimentary. However, it is now reported that in humans there are on average 600 foliate taste buds per papilla; each papilla consists of between two and nine folds. The taste buds in the more anterior folds of the

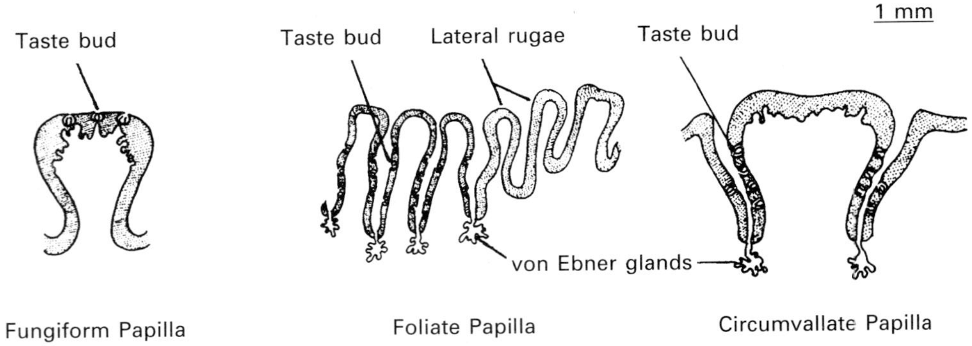

Fig. 13.2 The three types of gustatory papillae.

foliate papillae are innervated by the chorda tympani nerve and buds in the more posterior folds by the lingual branch of the glossopharyngeal nerve.

The circumvallate papillae are located on the dorsal surface of the tongue just anterior to the sulcus terminalis (Fig. 13.1). They number between 8 and 12 in humans, are arranged in a V-shaped formation, with the apex pointing caudally, and are reported to support on average 250 taste buds each. Circumvallate papillae are large mushroom-shaped structures surrounded by a sulcus and secretions from lingual salivary glands (von Ebner glands) are released from ducts located in the base of the sulcus (Fig. 13.2). In humans the taste buds are located along both walls of the circular sulcus, both in the papillae and the adjacent epithelium. The circumvallate papillae taste buds are innervated by the glossopharyngeal nerve. The glossopharyngeal nerve also innervates the taste buds on the pharyngeal part of the tongue, the palatoglossal arches, the oral part of the pharynx and the remaining posterior foliate papillae. Taste buds on the extreme posterior part of the tongue, the rest of the pharynx, the larynx and the epiglottis are innervated by the superior laryngeal branch of the vagus nerve. The superior petrosal nerve, a branch of the facial nerve, supplies most of the taste buds in the soft palate.

Morphology of the taste bud

Each taste bud consists of 50–150 neuro-epithelial cells arranged in a compact, pear-shaped structure (Fig. 13.3). They extend from the basal lamina of the epithelial layer to the epithelial surface and the cells are arranged within the taste bud like the segments of an orange. A single taste bud is about 70 μm high and has a diameter of 40 μm. There is a small 2–10 μm opening in the epithelial surface called the taste pore which allows direct access of gustatory stimuli to the apical membranes of the exposed receptor cells. The cells within the taste bud are called intragemmal cells and cells adjacent to or on the periphery of the bud are called perigemmal cells. Those cells found outside the taste bud are extragemmal cells. There are bundles of filamentous material associated with the perigemmal epithelial cells.

Recent ultrastructural studies have shed new light and controversy on the morphology of the intragemmal cells. It is generally agreed that the taste bud is made up of cells of varying morphological types but there is still no firm agreement in the literature about the functions or classifications of these types. It is generally agreed that there are four types of intragemmal cell: basal cells, type I (dark cells), intermediate cells and type II (light cells). The basal cell is a small, undifferentiated, round cell from which it is thought that the other cells are derived. The non-basal cell types are elongated, bipolar cells and have been collectively termed gustatory or taste receptor cells because they extend from the basal part of the bud where they synapse with the afferent fibres to the apex of the taste bud where they have microvilli processes that project into the taste pore. The apices of these receptor cells are recessed within the pore and tight junctions between the receptor cells restrict the access of the gustatory stimuli to the

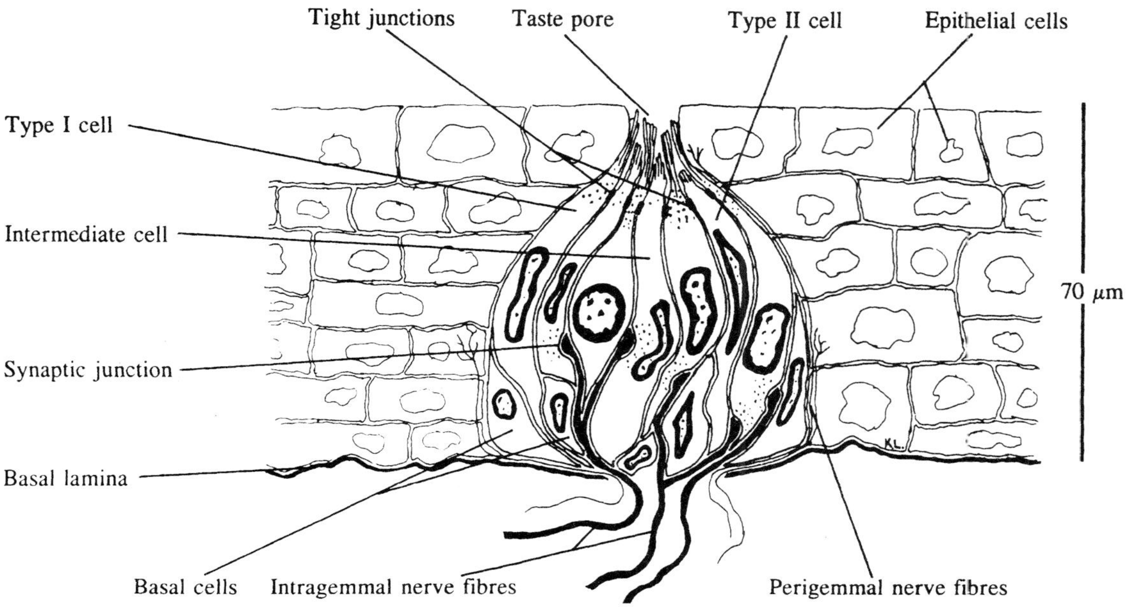

Fig. 13.3 A taste bud.

apical microvilli. Over half of the receptor cells are type I cells. These have long microvilli and dense, membrane-bound granules near the cell apex. The lighter, type II cells have an electron-lucent membrane and have shorter microvilli. The intermediate cell types have morphological characteristics of both type I and type II cells.

The existence and classification of these different morphological cell types do not necessarily imply that they have different functions or that they come from different cell lineages. There is no common agreement at present concerning the classification into different cell types or whether the different cell types are derived from one or more cell lines. Consequently, at present, it is not possible to do anything but speculate on the different functions of these so-called cell types. Recent evidence suggests that the different morphological types of cells represent different stages of cell development, with basal cells differentiating into dark cells which, in turn, develop into light cells. The intermediate cells are stages midway between the development of light from dark cells. However, other evidence suggests that light cells are a separate cell line.

The taste bud complex is a dynamic system in which there is a rapid turnover of cells within each bud. The life span of an individual receptor cell is about 10 days. Cells are continually being born, maturing, performing their gustatory function and eventually dying.

Primary afferent innervation

There are two groups of sensory nerve fibres associated with the taste bud – an intragemmal and a perigemmal plexus. The intragemmal neurons penetrate the basal lamina at the base of the taste bud, branch extensively and synapse with the receptor cells. A single taste bud is innervated by more than one nerve fibre and a single nerve fibre can innervate a number of receptor cells, taste buds or even papillae. This suggests a high degree of convergence of taste bud input on to the afferent fibres.

The synaptic connections between the neuron and the receptor cells is complex partly because of the rapid turnover of cells. The nerves are continually sprouting new processes, forming new synapses with young cells and retracting synaptic connections with dying cells. It is because of this that morphological snap shots often produce confusing results and conclusions. However, there is agreement that, although a single receptor cell can have multiple synapses, fewer than one-third of the receptor cells within a single bud are innervated. Synapses have been observed on type I (dark) cells, type II (light) cells and intermediate cells. A single nerve fibre contacts a small group of receptor cells of similar morphology; i.e. either type I or type II cells, but not both. All of these synapses appear to be of the chemical type. However, electrical synapses have been observed in lower vertebrate taste buds. The perigemmal neurons penetrate the basal lamina near to the taste buds and surround the taste buds *en route* to the epithelial surface. It has been shown that many of these fibres contain substance P, suggesting their involvement in nociception (see section on common chemical sense, below). Other perigemmal fibres have been shown to contain some calcitonin gene-related peptide (CGRP).

An intact nerve supply is necessary for the normal function of taste buds. It has been shown that, if the nerves innervating mammalian taste buds are damaged, the taste buds degenerate and presumably slough off. Following regeneration of the appropriate nerves, the taste buds reappear and assume normal function.

Basic tastes

Since the days of Aristotle (384–322 BC) people have tried to categorize taste into primary tastes. The four basic tastes of sweet, sour, salt and bitter have stood the test of time but there is still controversy as to whether these four qualities of taste adequately describe all taste experiences. In the past metallic and astringent have been suggested as primary tastes, but have since fallen out of favour. There is at present a primary taste that has been suggested by Japanese workers to describe the characteristic taste of monosodium glutamate and that is *umami*, meaning 'delicious or essence of taste'. Monosodium glutamate is used as a taste enhancer by the food industry.

Thresholds and adaptation to gustatory stimuli

The detection threshold for a particular gustatory stimulus is the lowest concentration that can be tasted. It is assumed to be the concentration at which the subject can detect a difference between the test solution and water. Water is used because there is sufficient sodium chloride in saliva to influence threshold measurements of sodium chloride. The recognition threshold is slightly higher than the detection threshold and is that at which the subject can not only taste the difference between water and the test solution but can also recognize the basic taste, i.e. whether it is salt, sour, sweet or bitter.

One of the major problems with threshold studies is that most solutions also produce non-taste sensations that can be detected by subjects. For example, sodium chloride, citric acid and quinine all produce tactile stinging sensations as well as taste sensations and these can easily be mistaken for detection thresholds by subjects. For this reason scaling techniques, which quantify the perception of stimulus intensities over a range of concentrations, from threshold to very intense, have been developed. These scales of perceived taste intensity have proved more valuable than threshold measurements in clinical studies.

If a concentrated solution of a gustatory stimulus is flowed across the extended tongue, the taste is initially very strong but fades to almost nothing in seconds. This demonstrates that taste exhibits almost complete adaptation. Adaptation to a citric acid stimulus has been shown to reduce the sourness of all other acids, and adaptation to sodium chloride reduces the saltiness of all other salts. Results for sweet and bitter are somewhat different: cross-adaptation does not occur for all bitter or for all sweet stimuli. This suggests that there are at least two receptor mechanisms involved in the transduction of these basic tastes.

Receptor mechanisms of transduction

The mechanisms involved in the process of transduction of the signals that produce these basic taste sensations are only now being unravelled. Modern physiological and biochemical techniques have allowed research workers to study these small and relatively inaccessible receptor cells. Unfortunately, because the work involves recording from single cells and neurons, most of the work has been performed on animal tissues and there is already some variation in mechanisms between different species. However, because of the work reported over the last few years, many generalities can now be stated with confidence, although this exciting field continues to produce greater understanding of this complex mechanism. Gustatory receptor cells, in common with many other receptor cells, use specifically localized ion channels and receptor sites for sensory transduction. In the case of gustatory cells they are apically located.

Unlike many other receptor cells, there is no single membrane transduction event and the different basic tastes utilize different ionic mechanisms. Most gustatory stimuli are water-soluble and non-volatile. These hydrophilic compounds are either already dissolved or are dissolved in saliva during mastication. A sour taste is mediated by protons, with the degree of taste depending on H^+ concentration. Virtually all acids taste sour. Salt taste is produced by monovalent cations such as Na^+ and K^+. However, it has been shown that anions like chloride inhibit the cation, and the larger the anion, the greater the inhibition. The taste of the cation is therefore reduced as the anion size increases. This is why sodium chloride tastes saltier than sodium acetate at the same concentrations. As anions get larger they not only inhibit cations but they take on bitter and sweet tastes depending on their structures. For instance, sodium saccharin tastes sweet. In addition, as cations get larger they tend to take on a bitter taste. This explains why no suitable salt substitute has been found. Lithium, the only cation smaller than sodium, is lethal, and potassium, the next cation up from sodium in the periodic table, is found to be bitter in taste to a number of people. Sweet and bitter tastes are typically produced by organic compounds. Sweet-tasting compounds include carbohydrates and some amino acids, whilst bitter-tasting compounds include alkaloids, some amino acids, denatonium (the most bitter substance known) and divalent cations. *Umami* taste is elicited by monosodium glutamate and disodium guanylate; both compounds act as taste enhancers.

In view of the wide range of chemicals that produce taste sensations, it is not surprising therefore that there is more than one mechanism involved in chemoreceptor transduction. Some of these mechanisms include direct ion permeation through open ion channels, activation of ligand-gated ion channels, ion channel modulation, G-protein activation and intracellular Ca^{2+} release, as well as combinations of these events. Although different mechanisms are involved in the transduction of each of the basic tastes, it is still not known if individual gustatory receptor cells have a predominance of one membrane mechanism, so that they can be 'tuned' to a particular basic taste or if they have a mixture of mechanisms and therefore respond to more than one basic taste.

The solutions around and within the taste pore consist of saliva from the major and minor salivary glands, combined with taste pore mucus which is thought to be secreted from the apical processes of gustatory receptor cells. This mucus contains mucopolysaccharide material similar to that found in the membrane-bound granules of the dark (type I) receptor cells. As mentioned earlier, most gustatory stimuli are hydrophilic; however, some are lipophilic, such as bitter-tasting quinine and caffeine. The detection thresholds for lipophilic molecules tend to be lower than for hydrophilic compounds. It has been suggested that a carrier protein assists in the transport of these lipophilic molecules to the taste pore. Recently, a protein named VEG (von Ebner gland) protein has been cloned from rat von Ebner glands. Proline-rich proteins have also been suggested as carrier molecules and these are also expressed in saliva from von Ebner glands.

Once the tastant chemicals are in the solutions surrounding the taste pore, they diffuse or are possibly transported to the apical membrane of the receptor cells. It is believed that the gustatory stimuli are restricted to the apical membrane by tight junctions between receptor cells just below the microvilli. However, recent studies have suggested that low-molecular-weight substances can permeate these junctions. This may explain why some gustatory stimuli elicit taste sensations when given intravenously. The possible mechanisms involved in the transduction of the various basic gustatory stimuli into receptor potentials are outlined below. It appears that there are direct interactions between gustatory stimuli and apically located ion channels involved in the transduction of monovalent salts, sour and some bitter stimuli. In the case of sweet stimuli, amino acids and some bitter-tasting compounds, specific apically located membrane receptors are involved in the transduction mechanism. It must be emphasized that the recent use of patch-clamp recording techniques has allowed us to

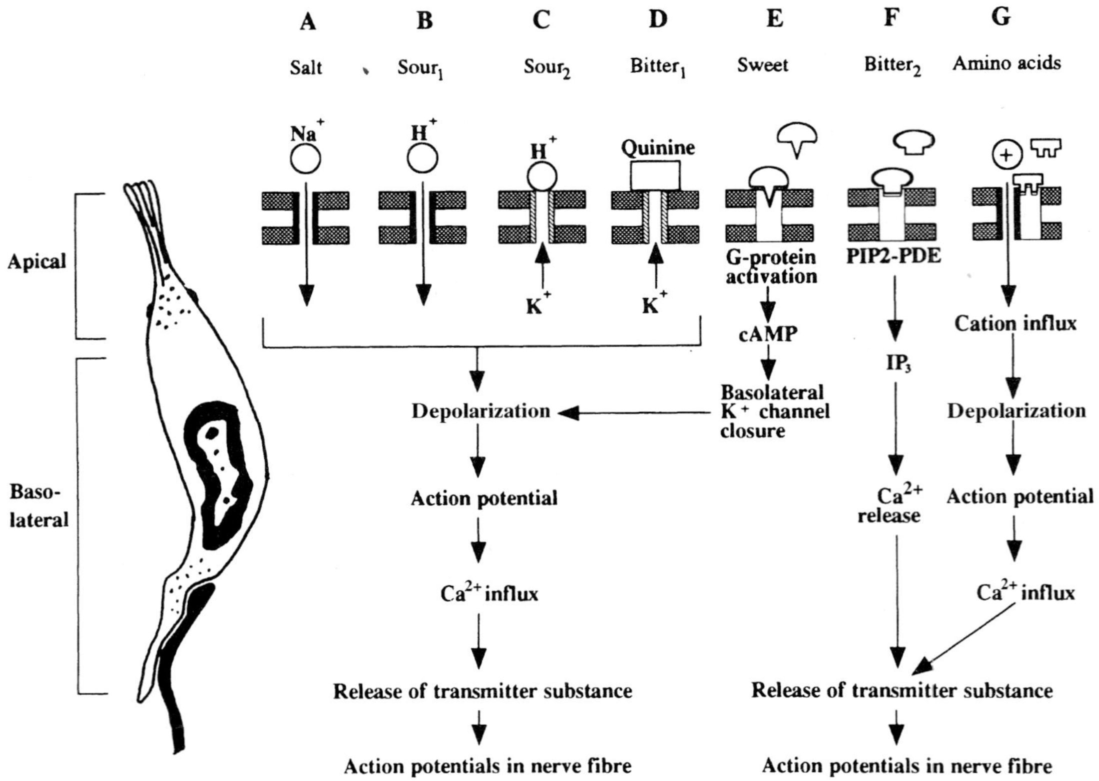

Fig. 13.4 Schematic diagram showing the proposed mechanisms of transduction in gustatory receptor cells. (See text for explanation and abbreviations.)

appreciate some of the mechanisms involved in the transduction of the various stimuli. It is very likely that new mechanisms will be discovered which may not exist in all species and that more than one mechanism is involved in the transduction of a single type of stimulus.

Present knowledge suggests that salt is mediated by amiloride-sensitive Na^+ channels found in the apical membrane (Fig. 13.4A). Passive influx of Na^+ generates a depolarizing receptor potential which in turn triggers action potentials in the cell. Two mechanisms have been postulated for sour. The first involves the influx of H^+ through the same amiloride-sensitive Na^+ channels (Fig. 13.4B), and the second involves the blocking of apically located voltage-dependent K^+ channels by the H^+ (Fig. 13.4C). The K^+ channels exhibit a significant permeability at rest with the constant efflux of K^+ and therefore when blocked they produce membrane depolarization. Blocking of K^+ channels has also been suggested in the transduction of some bitter tastes, particularly quinine (Fig. 13.4D). Biochemical studies have suggested the activation of a G-protein in the transduction of sweet stimuli. Guanosine triphosphate (GTP) binding proteins, G_s and G_o, and the second messenger-generating enzymes adenylate cyclase and phosphatidylinositol 4,5-bisphosphate phosphodiesterase (PIP_2-PDE) have been identified in gustatory receptor cells. It is postulated that sugars bind to specific receptors (Fig. 13.4E), activate a G protein, cause an increase in intracellular cyclic adenosine monophosphate (cAMP), which then causes a closure of basolateral K^+ channels leading to a depolarization of the cell.

The transduction of some bitter stimuli is also said to involve binding of the stimulus to apical receptors (Fig. 13.4F) that are coupled with PIP_2-PDE, which in turn causes inositol trisphosphate (IP_3) to be produced. This increase in IP_3 then causes the release of Ca^{2+} from intracellular stores. The Ca^{2+} directly mediates the release of the transmitter substance. Direct ligand-gated cation channels are thought to mediate transduction of some of the amino acids (L-arginine and L-proline; Fig. 13.4G). These amino acids bind to separate receptor sites and the associated cation channel is opened, leading to an influx of the ions. There is some evidence for the involvement of ligand-gated channels in sucrose transduction.

Taste interaction and anomalies

The interaction of tastes is of great interest to the manufacturers of foods and drinks. If substances of different tastes are mixed, there is often suppression of one or both components. This suppression can often take a taste below its perceived threshold. For example, if sucrose and quinine are mixed, the bitterness of the quinine is suppressed. It is not known if these effects occur at a peripheral level or a more central level. There are a number of substances that produce anomalies of taste; amongst these are miracle fruit (the berries of *Synsepalum dulcificum*), the leaves of *Gymnema sylvestre, Ziziphus jujuba* and *Hovenia dulcis*, and artichokes (*Cynara scolymus*). Miracle fruit has the effect of making sour substances taste sweet. It was first thought that the effect of the berry was to paralyse the sour receptors. However, this is now known to be untrue: a glycoprotein in the berry adds a sweet taste to acidic substances and the sourness is suppressed by the sweet taste. Leaves from *G. sylvestre, Z. jujuba* and *H. dulcis* temporarily reduce the ability to taste sweet. The underlying mechanisms for this are still unclear. Artichoke has the effect in some individuals of causing other substances to taste sweet. This sensitivity is thought to be inherited. It is for this reason that it is not recommended for wine to be served with artichoke. The effect is believed to be due to potassium salts of cholinergic acid and cynarin found in the artichoke which are thought to inhibit some sweet receptors.

Genetically derived mechanisms have been shown to be involved in the phenomenon of taste blindness in which a number of people cannot taste the bitter substance phenylthiocarbamide. About one-third of people cannot taste this substance and it has been demonstrated that non-tasting is a simple Mendelian recessive trait. Finally, dentists are often told by their patients that orange juice tastes awful after cleaning their teeth in the morning. This is due to the detergent used in toothpaste, sodium lauryl sulphate. Its effects are to reduce the subject's ability to taste sweetness and to add a bitter taste to acids. Once again, the underlying mechanisms are unknown.

Generation potentials, action potentials and transmitter release

For many years it was thought that gustatory receptor cells were passive transducers that generated receptor potentials only. It is now accepted that they generate both receptor potentials and action potentials in response to stimulation. The role of the action potential is unknown. It has been suggested that the action potential may be involved in coding the stimulus intensity, providing a rapid transient excitation at the onset of stimulation or that it may be necessary to activate the Ca^{2+} currents underlying transmitter release.

There is very little information concerning the release of the transmitter substances from the basolateral membranes of the receptor cells. There is thought to be some tonic release of transmitters since the afferent nerve fibres often show small amounts of spontaneous activity. This discharge is increased with an increase in concentrations of most gustatory stimulants. A number of different neurotransmitters have been identified as being involved in gustatory receptor functions; amongst these are acetylcholine, noradrenaline, serotonin and neuropeptides such as vasoactive intestinal peptide (VIP), bombesin, CGRP and many others. There is also some evidence for electrical synaptic connections between cells within the taste bud.

Response characteristics of first-order gustatory neurons

The response or taste profiles of particular neurons have been obtained by recording from primary afferent fibres in the cranial nerves VII, IX or X whilst applying different stimuli with variable concentrations to the taste areas of the mouth. From these studies it has been demonstrated that most single neurons respond to a wide range of sapid stimuli. The fibres have conduction velocities of 5–30 m/s with diameters of 1–5 μm, suggesting that they are all myelinated fibres. Attempts have been made to classify groups of neurons according to their response characteristics.

Neurons have been described as salt or sweet 'best', meaning the basic gustatory stimulus that they appear to fire most strongly to – in other words, the taste they are more finely tuned to. The classification of neurons into these neuronal types forms the basis of the 'labelled line' theory, which contends that the function of any one type of neuron is to signal the arrival of its associated basic taste. It must be remembered that these responses are not the result of stimulation of just one gustatory receptor cell but an unknown number, which could be in both the same taste bud and adjacent taste buds. Until intracellular recording can be made from gustatory receptor cells whilst recording from primary afferent neurons, the relative roles of the individual receptor cells to the overall response will not be discovered.

The major problem with the labelled line theory is that a large proportion of mammalian gustatory neurons respond almost equally to two or more of the basic tastes. Due to this observation an across-fibre pattern theory was proposed. The basis of this theory is that all neurons contribute to the quality code through their relative rates of activity. A particular stimulus elicits a certain rate of discharge from each of a population of cells; this would determine a pattern of impulses that is unique to the quality and intensity of that stimulus. The quality would be coded by the shape of the response profile whilst the cumulative discharge rate would code the intensity. Each neuron would contribute to the response and consequently would be of equal importance to the neural code. It is possible that the process of gustatory neural coding utilizes both labelled line and across-fibre pattern processes. Basic taste categories may be identified through labelled lines and quality discrimination within each category may depend on patterns of activity.

Central connections of gustatory neurons

The human gustatory system resembles that of non-human primates with regard to its central

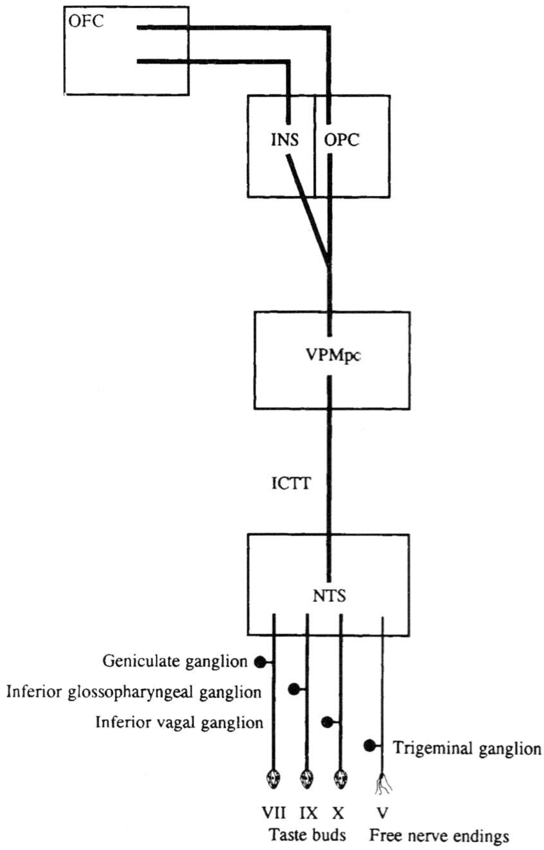

Fig. 13.5 Schematic diagram showing the central neural connections involved in the sensation of taste from the oral cavity. OFC = caudolateral orbitofrontal cortex; INS = anterior insula of the primary cortex; OPC = frontal operculum of the primary cortex; VPMpc = parvicellular division of the ventroposteromedial nucleus of the thalamus; ICTT = ipsilateral central tegmental tract; NTS = nucleus of the solitary tract. (See text for details.)

connections (Fig. 13.5). The first-order gustatory neurons of the cranial nerves VII, IX and X, with their cell bodies in the geniculate, the inferior glossopharyngeal and the inferior vagal ganglia respectively, project to the rostral part of the nucleus of the solitary tract (NTS) of the medulla. It is here in the NTS that they form their first synaptic connections. The axons from the neurons of this gustatory region of the NTS enter the ipsilateral central tegmental tract (ICTT) and bypass the pontine parabrachial nuclei (which are known to be relay points in rat and cat) and terminate in the parvicellular division of the ventroposteromedial nucleus of the thalamus (VPMpc). The gustatory system appears to be represented in the ipsilateral thalamus. Gustatory neurons from the VPMpc then project to two areas of the primary cortex, the frontal operculum (OPC) and the anterior insula (INS). There is also a secondary cortical taste area, the caudolateral orbitofrontal cortex (OFC), which receives its connections from both the frontal opercular taste cortex and the insular taste cortex but not from the thalamic taste area (VPMpc). On the other hand it has been shown that it receives thalamic projections from the mediodorsal nucleus of the thalamus (pars magnocellularis) and is therefore part of the prefrontal cortex.

Electrophysiological studies in the NTS, OPC, INS and OFC of macaque monkey have demonstrated that, as single neuron recordings are made higher in the central nervous system, the neurons encountered become more and more specific to a single basic taste, with almost no neurons responding to one taste in the NTS, the majority (82%) responding to three or four gustatory stimuli. Whereas in the OPC and INS approximately 25% of neurons respond to a single stimulus and in the OFC 74% respond to a single stimulus with only 4% responding to three or four gustatory stimuli. This suggests that the neurons of the caudolateral orbitofrontal cortex are more sharply tuned to the basic tastes than those of the primary frontal opercular and insular taste cortices which are, in turn, more finely tuned than those in the solitary tract nucleus. It has been suggested that the gustatory neurons in the orbitofrontal cortex may be involved with learning and other associated processes.

Gustatory stimuli produce copious secretions of saliva from all the major and minor salivary glands through a reflex pathway involving the first-order gustatory neurons of cranial nerves VII, IX and X, the NTS and the inferior and superior salivary nuclei. Sour stimuli are the most effective, followed by salt and then sweet, and bitter the least effective. Gustatory stimuli are also known to be involved in the cephalic phase of gastric acid and pancreatic secretions. However, it has been suggested that the vagus nerve is the primary mediator of cephalic-phase stimuli. The pathways involve the vagus nerve, the NTS and the dorsal vagal nucleus. Again, sour seems to be the most effective stimulus.

Common chemical sense

Common chemical sense has been defined as the sensation caused by the stimulation of epithelial or mucosal free nerve endings by chemicals. The evidence suggests that the receptors involved in this sense are polymodal nociceptors, which are free nerve endings containing substance P. The major contributor to the common chemical sense in the oral structures is the trigeminal nerve. The trigeminal branches that innervate the oral cavity are the lingual nerve, which innervates the tongue and the floor of the mouth; the nasopalatine nerve, which innervates the hard palate; the posterior palatine nerve, which innervates the soft palate; and the buccal nerve, which innervates the cheek mucosa.

The extensive trigeminal innervation is illustrated by the observation that 75% of the innervation of the fungiform papillae is accounted for by the trigeminal fibres, with the remainder accounted for by the chorda tympani fibres. Free nerve endings are found throughout the oral cavity. However, they appear to be most numerous in the anterior part of the mouth. The nerve endings are mostly confined to the deeper layers of the oral epithelium, except in the palate where they are also found superficially. Stimulation of these fibres does not necessarily produce the sensation of pain but is often described as an irritating or burning sensation. However, chemicals such as menthol, peppermint and phenethyl alcohol which are non-irritating also elicit responses from the trigeminal nerve. The fibres are thought to be finely myelinated fibres ($A\delta$) and unmyelinated (C) fibres.

A number of reflex responses have been reported when oral chemoreceptors are stimulated. Amongst these reflexes are increased salivation, vasodilatation (flushing of face and neck, reddening of the conjunctiva), increased nasal secretion, lacrimation and perspiration (gustatory sweating) in the regions of the head and neck.

Irritation itself has been shown to alter significantly the perceived intensities of the basic taste qualities. How it does so is still open to speculation. There are a number of ways in which trigeminal stimulation could affect gustatory perception: it could alter salivary flow; it could modulate central gustatory activity, since both trigeminal and gustatory neurons synapse in the nuclei of the solitary tract. It could alter the secretions around the pore, or even alter the size of the pore and limit the amount of gustatory stimulus reaching the receptor cells, and finally, it could alter the gustatory receptor cell transduction or transmission characteristics. Any one or a combination of these processes could account for the interactions between trigeminal and gustatory stimuli. Other, as yet unknown, processes could additionally be implicated.

Tongue maps

Many textbooks and detailed reviews contain pictures of the dorsal surface of the tongue showing sweet on the tip, salt on the front edges, sour on the rear edges and bitter on the back. According to Millar and Bartoshuk,[1] tongue maps are incorrect, as they owe their origin to a misunderstanding of the work of Hänig in 1901, concerning the thresholds of the four basic tastes on various loci: front, edges and rear of the tongue. Hänig showed that the thresholds did not remain constant as the locus was varied. For instance, the threshold for sweet was slightly lower on the front of the tongue, whereas the threshold for bitter was slightly lower on the rear of the tongue. Hänig never meant that perception of sweetness occurred exclusively on the front of the tongue. An application of moderate concentrations of substances with the four basic tastes shows that all four tastes are perceived well on all loci with taste receptors.

It is the present author's hope that he has not perpetuated any similar misunderstandings during the course of this review.

Acknowledgements

I am very grateful to Kate Linden for all the illustrations in this article. I would like to thank Vivienne Lee, Chris Louca and Brendan Scott for comments and suggestions.

Reference

1. Millar IJ, Bartoshuk LM. Taste perception, taste bud distribution, and spatial relationships. In: Getchell TV, Doty RL, Bartoshuk LM, Snow JB (eds) *Smell and Taste in Health and Disease*. New York: Raven Press, 1991.

Further reading

Finger TE, Silver WL (eds) *Neurobiology of Taste and Smell*. New York: John Wiley, 1987.

Getchell TV, Doty RL, Bartoshuk LM, Snow JB (eds) *Smell and Taste in Health and Disease*. New York: Raven Press, 1991.

Keverne EB. Chemical senses: taste. In: Barlow HB, Mollon JD (eds) *The Senses*, pp. 428–447. Cambridge: Cambridge University Press, 1982.

Kinnamon SC. Taste transduction: a diversity of mechanisms. *Trends Neurosci* 1988; **11**: 491–496.

Kinnamon SC, Cummings TA. Chemosensory transduction mechanisms in taste. *Annu Rev Physiol* 1992; **54**: 715–731.

Rolls ET, Yaxley S, Sienkiewicz ZJ. Gustatory responses of single neurons in the caudolateral orbitofrontal cortex of the macaque monkey. *J Neurophysiol* 1990; **64**: 1055–1066.

Roper SD. The microphysiology of peripheral taste organs. *J Neurosci* 1992; **12**: 1127–1134.

14

Saliva: its secretion, composition and functions

Michael Edgar

Sources of saliva

Saliva is a complex mixture of fluids, with contributions from the major salivary glands (parotid, submandibular and sublingual), the minor or accessory glands, and the gingival crevicular fluid. Additionally, it contains a high population of bacteria normally resident in the mouth, desquamated epithelial cells, and transient residues of food or drink, following their ingestion. When referring to the fluid normally present in the mouth, the term whole saliva is commonly used, as distinct from duct saliva, which is that flowing from the individual glands. The several sources of whole saliva complicate its composition, as the contribution from different sources can vary. For example, stimulated whole saliva contains a higher proportion of fluid from the parotid gland than does unstimulated saliva.

Control of salivation

The salivary glands are unusual among the glands of the digestive tract in being under purely nervous control; hormonal influences can alter the composition of saliva, but are not responsible for its secretion. The nerve supply to the major glands is derived from both sympathetic and parasympathetic branches of the autonomic nervous system. In humans, the sympathetic supply (derived from T1–T4 via the superior sympathetic ganglion) is trophic; in other words, stimulation leads to the release of secretory proteins such as amylase, and vasoconstrictor. The parasympathetic nerves (from the seventh and ninth cranial nerves) are secretomotor and vasodilator. The nerves innervate the acinar cells, the duct cells, blood vessels and myoepithelial cells.

Resting flow

Under resting conditions, without the exogenous stimulation associated with feeding, there is a slow flow of saliva (Table 14.1), which keeps the mouth moist and lubricates the mucous membranes. This unstimulated flow, which is present most of the time, is very

Table 14.1 Flow rates of saliva (ml/min)

	Unstimulated		*Stimulated*	
	Mean	*Range*	*Mean*	*Range*
Whole saliva	0.32	0.1–0.5	1.7*	1.1–3.0
Parotid saliva (each gland)	0.04	0.01–0.07	1.5†	0.7–2.3
Submandibular/sublingual saliva	0.10	0.02–0.20	0.8†	0.4–1.3

* Masticatory stimulus.
† Gustatory stimulus (acid).

important for the health and well-being of the oral cavity (see below).

The unstimulated flow rate varies considerably during the day, and is influenced by a number of factors.

Circadian variation

Unstimulated flow peaks at approximately 5 p.m. in most individuals, with a minimum flow during the night. This variation is independent of eating and sleeping behaviour.

Light and arousal

If one is blind-folded, or in an unlit room, the unstimulated flow rate falls. This is probably associated with the effect of visual input in maintaining a state of arousal. Saliva flow is much reduced during sleep.

Hydration

A loss of 8% of body water results in a cessation of saliva flow. The resultant drying of the oral cavity is a feature of thirst, although thirst and water intake are under hypothalamic control and not dependent upon oral dryness.

Exercise and stress

A dry mouth is a feature of the 'fright and flight' response. This is probably not a direct action of the sympathetic supply to the gland, but rather is due to inhibitory influences on the salivary nuclei arising from the hypothalamus.

Psychic flow

A mouth-watering sensation is a universal experience on the anticipation or sight of food, especially if temptingly presented when hungry. However, although the sensation is of a sudden flow of saliva into the mouth, it has not proved possible to demonstrate a large increase in flow rate in humans arising from such psychic stimuli.

This is in contrast to the well-established conditioned reflex effect in dogs, first demonstrated by Pavlov, who noted that the animals learned to associate the chiming of church bells with meal-times and would salivate on hearing the bells even if food was withheld.

In humans, a small increase in flow can usually be demonstrated on thinking about food, or seeing it being prepared, but this does not correspond in amount with the sensation of mouth-watering. It has been suggested that the latter is due to a sudden awareness of saliva already present in the mouth, or a momentary contraction of myoepithelial elements to express ready-formed saliva into the mouth without increasing the overall amount of saliva formed.

Unconditioned reflexes

The most important stimuli to salivation are those associated with feeding: masticatory movement and, especially, taste (Fig. 14.1).

Mastication

Chewing a flavourless bolus such as wax or chewing-gum base leads to an increase in saliva flow of about three fold. This is a reflex response: receptors in the muscles of mastication, temporomandibular joint, periodontal

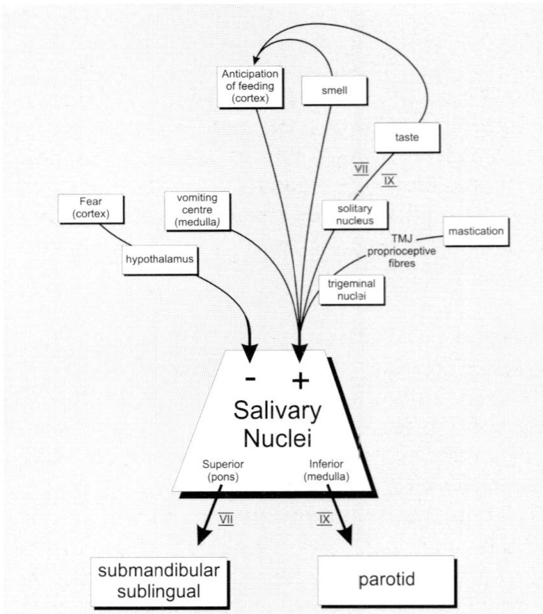

Fig. 14.1 Diagrammatic representation of parasympathetic reflexes controlling the flow rate of saliva. VII, IX = Facial and glossopharyngeal nerves; TMJ = temporomandibular joint.

ligament and mucosae detect the presence of a bolus and its mastication, and stimulate the salivary nuclei to increase the parasympathetic secretomotor discharge.

Gustatory stimuli

The reflex effects of taste stimuli are more dramatic, giving rise to perhaps a 10-fold increase in saliva flow (Table 14.1). Sour stimuli are most effective, followed by sweet, salt and bitter.

Most foods also elicit olfactory stimuli, and a reflex response to smell can be demonstrated.

Other stimuli

The inhibitory action of stress on the salivary nuclei has already been mentioned. On the other hand, there appear to be connections between the salivary nuclei and the vomiting centre in the medulla, since copious reflex salivation as well as nausea frequently occur just before vomiting, perhaps as an attempt to dilute or neutralize the irritant which is giving rise to the nausea.

Hypersalivation (ptyalism) is also described in pregnancy, but the physiological basis is unclear; perhaps it stems from morning sickness, or oesophageal irritation following reflux of gastric contents due to raised abdominal pressure in late pregnancy. Complaints of excess salivation other than under the above circumstances are usually associated with motor disturbances of the orofacial musculature, and are rarely substantiated by measurement of flow rates.

Formation of saliva

Saliva is formed in two stages: a primary secretion occurs in the acini, then modified as it passes through the ducts. The primary secretion is formed actively by the movement of sodium and chloride ions into the lumen, creating an osmotic gradient which leads to the passive movement of water. Other acinar components are added here, before the fluid enters the duct, where sodium ions are actively reabsorbed (chloride ions follow passively to maintain electrical equilibrium), and potassium and bicarbonate ions are secreted.

The macromolecular components (amylase, mucous glycoproteins, etc.) are formed in the usual way in the acinar cell endoplasmic reticulum, processed into secretory vesicles in the Golgi apparatus and exported from the cell by exocytosis.

Signal transduction

When a nerve to the salivary gland is stimulated, the transduction of this signal to increase the formation of saliva is first brought about by the release of neurotransmitter substances. These include noradrenaline (sympathetic) and acetylcholine, substance P and vasointestinal polypeptide (parasympathetic).

When the neurotransmitter (agonist) arrives at a secretory cell membrane it binds to and activates a receptor (which may be stimulatory or inhibitory) on the external surface of the membrane. This activates an intermediate guanine nucleotide-dependent membrane protein known as a G protein, which in turn activates an effector enzyme on the inner cytoplasmic surface of the cell (Fig. 14.2). The effector enzyme may be either phospholipase C or adenyl cyclase (AC).

Phospholipase C pathway (Fig. 14.3)

This enzyme (PLC) is activated on binding of acetylcholine at muscarinic receptors, substance P at peptidergic receptors, or noradrenaline at α-adrenergic receptors on the acinar cell membrane. It controls the intracellular pathway, leading to the secretion of water and electrolytes.

The pathway is rather complex. PLC is responsible for hydrolysing a membrane phospholipid (phosphatidyl inositol bisphosphate, PIP_2) to form diacylglycerol (DAG) and inositol triphosphate (IP_3). The latter stimulates the release of calcium ions from a cytoplasmic storage site – not yet fully identified. This rise in cytoplasmic calcium ion concentrations causes the opening of chloride channels in the luminal membrane of the cell, allowing chloride ions to pass out of the cell down an electrochemical gradient. The presence of chloride ions in the lumen triggers the movement of sodium ions from the intercellular canaliculi across the tight junction between the cells. The sodium chloride so formed creates an osmotic

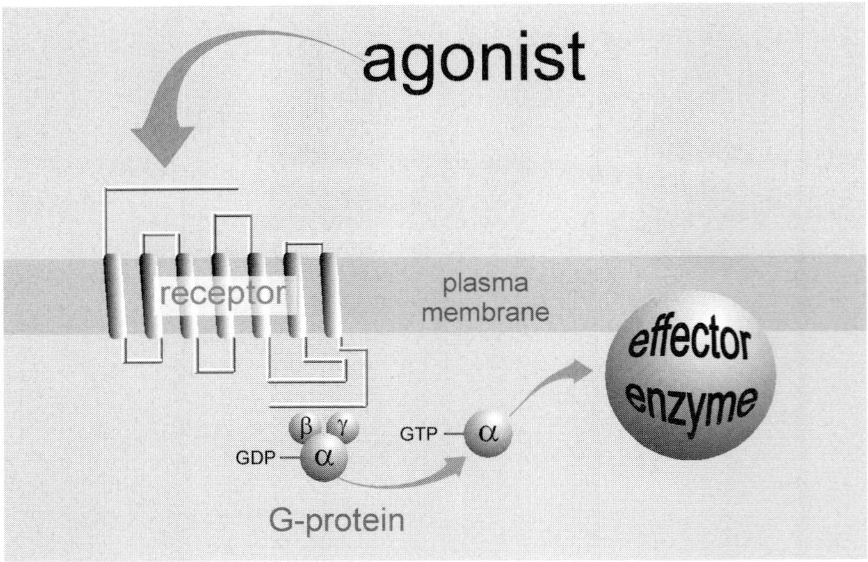

Fig. 14.2 Coupling of acinar membrane receptors. The receptor is a protein which crosses the cell membrane seven times. When an agonist (neurotransmitter) binds to and activates the receptor, this causes a guanine nucleotide-dependent protein (G protein) to become active. The G protein now activates an effector enzyme, leading to initiation of secretion of water and electrolytes, and of proteins. GDP = Guanosine diphosphate; GTP = guanosine triphosphate.

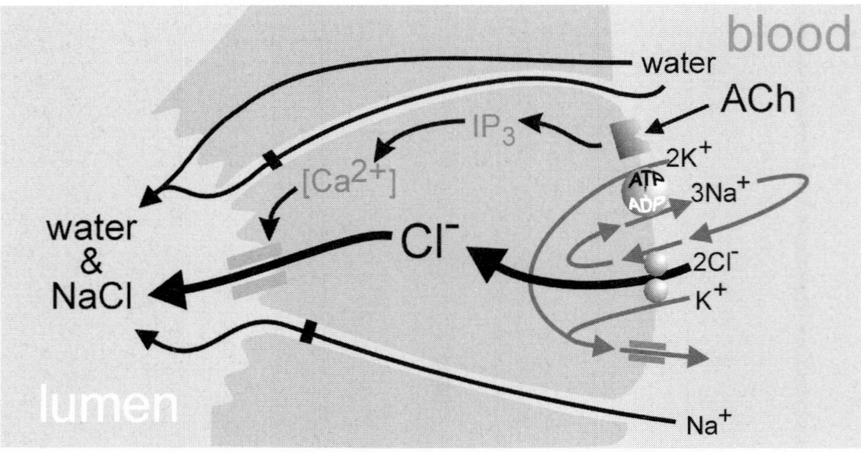

Fig. 14.3 Activation by muscarinic cholinergic receptors of fluid and electrolyte secretion. ACh = Acetyl choline; ADP = adenosine diphosphate; ATP = adenosine triphosphate; IP_3 = inositol triphosphate. Activation of the effector enzyme phospholipase C causes hydrolysis of a membrane phospholipid to form IP_3, which acts upon an intracellular Ca^{2+} store to release Ca^{2+}. This acts as a second messenger to open chloride channels in the apical membrane, leading to secretion of water and electrolytes into the lumen.

gradient, attracting water into the lumen to form the primary secretion.

The chloride ions, whose movement is responsible for secretion, enter the cell via a cotransporter mechanism in the basolateral membrane. This cotransporter allows the entry of Na^+ and K^+ and $2Cl^-$ ions into the cell – all ions must be present simultaneously for transport to occur. The driving force for the cotransporter is the Na^+/K^+ pump in the

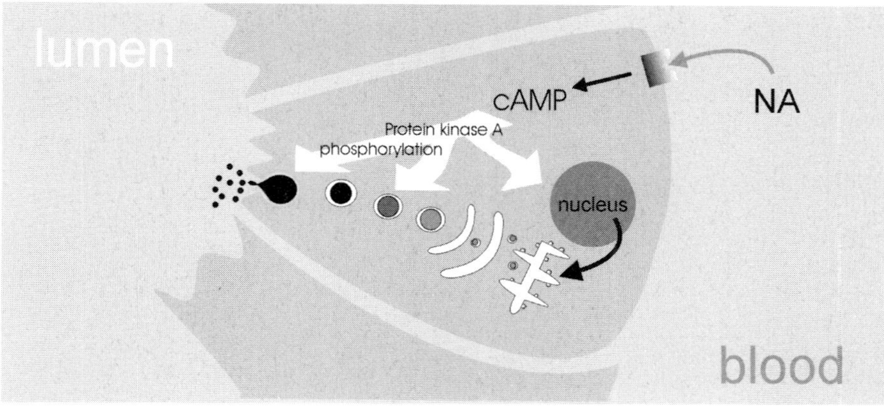

Fig. 14.4 Activation by β-adrenergic receptors of protein secretion. The effector enzyme, adenyl cyclase, is activated when noradrenaline (NA) binds to β-adrenergic receptors. Its action is to convert adenosine triphosphate to cyclic adenosine monophosphate (cAMP), which in turn activates by phosphorylation the enzyme systems, leading to increased synthesis, packaging and exocytosis of protein.

basolateral membrane, which actively exports Na^+ from the cell using energy derived from adenosine triphosphate (ATP). The K^+ entering via the cotransporter is extruded from the cell via a Ca^{2+}-sensitive K^+ channel, in order to preserve the membrane potential.

Adenyl cyclase pathway (Fig. 14.4)

AC is activated when noradrenaline binds to β-adrenergic acinar receptors, or vasoactive intestinal peptide (VIP) binds to peptidergic receptors. Activation leads to exocytosis of secretory proteins.

AC causes the intracellular formation of 3,5-cyclic AMP (cAMP) from ATP. cAMP activates a second enzyme, cAMP-dependent protein kinase (protein kinase A), which exists in four subunits. Two subunits are receptor molecules which bind with cAMP, thereby liberating the other two catalytic subunits to activate effector proteins by phosphorylation. The activated effector proteins then stimulate protein synthesis and exocytosis. Diacylglycerol (from the phospholipase C pathway, see above) also promotes exocytosis.

This complex sequence of intracellular events thus leads to the formation of the primary fluid.

Composition of saliva

Saliva is a dilute fluid, over 99% being made up of water. The concentrations of dissolved solids (organic and inorganic) are characterized by wide variation, both between individuals and within a single individual. Average concentrations quoted below thus disguise a wide range of normal values.

Protein

The proteins of saliva comprise approximately 200 mg per 100 ml – only about 3% of the protein concentration in plasma. They include enzymes, immunoglobulins and other antibacterial factors, mucous glycoproteins (mucins), traces of albumin, and certain polypeptides and oligopeptides of importance in oral health.

α-Amylase

The major digestive enzyme of saliva, α-amylase is present in parotid saliva at concentrations of 60–120 mg/100 ml, and in submandibular saliva at approximately 25 mg/100 ml. It is a glycoprotein, with a relative molecular mass of 62–67 kD. Six isoenzyme forms exist; the distribution of isoenzymes from saliva differs from that of pancreatic juice. The enzyme hydrolyses the α1:4 glycosidic bond between glucose units in the polysaccharide chain of starch; hydrolysis takes place anywhere along the chain (except where branching occurs), but is very slow for terminal glucose units. Thus the end-products of amylase digestion are mainly maltose, together with oligosaccharides as well as some free glucose. The optimum pH is in the region of 6.8, and chloride is required as a cofactor.

Immunoglobulins

Secretory immunoglobulin A (IgA) is the predominant immunoglobulin, at approximately 20 mg/100 ml, with IgG (1.5 mg/100 ml) and IgM (0.2 mg/100 ml) present in low amounts, possibly arising from the gingival crevice.

Antibacterial proteins

Three separate factors are found in saliva, as with many other secretions. *Lysozyme* is an antibacterial enzyme which attacks components of the cell wall of certain bacteria leading to lysis: its effects may be potentiated by certain anions. *Lactoferrin* is an iron-binding protein which removes free iron from saliva, depleting the supply of iron needed for bacterial growth. Some bacteria can, however, digest lactoferrin and use it as a source of iron. *Sialoperoxidase* oxidizes salivary thiocyanate ion (SCN^-) to hypothiocyanite ($OSCN^-$), a potent antibacterial substance, using hydrogen peroxide produced by oral bacteria as an oxidant.

Glycoproteins

The major groups of glycoproteins consist of two classes of mucous glycoprotein (MG1 and MG2) found in submandibular and sublingual saliva, and a group of proline-rich glycoproteins (PRPs) found in parotid saliva. Their characteristics are shown in Table 14.2. All consist of a polypeptide core with oligosaccharide side chains; the proportion of protein to carbohydrate varies between the different groups.

Table 14.2 Characteristics of principal salivary glycoproteins

	MG1	*MG2*	*PRP*
Relative molecular mass (kDa)	$>10^3$	200–500	40
Percentage polypeptide	15	30	60
Percentage carbohydrate	75	68	30
Subunit structure	Yes	No	No
Bound sulphate	Yes	?	No
Bound phosphate	No	?	Yes
Bound sialic acid	Yes	Yes	?
Blood group activity	Yes	Yes	No

MG1, MG2 = Mucous glycoproteins; PRP = proline-rich glycoproteins.
? = Variable or uncertain.

The oligosaccharide side chains are shorter and more variable than those of glycosaminoglycans. They contain amino sugars and their *N*-acetylated derivatives fucose, galactose, mannose and sialic acid. The terminal unit is often fucose or sialic acid, or a sulphated sugar derivative. The glycopeptide link between the side chain and the protein core is, for the mucous glycoproteins, between *N*-acetyl galactosamine and serine or threonine residues, and for the proline-rich glycoproteins, between *N*-acetyl galactosamine and asparagine residues.

Other polypeptides

Statherin is a small phosphoprotein (12 kDa) relatively rich in tyrosine and proline, which has the property of inhibiting hydroxyapatite crystal growth. It also prevents the precipitation of calcium phosphates from supersaturated solutions, and may be important as an inhibitor of calculus formation, both in the glands and on the teeth. Similar behaviour is seen with the proline-rich proteins, which have the ability to bind to hydroxyapatite.

Sialin, a tetrapeptide (glycine–glycine–lysine–arginine) can be utilized by several bacteria, leading to the formation of alkaline end products (amines) which are believed to help regulate the pH of plaque.

Other organic compounds

Many free amino acids are present at low concentrations (below 0.1 mg/100 ml). While saliva can be used by some oral bacteria as a sole source of nutrient, the amino acid content is too low to provide a rich growth medium. Some microorganisms possess hydrolytic enzymes by which they can degrade salivary glycoproteins, using both the carbohydrate side chains as an energy source, and the polypeptide core as a source of nitrogen.

Urea is present at levels of about 12–20 mg/100 ml. It is hydrolysed by many bacteria with the release of ammonia, leading to a rise in pH. *Glucose* concentrations (0.5–1 mg/100 ml) are too low to support extensive growth, but may be raised in diabetics. Much higher sugar concentrations in saliva

Table 14.3 Inorganic constituents of whole saliva (mg/100 ml)

	Range	*Mean*
Sodium	0–80	15 resting 60 stimulated
Potassium	60–100	80
Calcium	2–11	6
Phosphorus (inorganic)	6–71	17 resting 12 stimulated
Chloride	50–100	
Thiocyanate		9 (smokers) 2 (non-smokers)
Fluoride (parts/10^6)	0.01–0.04	0.03 resting 0.01 stimulated
Bicarbonate	0–40	6 resting 36 stimulated
pH	5.0–8.0	

follow ingestion of food and drinks; oral sugar clearance is described below.

Inorganic constituents

The inorganic composition of saliva is summarized in Table 14.3, which demonstrates the wide range of values for most components. The table also indicates some factors affecting the inorganic composition, and these are discussed below.

The major ions (sodium, potassium, chloride and bicarbonate) are the main contributors to the osmolarity of saliva, which is approximately half that of plasma. Bicarbonate is also the principal buffer in saliva. Thiocyanate has been referred to above in relation to the antibacterial effects of sialoperoxidase.

The fluoride content is approximately similar to that of plasma, but is elevated slightly in those who drink fluoridated water, or use fluoridated toothpaste (owing to the prolonged release of fluoride into the saliva from sparingly soluble deposits on the teeth and soft tissues). These small elevations in salivary levels are believed to be very important in the anticaries action of fluorides.

Calcium and phosphate in saliva

Not all of the calcium and phosphate in saliva is present free in solution; part of the calcium is bound to protein, and part is in soluble complexes with carbonate, phosphate or lactate. About 10% of the phosphate is in ester form, mainly in phosphoproteins, but traces of pyrophosphate ($P_2O_7^{4-}$) are also present.

These non-ionic forms notwithstanding, the levels of calcium and phosphate are such that saliva is supersaturated with respect to hydroxyapatite at normal intraoral pH, submandibular saliva to a greater degree than parotid saliva. The equilibrium for the dissolution of hydroxyapatite is described by the formula:

$$Ca_{10}(PO_4)_6(OH)_2 \longleftrightarrow 10Ca^{2+} + 6PO_4^{3-} + 2OH^-$$

If the pH falls (i.e. the H^+ concentration rises), the PO_4^{3-} ions are converted to HPO_4^{2-} or $H_2PO_4^-$, and the OH^- ions are neutralized to form water. This causes the saliva to be no longer supersaturated, and drives the reaction to the right (dissolution). If, however, the pH rises, the reaction is driven to the left (remineralization), because the degree of supersaturation increases. The pH at which the forces during the reaction on right and left are exactly balanced is called the critical pH.

Factors influencing the composition of saliva

Flow rate

As the flow rate increases, the concentrations of proteins, sodium, chloride and bicarbonate rise, while the levels of phosphate and magnesium fall. This is true for duct saliva as well as whole saliva. For sodium and chloride, this can be explained on the basis of the two-stage secretory mechanism: as the amount of primary secretion increases, the time during which the fluid is passing through the duct (and this the amount of ductal modification) is reduced. At very high flow rates, the composition of the ductal fluid therefore approaches that of the primary acinar secretion.

With other components, this process cannot explain the effect of flow rate. For example, bicarbonate is secreted by the duct, and its concentration should therefore fall with increased flow. In fact, bicarbonate levels rise dramatically at high flow rates, probably due to the secretion of the raised levels of bicarbonate formed by metabolically active gland cells.

Differential gland contributions

In unstimulated whole saliva, the parotid glands contribute only about 10% of the fluid volume, whereas in stimulated saliva they become predominant. Thus, the composition of the mixed fluid approaches that of parotid saliva at high flow rates. As the calcium concentration in parotid saliva is lower than that in submandibular saliva, stimulated whole saliva often contains lower levels of calcium than the unstimulated secretion, despite the fact that the levels may rise in both duct salivas as their flow rates increase.

Circadian rhythm

As well as the circadian rhythm in flow rate, rhythmic variations in the concentrations of many salivary constituents are seen. For example, the levels of calcium and phosphate ions are low in the early morning.

Duration of stimulus

At a constant rate of flow, the composition may vary with the duration of stimulation.

Nature of stimulus

If the flow rate is held constant, the secretions elicited with sour, salt, sweet or bitter stimuli are similar in electrolyte composition; however, salt stimulates a higher protein content. It has been claimed that sugar stimuli give rise to a high amylase content in saliva. Neither of these effects would appear to be biologically significant.

Diet

Long-term changes in diet do not appear to have a dramatic effect on salivary composition. It has been suggested, however, that changes in plasma phosphate and urea concentrations induced by dietary alterations may be reflected in the saliva.

The rise in fluoride concentrations in subjects drinking fluoridated water may be in part due to increased fluoride in the duct secretions, and also to the retention of fluoride in the mouth after ingestion.

Properties and functions of saliva

Digestion

Salivary amylase initiates the digestion of starch, but is inactivated in the stomach because of the low pH and proteolytic activity there. However, the rate of inactivation may be retarded if the meal is large and gastric juice fails to diffuse throughout the stomach contents. There is evidence that considerable breakdown of starch can occur prior to inactivation of salivary amylase and, especially after a heavy meal, this may account for a significant fraction of starch digestion by the body as a whole.

Salivary amylase has been considered to be of significance for dental health because of its intraoral actions. However, starch digestion in the mouth may either be beneficial in aiding starch clearance, or detrimental in liberating maltose for fermentation by oral bacteria to form acid. The overall effect on caries is still undecided.

Starch in cereal and potatoes is present in the form of granules which are resistant to amylase action. On cooking, however, the granules are disrupted and digestion can take place. Cooked starch has been shown to be cariogenic in rats, and to give rise to acid production in human plaque pH experiments, presumably because digestion by salivary amylase releases sufficient maltose to constitute a cariogenic challenge. The role of starch as a cause of caries in humans is, however, very limited.

Lubrication

The lubrication of the hard and soft oral surfaces is very important for speech, mastication and swallowing, and for general oral health and comfort. Saliva provides a tissue-coating film which is responsible for lubrication and bolus formation, a property which is due to the water and mucous glycoproteins it contains.

These glycoproteins are at high concentrations in the minor mucous gland and sublingual gland secretions, intermediate in submandibular saliva, and very low in parotid saliva; the viscosity of the different secretions varies accordingly. The viscosity of saliva is non-Newtonian. It exhibits different viscosities at different rates of shear, and has viscoelastic properties. The ability to draw out a thread of saliva is typical of a viscoelastic fluid, and is known as spinnbarkeit.

The viscous behaviour of whole saliva changes with time after secretion, partly because of its non-Newtonian properties, but also because of post-secretory degradation of mucous glycoproteins by bacterial enzymes.

Dilution and clearance

Another effect of the water content of saliva is the dilution of substances introduced into the mouth, and their subsequent removal by swallowing or spitting. Food solids are first dissolved (whereby they can be tasted) and then diluted as the saliva flows into the mouth. After swallowing the bulk of the food and drink, the food residues are cleared slowly by the continuing flow of unstimulated saliva. If the substance is noxious or distasteful, clearance may be achieved by spitting.

Clearance of sucrose has been modelled successfully by a computed simulation based on the principle of an incomplete syphon (Fig. 14.5). Saliva flows into the mouth until a swallow is triggered, leaving a residue of saliva (with dissolved sugar) to be further diluted until another swallow ensues. This repeating syphon effect implies that the flow rate of (unstimulated) saliva, and the volume of saliva remaining after a swallow, are especially important in determining the rate of clearance of sugar.

Clearance is more rapid from some parts of the mouth than others. Unstimulated saliva is present as a thin film covering the hard and soft tissues of the mouth, and the velocity with which this film moves over the surface determines the rate of clearance of a substance from different sites. Areas close to the ducts of the major glands (e.g. lower anterior teeth, upper posterior teeth) show more rapid clearance and a higher salivary film velocity. These sites are those which are also less prone to caries.

Clearance studies can be of value in considering the rate of removal both of potentially harmful substances (e.g. sugars, plaque, acids), and of preventive agents such as fluoride. Fortunately, individuals (or tooth sites) in which removal of harmful substances is low are those in which clearance of protective agents is also delayed.

Neutralization and buffering

Whole saliva is usually slightly alkaline and is an effective buffer system. These properties protect the oral tissues against acids from food or from plaque. The principal constituent responsible for these properties (especially in stimulated saliva) is bicarbonate. If, after

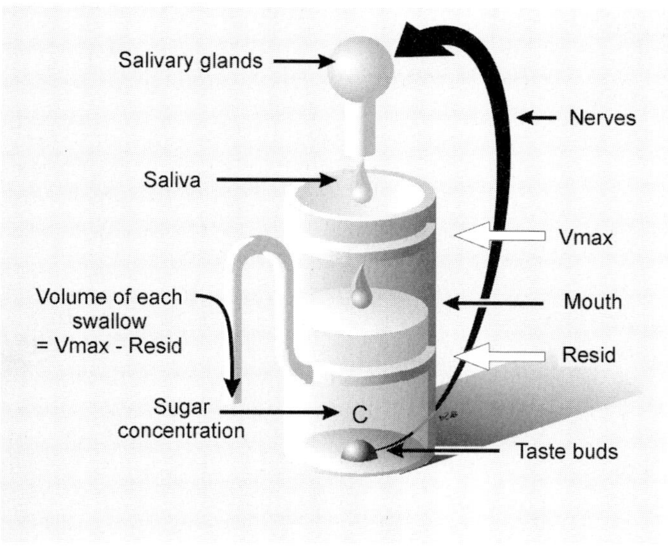

Fig. 14.5 The 'incomplete syphon' model of sugar clearance. Saliva enters the mouth at a rate determined by the gustatory reflex drive from the taste buds as a function of the sugar concentration in saliva. A swallow is triggered when the salivary volume reaches a particular volume (Vmax). After swallowing, the concentration of sugar in the residual saliva (Resid) is further diluted by saliva until a further swallow is triggered.

eating a sugary food, saliva is stimulated by chewing substances such as wax or sugar-free chewing gum, the drop in pH in plaque which would have occurred is reduced or even eliminated. This salivary neutralization and buffering effect can markedly reduce the cariogenic potential of foods.

Besides bicarbonate, a small amount of buffering is provided by the phosphate and proteins of saliva; these contributions may be appreciable in unstimulated saliva but are overwhelmed by that of bicarbonate in stimulated saliva.

Saturation

As previously mentioned, saliva is supersaturated with respect to tooth mineral. This is responsible for the growth of hydroxyapatite crystals during the remineralization phase of the caries process. Indeed, were it not for this saturation, the teeth would slowly dissolve in saliva (i.e. the critical pH would be at or above the pH of saliva).

In addition, salivary calcium and phosphate are the source of minerals for calculus formation. The presence in saliva of inhibitors of precipitation such as statherin and the proline-rich proteins is presumably a major factor preventing excessive calcification in the mouth. However, in plaque, where these proteins cannot penetrate owing to their relatively large molecular size (or perhaps due to proteolysis by oral bacteria), they are unable to prevent seeding and growth of calcium phosphate crystals, and hence calculus formation.

Saliva is also a source of fluoride for plaque, and for uptake into carious lesions during de- and remineralization.

Antibacterial effects

Immunoglobulins

Salivary antibodies are mainly of the IgA class, whose principal action is to aggregate specific bacteria and prevent their adhesion to oral hard and soft tissues. Bacterial lysis due to complement activation may occur in the gingival crevice as a result of the effects of IgG in crevicular fluid, which may also opsonize bacteria to assist phagocytosis by polymorphonuclear leukocytes.

Bacterial aggregation can also occur non-specifically by means of interactions between mucous glycoproteins and bacterial surface receptor molecules, known as *adhesins*.

Non-specific antibacterial proteins

The actions of sialoperoxidase, lactoferrin and lysozyme have already been described. Although the saliva contains a very large bacterial population (indicating that these systems are incapable of controlling many of the normal residents of the mouth), they may be of importance in preventing colonization by transient pathogens.

The classical descriptions of the actions of those molecules are being expanded as new information indicates cooperative activity between these and other agents. Further proteins (called histatins) have been described, which may be important antifungal components. It has even been shown that amylase, in addition to its digestive function, may have antibacterial properties; it is present in tears and other situations where its digestive action is irrelevant (such as bronchial and urogenital secretions).

Bacterial competition

Because of the large number of bacteria in saliva, competition for scarce nutrients is fierce, and pathogens (normally fastidious in their nutritional requirements) may thus be unable to survive. The products of metabolism of one species may be toxic to another; a good example of this is provided by acidogenic, aciduric organisms which thrive at the low pH levels resulting from the accumulation of their own metabolic end-products.

Bacterial competition is also demonstrated by the synthesis of bacteriocins by certain species. These are inhibitory molecules by which an organism can establish dominance over susceptible neighbours.

In addition to these competitive mechanisms, certain species are adapted to utilize salivary glycoproteins as sources of energy and nitrogen. This appears to be related to their ability to synthesize extracellular glycosidase enzymes to break down the oligosaccharide side chains. Saliva can thus play a role in the control of the bacterial flora by acting as a selective growth medium.

Pellicle and plaque formation

Both pellicle and plaque matrix contain proteins predominantly derived from saliva. Pellicle formation is a physicochemical process involving selective, sequential adsorption of salivary glycoproteins to the tooth surface; other proteins from bacteria (e.g. glucosyl transferase) and gingival crevicular fluid (e.g. albumin, IgG) are also present. The proteins with the highest affinity appear to be a group of acidic proline-rich proteins, but early (2 h) pellicle also contains high-molecular-weight proteins with blood group activity similar to MG1.

Pellicle protects the teeth against both chemical and mechanical insult. In addition, however, it acts as a substrate for colonization by bacteria, many of which have developed mechanisms of attachment involving the synthesis of adhesins, molecules which bind to oligosaccharide groups of mucous glycoproteins. Other organisms appear to attach by means of glucans synthesized by cell-bound as well as pellicle-bound glucosyl transferase enzymes.

Plaque formation involves incorporation of salivary proteins, but their characterization is difficult because they are extensively degraded in plaque. They are believed to be incorporated by electrostatic bonds and hydrophobic interactions. Plaque matrix proteins may have a limited structural role in holding plaque together, but more important in promoting cohesion is the synthesis of extracellular glucans.

Salivary gland dysfunction

The importance of saliva in oral health is dramatically revealed in patients with salivary gland dysfunction, leading to the subjective complaint of xerostomia (dry mouth), which includes difficulty with speech and mastication, a tendency towards mucositis often associated with candidal infection, atrophic changes in the mucosa of the tongue, and (when teeth are present) a tendency to rapid carious destruction as well as periodontal disease. Diagnosis of salivary gland dysfunction can be made in the first instance by sialometry (measurement of salivary flow), followed later by more sophisticated radiological investigation.

Table 14.4 Some drugs which cause dry mouth

Category	*Example*
Anorectics	Amphetamine
Anticholinergic	Atropine, scopolamine
Antidepressants	Amitriptyline, nortriptyline
Antipsychotics	Phenothiazine
Antihypertensive	Clonidine
Antiparkinsonism	Benztropine

While the range of normal flow rates is very wide, so that a value which would be low for one patient may be normal for another, flow rates for whole saliva of less than 0.1 ml/min (unstimulated) would be regarded as abnormally low. The prevalence of dry mouth is probably much higher than previously considered – a recent survey in the USA found that 30% of patients attending a general medical practice clinic had unstimulated flow rates below 0.1 ml/min. A similar proportion of the general adult population had symptoms of dry mouth.

The most common cause of salivary dysfunction is as a side- effect of drugs (Table 14.4). Other causes are associated with local or systemic disease, for example, surgery or irradiation of the salivary glands, diabetes and especially the autoimmune condition Sjögren's syndrome.

Treatment is principally focused on the relief of symptoms by saliva substitutes and, where relevant, the prevention of caries and periodontal disease by intensive fluoride therapy and oral hygiene. If functional gland tissue remains, it can be stimulated by chewing non-cariogenic foods such as raw vegetables or sugar-free chewing gum. Alternatively, parasympathomimetic drugs (e.g. pilocarpine) have been used with success in selected patients under medical supervision.

Further reading

Edgar WM, O'Mullane DM. *Saliva and Oral Health*, 2nd edn. London: British Dental Association, 1996.

Proceedings, 10th International conference on Oral Biology on Saliva and Salivary Glands. *J Dent Res* 1987; **66**: 385–618.

Proceedings, Conference on the Evaluation and Management of Salivary Gland Dysfunction. *J Dent Res* 1987; **66**: 623–708.

Sreebny LM (ed.) *The Salivary System*. Boca Raton: CRC Press, 1987.

15

The essential features of microorganisms and the rationale for antimicrobial therapy

C. W. Ian Douglas

Summary

Antimicrobial agents have had a major impact on the control of most bacterial diseases. However, generally viral, fungal, protozoal and helminthic diseases have been less amenable to drug therapy. The reason for this lies in the different structural and physiological features of each group of microorganisms. This chapter will outline the basic features of the various types of microorganisms and relate these to the mechanisms of action of commonly used antimicrobial agents.

Basic features of microorganisms

The microbial world is divided into viruses, prokaryotes and eukaryotes. With the exception of the viruses, microorganisms consist of cells but the structure and physiology of some of them show significant differences from mammalian cells, making it possible selectively to target these differences with drugs. To understand what the potential targets for drugs are, the features of the various types of microorganism will be described briefly.

Viruses

Viruses are absolutely dependent upon other cells for their reproduction because they have no metabolism of their own; thus, they are obligate intracellular parasites. A complete virus particle or virion consists of one or more molecules of DNA or RNA enclosed in a protein coat, the nucleocapsid, and sometimes also within a phospholipid membrane. The latter is, in fact, a small part of the cytoplasmic or nuclear membrane of the last cell that the virus infected. The viral nucleic acid varies in complexity between different viruses. Some viruses have a genome only large enough to code for three or four proteins, while others have genomes capable of directing the synthesis of over 100 proteins.

To classify viruses, several features are taken into account, including type of nucleic acid, whether the virus is enveloped or not, the symmetry of the capsid and the site of its assembly (cytoplasm or nucleus), sensitivity of the virus to ether and size of the virus. A summary of the main groups of viruses infecting humans is given in Table 15.1.

Life cycle

Adsorption

For a virus to infect a cell, it must first attach to the cell surface. The virus uses a specialized adhesin molecule, which is a capsid structural protein or a spike-like structure projecting from the capsid or membrane envelope. This adhesin attaches to a cell membrane receptor, the distribution of which is crucial in determining the tissue and host specificity of the virus. For example, poliovirus receptors are found only in the human nasopharynx, gut and

Table 15.1 Classification of viruses

Virus	*Capsid*	*Envelope*	*Example*
RNA viruses			
Picornavirus	Icosahedral	−	Poliovirus
Reovirus	Icosahedral	−	Rotavirus
Togavirus	Icosahedral	+	Rubella
Orthomyxovirus	Icosahedral	+	Influenza
Paramyxovirus	Helical	+	Mumps, measles
Rhabdovirus	Helical	+	Rabies
Arenavirus	Coiled	+	Lassa fever
Retrovirus	Uncertain	+	Human immunodeficiency virus (HIV)
DNA viruses			
Herpesvirus	Icosahedral	+	Herpes simplex
Hepadnaviruses	Icosahedral	+	Hepatitis B
Adenovirus	Icosahedral	−	Respiratory infections
Papovavirus	Icosahedral	−	Papillomaviruses
Poxvirus	Complex	+	Smallpox

spinal cord anterior horn cells, whereas measles virus receptors are present in most tissues.

Penetration and uncoating

The mechanism of penetrating the cell membrane varies with the type of virus. It is thought that naked viruses either directly inject their nucleic acid into the host cell or take advantage of a phagocytic-like process that the majority of mammalian cells perform, called endocytosis. Membrane-bound viruses either use endocytosis or fuse directly with the host cell membrane. Most viruses are uncoated by the action of lysosomal enzymes, which releases their nucleic acid into the cytoplasm of the cell.

Replication

This part of the cycle varies according to the type of nucleic acid within the virus. Positive-stranded RNA viruses (e.g. poliovirus) can use their genome directly to transcribe an enormous peptide, which is subsequently cleaved into functional proteins. Retroviruses, such as human immunodeficiency virus (HIV), employ a viral reverse transcriptase to synthesize a DNA mirror image (complementary DNA) of their RNA; this is then made double-stranded and integrated into the genome of the infected cell. Negative-stranded RNA viruses (e.g. mumps, measles and influenza viruses) must first convert their genome into a complementary messenger RNA sequence using a viral transcriptase. Subsequently, products of viral gene translation take over the cell's synthetic machinery for the purposes of manufacturing new virions.

Release

Again, mechanisms of virion release differ between different virus types. Naked viruses appear to be released mostly by host cell lysis, whereas enveloped viruses are usually released by budding through the membrane, taking a part of it with them. The above stages are represented diagrammatically in Figure 15.1.

Antiviral drugs

All stages of the life cycle of viruses are theoretically open to selective attack. However, although numerous agents have been described which interfere with one or other of those stages, few have been found that are sufficiently selective in their action to be therapeutically useful because viruses utilize the host's metabolic machinery. The main agents that are in regular therapeutic use are shown in Table 15.2. Most are nucleoside analogues which, after phosphorylation, are mistakenly inserted into the newly synthesized viral nucleic acid, rendering its code unreadable.

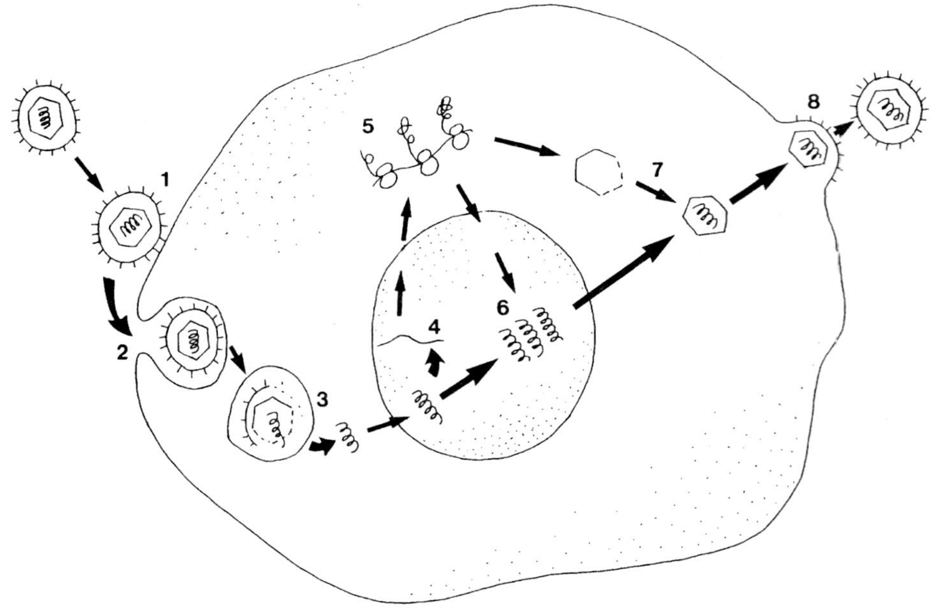

Fig. 15.1 Viral replication involves: (1) adsorption; (2) penetration into the cell; (3) uncoating of the virus and release of the nucleic acid; (4) transcription into messenger RNA; (5) translation into proteins; (6) nucleic acid replication; (7) assembly of the capsid and packaging of the nucleic acid; and (8) release of the new viruses.

Table 15.2 Main antiviral agents

Drug	*Virus*	*Mode of action*
Acyclovir	Herpes simplex	Nucleoside analogue
Amantadine	Influenza A	Uncoating virus
Idoxuridine	Herpes simplex	Nucleoside analogue
Vidarabine	Herpesviruses	Nucleoside analogue
Zidovudine	Human immunodeficiency virus	Nucleoside analogue

Acyclovir

Acyclovir is the only antiviral agent available that exhibits true selective toxicity. It is an analogue of guanosine and is unique in that it is phosphorylated by a viral-coded enzyme; the corresponding host cell enzyme is much less efficient at phosphorylating acyclovir. Consequently, the drug is only activated in virus-infected cells.

Zidovudine (AZT)

This is a dideoxynucleoside in which one of the hydroxyl groups has been replaced by an azido group. Since, during nucleic acid synthesis, the nucleosides are joined by their hydroxyl groups, insertion of AZT effectively terminates nucleic acid-chain elongation. AZT inhibits the reverse transcriptase of retroviruses at much lower concentrations than that required to inhibit host DNA synthesis.

Prokaryotic cells

These are bacteria, mycoplasmas, *Chlamydia* and *Rickettsia*. They lack complex internal membrane systems and there is no compartmentation of cellular functions. All except *Chlamydia* and *Mycoplasma* have a complex cell wall and many have polysaccharide capsules, surface fibrils and flagellae. Some bacteria form resistant endospores to survive harsh environmental conditions.

Cell wall structure

The cell walls of bacteria are rigid structures conferring shape and enabling them to survive the osmotic intake of solutes in hypotonic environments. The rigidity of the cell wall is due to the presence of peptidoglycan, a polymer comprising strands of sugar units cross-linked to each other by short peptide chains. Although most bacteria contain peptidoglycan, they do not all have the same overall cell wall structure. Gram-positive organisms have a dense peptidoglycan layer overlying the cytoplasmic membrane, with one or a number of accessory polymers (e.g. teichoic acids) linked to the peptidoglycan. Gram-negative bacteria, on the other hand, have a thinner peptidoglycan layer, which is covered by an outer phospholipid membrane; other accessory molecules are attached to either the peptidoglycan or the outer membrane (e.g. lipoprotein and lipopolysaccharide respectively). Pores in the outer membrane control the access of molecules to the deeper layers of the cell wall and cytoplasmic membrane, including certain antimicrobial agents. Some prokaryotes, *Chlamydia* and *Mycoplasma*, lack a peptidoglycan layer and are bound only by a phospholipid membrane.

Because there is no structure in mammalian cells that is comparable to the peptidoglycan of bacteria, it is a useful target for antimicrobial drugs. A scheme illustrating the synthesis of the peptidoglycan layer and the points at which several antibiotics act is shown in Figure 15.2. Clearly, such drugs will not affect microorganisms which lack a peptidoglycan

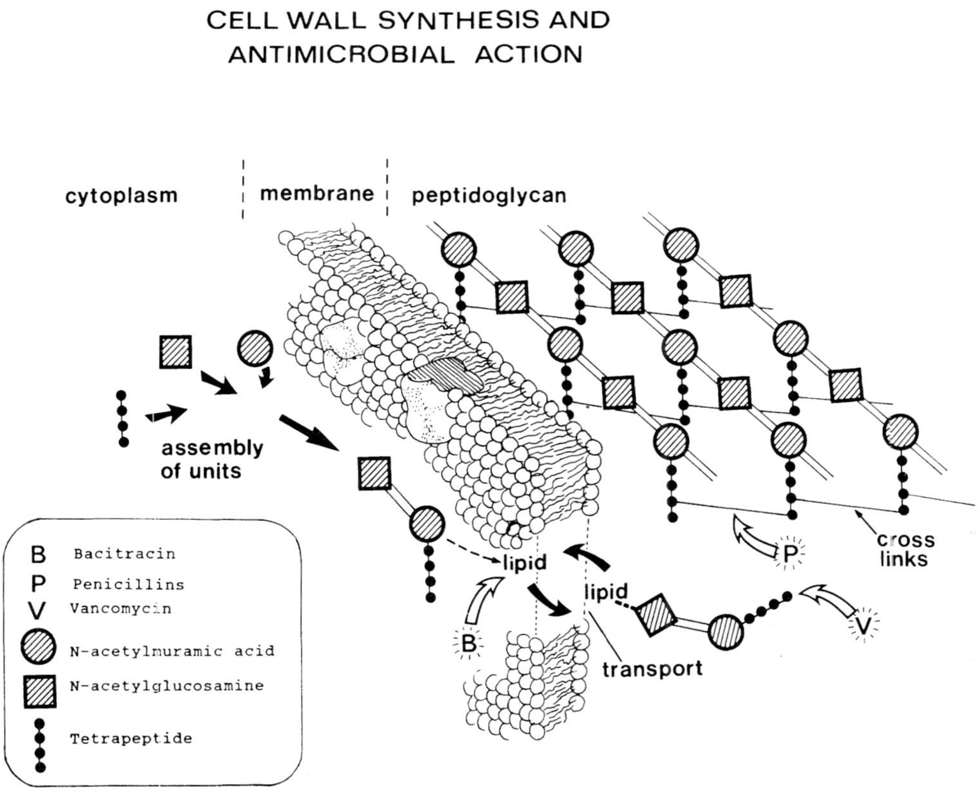

Fig. 15.2 Peptidoglycan synthesis involves (1) assembly of a peptide of five amino acids, a molecule of *N*-acetylmuramic acid (NAM) and *N*-acetylglucosamine into a unit in the cytoplasm; (2) transport of this unit across the membrane via a lipid carrier; (3) insertion of the unit into the peptidoglycan structure; and (4) cross-linking of the peptide chain, with resultant loss of an amino acid, to an adjacent tetrapeptide. The open arrows show the points in the process which are inhibited by antibiotics.

layer, such as *Chlamydia*, *Mycoplasma*, viruses, fungi or protozoa.

Penicillins and cephalosporins (β-lactams)

These drugs were thought for many years to work simply by inhibiting the cross-linking reaction between peptide side chains in the peptidoglycan, rendering the cell osmotically fragile. However, it is now known that β-lactam drugs bind to several proteins in bacterial cell membranes, called penicillin-binding proteins (PBP). *Escherichia coli* has seven PBPs; 1a,b,2 and 3 are transpeptidases involved in cell elongation and cross-wall formation; 4–6 are carboxypeptidases involved in lipoprotein attachment and controlling the extent of cross-linking. Both types of drugs contain a β-lactam ring as part of their structure, which is an analogue of alanyl-alanine, the terminal part of the peptide side chain.

Protein synthesis

Unlike viruses, prokaryotic cells have complex metabolic pathways, including the ability to synthesize protein. Although the basic mechanism of protein synthesis is thought to be universal, bacteria differ from mammalian cells in having differently structured ribosomes and it is by preferentially binding to bacterial ribosomes that certain drugs can inhibit protein synthesis without being too toxic. The essential steps in the protein synthetic process are shown in Figure 15.3, along with the site of action of some antibiotics.

Chloramphenicol

Chloramphenicol acts by inhibiting peptide bond formation (peptidyl transferase reaction) on the ribosome. It has a wide spectrum of activity extending to the strictly intracellular parasites, *Chlamydia* and *Rickettsia*, by virtue of its ability to penetrate readily into mammalian cells.

Tetracyclines

Tetracyclines have a very broad spectrum of activity but their therapeutic usefulness has declined because of the increase in microbial resistance. They act by interfering with the

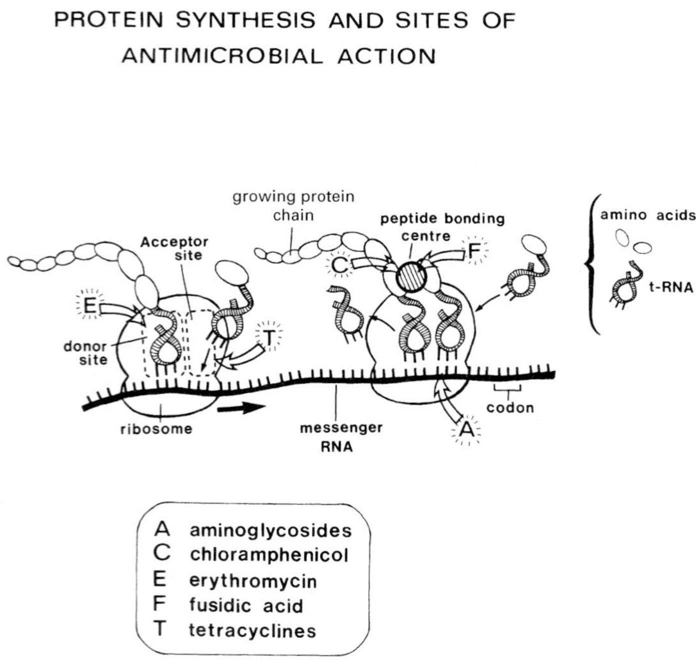

Fig. 15.3 The process of protein synthesis involves: (1) ribosomes binding to messenger RNA; (2) attachment of two transfer-RNA (t-RNA) molecules, carrying the amino acids determined by the messenger RNA code, to the ribosome; the first at the donor site, the next at the acceptor site, (3) formation of a peptide bond between the two amino acids by the action of peptidyl-transferase; (4) ejection of the t-RNA from the donor site; the second t-RNA with peptide then moves across into the donor site by the action of a translocase; the ribosome moves along the messenger RNA and the process is repeated. The open arrows show the points in the process which are inhibited by antibiotics.

binding of amino acid-transfer RNA (t-RNA) complexes to the acceptor site on the ribosome, thus preventing addition of new amino acids to the growing peptide chain.

Fusidic acid

Fusidic acid is a steroid-like agent which prevents the transfer of the growing peptide chain from the acceptor site to the donor site, by binding to the translocase enzyme, 'G' factor. Fusidic acid fails to penetrate the Gram-negative outer membrane and so its activity is restricted to Gram-positive bacteria.

Erythromycin

Erythromycin belongs to a group known as the macrolides, which also act by inhibiting peptide translocation. However, erythromycin binds to the donor site on the ribosome, preventing the transfer of the peptide chain from the acceptor site.

Aminoglycosides

Aminoglycosides (e.g. gentamicin, kanamycin) have a fairly broad spectrum of activity but have no effect on anaerobic organisms. This is because they are taken into cells by first complexing with respiratory quinones in the cell membrane; anaerobes lack quinones. Once inside cells, they bind to a ribosomal protein causing misreading of the messenger RNA code and resulting in the insertion of the wrong amino acids into the growing peptide chain. The aminoglycosides are not absorbed from the gastointestinal tract and so must be administered parenterally.

Miscellaneous antibacterial agents

Various targets other than the cell wall and bacterial ribosome are available for selective attack by chemotherapeutic agents. These include the cell membrane, nucleic acid synthesis and several essential metabolic activities taking place within the bacterial cell. However, most of the agents acting in these ways are not strictly antibiotics because they are synthetic substances, rather than naturally occurring compounds.

Sulphonamides

Sulphonamides are analogues of *p*-aminobenzoic acid and competitively inhibit dihydrofolate reductase, an enzyme involved in the synthesis of folic acid by bacteria. Mammalian cells cannot make their own folic acid and so lack dihydrofolate reductase. Folic acid is a precursor in the synthesis of purines and pyrimidines.

Quinolones

Quinolones act by inhibiting DNA gyrase, an enzyme responsible for unwinding the supercoiled DNA helix before transcription and replication. Nalidixic acid is the best known of this group of drugs and is virtually restricted to Gram-negative organisms in its activity, but the newer quinolones (e.g. ciprofloxacin) have a much broader spectrum of activity.

Imidazoles

Imidazoles can affect a wide spectrum of microorganisms, including bacteria, fungi, viruses and protozoa. The derivatives with antibacterial activity are 5-nitroimidazoles, of which metronidazole is the best known. Metronidazole was discovered to affect anaerobic bacteria when a patient's acute ulcerative gingivitis improved during treatment for a *Trichomonas* infection. Metronidazole is inactive itself, but becomes reduced to an active form in the low-redox conditions prevailing within anaerobic organisms. It is thought to work by inducing strand breakage of DNA.

Eukaryotic cells

Eukaryotic cells differ most obviously from prokaryotic cells in first, having a variety of complex membranous organelles in the cytoplasm (e.g. mitochondria and Golgi bodies); second, in having sterols in the cytoplasmic membrane; and third, having their genetic material within a membrane-bound nucleus. Fungi, protozoa and higher plants and animals, including humans, are eukaryotes. Thus, because they are all biochemically very similar, it has been difficult to devise many drugs which are sufficiently selectively toxic for treatment of infections caused by eukaryotic microorganisms.

Fungi

The fungi vary in complexity and size, ranging from single-celled microscopic yeasts to the multicellular moulds and mushrooms. Many fungi, especially the medically important ones, are dimorphic, that is, they can change between a yeast and a filamentous (hyphal) form, which allows them to penetrate tissue more readily.

The cell walls of fungi consist of a network of microfibrils of chitin, mannan, cellulose or other glucans in a matrix of polysaccharides, protein and lipids. Despite the difference in structure from mammalian cell envelopes, fungal cell wall synthesis does not appear to be a useful target for antifungal drugs. Instead, the main groups of antifungals have an affinity for sterols in cell membranes, particularly ergosterol; the major sterol in mammalian cell membranes is cholesterol. Most of the toxic effects of such drugs are probably due to the ability of the drug to bind to cholesterol, although with a lower affinity.

Polyenes

Polyenes act by binding to ergosterol, altering the permeability of the membrane of the cell and leading to leakage of essential metabolites. The most commonly used are nystatin and amphotericin B. The latter has also been observed to induce ultrastructural and biochemical changes in the lipoprotein coat of hepatitis B virus.

Imidazoles

Imidazoles are fungistatic at low concentrations by interfering with ergosterol synthesis in growing organisms, whereas at high concentrations they are fungicidal due to membrane damage induced by direct binding to sterols.

Some antifungal imidazoles also show activity against Gram-positive bacteria (e.g. miconazole); however, their mode of action in this case is not clear, since sterols are not structurally important in bacteria.

5-Fluorocytosine

This is a pyrimidine analogue, originally developed as an anticancer drug, but it was found to have activity against yeasts. In the yeast cell, the compound is deaminated by cytosine deaminase to 5-fluorouracil and incorporated into fungal RNA, leading to misreading of the code. Mammalian cells lack cytosine deaminase, explaining the low toxicity of this drug.

Protozoa

Protozoa are eukaryotic, usually motile, unicellular organisms. They are bound by a cytoplasmic membrane of similar type to our own but the cytoplasm immediately underneath the membrane is often semisolid or gelatinous, probably to provide some rigidity to the body of the organism. Osmoregulation in these cells is achieved by the action of contractile vacuoles, which continuously expel water. Some protozoa are anaerobic and, unlike mammalian cells, lack mitochondria, cytochromes and a functional tricarboxylic acid cycle. Many reproduce by a multistage life cycle, including the production of a cyst or resting stage, which provides protection against adverse conditions. In parasitic species, the cyst is the means of transfer from one host to another.

Pathogenic protozoa are among the most important causes of morbidity and mortality in the world, accounting for infection in about 700 million people. Examples of such infections are malaria, amoebic dysentery, sleeping sickness, *Trichomonas* vaginitis and toxoplasmosis. Some of these diseases have been treated successfully with specific drugs for centuries but the range of drugs available for treating this group of microorganisms, even today, is small.

Quinine

Quinine is the traditional mainstay of treatment for malaria but a variety of derivatives of this drug have now been developed. Their mechanism of action is not entirely clear but it is thought that quinines raise the pH of acidic vesicles in the erythrocytic stage of the disease. Acidic vesicles appear to be important in a variety of eukaryotic intracellular functions, including endocytosis, membrane movement and targeting of lysosomal enzymes. Our cells seem to be less sensitive to the effects of quinines than those of *Plasmodium* species.

Microbial resistance to drugs

The introduction of sulphonamides into clinical practice in 1935 heralded the beginning of effective treatment of bacterial infections, but it also heralded the emergence of drug resistance as a practical clinical problem. Within a few years sulphonamide-resistant strains of organisms were common. When penicillin came into use in 1941, less than 1% of *Staphylococcus aureus* were resistant. By 1946, the proportion of penicillin-resistant strains in hospitals was 14% and now it is over 90%. While drug resistance in some organisms has been problematic, it has not been the case with all organisms; *Streptococcus pyogenes* has remained fully sensitive to penicillin.

Generally, organisms are intrinsically resistant to a particular antimicrobial drug or become resistant by one or more of the following mechanisms:

1. The target for the drug is absent from the organism.
2. The target for the drug has become insensitive.
3. The target for the drug is overproduced.
4. The drug is prevented from reaching its target:
   (a) because of limited membrane permeability.
   (b) because it is destroyed by enzymes.
   (c) because it is expelled from the cell.
5. The drug is not activated in the organism.

Examples of the above include:

1. β-Lactam antibiotics having no effect on viruses, fungi or protozoa because they lack the target, peptidoglycan. Similarly, the antiviral agent acyclovir is not active against viruses that do not have a gene coding for the production of a sensitive thymidine kinase.
2. Drug resistance due to alteration of the target molecule usually arises by chance mutation, but may also arise by acquisition of a foreign gene from another organism, which codes for an altered target molecule, or by enzymic modification of the target molecule. For example:
   (a) A single amino acid change in the ribosomal protein designated S12 entirely prevents streptomycin binding and confers resistance to high levels of this drug.
   (b) Mutation of the enzyme dihydropteroate synthetase decreases its affinity for sulphonamides.
   (c) Erythromycin resistance in staphylococci and streptococci usually arises by methylation of the ribosomal RNA by an inducible plasmid-mediated enzyme.
3. Some *E. coli* mutants produce 25-fold more dihydrofolate reductase, the target for trimethoprim, than their normal counterparts. These strains would, therefore, require a much higher concentration of drug to be present in their cytoplasm if the folate pathway was to be effectively blocked.
4. (a) The outer membrane of Gram-negative bacteria is full of holes or pores, through which substances diffuse to reach the underlying cell. Several drugs are unable to pass through these pores, preventing access of many antibiotics to the cell interior, and in *Pseudomonas aeruginosa*, a notoriously resistant organism, it seems that many of the pores are blocked.
   (b) The classic example of a drug-destroying enzyme is the β-lactamase produced by *Staphylococcus aureus*, which is a plasmid-coded, inducible exoenzyme. A plasmid is a piece of DNA, not part of the chromosome of the cell, which is transferable from one organism to another. Plasmids also code for a variety of other drug resistance mechanisms.
   (c) Tetracyclines are actively transported into the bacterium, resulting in the accumulation of the drug in the cytoplasm. A plasmid codes for the production of a protein which then

actively expels the drug, so that drug entering the cell is simultaneously removed and never reaches an inhibitory concentration.

5. Metronidazole diffuses into both aerobic and anaerobic bacteria equally well, but in the former it remains unchanged, while in the latter it is reduced by nitroreductases. Thus, the drug is only activated in anaerobic organisms.

Conclusions

Because of the inherent differences between various types of microorganisms, the proper choice of antimicrobial drug depends upon identifying the infecting organism. An alternative strategy is to use a 'shotgun' approach but there are several drawbacks to this, including failure to cover the pathogen, antagonism or toxicity if multiple drugs are used, increased likelihood of superinfection and increased cost of therapy. With definition of the microorganism, specific drugs may be substituted for broad antimicrobial therapy.

Further reading

Garrod LP, Lambert HP, O'Grady F. *Antibiotic and Chemotherapy*, 6th edn. Edinburgh: Churchill Livingstone, 1989.

Kucers A, McK Bennet N. *The Use of Antibiotics: A Comprehensive Review with Clinical Emphasis*, 4th edn London: Heinemann, 1987.

Prescott LM, Harley JP, Klein DA. *Microbiology*. Dubuque, USA: WC Brown, 1990.

Schaechter M, Medoff G, Schlessinger D. *Mechanisms of Microbial Disease*. Baltimore, USA: Williams & Wilkins, 1989.

16

The microbiology of dental caries and periodontal disease

Jeremy M. Hardie

Summary

The microbial flora of the mouth is highly complex, containing a wide variety of bacterial species. The most common types of oral disease, dental caries and periodontal disease, are both related to dental plaque and seem to occur when the normal balance between the microorganisms and the host is disturbed in some way. Dental caries is usually associated with increased numbers of mutans streptococci and lactobacilli at the sites of disease; estimation of salivary levels of these organisms may be useful for assessing caries risk in patients and for monitoring their response to preventive measures. A large number of 'candidate pathogens' have been identified as potential aetiological agents in different types of periodontal disease, although the specific plaque hypothesis may still be controversial. *Porphyromonas gingivalis*, *Prevotella intermedia*, *Actinobacillus actinomycetemcomitans*, together with the poorly understood spirochaetes, have most frequently been reported as significant periodontopathogens and a number of possible virulence factors have been described. Application of modern molecular techniques to the study of the microbiology of oral diseases should allow rapid further progress to be made and will lead, hopefully, to improved methods of diagnosis, risk assessment and treatment.

Introduction

Oral microbiology occupies a central role in understanding the aetiology, prevention and treatment of many of the more common oral and dental diseases.[1] For example, purulent conditions such as dentoalveolar abscesses, pericoronitis and actinomycosis are usually endogenous infections caused by bacteria that make up part of the resident, commensal flora of the mouth; many of these are obligate anaerobes.[2] Similarly, oral candidosis is due to yeasts that are commonly present in the mouths of healthy individuals which may assume a more aggressive role when local or systemic defence mechanisms have been altered or compromised in some way.[3]

The two most common types of dental disease, dental caries and periodontal disease, are known to be associated with microorganisms present on the tooth surface in dental plaque. Thus, these diseases may be regarded as plaque-related infections, although their aetiologies are often complex and can be affected by a number of host and environmental factors in addition to any microbial activities.[2–4]

In this short chapter, some of the current ideas about the role of microorganisms in dental caries and various types of periodontal disease are discussed. In view of the extensive published literature on these topics, references have been confined mainly to major reviews and books, together with a few original papers. As with other aspects of microbiology, supplementation of conventional laboratory methods by the newer molecular biological techniques such as gene cloning and analysis, nucleic acid hybridization and sequencing, development of gene probes, and application of polymerase chain reaction (PCR) is having a considerable impact on oral microbiology and further rapid advances can be anticipated over the next few years.[5,6]

The microflora of the mouth

The oral cavity provides a variety of surfaces and microenvironments which become colonized by microorganisms, commencing immediately after birth and continuing thereafter.[7] When the intraoral environment changes in some way as, for example, during the eruption of the first teeth into the infant's mouth or, later in life, when teeth are lost, new opportunities and challenges are presented to would-be colonizers. Within the oral cavity potential habitats include either non-shedding hard tooth surfaces or soft, constantly replaced epithelial surfaces for attachment, and a variety of conditions with respect to oxygen levels and anaerobiosis, availability of nutrients, exposure to salivary secretions or gingival crevicular fluid, masticatory forces and other variables such as oral hygiene procedures.[8,9]

As a result of all these and other variables, the composition of the microbial flora of the mouth varies considerably from site to site and at different times. Thus, for example, the predominant types and relative numbers of bacteria in supragingival dental plaque usually differ from those found on soft-tissue surfaces or in whole saliva. Even within dental plaque itself, marked variations can be demonstrated between different sites on the teeth. The characteristics of subgingival plaque are generally different from those of supragingival plaque, the former being richer in anaerobes, motile organisms and predominantly Gram-negative bacteria.[8,9]

The composition of the oral microflora, in addition to being variable, is highly complex. At least 30 bacterial genera are commonly isolated from the mouth (Table 16.1), and many of these genera are represented by several species.[8–10] To give just a few examples, more than 15 species of oral streptococci are now recognized amongst the group often referred to in the past simply as *Streptococcus viridans*.[11,12] Similarly, the organisms previously called black-pigmented *Bacteroides* are now considered to represent at least 11 different species which fall into two distinct genera, *Porphyromonas* and *Prevotella*.[13,14] The total number of bacterial species known to be associated with the mouth is over 300, but in any particular individual there are likely to be 50–100 species present. In addition to the known bacterial species which can be isolated and identified, there are others which can be seen microscopically but have yet to be cultured in the laboratory. Yeasts, usually *Candida* species, are also commonly present, and other kinds of microorganisms such as mycoplasmas

Table 16.1 Some bacterial genera commonly present in the mouth

Gram-positive		*Gram-negative*		
Cocci	*Rods and filaments*	*Cocci*	*Rods and filaments*	*Spirals*
Enterococcus	*Actinomyces*	*Branhamella*	*Actinobacillus*	*Treponema*
Peptostreptococcus	*Arachnia*	*Neisseria*	*Campylobacter*	
Stomatococcus	*Bifidobacterium*	*Veillonella*	*Capnocytophaga*	
Streptococcus	*Corynebacterium*		*Centipeda*	
	Eubacterium		*Eikenella*	
	Lactobacillus		*Fusobacterium*	
	Propionibacterium		*Haemophilus*	
	Rothia		*Leptotrichia*	
			*Mitsuokella**	
			*Prevotella**	
			*Porphyromonas**	
			Selenomonas	
			Simonsiella	
			Wolinella	

*Formerly in genus *Bacteroides*.

and protozoa may also be found as part of the oral flora.[8,9]

Many factors, both intrinsic and extrinsic, can have an effect on the composition and metabolic activities of the microflora of the mouth.[15] Under stable or constant conditions there is an equilibrium between the host and the microorganisms which is thought to be mutually beneficial, but disturbances of this steady state can have adverse effects, as reviewed by Marsh.[10] Such ecological perturbations may lead to one or other of the two main disease processes associated with dental plaque, dental caries and periodontal disease.

Dental caries

Theories about aetiology

These days most people accept that dental caries is caused by bacteria which ferment dietary carbohydrates, notably sucrose, to produce acids, and that these acids initiate dissolution of the tooth enamel. This view has been around since at least 1890, when Miller first proposed the chemico-parasitic theory[16] for the aetiology of caries, and it is supported by a large body of experimental evidence.[17] There have been several other theories over the centuries, including worms, disproportions of the body humours, proteolysis, chelation and autoimmunity, but these are generally lacking in supporting scientific evidence.[17]

Cariogenic bacteria in animals

The demonstration by Orland and colleagues[18] that single strains of bacteria could induce dental caries when inoculated into the mouths of germ-free animals allowed the development of experimental models for testing the cariogenic potential of different bacteria.[19] Since the late 1950s many strains, representing several species of bacteria, have been shown to be capable of inducing caries in such animal models, commonly in rats or hamsters[20] (Table 16.2). The wide range of organisms listed in Table 16.2 demonstrates that caries-inducing potential, at least in experimental animals, is not confined to a single species. However, not all bacteria tested cause equal amounts of disease; *Streptococcus mutans* and other mutans streptococci certainly head the league table of cariogenic bacteria, both in terms of the number of strains shown to induce caries, and the number and extent of carious lesions produced in infected animals. Thus, strains of *S. mutans* often induce caries in both fissures and smooth surfaces, whereas other species may be associated only with fissure lesions or, in the case of *Actinomyces* species, root surface caries.[20]

In view of the known complexity of the natural plaque flora, it can be appreciated that the monoinfected animal maintained on a high-sucrose diet is a highly artificial model system. The few studies that have been reported on defined mixtures of bacteria indicate that the cariogenic potential of an organism like *S. mutans* can be modified by

Table 16.2 Bacterial species shown to be cariogenic in animals

	Streptococcus	*Lactobacillus*	*Actinomyces*
Mutans streptococci	*S. mutans*	*L. acidophilus*	*A. naeslundii*
Mutans streptococci	*S. cricetus*	*L. casei*	*A. viscosus*
Mutans streptococci	*S. rattus*	*L. salivarius*	*A. israelii*
Mutans streptococci	*S. sobrinus*	*L. fermentum*	
Mutans streptococci	*S. ferus*		
	*S. faecalis**		
	S. milleri†		
	S. oralis‡		
	S. salivarius		
	S. sanguis§		

**Streptococcus faecalis* is now called *Enterococcus faecalis*.
†The '*S. milleri* group' of streptococci now comprises three distinct species: *S. anginosus*, *S. constellatus* and *S. intermedius*.
‡*S. oralis* includes strains previously described as '*S. mitior*'.
§Strains formerly classified as *S. sanguis* have now been divided into two species: *S. sanguis* and *S. gordonii*.

the presence of a second bacterium, such as *Veillonella alcalescens*.[21] Such studies have been complemented by laboratory experiments in which these organisms have been grown together symbiotically in continuous culture.[22] The *Veillonella* species utilizes lactic acid produced by the *Streptococcus* and this explains why, *in vivo*, there is less net acid available for enamel demineralization. This is just one example of the importance of microbial interactions in complex ecological systems, like those which exist on the tooth surface.

Microbiology of human caries

Much attention has been focused on the role of the mutans streptococci in human caries and the extensive literature has been reviewed by several authors.[23,24] The term mutans streptococci (MS) is now widely used to describe the group of streptococci which includes *S. mutans*, *S. sobrinus*, *S. cricetus*, *S. rattus*, *S. ferus*, *S. downei* and *S. macacae*. Initially, these were considered to be serovars or biovars of *S. mutans*, but detailed taxonomic studies have clearly shown that they represent separate species.[25,26] Only *S. mutans* and *S. sobrinus* are regularly isolated from humans, the remaining species being confined mainly to other animals, including rats, hamsters and monkeys.

As pointed out by Bowden,[27] there may be other bacteria involved in human caries, in addition to the MS (Table 16.3). These include other streptococci, lactobacilli and *Actinomyces*, which have been found in association with carious lesions. The disease process in dental caries goes through a number of stages, from the earliest initial demineralization (which may be reversible), through to obvious cavitation and involvement of the deeper dental tissues. The predominant bacterial flora undergoes changes in parallel with these different stages, demonstrating the phenomenon known as microbial succession.

Table 16.3 Bacterial species considered to be cariogenic in humans

Strongly implicated	*Possible association*
Mutans streptococci	Other streptococci
S. mutans	*S. mitis*
S. sobrinus	
Lactobacilli	Actinomyces
L. casei	*A. viscosus* (serovar 2)
L. fermentum	
L. plantarum	
L. acidophilus	

According to the ecological view of events which occur during the development of dental caries, the delicate balance between the normal resident flora on the tooth surface (i.e. supragingival dental plaque) and the host is disturbed in some way (for example, by dietary pressures or some perturbation of the host's defences), leading to initial demineralization of the enamel by acidogenic bacteria. This results in shifts in the microbial population at the affected site, with an increase in the numbers of bacteria such as MS and lactobacilli, probably related to the lowering of pH. As these organisms increase, the relative numbers of other bacteria like *S. sanguis* and *A. naeslundii* diminish. By the time a definite white spot lesion has developed, the carious site may be dominated by *S. mutans*, colonized by *Lactobacillus* species, and reveal increased numbers of other species such as *S. mitis* and *A. viscosus*.[28,29] Isolation of both *S. mutans* and lactobacilli is thought to be indicative of progressive lesions.[29] Thus, the detection of different combinations of bacteria at carious sites may give an indication of the state of a lesion and the likelihood of its progression.[27]

Although the association between MS in plaque and the development of caries has been demonstrated in many studies, both cross-sectional and longitudinal, several investigators have shown that lesions can occasionally develop in the apparent absence of these organisms.[30] This suggests that other bacteria may also be capable of inducing the disease in humans, as might be predicted from the animal studies described earlier. In addition, individuals can be found in some populations who harbour large numbers of MS, without the development of caries.[31] Thus, the disease should perhaps be regarded as the outcome of events determined by a 'cariogenic community' of microorganisms, rather than the direct activity of any single species or type.[27]

Whether root surface caries has a different microbial aetiology to coronal caries has yet to be clearly established. Despite some indications that *Actinomyces* species might be involved, other studies have indicated an association with MS and lactobacilli.[20] In one recent study, significant differences were demonstrated between the microbial composition of dental plaque over root surface lesions and that found in samples from the underlying carious dentine.[32] In particular, there were significantly higher proportions of lactobacilli and pleomorphic Gram-positive rods in the infected dentine. Other recently published investigations have shown that the bacteria overlying human root caries are similar to those associated with gingivitis, with a predominance of *Actinomyces* species and a variety of other Gram-positive and Gram-negative genera – findings which tend to support a polymicrobial aetiology for the initiation of root surface caries.[33] Further examination of root surface lesions of varying severity revealed a higher proportion of *A. naeslundii* and other *Actinomyces* species in initial rather than advanced lesions, whereas with *S. mutans* the reverse trend was observed.[34] Although Gram-positive bacteria accounted for about 90% of the viable organisms recovered from lesions of all levels of severity in this study, the presence of Gram-negative anaerobes such as *Prevotella*, *Selenomonas* and *Bacteroides* was also noted.[34] Further work is required to clarify the microbial aetiology of human root surface caries, but it does appear that this type of caries is associated with a polymicrobial microflora and that successional changes in its composition occur as the disease progresses from initiation to the development of deeper lesions.

Prediction of caries risk

Although dental caries occurs as a result of microbial activities at the dental plaque–tooth surface interface, an idea of the level of potentially cariogenic bacteria in the mouth can be gained from examination of whole saliva.[35] Salivary *Lactobacillus* counts were used many years ago as a means of assessing caries risk but, more recently, these have been either replaced or supplemented by estimates of MS. In most cross-sectional studies, there is a correlation between both these types of bacteria and the prevalence of caries; higher counts are found when there are more lesions present.[36] Such associations, however, do not necessarily indicate a cause-and-effect relationship between the bacteria and the observed amount of caries.

Table 16.4 Threshold values of cariogenic bacteria in saliva in relation to caries risk*

	Low risk	*High risk*
Mutans streptococci	$< 10^5$	$\geqslant 10^5$
Lactobacilli	$< 10^4$	$\geqslant 10^5$

*Values expressed as colony-forming units (cfu) per millilitre of saliva.

In longitudinal studies, the presence of high salivary levels of cariogenic bacteria has been shown to have some predictive value in determining future caries risk.[36,37] The ability to assess patients in this way has enabled researchers to suggest possible threshold values for potentially high-risk (HR) and low-risk (LR) patients, and this has obvious advantages when deciding priorities for the application of intensive preventive programmes, both for the individual and for groups of patients. However, as pointed out by Beighton,[36] the actual levels of bacteria which indicate increased caries risk will vary for different populations and in relation to other variables such as age and dental status. Thus, it is difficult to define the microbial thresholds with absolute certainty. None the less, some suggested values which may be useful in clinical studies are shown in Table 16.4.

One aspect of caries risk assessment of particular interest is the relationship between salivary levels of MS in mothers and the subsequent colonization of their newborn children. Studies in Scandinavia have shown that the children of HR mothers with MS levels of $\geqslant 10^6$/ml acquire these organisms at an earlier age than those of LR mothers and, subsequently, develop more carious lesions.[37,38] The correlation between levels of these potentially cariogenic bacteria in the saliva of mothers and their 2–5-year-old children was found to be low in a recent longitudinal study in the Netherlands.[39] However, highly significant correlations between lactobacillus and MS levels and clinical caries scores were noted in children from the age of 2½ years and above.

Use of strain-typing systems, such as bacteriocin typing[40] or, more recently, DNA restriction fragment polymorphism,[41] has shown that infants usually become colonized by the same types of MS as are found in their mothers' mouths. Such techniques are extremely useful for studies on transmission of such bacteria within family groups. In one detailed study on

46 mother–child pairs in the USA, observed for the first 5 years of the infants' lives, initial acquisition of MS was found to occur between 19 and 31 months in 38 of the children, with a median age of 26 months. This time period was referred to by the authors as 'a discrete window of infectivity'.[42] The remaining 8 children (17%) remained free of MS until the end of the study period. Whether the same window of infectivity applies to other populations remains to be determined, and may be a significant factor when planning caries-preventive strategies for infants.

It is recognized that, despite the general decrease in caries levels in the UK and elsewhere over recent years, there are particular groups within the population who still experience high levels of the disease.[43–45] The use of salivary counts of cariogenic bacteria is one way in which such HR groups could be recognized and appropriate preventive regimens instituted.[46] In particular, it would be useful to screen mothers at antenatal clinics in the hope of improving the subsequent dental health of their offspring.[37] The bacterial counts, in addition to facilitating the recognition of HR and LR patients, can also be used as a means of monitoring the efficacy of dietary control, oral hygiene and other preventive procedures and can be an effective aid for patient motivation.

Interpretation of salivary counts may be problematical, and these tests are possibly more reliable for the recognition of LR rather than HR. An individual with zero or low detectable levels of both MS and lactobacilli can confidently be regarded as an LR person. Conversely, someone with 10^6 MS/ml and over 10^5/ml lactobacilli is clearly in the HR category. Intermediate values, or contradictory levels of the two indicator organisms, are less conclusive and suggest intermediate or uncertain levels of risk. As discussed by Krasse,[46] the best prediction of future caries is probably obtained by taking into consideration a variety of factors, including salivary bacterial counts. It has long been recognized that past caries experience is also a key factor in determining caries susceptibility.

The estimation of salivary levels of cariogenic bacteria does not necessarily require the services of a fully equipped microbiology laboratory. Chairside kits are now available for the measurement of both lactobacilli and MS, as well as for *Candida*.[47–51] In addition, tests for salivary-buffering capacity can also be obtained commercially.

Microbiological approaches to caries prevention

The three time-honoured approaches to caries prevention, based on the multifactorial nature of the disease, may be summarized as follows:[17]

1. To increase the resistance of the tooth.
2. To reduce the intake of carbohydrate in the diet.
3. To reduce or inhibit the microbial challenge.

In practice, some of the measures used to increase tooth resistance – notably the application of fluoride in various ways – may also have some antibacterial effects. Similarly, restriction of carbohydrate intake or substitution of sucrose by other, non-fermentable substrates (such as xylitol) are likely to have an effect on the oral microflora.

Attempts to control dental caries by mechanical plaque control have generally proved ineffective, despite a few encouraging reports.[52,53] Chemical agents, notably chlorhexidine,[54] have been shown to reduce levels of MS in the mouth and may be particularly useful for short-term prophylactic use in HR patients, in combination with topical fluoride application. One specific situation where such regimes are of considerable value is in the management of patients with xerostomia following irradiation of head and neck tumours.[55]

The development of a caries vaccine, based on active immunization against *Streptococcus mutans*, has been an interesting area of intense activity in several laboratories.[56–58] Although a great deal has been discovered from such studies about immune responses to various antigen preparations,[59] and immunization of both rodents and primates has been shown to be protective against caries in some experiments, it has not yet proved possible to carry out clinical trials in children. Because of concern about the theoretical risks of any such immunization procedure, the availability of tried and tested alternative preventive measures, and the almost negligible mortality of dental caries, the future application of such vaccines seems uncertain at present.

However, the detailed studies generated by the quest for further information about the antigenic composition of cariogenic bacteria, the systemic and mucosal immune responses which they may induce, and the possible biological functions of antigens such as the I/II antigen of *S. mutans*,[60] have led to a rapid increase in knowledge within the fields of oral microbiology and oral immunology.[59,61] One interesting development is the possibility of passive immunization by applying preformed antibodies to the teeth.[62] If this approach is found to be effective in preventing caries in humans it would overcome many of the problems associated with active immunization.

Periodontal diseases

Theories of aetiology

There is no way of disguising the fact that the microbiology of periodontal disease is highly complex. The literature is very extensive, but two books published in 1991 provide useful reviews of the background to this large mass of information.[63,64] Some of the theories about the involvement of particular bacteria are controversial and there is disagreement in the literature about the correct interpretation of much of the published data.[65] However, it is generally accepted that the gingival crevice and periodontal pocket contain a large variety of bacterial species, that many of these organisms are obligate anaerobes, and that some, at least, are thought to be implicated in disease processes affecting the periodontal tissue.[2]

One issue of controversy is that of the specific plaque hypothesis versus the non-specific plaque hypothesis. According to the latter, periodontal diseases result from the excessive accumulation of dental plaque, regardless of the particular types of bacteria present.[66] This implies that all dental plaque is potentially harmful. Conversely, the rival theory maintains that there are specific associations between particular microorganisms and different types of periodontal disease.[67,68] Most workers in the field have taken the view that periodontal diseases result from local events in the crevicular area, either due to the activities of the microorganisms themselves, or to the host response to their presence. However, in contrast, it has been suggested that the some conditions could arise from the spread of pulpal inflammation to the adjacent periodontal tissues.[65] There is clearly a need for further studies to answer unresolved questions about the aetiology of periodontal diseases.

Developments in periodontal research

It is well-recognized that a variety of types of periodontal disease occur clinically and that these may have different aetiologies.[63,64] Different manifestations of gingivitis and periodontitis, including experimental, acute and chronic, localized or generalized, adult and juvenile, slowly or rapidly progressing, active or quiescent, refractory to treatment, and other forms related to underlying systemic conditions (including human immunodeficiency virus (HIV) infection), have all been studied. As a result of the diversity of conditions investigated, coupled with the problems of making an accurate and reproducible clinical diagnosis, and the variety of laboratory methods employed, it is often difficult to compare the results from different studies.[69]

The idea that periodontal disease proceeds inexorably throughout life at a steady rate, starting as a mild, chronic gingivitis which progresses inevitably to periodontitis, is no longer accepted. In fact, the direct progression of gingivitis to periodontitis has not been clearly established in well-controlled longitudinal studies. In contrast, it has been demonstrated that periodontal destruction in individual pockets tends to be episodic, with active bursts of tissue-damaging activity occurring from time to time, followed by periods of remission.[70,71] Detection of such bursts of activity and analysis of what actually transforms an inactive to a disease-active site is one of the central issues in periodontal research.[72]

Development in clinical sampling methods, in culture and isolation techniques in the laboratory (especially with respect to obligate anaerobes) and in the taxonomy and identification of microorganisms from the mouth, have all contributed to the enormous increase in factual information that is now available. Non-cultural methods, such as the microscopic examination of plaque material by dark-field or phase-contrast microscopy can provide some useful information and may indicate major shifts in the microbial flora associated with diseased sites when compared to healthy sites.[73] Such examination also illustrates clearly the presence of microorganisms, such as spirochaetes and some other motile forms, which are not routinely cultivated in the laboratory. Thus, whatever is revealed on the microbiologist's culture plates is almost invariably a distorted view of the actual range of organisms present and their relative numbers at the original sample site.

Association of bacteria with different types of periodontal disease

Notwithstanding the technical and logistic problems implicit in trying to prove causal relationships between particular microorganisms and the aetiology of periodontal diseases, many investigators have published reports of observed associations. In experimental gingivitis, it is not clear whether any specific organisms are implicated, although some workers have suggested that *Actinomyces israelii*, *A. viscosus* and some black-pigmented anaerobes may be involved, especially when gingival bleeding occurs.[74] Others have demonstrated elevated numbers of *A. naeslundii*, *A. odontolyticus*, *Fusobacterium nucleatum*, *Lactobacillus* species, *Streptococcus anginosus*, *Veillonella parvula* and a *Treponema* species (amongst 166 bacteria species and subspecies identified from 96 samples in 4 subjects) and suggested that these might be aetiological agents.[75]

There have been few detailed studies on the bacteriology of acute necrotizing ulcerative gingivitis (ANUG), which is traditionally thought of as fusospirochaetal in origin. In one study, microscopic examination of samples from 22 ulcerated sites showed high levels of *Treponema* (32%) and *Selenomonas* (6%), whilst viable counts yielded significant levels of *Bacteroides* (now *Prevotella*) *intermedius* (24%) and *Fusobacterium* spp. (3%).[76]

Most attention has been directed towards studying various forms of periodontitis, particularly in an attempt to identify which bacteria are associated with 'active' lesions.[77–86] A summary of some of the reported associations is shown in Table 16.5. It can be seen from this table that there is a long list of 'candidate pathogens', but evidence for a definite cause-and-effect relationship between most of these and the various types of periodontal disease is not available. Of the organisms most frequently reported from disease-active sites, considerable attention has been paid to *Porphyromonas gingivalis*, which is one of the

Table 16.5 Bacteria reported to be associated with various types of periodontitis

Frequently reported	*Occasionally reported*
Porphyromonas gingivalis	*Prevotella denticola*
Prevotella intermedia	*Prevotella oris*
Actinobacillus actinomycetemcomitans	*Prevotella melaninogenica*
	Bacteroides forsythus
Spirochaetes (*Treponema* spp.)	*Bacteroides gracilis*
	Fusobacterium nucleatum
	Fusobacterium alocis
	Fusobacterium periodonticum
	Eikenella corrodens
	Wolinella recta
	Selenomonas spp.
	Capnocytophaga spp.
	Campylobacter spp.
	Treponema denticola
	Eubacterium brachy
	Eubacterium nodatium
	Eubacterium timidum
	Lactobacillus spp.
	Peptostreptococcus spp.
	Streptococcus spp.

black-pigmented anaerobes,[87] and *Actinobacillus actinomycetemcomitans*, a microaerophilic Gram-negative rod found in several types of periodontal lesion but particularly associated with localized juvenile periodontitis.[88] These two species, together with another black-pigmented anaerobe, *Prevotella intermedia* and the spirochaetes, are the current favourites as potential microbiological markers of disease activity, but the complexity of the subgingival flora makes it difficult to be certain of the contribution that each species makes to the disease process.[69,83,89]

Nothwithstanding any inherent technical difficulties in establishing unequivocal causal relationships, reports continue to appear showing the association between *P. gingivalis*, *P. intermedia*, *A. actinomycetemcomitans*, together with some of the other putative pathogens, and periodontal disease in various populations.[90] Molecular-typing methods have also been employed effectively to demonstrate transmission of these bacteria between spouses and other family members.[91–93] Such intrafamilial spread may be a significant factor in the subsequent development of disease, since it has been shown that spouses of patients with advanced periodontitis have a worse periodontal condition than the spouses of periodontally healthy individuals.[92]

Pathogenicity and virulence of putative periodontal pathogens

The exact mechanisms by which subgingival microorganisms evade host defence mechanisms and cause damage to the periodontal tissues, either acting alone or in consortia, are not fully understood but a number of factors may be involved,[63,89,94,95] some of which are listed in Table 16.6. The role of invasion of tissues by periodontopathic bacteria has not, until recently, been thought of as particularly important, but there is some evidence that such penetration does occur.[96]

Several putative periodontal pathogens, including *P. gingivalis*, *A. actinomycetemcomitans* and *Eikenella corrodens*, have been shown to possess surface-associated material (SAM) which has important biological activity, such as induction of bone resorption.[97] The nature of the active molecules involved and their mechanisms of action during bone resorption differ from one species to another, but the activity is unlikely to be due to lipopolysaccharide.[97] *A. actinomycetemcomitans* is also known to produce a potent leukotoxin which lyses human polymorphonuclear leukocytes and may therefore help the organisms to evade host defence mechanisms.[98,99] A

Table 16.6 Some bacterial factors which may be related to virulence of periodontal pathogens

Function	*Specific bacterial factors*	
Adherence	Adhesins (fimbriae, fibrils)	
	Coaggregation factors	
Evasion of host defence mechanisms	Capsules, slime layers	
	Leukotoxin	
	Immunoglobulin proteases	
	Complement proteases	
	Suppression of T-cells	
Direct tissue damage	*Enzymes*	Trypsin-like proteases
		Chymotrypsin
		Collagenase
		Hyaluronidase
		Chondroitin sulphatase
		Heparinase
	Metabolic products	Volatile fatty acids
		Indole
		Amines, ammonia
		Volatile sulphur compounds
Induction of bone resorption	Lipoteichoic acid	
	Lipopolysaccharide	
	Capsules	
	Surface-associated material (SAM)	
Indirect tissue damage	Antigenic stimulation, leading to immune responses and inflammation	
	Activation of alternative complement pathway	

number of pathogenic strategies have been attributed to *P. gingivalis*, including the possession of fimbriae, haemagglutin(s), capsules and coaggregation factors, all of which may be involved in adherence to oral tissues.[100]

Considerable attention has been given in recent years to the production of various proteinase enzymes by *P. gingivalis*,[101] including the so-called 'trypsin-like proteases' such as one described some years ago as gingivain.[102] Unfortunately, several other names have been proposed, and the nomenclature of the enzymes described by different groups of research workers, as well as the genes which encode for them, has become somewhat complex and in need of clarification.[103] The demonstration that a genetically altered mutant of *P. gingivalis*, defective in the prt H gene which specifies a 97-kDa protease, was less virulent than the parent strain underlies the potential importance of such enzymes.[104] This is an important and active area of periodontal research, not only because of the probable significance of *P. gingivalis* proteinases as virulence factors in disease, but also because the development of carefully targeted enzyme inhibitors may offer a novel approach to prevention of periodontal disease.[105]

Diagnostic screening for periodontal pathogens

As a result of the many studies indicating possible associations between bacterial species and different types of periodontal disease, diagnostic tests have been sought that might be of value as markers of disease activity and for monitoring the effects of therapy. Conventional cultural techniques can be used to detect and quantify putative pathogens, but these are rather slow, labour-intensive and expensive, requiring the facilities of a well-equipped microbiology laboratory. Increasingly, use is being made of gene probes, PCR, immunological blotting and other more sophisticated methods for detection of such organisms in periodontal pocket samples, and access of some to these approaches is now commercially available.[106,107] However, interpretation of the results of such approaches may continue to be a problem until the postulated aetiological associations between the various organisms and periodontal disease have been fully validated.

Conclusions

As will be clear from this brief review, the microbiology of the mouth is complex. Much has been learned about the microorganisms in dental plaque which are associated with dental caries and periodontal diseases. In each case, it is likely that some ecological perturbation occurs which disturbs the normal balance between the indigenous microorganisms and the host at specific sites, resulting in disease. Further investigation of the properties of these microorganisms and their interactions, particularly with the rapidly increasing application of modern molecular methods of study, should lead to a better understanding of these important plaque-related diseases. Hopefully such understanding will rapidly be converted into useful clinical applications, including improved diagnostic methods and treatment.

References

1. MacFarlane TW, Samaranayake LP. *Clinical Oral Microbiology*. London: Wright, 1989.
2. Hardie JM. Dental and oral infection. In: Duerden BI, Drasar BS (eds) *Anaerobes in Human Disease*, pp. 245–267. London: Edward Arnold, 1991.
3. Samaranayake LP, MacFarlane TW (eds) *Oral Candidosis*. London: Wright, 1990.
4. MacFarlane TW. Plaque-related infections. *J Med Microbiol* 1989; **29**: 161–170.
5. Russell RRB. Genetic analysis and genetic probes for oral bacteria. In Ferguson DB (ed) *Aspects of Oral Molecular Biology*, pp. 57–76. Basel: Karger, 1990.
6. Myers HM (ed) *New biotechnology in Oral Research*. Basel: Karger, 1989.
7. Socransky SS, Manganiello SD. The oral microbiota of man from birth to senility. *J Periodontol* 1971; **42**: 485–494.
8. Marsh PD, Martin MV. *Oral Microbiology*, 3rd edn. London: Chapman & Hall, 1992.
9. Hardie JM, Bowden GHW. The normal microbial flora of the mouth. In: Skinner FA, Carr JG (eds) *The Normal Microbial Flora of Man*. pp. 47–83. London: Academic Press, 1974.
10. Marsh PD. The significance of maintaining the stability of the natural microflora of the mouth. *Br Dent J* 1991; **171**: 174–177.

11. Hardie JM, Whiley RA. The genus *Streptococcus-oral*. In: Balows A, Truper HG, Dworkin M, Harder W, Schleifer K-H (eds) *The Prokaryotes*, vol. 2, 2nd edn. New York: Springer-Verlag, 1991.
12. Beighton D, Hardie JM, Whiley RA. A scheme for the identification of viridans streptococci. *J Med Microbiol* 1991; **35**: 367–372.
13. Shah HN, Collins MD. Proposal for reclassification of *Bacteroides asaccharolyticus*, *Bacteroides gingivalis* and *Bacteroides endodontalis* in a new genus, *Porphyromonas*. *Int J Syst Bacteriol* 1988; **38**: 128–131.
14. Shah HN, Collin MD. *Prevotella*, a new genus to include *Bacteroides melaninogenicus* and related species formerly classified in the genus *Bacteroides*. *Int J Syst Bacteriol* 1990; **40**: 205–208.
15. Hardie JM, Shah HN. Factors controlling the microbial flora of the mouth. *Eur J Chemother Antibiot* 1982; **2**: 3–11.
16. Miller WD. *The Micro-organisms of the Human Mouth*. Originally published in Philadelphia, 1890. Reprinted; Basel: S. Karger, 1973.
17. Silverstone LM, Johnson NW, Hardie JM, Williams RAD. *Dental Caries; Aetiology, Pathology and Prevention*. London: Macmillan, 1981.
18. Orland FJ, Blayney JR, Harrison R *et al*. Use of the germfree animal technic in the study of experimental dental caries. *J Dent Res* 1954; **33**:147–174.
19. Tanzer JM (ed) *Animal Models in Cariology*. Washington, DC: Information Retrieval, 1981.
20. Edwardsson E. Microorganisms associated with dental caries. In: Thylstrup A, Fejerskov O (eds) *Textbook of Cariology*, pp. 107–130. Copenhagen: Munksgaard, 1986.
21. Mikx FHM, van der Hoeven JS, Konig KG *et al*. Establishment of defined microbial ecosystems in germfree rats. 1. Effect of the interaction of *Streptococcus mutans* or *Streptococcus sanguis* with *Veillonella alcalescens* on plaque formation and caries activity. *Caries Res* 1972; **6**: 211–221.
22. Mikx FHM, van der Hoeven JS. Symbiosis of *Streptococcus mutans* and *Veillonella alcalescens* in mixed continuous culture. *Arch Oral Biol* 1975; **20**: 407–410.
23. Hamada S, Slade HD. Biology, immunology and cariogenicity of *Streptococcus mutans*. *Microbiol Rev* 1980; **44**: 331–384.
24. Loesche WJ. The role of *Streptococcus mutans* in human dental decay. *Microbiol Rev* 1986; **50**: 353–380.
25. Schleifer K-H, Kilpper-Balz R, Kraus J, Gehring F. Relatedness and classification of *Streptococcus mutans* and 'mutans-like' streptococci. *J Dent Res* 1984; **63**: 1047–1050.
26. Coykendall AL. Classification and identification of the viridans streptococci. *Clin Microbiol Rev* 1989; **2**: 315–328.
27. Bowden GHW. Which bacteria are cariogenic in humans? In: Johnson NW (ed) *Risk Markers for Oral Diseases, vol. 1. Dental Caries*, pp. 266–286. Cambridge: Cambridge University Press, 1991.
28. Milnes AR, Bowden GHW. The microflora associated with the developing lesions of nursing caries. *Caries Res* 1985; **19**: 289–297.
29. Boyar RM, Bowden GHW. The microflora associated with the progression of incipient caries lesions in teeth of children living in a water-fluoridated area. *Caries Res* 1985; **19**: 298–306.
30. Hardie JM, Thomson PL, South RJ *et al*. A longitudinal epidemiological study on dental plaque and the development of dental caries – interim results after two years. *J Dent Res* 1977; **56**: c90–c98.
31. Lang KP, Hotz PR, Gusberti F, Joss A. Longitudinal, clinical and microbiological study on the relationship between infection with *Streptococcus mutans* and the development of caries in humans. *Oral Microbiol Immunol* 1987; **2**: 39–47.
32. Beighton D, Lynch E. Comparison of selected microflora of plaque and underlying carious dentine associated with primary root caries lesions. *Caries Res* 1995; **29**: 154–158.
33. Schübach P, Osterwalder V, Guggenheim B. Human root caries: microbiota in plaque covering sound, carious and arrested carious root surfaces. *Caries Res* 1995; **29**: 383–395.
34. Schübach P, Osterwalder V, Guggenheim B. Human root caries: microbiota of a limited number of root caries lesions. *Caries Res* 1996; **30**: 52–64.
35. Togelius J, Kristoffersson K, Anderson H, Bratthall D. *Streptococcus mutans* in saliva: intra-individual variations and relation to number of colonized sites. *Acta Odont Scand* 1984; **42**: 157–163.
36. Beighton D. The value of salivary bacterial counts in the prediction of caries activity. In: Johnson NW (ed) *Risk Markers for Oral Diseases*, vol. 1. Dental Caries pp. 313–326. Cambridge: Cambridge University Press, 1991.
37. Kohler B, Bratthall D, Krasse B. Preventive measures in mothers influence the establishment of the bacterium *Streptococcus mutans* in their infants. *Arch Oral Biol* 1983; **28**: 225–231.
38. Kohler B, Andreen I, Johnsson B. The earlier colonization of mutans streptococci, the higher the caries prevalence at 4 years of age. *Oral Microbiol Immunol* 1988; **3**: 14–17.
39. Roeters FJM, Van der Hoeven JS, Burgersdijk RCW, Schaeken MJM. Lactobacilli, mutans streptococci and dental caries: a longitudinal study in 2-year old children up to the age of 5 years. *Caries Res* 1995; **29**: 272–279.
40. Berkowitz RJ, Jordan HV. Similarity of bacteriocins of *Streptococcus mutans* from mothers and infant. *Arch Oral Biol* 1975; **20**: 1–6.
41. Caufield PW, Walker TM. Genetic diversity within *Streptococcus mutans* evident from chromosomal DNA restriction fragment polymorphisms. *J Clin Microbiol* 1989; **27**: 274–278.
42. Caufield PW, Cutter GR, Dasanayake AP. Initial acquisition of mutans streptococci by infants: evidence for a discrete window of infectivity. *J Dent Res* 1993; **73**: 37–45.

43. Holt RD, Joels D, Bulman J, Maddick IH. A third study of caries in preschool aged children in Camden. *Br Dent J* 1988; **45**: 87–91.
44. Frencken JE, Kalsbeek H, Verrips GH. Has the decline in dental caries been halted? Changes in caries prevalence among 6- and 12-year-old children in Friesland, 1973–1988. *Int Dent J* 1990; **40**: 225–230.
45. Johnson NW (ed) *Risk Markers for Oral Diseases, vol. 1. Dental Caries*. Cambridge: Cambridge University Press, 1991.
46. Krasse B. Biological factors as indicators of future caries. *Int Dent J* 1988; **38**: 219–225.
47. Larmas M. A new dip-slide test for the counting of salivary lactobacilli. *Proc Finn Dent Soc* 1975; **71**: 31–35.
48. Alaluusua S, Savolainen J, Tuompo H, Gronroos L. Slide scoring method for estimation of *Streptococcus mutans*. *Scand J Dent Res* 1984; **92**: 127–133.
49. Crossner C-G, Unel L. Salivary lactobacillus counts as a diagnostic and didactic tool in caries prevention. *Community Dent Oral Epidemiol* 1986; **14**: 156–160.
50. Twetman S, Frostner N. Salivary mutans streptococci and caries prevalence in 8-year-old Swedish schoolchildren. *Swed Dent J* 1991; **15**: 145–151.
51. Russell JI, MacFarlane TW, Aitchison TC *et al.* Caries prevalence and microbiological and salivary caries activity tests in Scottish adolescents. *Community Dent Oral Epidemiol* 1990; **18**: 120–125.
52. Lindhe J, Axelsson P, Tollskog G. The effect of proper oral hygiene on gingivitis and dental caries in schoolchildren. *Community Dent Oral Epidemiol* 1975; **3**: 150–155.
53. King J, Hardie JM, Duckworth R. Dental caries and periodontal health following a professionally administered plaque control programme in adolescents. *Br Dent J* 1985; **158**: 52–54.
54. Zickert I, Emilson C-G, Krasse B. Effect of caries preventive measures in children highly infected with the bacterium *Streptococcus mutans*. *Arch Oral Biol* 1982; **27**: 861–868.
55. Joyston-Bechal S, Hayes K, Davenport ES, Hardie JM. Caries incidence, mutans streptococci and lactobacilli in irradiated patients during a 12-month preventive programme using chlorhexidine and fluoride. *Caries Res* 1992; **26**: 384–390.
56. Krasse B, Emilson C-G, Gahnberg L. An anticaries vaccine; report on the status of research. *Caries Res* 1987; **21**: 255–276.
57. Russell RRB, Johnson NW. The prospects for vaccination against dental caries. *Br Dent J* 1987; **162**: 29–34.
58. Klein JP, Scholler M. Recent advances in the development of a *Streptococcus mutans* vaccine. *Eur J Epidemiol* 1988; **4**: 419–425.
59. Hamada S, Michalek SM, Kiyono M *et al* (eds) *Molecular Microbiology and Immunobiology of Streptococcus mutans*. Amsterdam: Elsevier, 1986.
60. Ma J K-C, Kelly CG, Munro G *et al.* Conservation of the gene encoding streptococcal antigen I/II in oral streptococci. *Infect Immunol* 1991; **59**: 2686–2694.
61. Russell MW. Immunization against dental caries. *Oral Maxillofacial Surg Infect* 1992; **2**: 72–80.
62. Lehner T, Ma JK, Kelly CG. A mechanism of passive immunization with monoclonal antibodies to a 185,000 M(r) streptococcal antigen. *Adv Exp Med Biol* 1992; **327**: 151–163.
63. Hamada S, Holt SC, McGhee JR. *Periodontal Disease: Pathogens and Host Immune Responses.* Tokyo: Quintessence, 1991.
64. Johnson NW. *Risk Markers for Oral Diseases, vol. 3. Periodontal Diseases.* Cambridge: Cambridge University Press, 1991.
65. Hirsch RS, Clarke NG. Infection and periodontal diseases. *Rev Infect Dis* 1989; **11**: 707–715.
66. Theilade E. The non-specific theory in microbial etiology of inflammatory periodontal diseases. *J Clin Periodontol* 1986; **13**: 905–911.
67. Slots J, Listgarten MA. *Bacteroides gingivalis, Bacteroides intermedius* and *Actinobacillus actinomycetemcomitans* in human periodontal diseases. *J Clin Periodontol* 1988; **15**: 85–93.
68. Loesche WJ. The bacterial etiology of periodontal disease: the specific plaque hypothesis. In: Clark JW (ed) *Clincial Dentistry*. Philadelphia: Harper & Row, 1987.
69. Moore WEC. Microbiology of periodontal disease. *J Periodont Res* 1987; **22**: 335–341.
70. Goodson JM, Tanner AC, Haffajee AD *et al.* Patterns of progression and regression of advanced destructive periodontal disease. *J Clin Periodontol* 1982; **9**: 472–481.
71. Haffajee AD, Socransky SS. Attachment level changes in destructive periodontal diseases. *J Clin Periodontol* 1986; **13**: 461–475.
72. Dzink JL, Haffajee AD, Socransky SS. The predominant cultivable microbiota of active and inactive periodontal lesions. *J Clin Periodontol* 1988; **15**: 316–323.
73. Listgarten MA, Hellden L. Relative distribution of bacteria at clinically healthy and periodontally diseased sites in humans. *J Periodont Res* 1978; **5**: 115–132.
74. Loesche WJ, Syed SA. Bacteriology of human experimental gingivitis: effect of plaque and gingivitis score. *Infect Immun* 1978; **21**: 830–839.
75. Moore WEC, Holdeman LV, Smibert RM *et al.* Bacteriology of experimental gingivitis in young adult humans. *Infect Immun* 1982; **38**: 651–667.
76. Loesche WJ, Syed SA, Laughon BE, Stoll J. The bacteriology of acute necrotizing ulcerative gingivitis. *J Periodontol* 1982; **53**: 223–230.
77. Mandell RL. A longitudinal microbiological investigation of *Actinobacillus actinomycetemcomitans* and *Eikenella corrodens* in juvenile periodontitis. *Infect Immun* 1984; **45**: 778–780.
78. Tanner ACR, Dzink JL, Ebersole JL, Socransky SS. *Wolinella recta, Campylobacter concisus, Bacteroides*

gracilis and *Eikenella corrodens* from periodontal lesions. *J Periodontol Res* 1987; **22**: 327–330.
79. Dzink JL, Tanner ACR, Haffajee AD, Socransky SS. Gram negative species associated with active destructive periodontal lesions. *J Clin Periodontol* 1985; **12**: 648–659.
80. Slots J, Bradg L, Wikstrom M, Dahlen G. The occurrence of *Actinobacillus actinomycetemcomitans*, *Bacteroides gingivalis* and *Bacteroides intermedius* in destructive periodontal disease in adults. *J Clin Periodontol* 1986; **13**: 570–577.
81. Lai C-H, Listgarten MA, Shirakawa M, Slots J. *Bacteroides forsythus* in adult gingivitis and periodontitis. *Oral Microbiol Immunol* 1987; **2**: 152–157.
82. Haffajee AD, Socransky SS, Dzink JL *et al.* Clinical, microbiological and immunological features of subjects with destructive periodontal diseases. *J Clin Periodontol* 1988; **15**: 240–246.
83. Socransky SS, Haffajee AD, Smith GL, Dzink JL. Difficulties encountered in the search for the etiologic agents of destructive periodontal diseases. *J Clin Periodontol* 1987; **14**: 588–593.
84. Moore WEC, Holdeman LV, Smibert RM *et al.* Bacteriology of severe periodontitis in young adult humans. *Infect Immun* 1982; **38**: 1137–1148.
85. Moore WEC, Holdeman LV, Cato EP *et al.* Bacteriology of moderate (chronic) periodontitis in mature adult humans. *Infect Immun* 1983; **42**: 510–515.
86. Zambon JJ. *Actinobacillus actinomycetemcomitans* in human periodontal disease. *J Clin Periodontol* 1985; **12**: 1–20.
87. van Steenbergen TJM, van Winklehoff AJ, de Graaff J. Black-pigmented oral anaerobic rods: classification and role in periodontal disease. In: Hamada S, Holt SC, McGhee JR (eds) *Periodontal Disease: Pathogens and Host Immune Responses*, pp. 41–52. Tokyo: Quintessence, 1991.
88. Slots J, Schonfeld SE. *Actinobacillus actinomycetemcomitans* in localized juvenile periodontitis. In: Hamada S, Holt SC, McGhee JR (eds) *Periodontal Disease: Pathogens and Host Immune Responses*, pp. 53–64. Tokyo: Quintessence, 1991.
89. Marsh PD. Do bacterial markers exist in subgingival plaque for predicting periodontal disease susceptibility? In: Johnson NW (ed) *Risk Markers for Oral Diseases, vol. 3. Periodontal Disease*, pp. 365–388. Cambridge: Cambridge University Press, 1991.
90. Preus HR, Ånerud Å, Boysen H, Dunford RG, Zambon JJ, Löe H. The natural history of periodontal disease. The correlation of selected microbiological parameters with disease severity in Sri Lankan tea workers. *J Clin Periodont* 1995; **22**: 674–678.
91. Könönen E, Jousimes-Somer H, Asikainen S. Relationship between oral Gram-negative anaerobic bacteria in saliva of the mother and the colonization of her edentulous infant. *Oral Microbiol Immunol* 1992; **7**: 273–276.
92. Von Troil-Lindén B, Torkko H, Alaulusua S, Wolf J, Jousimies-Somer H, Asikainen S. Periodontal findings in spouses. A clinical, radiographic and microbiological study. *J Clin Periodont* 1995; **22**: 93–99.
93. Van Steenbergen TJM, Petit MDA, Scholte LHM, Van der Velden U, De Graaff J. Transmission of *Porphyromonas gingivalis* between spouses. *J Clin Periodont* 1993; **20**: 340–345.
94. Slots J, Dahlen G. Subgingival microorganisms and bacterial virulence factors in periodontitis. *Scand J Dent Res* 1985; **93**: 119–127.
95. Listgarten MA. Nature of periodontal diseases: pathogenic mechanisms. *J Periodont Res* 1987; **22**: 172–178.
96. Saglie FR. Bacterial invasion and its role in the pathogenesis of periodontal disease. In: Hamada S, Holt SC, McGhee JR (eds) *Periodontal Disease: Pathogens and Host Immune Responses*, pp. 27–40. Tokyo: Quintessence, 1991.
97. Meghji S, Wilson M, Barber P, Henderson B. Bone resorbing activity of surface-associated material from *Actinobacillus actinomycetemcomitans* and *Eikenella corrodens*. *J Med Microbiol* 1994; **41**: 197–203.
98. Ohta H, Kato K. Leukotoxic activity of *Actinobacillus actinomycetemcomitans*. In: Hamada S, Holt SC, McGhee JR (eds). *Periodontal Disease: Pathogens and Host Immune Responses*, pp. 143–154. Tokyo: Quintessence, 1991.
99. Baehni P, Tsai C-C, McArthur WP, Hammond BJ, Taichman NS. Detection of leukotoxic activity of a plaque-derived Gram-negative microorganism. *Infect Immun* 1979; **24**: 233–243.
100. Cutler CW, Kalmar JR, Genco CA. Pathogenic strategies of the oral anaerobe, *Porphyromonas gingivalis*. *Trends Microbiol* 1995; **3**: 45–51.
101. Nakamura R, Hinode H, Terai H, Morioka M. Extracellular enzymes of *Porphyromonas (Bacteroides) gingivalis* in relation to periodontal destruction. In: Hamada S, Holt SC, McGhee JR (eds) *Periodontal Disease: Pathogens and Host Immune Responses*, pp. 129–142. Tokyo: Quintessence, 1991.
102. Shah HN, Gharbia SE, Knowlessur D *et al.* Gingivain: a cysteine proteinase isolated from *Porphyromonas gingivalis*. *Microb Ecol Health Dis* 1991; **4**: 319–328.
103. Potempa J, Pavloff N, Travis J. *Porphyromonas gingivalis:* a proteinase/gene accounting audit. *Trends Microbiol* 1995; **3**: 430–434.
104. Fletcher HM, Schenkein HM, Morgan RM, Bailey KA, Berry CR, Macrina FL. Virulence of *Porphyromonas gingivalis* W83 mutant defective in the prt H gene. *Infect Immun* 1995; **63**: 1521–1528.
105. Travis J, Potempa J, Maeda H. Are bacterial proteinases pathogenic factors? *Trends Microbiol* 1995; **3**: 405–407.
106. Tanner A, Lai C-H, Maiden M. New methods for microbial screening in the diagnosis of periodontal infections: cultural, immunological, gene probes. In: Johnson NW (ed) *Risk Markers for Oral Diseases,*

vol. 3. Periodontal Diseases, pp. 389–413. Cambridge: Cambridge University Press, 1991.

107. Loesche WJ, Hujoel P. Microbiologically based diagnostic tests for periodontitis. Considerations of sensitivity, specificity and accuracy. In: Johnson NW (ed) *Risk Markers for Oral Diseases, vol. 3. Periodontal Diseases*, pp. 417–440. Cambridge: Cambridge University Press, 1991.

17

Infective endocarditis: a review of the aetiology, epidemiology and pathogenesis

Christopher Franklin

It is over 100 years since William Osler reported on malignant endocarditis to the Royal College of Physicians[1] and, for at least 50 years, it has been a long-held belief by doctors and dentists that dental procedures carried out on susceptible patients are a major cause of infective endocarditis (IE).[2] In the past, IE has usually been classified as acute or subacute. There is, however, considerable overlap and it is probably best to consider this condition as a spectrum of clinical features ranging between these two extremes. It is possibly more important to identify the causative organisms than to classify the disease as acute or subacute and so the convention of IE to include the changes seen in this spectrum is generally used.

Aetiology and epidemiology

During the last 50 years, the number of deaths due to IE has fallen by 80% but IE remains a life-threatening infection. It is thought that there are approximately 200 deaths a year and, of these, deaths in males exceed those in females; unfortunately, it is difficult to obtain precise data on a national basis. Similarly, the incidence is not precisely known, since IE is not a notifiable disease. Estimates vary from 11–16 cases per million to as many as 30 per million. In a recent study, at regional level, Skehan *et al.*[3] reported on 182 cases occurring over a 30-month period. Extrapolating from their figures for the population gives an annual incidence of 21 cases per million; this provides an incidence of about 1000 new cases per year for England and Wales.[4] However, Oakley,[5] who previously estimated that there would be about 1500 cases a year, believes that even this is an underestimate.

In a special survey for the Royal College of Physicians (RCP) Research Unit,[6] the age of 577 patients with IE ranged from 2 to 87 years (M:F=2) and 83 (14%) died. This is lower than the often-quoted mortality of between 20% and 40%[7] and it may be that the general mortality is lower than this.[8] Hospital In-patient Enquiry (HIPE) data has provided information for the 5-year period 1977–1981 that shows a similar M:F ratio. Three per cent of the sample was less than 15 years, 64% were aged 15–64 and 33% were 65 and over[4] (Table 17.1). Reports from microbiologists to the Communicable Disease Surveillance Centre (CDSC) increased from 366 in 1976 to 571 in 1985. However, the reporting system is voluntary and patients with culture-negative endocarditis are not reported, so that the figures reported to CDSC underestimate the true incidence of IE.

Table 17.1 Survey of patients with infective endocarditis compiled from the Royal College of Physicians survey[6] and Hospital In-patient Enquiry data[4]

Male:female ratio	2:1
Age range	2–87 years
Mortality rate	14%
Patients < 15 years	3%
Patients aged 15–64	64%
Patients over 64 years	33%

Table 17.2 Microorganisms most commonly causing infective endocarditis

Streptococci	63%
Staphylococci	26%
Coxiella burnetii (Q fever)	3%
Various others	8%

Staphylococcus aureus accounts for >50% of staphylococcal cases.
Of the streptococci, almost 50% are of the *Streptococcus viridans* group.

Table 17.3 Predisposing conditions for infective endocarditis*

Congenital heart lesions	19%
Predisposing rheumatic heart disease	24%
Other cardiac abnormalities, e.g. mitral valve prolapse, calcifying aortic valves	25%
No previous known cardiac abnormality	32%
Intravenous drug abusers	2–7%

*Figures from various studies.

Table 17.4 Sources of causal organisms in infective endocarditis

Possibly dental	19%
Alimentary tract	4%
Genitourinary tract	4%
Respiratory tract	3%
Skin	3%
Drug addiction	1%
Pregnancy and parturition	1%
Related to cardiac or vascular procedures	5%
Portal of entry unknown	60%

From Bayliss *et al.*[8] with permission.

The types of organisms isolated, from those reported to CDSC, were similar to those for the RCP survey (Table 17.2). Streptococci accounted for 63% of the total cases, staphylococci 26%, *Coxiella burnetii* (Q fever) for 3% and a wide variety of organisms for 8%. Of the streptococci, almost 50% were of the viridans group. Overall, *Streptococcus sanguis* was the most commonly reported, followed by *S. mitior/mitis* and *S. mutans. Staphylococcus aureus* accounted for more than half of staphylococcal cases.

According to Bayliss *et al.*,[6] 19% of patients had congenital heart lesions, 24% had pre-existing rheumatic heart disease and 25% had other cardiac abnormalities, mainly mitral valve prolapse and calcific aortic valves. In all, 32% were not thought to have any previous cardiac abnormality. Of the 577 patients, 9 (2%) were known to be intravenous drug abusers, whereas in the CSDC returns almost 7% were intravenous drug abusers (Table 17.3). Some of the most vulnerable patients appear to be those with prosthetic heart valves, those who have had other cardiac surgery and patients with previous episodes of IE; these three groups comprise 21% of patients with IE.

Over the last 80 years, many studies have shown a changing pattern of the disease and, although there have been many advances, particularly with regard to the microbiological aspects, the source of the infection is often not known. In addition, it has been confirmed[8] that the proportion of cases which are apparently dentally related is probably smaller than previously believed.

Table 17.4 shows the source of causal organisms as reported by Bayliss *et al.*[8] In this study, the mean age of the patients is high, at about 50, and the authors report that the current trend is for the disease to present in an older age group than previously. For example, in the classic description by Horder,[9] in 1909, of 150 cases, there were only 12 over the age of 50 while 40 years ago[10] most patients were between the ages of 15 and 35. In the study by Bayliss *et al.*[8] only 14% were in this lower age range. Many factors have probably contributed to this changing pattern; of these, the use of antibiotics, decline in acute rheumatic fever and hence rheumatic heart disease, longer survival of patients operated on for congenital heart disease and the greater longevity of the population are probably the most important. Men are increasingly more often affected than women, which is a trend reported in many studies. The reasons for this, although uncertain, may be the higher incidence of bicuspid aortic valves and calcific aortic stenosis in men and to the decreasing incidence of rheumatic heart disease, which is more common in women.[8]

Mortality appears to be age- and organism-related as well as whether the patient has had previous cardiac surgery.[8] For example, the age of those who die (mean age 59.0) appears to be almost a decade older than those who survive (mean age 51). The mortality reported in this study, which is in broad agreement with other workers, was 30% in staphylococcal infections, 14% in infections due to bowel organisms and only 6% in other streptococcal infections. While childhood IE remains uncommon, it appears to be associated with a poor prognosis and higher mortality (27%).[11]

Dental aspects of IE

It is well-known that a streptococcal bacteraemia may occur following dental extraction and other minor oral surgical procedures. There is good evidence[12] that oral streptococci of the viridans group (e.g. *Streptococcus mitis, S. mutans*) can be recovered from heart lesions in rabbits that have experimentally induced endocarditis, following inoculation of the organisms into fresh tooth sockets. However, an important factor appeared to be the critical mass of organisms inoculated. If the number of organisms was above the threshold level of 10^7 there was a 94% yield of IE. The authors[12] contended that their work supported a possible dental aetiology of IE and that such infection may be proportional to the systemic level of organisms attained.

It has been difficult to establish why the viridans group of streptococci, in particular, are so important in IE and why they should account for half of the cases. It may simply be that the association reflects the large proportions of these organisms in the oral flora and the frequency of subsequent bacteraemias in comparison with those that arise elsewhere. The specificity of infection, however, may also reflect special virulence traits of these bacteria.[13] For example, it has been suggested that synthesis of dextrans by streptococci may be an important virulence factor in IE; such dextrans may increase adhesion of bacteria to valvular tissue.[14] Certain strains of *S. sanguis* from dental plaque and blood cultures have been shown *in vitro* to adhere to and induce thrombotic aggregation of human platelets; this appears to be independent of the role of dextrans.[13] A further complication in the clarification of which organisms are particularly involved in IE is that recently the *viridans* streptococci have been undergoing reclassification in order to improve the characterization of this group of bacteria.[15,16] Consequently, *S. sanguis* has been split into *S. sanguis*, *S. parasanguis* and *S. gordonii*; *S. mitis* into *S. mitis* and *S.oralis* and *S. salivarius* into *S. salivarius* and *S. vestibularis*. It may be that a particular species is more capable of aggregating platelets and that this may be a factor in its virulence[17–19] or that dextran production is associated with a greater propensity to cause disease.[20] Putative virulence factors include microbial adhesins other than dextran such as lipoteichoic acid (LTA) and surface proteins; receptors for plasma adhesive proteins including fibronectin, fibrinogen and vitronectin; and platelet-interactive molecules. As yet no single factor or combination has emerged as the most important in IE.[21] It has been suggested[22] that fibronectin may play a role in the adherence of *S. sanguis* to damaged endothelial cells.

Bayliss *et al.*[2] cite many papers which support the evidence that dental procedures may cause bacteraemia and that this may progress to IE. Figures vary from 5% to 40% of the patients with IE in whom a dental procedure or infection has been considered responsible, usually in the immediately preceding 3 months. However, in the most recently available survey by the RCP Research Unit,[6] only 19% of 544 episodes of IE were possibly due to dental procedures (12%) or dental infection (7%). However, of these patients, 42.5% were not known to have any pre-existing heart disease. *S. viridans* accounted for 82% of the episodes.

Since 1951, the suggestion[10] that the incubation period might be up to 3 months has become an often-quoted maxim. However, in staphylococcal and even viridans infections it is often shorter.[2] It has been estimated from Department of Health and Social Security data[2] that about a quarter of the general population will admit to having had a dental procedure (of some kind) in the last 3 months. This proportion is more than double that found in the patients with IE. It is likely, therefore, that IE is sometimes of dental origin and the proportion of viridans infections found in patients who had received dental treatment or who had dental infection in the 3 months prior to diagnosis supports this. The viridans group of streptococci, which is abundantly present in the oral cavity and nasopharynx, accounted for almost half of the cases in the RCP survey.[2,6] Clearly, many people are capable of sustaining a bacteraemia from brushing the teeth, or chewing or from minor and unrecognized periapical or periodontal infections; only a small proportion of these people would be considered at risk of developing IE.

Many other causative factors are much more firmly established, such as infective, malignant and other lesions in the respiratory, alimentary and genitourinary tracts as well as the procedures used in their investigation and treatment. Other important factors are skin lesions and injuries, drug addiction, fractures, orthopaedic surgery, pregnancy and parturition and any procedures involving the cardiovascular system, such as haemodialysis and cardiac catheterization.[8]

Pathogenesis

In order for the heart to become susceptible to IE, the endocardium usually has to be damaged as it is thought that normal endocardium is fairly resistant to infection by most organisms, with the exception, perhaps, of the more virulent ones. Injury to the endocardial surfaces results in so-called non-bacterial thrombotic vegetations (NBTV), a lesion comprising mainly fibrin and platelets. These vegetations arise mainly by the binding of plasma von Willebrand factor (vWF) to subendothelial components and, at high shear rates as might occur when blood flow is altered around a damaged valve, the immobilized vWF binds to glycoprotein Ib (GP Ib) on the membrane of platelets. Thus, platelets become attached to the endothelial wall and are activated; this leads to aggregation and further platelet deposition. Microorganisms that gain access to the circulation can attach to the NBTV and then become encased in more fibrin and platelets and subsequently multiply. This appears to protect the bacteria from contact with other cellular components. However, it seems that the bacteria can escape back into the circulation. It is this sequence of events in the heart that leads to IE.

The main events leading to IE can be reviewed under four headings:[23]

1. Damage to the endocardium with deposition of platelets and fibrin to form an NBTV.
2. A bacteraemia caused by discharge of microorganisms into the circulation from a peripheral site.
3. Adherence of microorganisms to the NBTV with additional deposition of fibrin and platelets.
4. Multiplication of microorganisms within the vegetation (Fig. 17.1).

Once such a lesion is established, the infection can progress in four main ways:

1. Discharge of the infecting agent into the circulation produces a constant bacteraemia, resulting in symptoms such as fever, fatigue, loss of appetite and weight as well as anaemia, antibody formation, splenomegaly and, depending on the organism, metastatic infection. The circulating organisms also continue to reseed the original vegetation.
2. Local infiltration of the vegetation by the bacteria within it results in abnormalities of cardiac conduction, valve ring abscesses, pericarditis and even fatal valvular incompetence.
3. Peripheral emboli are produced by dislodgement of the fragments of infected vegetations; these may be responsible for so-called mycotic aneurysms and septic infarcts. It is also possible for these infected vegetations to be yet another source of bacteraemia.
4. Circulating immune complexes result from the combination of circulating antibodies to the infecting microorganisms and the infecting organism (antigen) itself. These complexes are probably responsible for the skin manifestations of IE as well as arthritis and glomerulonephritis.

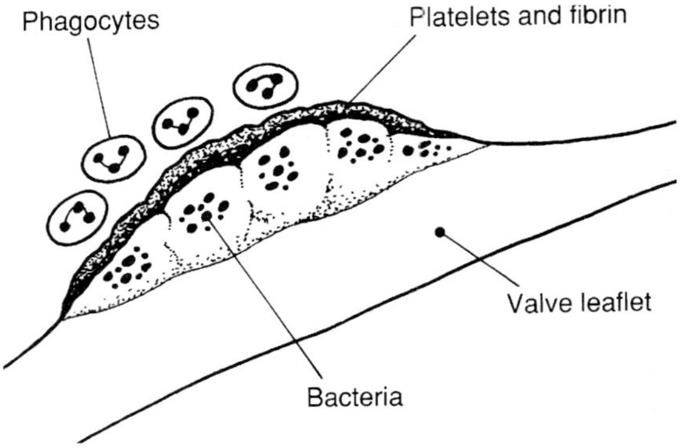

Fig 17.1 Formation of a vegetation on a valve leaflet in infective endocarditis. A focal area of injury to the endocardial surface is covered by deposits of platelets and fibrin. Bacteraemia produces circulating microorganisms which adhere to the damaged area. Further layers of platelets and fibrin are laid down. Bacteria proliferate to form colonies within the vegetation but are protected from phagocytes by the fibrin layer; however, this is not a barrier to nutrients.

Endocardial injury

The characteristic lesion of IE is the NBTV found on valve leaflets or on other sites on the endocardium, mainly on the downstream side of a jet lesion. Some cardiac abnormalities are more susceptible to infection than others and haemodynamic forces serve to explain the difference. IE is most likely to occur when blood jets from a high- to a low-pressure chamber. The infection develops downstream where the velocity of the blood is greatest and lateral pressure is lowest, thus causing sites of endothelial damage where blood-borne bacteria may be deposited.[23] For example, the infected regurgitant mitral valve infects the left atrial wall at the point of impact and there is a marked tendency to seeding of the mitral valve in aortic regurgitation.

Although normal hearts appear to be less susceptible to infection than damaged ones, some patients may have an underlying abnormality that was asymptomatic. For example, minor degenerative changes take place in the aortic and mitral valves of the elderly and in young men a condition that is sometimes missed clinically is that of bicuspid aortic valves which cause no symptoms. These factors of high-pressure gradients and jet effects together increase the likelihood of endocardial injury.

Even though rheumatic heart disease has decreased in incidence, it is still an important cause of endocardial abnormality. Before the antibiotic era, rheumatic heart disease accounted for 70% of cases; by the 1970s it was about 40%, whereas currently the figure is closer to 24%. The lesions of rheumatic endocarditis heal by fibrosis; this may occur in the free endocardium, most commonly in the posterior wall of the left atrium (McCallum's patch) or, more significantly, it involves the valves causing their dysfunction. The resultant effects are mitral incompetence and aortic valve disease.

On the other hand, the incidence of IE in patients with congenital heart disease has risen from about 16% in the 1970s to 19% currently.[6] This increase is almost certainly due to the improved survival of patients with congenital heart disease. Most commonly, a ventricular septal defect (VSD) or bicuspid valve gives rise to endocardial damage and the haemodynamic theory explains why a small VSD will become infected but not a large one.[24] Patients with prosthetic heart valves are among those who are particularly susceptible to IE and it is in these patients that staphylococcal and candidal IE are more likely to be seen.

Pathological aspects

Changes in the heart

The characteristic vegetations of IE are multiple, large and friable. They project from the endocardial surface, especially the valve cusps. These vegetations occur mainly on the valves of the left side of the heart following the distribution seen in chronic rheumatic heart disease (i.e. mitral > aortic > tricuspid > pulmonary). Right-sided IE is uncommon but may occur in intravenous drug abusers (when the tricuspid valve is affected), patients with indwelling venous catheters extending into the right atrium, patients with gonococcal endocarditis and patients with VSD (the jet of shunted blood causes endocardial injury in the right ventricle).

The infected vegetations usually develop along the lines of cuspal contact. The microorganisms eventually invade the underlying cusp tissue and cause necrosis; this may result in aneurysm formation or rupture of the cusp and, eventually, possible rupture of the chordae. However, these destructive changes are most likely to be seen in acute endocarditis.

The cusps become vascularized, thickened and fibrosed; they also become infiltrated with polymorphs and macrophages and, possibly, bacteria. In animals, at least, it is thought that the polymorphs play a role in causing tissue damage to the heart, possibly by causing softening and separation of valve tissue.[23] Large vegetations on the valve affect blood flow causing turbulence and cardiac murmurs. Progressive destruction of the valves can lead to valve perforation. Eventually, valve replacement may be necessary but this, of course, may bring still further problems.

Embolism

Embolic phenomena result from detachment of fragments of the vegetations. With left-sided IE, subsequent infarction of the brain, kidneys, spleen and intestine are common complications and minor or major myocardial infarction may also occur, particularly when the aortic valve is involved. With right-sided vegetations, embolism involves the pulmonary vessels.

In about 10% of cases of IE, the organisms in the emboli produce a local infection in the artery at the site where they become lodged; this can cause a weakening of the arterial wall and hence the formation of the mycotic aneurysms. These may rupture, causing massive haemorrhage.

Immune complexes

After some time, the presence of bacteria in the blood elicits an antibody response. When relatively large amounts of antigen are present, antigen–antibody complexes may form in sufficient quantity to cause immune complex disease; the results of this are often seen in the joints or kidneys. These immune complexes, together with products from activated complement can therefore cause vasculitis, synovitis, glomerulonephritis and skin lesions. Cutaneous immune complex-mediated vasculitis is responsible for the erythematous papules in the palms and soles (Janeway lesions) and the characteristic tender red nodules in the fingers and toes (Osler's nodes).

Clinical correlations and course of IE

The foregoing account of the pathogenesis and pathology of this disease provides the background which gives rise to the subsequent clinical signs and symptoms of the disease. Table 17.5 provides a list of possible signs and symptoms.[25]

IE often starts insidiously with irregular fever, malaise and mild anaemia. As it progresses, petechiae may appear, usually in small numbers, in the skin, mucous membranes and retina, and splinter haemorrhages may occur under the nails; these are probably embolic. The spleen may become palpable and cardiac murmurs can occur, either from previous disease, or may develop and change in quality as IE progresses. Clinical features may arise from embolic phenomena and cause subsequent infarction of the brain, myocardium, spleen and kidneys. Haematuria may result from renal infarction or glomerulonephritis. Heart failure eventually develops and is the commonest cause of death. It may be progressive, probably because of increasing valve damage, or it may deteriorate suddenly from rupture of a valve cusp or chordae; alternatively, it may arise from myocardial infarction. The other major causes of death are embolic phenomena and renal failure.

IE can be difficult to diagnose. Positive blood cultures are helpful and enable bacterial sensitivity testing to take place. However, up to 20% of patients with IE will have negative blood cultures. The usual reason is antibiotics given in the preceding month. Fungal endocarditis can give repeatedly negative blood cultures as the fungal vegetations only break off occasionally into the blood stream.

Echocardiography should be performed in all suspected cases of IE in order to detect vegetations and to confirm the structural diagnosis and severity of the disease.

Table 17.5 Possible signs and symptoms of infective endocarditis

Heart murmur
Fever, malaise or sweating
Unexplained heart failure
Embolic stroke or limb embolism
Anaemia, high ESR or C-reactive protein
Vasculitic rash
Unexplained nephritis or renal failure

ESR = Erythrocyte sedimentation rate.

Prophylaxis

The Endocarditis Working Party of the British Society for Antimicrobial Chemotherapy published its latest recommendations in January 1990;[26] however, since then modifcations have been made. The

Table 17.6 Risk categories for antibiotic prophylaxis

Chronic rheumatic heart disease or history of rheumatic fever
Congenital heart disease
Prosthetic heart valves
Mitral or aortic incompetence
Previous history of infective endocarditis
Hypertrophic cardiomyopathy
Heart murmurs, unless it is certain that they are innocent
Systolic murmurs, especially in the elderly
Intravenous drug abusers

The revised recommendations for prophylaxis are available from the British Heart Foundation, 102 Gloucester Place, London W1H 4DH, and are printed on cards to be carried by patients at risk of developing infective endocarditis

Table 17.7 Recommendations for infective endocarditis prophylaxis

1. **Dental extractions, scaling, or periodontal surgery**
A. Under local or no anaesthesia

(a) For patients not allergic to penicillin and not prescribed penicillin more than once in the previous month, but including those with a prosthetic valve (but not those who have had endocarditis, see special-risk patients below):
- Adults: Single dose of amoxycillin* 3 g by mouth taken under supervision 1 h before procedure
- Children 5–10: half adult dose
- Children under 5: quarter adult dose

(b) For patients allergic to penicillin or who have received penicillin more than once in the previous month, including those with a prosthetic valve (but not those who have had endocarditis, see special-risk patients below):
- Adults: Single dose of clindamycin† 600 mg by mouth taken under supervision 1 h before procedure
- Children 5–10: half adult dose
- Children under 5: quarter adult dose

B. Under general anaesthesia

(c) For patients not allergic to penicillin and not given penicillin more than once in the previous month (but not those with a prosthetic valve or who have had endocarditis; see special-risk patients below):
- Adults: amoxycillin 1 g by intramuscular or intravenous injection‡ at induction then 500 mg by mouth 6 h later
- Children 5–10: half adult dose§
- Children under 5: quarter adult dose§

or

- Adults: amoxycillin* 3 mg by mouth 4 h before induction then a further 3 g as soon as possible after procedure
- Children 5–10: half adult dose
- Children under 5: quarter adult dose§

or

- Adults: amoxycillin 3 mg by mouth and probenecid 1 g by mouth 4 h before procedure

Special-risk patients who should be referred to hospital:

(i) Patients with prosthetic valves who are to have a general anaesthetic
(ii) Patients who are allergic to penicillin and who are to have a general anaesthetic
(iii) Patients who have had penicillin more than once in the previous month and who are to have a general anesthetic
(iv) Patients who have had a previous attack of endocarditis

Recommendations for these patients are:

(d) For patients not allergic penicillin and who have not had penicillin more than once in the previous month:
- Adults: amoxycillin 1 g by intramuscular or intravenous injection at induction then 500 mg by mouth 6 h later plus 120 mg gentamicin by intramuscular or intravenous injection at induction, then 500 mg amoxycillin orally 6 h later
- Children 5–10: half adult dose amoxycillin§ *plus* gentamicin 2 mg/kg
- Children under 5: quarter adult dose amoxycillin§ *plus* gentamicin 2 mg/kg

(e) For patients allergic to penicillin or who have had penicillin more than once in the previous month:
- Adults: vancomycin 1 g by slow intravenous infusion over at least 100 min followed by gentamicin 120 mg intravenously at induction or 15 min before procedure
- Children under 10: vancomycin 20 mg/kg intravenously *plus* gentamicin 2 mg/kg intravenously

or

- Adults: teicoplanin 400 mg intravenously *plus* gentamicin 120 mg intravenously at induction or 15 min before procedure
- Children under 14: teicoplanin 6 mg/kg, gentamicin 2 mg/kg

or

- Adults: clindamycin 300 mg intravenously over at least 10 min at induction or 15 min before procedure then oral or intravenous clindamycin 150 mg 6 h later
- Children 5–10: half adult dose
- Children under 5: quarter adult dose

2. **Surgery or instrumentation of upper respiratory tract**
As for dental procedures; postoperative dose may be given parenterally if swallowing is painful

3. **Genitourinary procedures**
As for special-risk patients undergoing dental procedures under general anesthetic, except that clindamycin is not given (*see above*). If the urine is infected, prophylaxis should also cover infective organism

4. **Obstetric, gynaecological and gastrointestinal procedures**
As for genitourinary procedures (prophylaxis required for patients with prosthetic valves or those who have had endocarditis only)

Approved by the Endocarditis Working Party of the British Society for Antimicrobial Chemotherapy and the Dental Formulary Subcommittee.[27]

Notes

*Amoxycillin is liable to cause irritating rashes, especially in people with infectious mononucleosis, chronic lymphatic leukaemia and in human immunodeficiency virus (HIV) infection, in whom it should be avoided.

†If clindamycin is given, periodontal or other multistage procedures should not be repeated at intervals of less than 2 weeks.

‡If the intramuscular or intravenous route is considered necessary it may be preferable for the procedure to be carried out in hospital. To reduce the pain, intramuscular injection is given in 2.5 ml lignocaine hydrochloride 1% injection.

§Whenever possible, painful intramuscular injections should be avoided in children.

latest recommendations may be found in the *Dental Practitioners' Formulary/British National Formulary*.[27]

It is axiomatic that patients who fall into the risk categories should be well-informed and provided with regular preventive dental care. The maintenance of healthy teeth, gingival and periodontal tissue to reduce spontaneous bacteraemia may well be far more important than antibiotic prophylaxis in reducing the incidence of IE.[28] A recent study into the cost-effectiveness of antimicrobial prophylaxis[29] found that such prophylaxis is highly cost-effective before dental extractions, but that its value for other invasive dental procedures is unproved.

Table 17.6 provides a list of the risk categories. Patients with coronary heart disease, including those who have had coronary revascularization (e.g. coronary bypass surgery), are not at risk.[5] The current recommendations are set out in Table 17.7.

References

1. Osler W. The Gulstonian lectures on malignant endocarditis. *Br Med J* 1885; **i**: 467–470; 522–526; 577–579.
2. Bayliss R, Clarke C, Oakley C, Somerville W, Whitfield AGW. The teeth and infective endocarditis. *Br Heart J* 1983; **50**: 506–512.
3. Skehan JD, Murray M, Mills PG. Infective endocarditis, current incidence and mortality. *Br Heart J* 1985; **54**: 614.
4. Young SEJ. Aetiology and epidemiology of infective endocarditis in England and Wales. *J Antimicrob Chemother* 1987; **20** (suppl. A): 7–14.
5. Oakley CM. Controversies in the prophylaxis of infective endocarditis: a cardiological view. *J Antimicrob Chemother* 1987; **54**: 99–104.
6. Bayliss R, Clarke C, Oakley CM, Somerville W, Whitfield AGW, Young SEJ. Incidence, mortality and prevention of infective endocarditis. *J R Phys* 1986; **20**: 15–20.
7. Leading article. Infective endocarditis. *Br Med J* 1981; **282**: 677–678.
8. Bayliss R, Clarke C, Oakley CM, Somerville W, Whitfield AGW, Young SEJ. The microbiology and pathogenesis of infective endocarditis. *Br Heart J* 1983; **50**: 513–519.
9. Horder TJ. Infective endocarditis with an analysis of 150 cases with special reference to the chronic form of the disease. *Q J Med* 1909; **2**: 289–324.
10. Cates JE, Christie RV. Subacute bacterial endocarditis: a review of 442 patients in 14 centres appointed by the Penicillin Trials Committee of the Medical Research Council. *Q J Med* 1951; **20**: 93–130.
11. Coutlee F, Carceller AM, Deschamps L *et al*. The evolving pattern of pediatric endocarditis from 1960 to 1985. *Can J Cardiol* 1990; **6**: 164–170.
12. Bahn SL, Goveia G, Bitterman P, Bahn AN. Experimental endocarditis induced by dental manipulation and oral streptococci. *Oral Surg Oral Med Oral Pathol* 1978; **45**: 549–559
13. Herzberg MC, Gong K, MacFarlane GD *et al*. Phenotypic characterization of *Streptococcus sanguis* virulence factors associated with bacterial endocarditis. *Infect Immun* 1990; **58**: 515–522.
14. Erickson PR, Herzberg MC. Purification and partial characterization of a 65-kDa platelet aggregation-associated protein antigen from the surface of *Streptococcus sanguis*. *J Biol Chem* 1990; **256**: 14080–14087.
15. Kilian M, Mikkelsen L, Henrichsen J. Taxonomic study of viridans streptococci: description of *Streptococcus gordonii* sp. nov. and emended descriptions of *Streptococcus sanguis* (White and Niven 1946), *Streptococcus oralis* (Bridge and Sneath 1982), and *Streptococcus mitis* (Andrews and Horder 1906). *Int J Syst Bacteriol* 1989; **39**: 471–484.
16. Whiley RA, Fraser H Y, Douglas CWI, Hardie JM, Williams AM, Collins MD. *Streptococcus parasanguis* sp. nov., an atypical viridans *Streptococcus* from human clinical specimens. *FEMS Microbiol Lett* 1990; **68**: 115–122.
17. Douglas CWI, Brown PR, Preston FE. Platelet aggregation by oral streptococci. *FEMS Microbiol Lett* 1990; **72**: 62–68.
18. Ford I, Douglas CWI, Preston FE *et al*. Mechanisms of platelet aggregation by *Streptococcus sanguis*, a causative organism in infective endocarditis. *Br J Haematol* 1993; **84**: 95–100.
19. Manning JE, Hume EB, Hunter N, Knox KW. An appraisal of the virulence factors associated with streptococcal endocarditis. *J Med Microbiol* 1994; **40**: 110–114.
20. Baddour LM, Christensen GD, Lawrence JH, Simpson WA. Pathogenesis of experimental endocarditis. *Rev Infect Dis* 1989; **11**: 452–463.
21. Douglas CWI. Pathogenic mechanisms in infective endocarditis. *Rev Med Microbiol* 1993; **4**: 130–137.
22. Lowrance JH, Hasty DL, Simpson WA. Adherence of *Streptococcus sanguis* to conformationally specific determinants in fibronectin. *Infect Immun* 1988; **56**: 2279–2285.
23. Freedman LR. The pathogenesis of infective endocarditis. *J Antimicrob Chemother* 1987; **20** (suppl A): 1–6.
24. Oakley CM. Infective endocarditis. *Br J Hosp Med* 1980; **24**: 232–243.
25. Oakley CM. Treatment of infective endocarditis. *Prescribers J* 1990; **30**: 152–164.
26. Antibiotic prophylaxis of infective endocarditis. Recommendations from the Endocarditis Working

Party of the British Society for Antimicrobial Chemotherapy. *Lancet* 1990; **335**: 88–89.

27. *Dental Practitioners' Formulary/British National Formulary*, p. 215. London: British Medical Association and the Royal Pharmaceutical Company of Great Britain, 1994.

28. Shanson DC. Antibiotic prophylaxis of infective endocarditis in the United Kingdom and Europe. *J Antimicrob Chemother* 1987; **20**: 119–131.

29. Gould IM, Buckingham JK. Cost effectiveness of prophylaxis in dental practice to prevent infective endocarditis. *Br Heart J* 1993; **70**: 79–83.

18

Oral infections in the immunocompromised patient

Crispian Scully

Introduction

The number of immunocompromised patients is increasing because of iatrogenic immunosuppression and human immunodeficiency virus (HIV) infection. Most have T-lymphocyte defects and are prone to develop persistent and severe fungal and viral infections. Oral candidosis and herpes simplex infections are particularly common. Hairy leukoplakia, mouth ulceration, neoplasms and impaired periodontal health are less common.

Immunocompromising states

The last quarter of the 20th century is seeing a dramatic increase in numbers of immunocompromised persons in all communities. Formerly virtually a sole consequence of medical treatment such as immunosuppression with corticosteroids and other agents, the effects of the immune defects associated with infection by HIV are now a major cause of immune defect.[1,2] HIV-infected persons will soon be seen by every dental practitioner if, indeed, that is not already the situation. HIV seropositivity in the UK has now reached levels as high as 1 in 300 or so in some younger heterosexuals and higher in some groups at special risk.

Thus the main groups of immunocompromised persons are now organ transplant patients, persons receiving immunosuppressive treatment for other conditions and persons with HIV disease. These secondary immune defects are characterized by a predominantly T-lymphocyte immune defect. Other immunocompromising conditions are far less common but may involve a range of different immune defects, affecting B lymphocytes, neutrophils or other aspects of immune defences, and are usually genetically determined.

Consequences of T-lymphocyte immune defects

T lymphocytes (T cells) are a heterogeneous population of white cells originating in the thymus and a whole vocabulary has evolved with respect to the various types. Some T cells enhance the activity of B lymphocytes which are formed in the bone marrow and produce antibodies (T-helper cells – T_H or CD4 cells). Other CD4 cells are involved in the delayed type of hypersensitivity reaction (T_{DH}; see Chapter 19). T cells also suppress B-lymphocyte activity (T-suppressor – T_S or CD8 cells). Some of these T cells are capable of damaging or killing other cells (cytotoxic T cells – T_C). A simple way of looking at the function of T cells, but one which is useful in a clinical setting, is to regard T cells as essential for protection against infection with fungi, viruses, and some bacteria, mainly mycobacteria. This takes place when the infective agent is presented to them by the infected cell. This is a complex process whereby the infected cell foreign material such as a virus particle is bound to a specialized molecule within the target cell, termed the

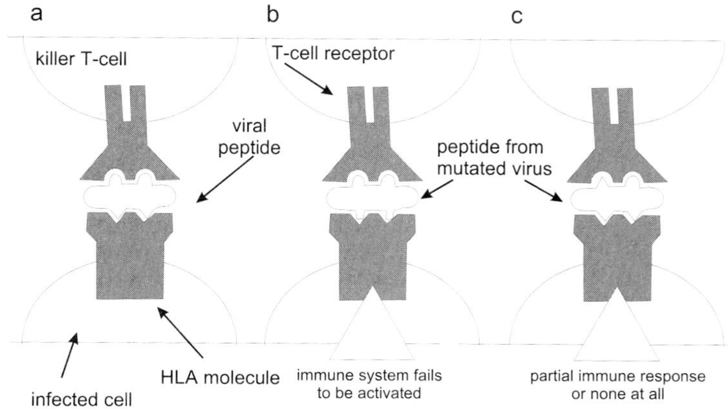

Fig. 18.1 (a) The target cell major histocompatibility complex (MHC) human leukocyte antigens (HLA) presenting ingested microbial or viral peptides to the T cells. The peptide is recognized and therefore fits. The CD4 receptor recognizes the MHC II antigen, whereas the CD8 receptor recognizes the MHC I antigen and their respective foreign peptides.
(b) The mutated virus peptide will not fit the HLA molecule and so the T cell is not activated.
(c) A partial fit may give a partial or no response.

major histocompatibility complex (MHC) antigen. There are three groups of genes encoding (producing) MHC molecules, which are therefore called class I, II and III antigens. In humans these are also called human leukocyte antigens (HLAs). The HLA/MHC molecule transports the viral fragment to the surface, where it will be detected by a T-cell receptor (Fig. 18.1a). The CD4 receptor of the helper T cell recognizes class II MHC antigens, whereas the CD8 receptor of the cytotoxic T cell recognizes the MHC class I antigens. These interactions activate the T cells, so that CD4 cells activate the CD8 cells to kill the target cell with its virus or microbe and also to activate B cells.

Acquired immunodeficiency syndrome (AIDS) arises when the HIV virus particles either overcome the T-helper cells or mutate so that they do not fit the HLA-presenting antigen (Fig. 18.1b) or are not recognized by the T cell (Fig. 18.1c) and also when the killer T cells destroy infected helper T cells.

Most immunocompromised patients are prone to infection with microorganisms (Table 18.1), some of which in the healthy immunocompetent person are purely commensals. Such infections are termed opportunistic – the microorganisms are opportunistic of the impaired host immunity. Immunocompromised patients are also more liable to infection with recognized pathogens.

Table 18.1 Some orofacial infections in immunocompromised persons*

Fungal	*Viral*	*Bacterial*
More common		
Candidosis	Herpes simplex virus	Destructive gingival and periodontal infections
	Varicella-zoster virus	
	Cytomegalovirus	
	Epstein–Barr virus	
	Human herpesvirus 6	
Uncommon		
Aspergillosis	Molluscum contagiosum	Tuberculosis
Cryptococcosis	Human papillomavirus	Atypical mycobacterioses
Zygomycosis	Human herpesvirus 8	Syphilis
Histoplasmosis		Epithelioid angiomatosis
Coccidioidomycosis		Gangrenous stomatitis
Blastomycoses		Various oral opportunists
Others		

*See also Table 18.2.

The oral cavity is both a common site of infection in the immunocompromised person and also often the source of considerable discomfort. Such oral infections tend to be recurrent or protracted, severe, sometimes resistant to treatment, and may occasionally spread systemically from the mouth. In general, the spectrum of infections is wider – and their severity greater – the more profound is the immune defect. Oral lesions may be localized, or part of more disseminated disease.

This chapter discusses mainly the more common fungal, viral and bacterial infections in secondary immune defects. Exotic organisms and parasites are not included, though they are beginning to become important.

Secondary immune defects

Oral fungal infections in the immunocompromised person

Superficial mycoses

Superficial oral fungal infections (mycoses) are extremely common in immunocompromised persons.[3–6] Oral candidosis (candidiasis) is by far the most common superficial mycosis of any significance[4] but other organisms are sometimes found (Table 18.2). *Candida* species account for nearly 80% of hospital-acquired fungal infections[5] and many patients die with undiagnosed invasive candidosis. Pathogenicity appears related to adherence and protease production.[5] Oral candidosis is a prominent and common early feature in HIV infection and also a prognostic indicator of progression to AIDS. Oral candidosis is also extremely common in other T-cell immune defects. Indeed, in view of the predilection for candidiosis in immunocompromised patients, antifungal prophylaxis may well be indicated.

Table 18.2 Fungi associated with superficial mycoses found in oral cavities of human immunodeficiency (HIV)-infected patients[6]

Candida species	*Others*
C. albicans	*Saccharomyces cerevisiae*
*C. glabrata**	*Rhodotorula rubra*
C. famata	*Rhodotorula piliminae*
C. kefyr	*Fonsecaea pedrosi*
C. krusei	*Prototheca stagnura*
C. rugosa	*Trichosporon pullulans*
C. guilliermondii	
C. tropicalis	

**Torulopsis glabrata.*

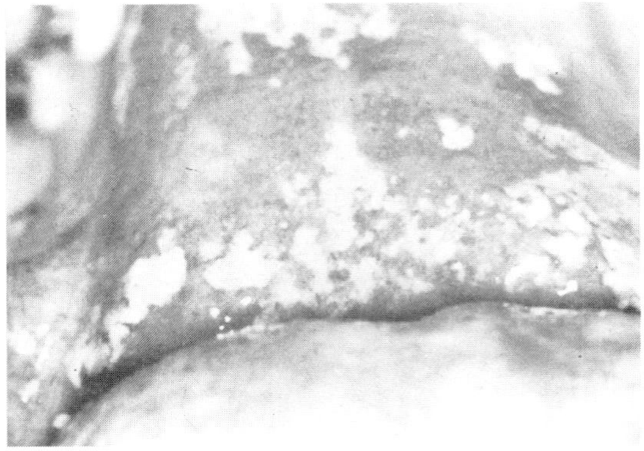

Fig. 18.2 Thrush on the palate.

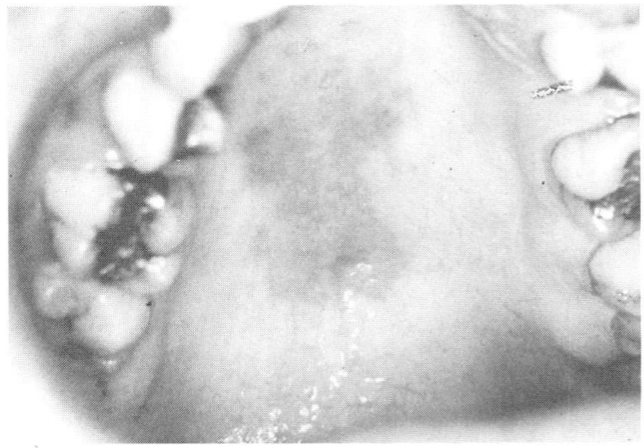

Fig. 18.3 Erythematous candidosis

Most infection is caused by *Candida albicans* and presents with or without soreness, as the typical white lesions of thrush (Fig. 18.2) on an erythematous background, or there may be purely an erythematous appearance (Fig. 18.3) sometimes in the palate, or as median rhomboid glossitis. Some patients may develop angular stomatitis, even if they are not wearing dentures.[6]

Oral candidosis in immunocompromised persons is usually responsive to standard antifungals such as topical nystatin or amphotericin, at least initially.[7,8] However, relapses are increasingly seen and there is consequently a trend towards the use of systemic imidazoles (ketoconazole) and bis-triazoles (fluconazole and itraconazole). Unfortunately, ketoconazole is hepatotoxic and, for this reason, fluconazole is currently often the antifungal of first choice. Fluconazole appears to act by interfering with fungal cell wall synthesis and by an effect on the epithelial cells themselves it inhibits fungal adherence to epithelium. Fluconazole resistance is now emerging as a clinical problem.[6] Invasive candidosis is best treated with intravenous amphotericin.[5]

Systemic mycoses

Several of the systemic mycoses are increasing in prevalence in immunocompromised individuals.[9–12] Aspergillosis, cryptococcosis, histoplasmosis and zygomycosis are increasingly seen, and reports of oral involvement are also increasing. Indeed, the oral cavity is often the most common site of fungal infection. This is the case, for example, in children being treated for cancer or other neoplasms.

Aspergillosis is second only to candidosis as an opportunistic mycosis. *Aspergillus fumigatus* and *A. flavus* are ubiquitous organisms and the predominant pathogens, typically causing maxillary antrum aspergillosis but sometimes presenting with yellow or black necrotic palatal or lingual ulcers. *A. niger* and other species may occasionally be involved. Since the organisms are ubiquitous, the diagnosis of aspergillosis must be confirmed by biopsy. Treatment is usually with systemic amphotericin and surgical debridement.[12,13]

Cryptococcus neoformans is also a ubiquitous organism. Oral cryptococcosis has now been described in HIV disease, presenting as palatal or lingual ulcers, or non-healing extraction wounds.[12] Diagnosis is confirmed histologically and the disease is treated with systemic amphotericin, ketoconazole or itraconazole.[14,15]

Histoplasmosis is increasingly reported in immunocompromised persons.[12] The main causal organism is *Histoplasma capsulatum* which, though found in a number of countries, is particularly common in the Mississippi and Ohio river valleys in the USA, and it is from those areas that most cases have originated. As in the systemic mycoses already discussed, oral lesions have been ulcerative or nodular; diagnosis is confirmed by microscopy; and systemic amphotericin or ketoconazole are the main treatments.

Mucormycosis (phycomycosis or zygomycosis) is caused by fungi of the family Mucoraceae – mainly by *Mucor* or *Rhizopus* species. Mucormycosis is almost exclusively seen in immunocompromised individuals, and oral involvement is usually associated with rhinocerebral mucormycosis.[12] It presents as chronic antral infection with pain and nasal discharge which invades the maxilla and involves the palate or the orbit, eventually spreading intracranially. Diagnosis is confirmed by smear and histology and treatment is with surgical debridement and systemic amphotericin.

Other systemic mycoses, such as coccidioidomycosis and paracoccidioidomycosis, might be expected to increase in prevalence in immunocompromised persons but oral lesions appear to be very rare as yet, presumably because of the restricted geographical distribution of the fungi.

Oral viral infections in the immunocompromised person

Herpesviruses account for most oral viral infections in the immunocompromised person.[16–19] Herpesviruses are all DNA viruses which remain latent after primary infection. Most infections result from reactivation of latent virus and the viruses are often shed in saliva. Antiviral prophylaxis therefore may be indicated in immunocompromised patients.

Herpes simplex virus (HSV) infections are the most commonly recognized oral viral infections.[20] HSV is latent in trigeminal ganglia. Over 50% and often up to 75% of immunocompromised patients develop oral HSV lesions. Chronic extensive and painful ulcers affecting especially the keratinized mucosa are the most common intraoral lesions (Fig. 18.4). Severe herpes labialis may be seen.[21–23] Acyclovir is the most reliable therapy but foscarnet may be indicated if viral resistance to acyclovir develops.[7]

Varicella-zoster virus (VZV) oral infections are less common than HSV infections. VZV is latent in sensory root ganglia and reactivation causes herpes zoster (shingles). This is extremely painful, may lead to scarring and postherpetic neuralgia and occasionally is associated with dissemination of VZV.[24] Acyclovir is the most reliable therapy and may reduce the incidence of postherpetic neuralgia, but acyclovir-resistant VZV are now being identified.

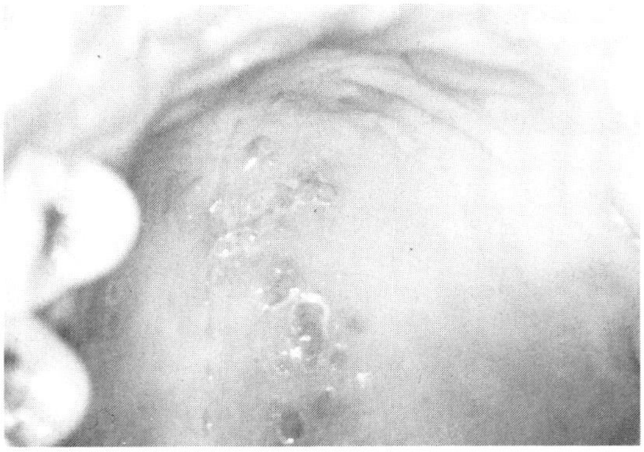

Fig. 18.4 Intraoral recurrent herpes simplex infection

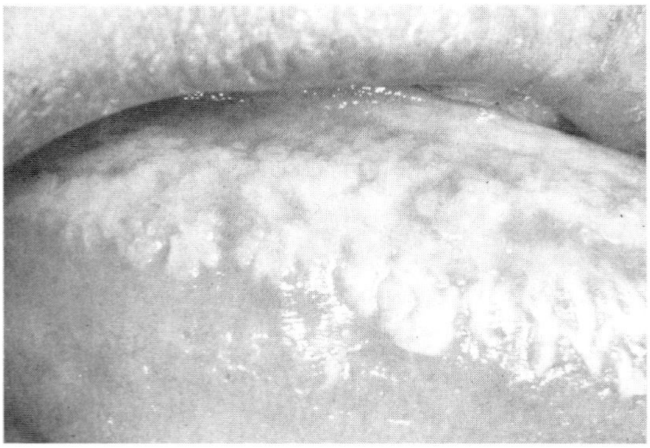

Fig. 18.5 Hairy leukoplakia of the lateral border of tongue

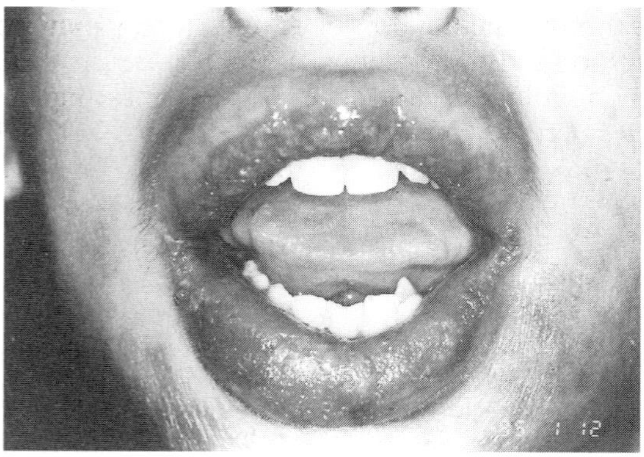

Fig. 18.6 Cheilitis and perioral dermatitis in chronic granulomatous disease.

Cytomegalovirus (CMV) is latent in salivary glands and is one of the leading causes of morbidity and mortality in immunocompromised patients. It is however only recently that CMV has been recognized as causing oral lesions which are usually chronic painful oral ulcers.[25] Unfortunately, acyclovir is not reliably effective against CMV; ganciclovir is preferred but is toxic, particularly to the kidneys and bone marrow.

Epstein–Barr virus (EBV) is latent in oropharyngeal epithelium and commonly reactivates in immunocompromised persons. High levels of EBV in the oropharynx appear to predict disease progression in HIV disease. EBV may produce oral ulcers, lymphoproliferative syndromes (typically non-Hodgkin's lymphomas in the faucial area), or oral hairy leukoplakia in immunocompromised persons.[26] First described in HIV disease, hairy leukoplakia has now been reported in various other immunocompromised patients including those immunosuppressed for renal, bone marrow, heart and liver transplants. Hairy leukoplakia typically presents as asymptomatic white lesions on the lateral margins of the tongue (Fig. 18.5). It has no known premalignant potential. Hairy leukoplakia may however, be a prognostic indicator for progression to AIDS and lymphoma. Treatment is not usually indicated but the lesion may clear with zidovudine, acyclovir or other agents.

Relatively recently, a new herpesvirus has been described, human herpesvirus 6 (HHV-6). Like the other herpesviruses noted above, it is a common infection and the virus remains latent in salivary glands. Reactivation is common in the immunocompromised patient but specific oral lesions have not been reported.[27,28] A further new herpesvirus, known as Kaposi's sarcoma herpesvirus (KSHV), herpesvirus may be implicated in Kaposi's sarcoma.[29]

Human papillomaviruses (HPV) are not herpesviruses. HPV are DNA viruses which commonly cause benign epithelial proliferative lesions such as warts.[30] Some 70 different HPV types have now been described, some associated with specific oral lesions. Oral lesions induced by HPV appear to be fairly uncommon but HPV have been identified in apparently healthy oral epithelium, and HPV-related lesions, usually warty in nature, are now increasing in prevalence in immunocompromised persons. Verrucae, genital warts (condylomata acuminata) and focal epithelial hyperplasia have been described. An increased incidence of labial carcinoma is recognized in immunocompromised patients and may possibly be related to HPV and/or HSV.[31]

Molluscum contagiosum is another DNA virus but it belongs to the poxvirus family. Labial and perioral molluscum contagiosum has been described in HIV-infected patients.[32,33] Several other viruses have also been reportedly associated with oral lesions in immunocompromised persons and the new technologies will undoubtedly shed further light in this expanding field.[19]

Bacterial infections in the immunocompromised person

A wide range of organisms can[34] occasionally colonize the mouth in immunocompromised patients and these may cause oral infections, presenting as ulcers which may even be the portal for septicaemia.[35] Reports have demonstrated the potential pathogenicity of bacteria that are part of the normal oral flora (viridans streptococci such as *Streptococcus mitis*, *S. sanguis* and *S. salivarius*)[36–44] and others that are typically found elsewhere, such as lower in the gastrointestinal tract (*Escherichia coli*, *Pseudomonas aeruginosa*, *Enterobacter cloacae*, *Klebsiella pneumoniae*, *Salmonella enteritidis*).[45–50] Septicaemias involving viridans streptococci or coagulase-negative staphylococci originating in the mouth are increasingly recognized in leukaemic or neutropenic patients.[45–50]

Mucositis following radiotherapy involving the oral mucosa may also have a bacterial component, and it now appears that Gram-negative bacilli may be implicated.[51,52]

Specific infections

Specific oral bacterial infections are rather uncommon in the immunocompromised person. Tuberculosis is, however, an increasing problem in immunocompromised persons and both infection by *Mycobacterium tuberculosis* and by atypical mycobacteria (usually *M. avium-intracellulare*) are more frequently seen than in immunocompetent persons, especially in HIV disease.[53] Oral lesions have been recorded – usually chronic oral ulcers, or chronically enlarged infected cervical lymph nodes.[54] Various atypical mycobacteria such as *M. kansasii*, *M. avium-intracellulare* and *M. xenopi* have caused outbreaks of infection emanating from water supplies, including those from health care facilities[55] and these sources may pose a particular hazard to immunocompromised patients. Diagnosis of these mycobacterial infections may be confirmed by histology and culture. Treatment is with combination antimicrobial chemotherapy but atypical mycobacteria in particular may be resistant to therapy.

A new rather bizarre vascular cutaneous pseudoneoplastic entity termed epithelioid angiomatosis which clinically resembles Kaposi's sarcoma or pyogenic granuloma has been described in HIV disease.[56,57] This may be seen periorally or orally.[58] Gram-negative bacilli which stain with the Warthin–Starry technique and antiserum against the cat-scratch disease bacillus have been described in the lesion[59] which may be a variant reaction to the cat-scratch bacillus but is more likely to be related to *Bartonella bacilliformis* or some other rickettsia such as *Rochalimaea quintana*.[60–64] It usually responds to erythromycin.

Non-specific infections

Gingival and periodontal disease

Destructive gingival and periodontal diseases are not uncommon in immunocompromised persons. But despite the observation that immunological defects can influence gingival and periodontal health,[1,2,65–67] studies of patients with rapidly progressive or severe periodontitis have as yet demonstrated little detectable, clinically significant systemic disease.[67,68]

A range of congenital (primary – see Table 18.3) and acquired (secondary) immune defects can predispose to periodontal disease,[1,2,69] but currently the periodontal diseases in infection with HIV and those associated with defects of polymorphonuclear leukocytes (PMNLs) are of greatest interest. Immune defects may underlie the predilection for periodontal disease found in diabetes mellitus, Crohn's disease and some other systemic disorders.[70] Primary immune defects are 'experiments of nature' that are fortunately rare but, since they often involve specific elements of the immune response,

Table 18.3 Defects of leukocyte function

Neutropenia
Cyclic neutropenia
Leukaemias
Drug-induced agranulocytosis
Disorders of microbial killing mechanism
Impaired H_2O_2 production – chronic granulomatous disease
Myeloperoxidase deficiency
Glucose-6-phosphate dehydrogenase deficiency
Drugs (e.g. sulphonamides)
Disorders of phagocytosis
Opsonin deficiencies
Hypogammaglobulinaemia
Complement deficiencies (C_3)
Sickle-cell disease
Impaired engulfment
Drugs which impair degranulation and liberation of lysosomal contents into phagosome
Chédiak–Higashi syndrome*
Disorders of migration and chemotaxis
Chédiak–Higashi syndrome
Lazy leukocyte syndrome
Drugs (e.g. corticosteroids)
Deficiencies of chemotactic factors
Complement deficiencies
Chemotactic factor inactivators in the serum
Diabetes mellitus

*Neutrophils contain lysosomal granules which are associated with impaired antibacterial activity.

they have helped outline the pathogenesis of many disorders.[1] Many of these very rare defects present with periodontal destruction and oral ulceration.[1,69–71]

It is also possible that subtle immune defects underlie some forms of early onset periodontitis where tissue destruction is disproportionate to the amount of bacterial plaque present. There may be a chemotactic defect affecting PMNLs in juvenile periodontitis,[72–74] though this is not always found.[75–77] A similar pattern has been found in rapidly progressive periodontitis.[73,76–78]

Mouth ulcers and periodontitis are the main oral manifestations in congenital neutropenia, chronic granulomatous disease and other PMNL defects.[69,78]

Agranulocytosis may manifest with mouth ulcers and periodontitis,[79–82] as may neutropenia.[83] Cytotoxic chemotherapy may induce neutropenia, directly damage the periodontium and alter the oral flora with an increase in *Candida albicans* and staphylococci.[84,85]

Ulcerative necrotizing gingival lesions and destructive lesions are common in infectious mononucleosis, preleukaemia,[86] leukaemias[87,88] and lymphomas.[89] Leukaemic infiltration may also cause loss of the lamina dura, widening of the periodontal space and loss of crypt outlines around unerupted teeth, especially in the premolar/molar region.[87,89]

Periodontal diseases are also common in HIV disease.[90–94] Two main distinct types of periodontal disease have been described in HIV-infected patients – an atypical gingivitis (HIV-G) and a rapidly progressive form of periodontitis (HIV-P). Gingivitis may be the precursor of the HIV-P which can be localized or generalized, and may be an early sign of HIV disease. HIV-G usually presents with spontaneous gingival bleeding and an erythematous band in the free gingiva. HIV-P may occur at any site but is often localized to a single aspect, typically causing necrosis, pocketing and a deep, boring pain. Free gingival and attached gingival erythema are common.

Gingival inflammation and destruction similar to acute necrotizing ulcerative gingivitis (ANUG) are more common in

HIV-infected individuals than in the general population[95,96] but analysis of microbiological cultures shows a flora distinct from that of ANUG.[97]

Studies of the plaque microflora in HIV-G and HIV-P suggest that the frequency of isolation of some black-pigmented anaerobic bacterial species (e.g. *Prevotella intermedius* and *Bacteroides* or *Porphyromonas gingivalis*) and levels of *Fusobacterium nucleatum* and *Actinobacillus actinomycetemcomitans* are higher than in controls. In addition, *Candida* spp., *Capnocytophaga* spp., *F. nucleatum*, *Eikenella corrodens*, *Wolinella* spp., *A. actinomycetemcomitans*, *P. gingivalis* and *P. intermedius* have been frequently isolated[97–101] and serum antibodies to these organisms and other black-pigmented anaerobes are increased.

Although little is yet known about the precise aetiology of HIV-G and HIV-P, the gingival lesions may appear before a dramatic decrease in CD4 numbers whereas, not surprisingly, HIV-P is seen mainly in those with low CD4/CD8 ratios and with other oral and extraoral lesions of HIV.[101]

Local debridement with the application of an antimicrobial such as povidone-iodine and the possible inclusion of antifungals to treat candidosis is a suggested regimen. Twice-daily rinses with aqueous 0.2% chlorhexidine gluconate also greatly help reduce gingival erythema, bleeding and pocket depths. Metronidazole can also be a useful adjunct for the anaerobes.

Gangrenous stomatitis (noma) has been described in several patients infected with HIV, the severity increasing with decreasing T4 (CD4) cell counts,[101–104] and has been seen in other severe immune defects.[105] The lesion is very resistant to treatment.

Iatrogenic immunosuppression can also influence periodontal health. Levamisole may increase gingivitis.[106] Corticosteroids, however, despite their immunosuppressive effects, appear not to have a significantly detrimental clinical effect on the periodontium[107,108] and in iatrogenically immunosuppressed patients there may actually sometimes be a *decrease* in clinical periodontal disease.[109–116] This should not be interpreted as a protective effect of immunosuppression but rather an inhibition of inflammation.

Wound infection

There is a liability to wound infection in immunocompromised patients, and non-healing extraction wounds, wound breakdown and actinomycosis are common if not prevented with antibiotics.[117–119]

Primary immune defects

Primary immune defects are rare, genetically determined, and present mainly with recurrent respiratory and skin infections. Oral lesions include ulcers, sinusitis and wound infections.[120–129] Leukocyte defects are listed in Table 18.3. Chronic granulomatous disease is an example of this group which present with oral and perioral infections (Figure 18.6). This is an inherited disorder of granulocyte function due to a lack of intracellular superoxide oxygen production. Oxygen normally dismutates to H_2O_2 in the activated neutrophil, which kills many strains of engulfed bacteria, hence patients suffer recurrent infections, especially due to *Staphylococcus aureus* and *Aspergillus* species. This condition should be considered even in adults with unexplained infections or granulomas.[130]

References

1. Scully C, Porter SR. Immunodeficiency. In: Ivanyi L (ed) *Immunology of Oral Diseases*, pp. 235–256. Lancaster: MTP Press, 1986.
2. Porter SR, Scully C. *Oral Healthcare for those with HIV and Other Special Needs*. Northwood: Science Reviews, 1995.
3. Samaranayake LP, MacFarlane TW (eds) *Oral Candidosis*. Bristol: Wright, 1990.
4. Holmstrup P, Axell T. Classification and clinical manifestations of oral yeast infections. *Acta Odontol Scand* 1990; **48**: 57–59.
5. Edwards JE. Invasive *Candida* infections. *N Engl J Med* 1991; **324**: 1060–1062.
6. Scully C, Elkabir M, Samaranayake LP. *Candida* and oral candidosis. *Crit Rev Oral Biol Med* 1994; **5**: 124–158.
7. Scully C, McCarthy G. Management of oral health in persons with HIV infection. *Oral Surg* 1992; **73**: 215–225.
8. Scully C, Porter SR. An ABC of oral health care in patients with HIV infection. *Br Dent J* 1991; **170**: 149–150.

9. Scully C, Almeida OP, Sposto MR. Systemic mycoses. In: Millard HD, Mason DK (eds) *1993 World Workshop on Oral Medicine*. pp. 61–70. Michigan: University of Michigan, 1995.
10. Bodey GP. The emergence of fungi as major hospital pathogens. *J Hosp Infect* 1988; **11** (suppl A): 411–426.
11. Pizzo PA, Walsh TJ. Fungal infections in the pediatric cancer patient. *Semin Oncol* 1990; **17** (suppl 3): 6–9.
12. Scully C, Almeida OP, Sposto MR. Deep mycoses in HIV infection. *Oral Dis* 1997; **3** (suppl 1): 5200–5207.
13. Denning DW, Stevens DA. Antifungal and surgical treatment of invasive aspergillosis: review of 2121 published cases. *Rev Infect Dis* 1990; **12**: 1147–1201.
14. Viviani MA, Tortorano AM, Pagano A *et al.* European experience with itraconazole in systemic mycoses. *J Am Acad Dermatol* 1990; **23**: 587–593.
15. Klein RS. Prophylaxis of opportunistic infections in individuals infected with HIV. *AIDS* 1989; **3** (suppl 1): 5161–5173.
16. Scully C. Infectious diseases in oral medicine. In: Millard D, Mason DK (eds) *Perspectives on 1988 World Workshop on Oral Medicine*. pp. 131–212. Chicago: Year Book, 1989.
17. Scully C. Infectious diseases. In: Millard HD, Mason DK. (eds) *World Workshop on Oral Medicine*, pp. 7–82. Michigan: University of Michigan, 1995.
18. Schubert MM. Oral manifestations of viral infections in immunocompromised patients. *Curr Opin Dent* 1991; **1**: 384–397.
19. Scully C, Samaranayake LP. *Clinical Virology in Oral Medicine and Dentistry*. Cambridge: Cambridge University Press, 1992.
20. Scully C. Orofacial herpes simplex virus infections: current concepts in the epidemiology pathogenesis and treatment and disorders in which the virus may be implicated. *Oral Surg* 1989; **68**: 701–710.
21. Schubert MM, Peterson DE, Flournoy N, Meyers JD, Truelove EL. Oral and pharyngeal herpes simplex virus infection after allogeneic bone marrow transplantation: analysis of factors associated with infection. *Oral Surg* 1990; **70**: 286–293.
22. Greenberg MS, Friedman H, Cohen SG, Oh SH, Laster L, Starr S. A comparative study of herpes simplex infections in renal transplant and leukemic patients. *J Infect Dis* 1987; **156**: 280–287.
23. Epstein JB, Sherlock C, Page JL, Spinelli J, Phillips G. Clinical study of herpes simplex virus infection in leukemia. *Oral Surg* 1990; **70**: 38–43.
24. Scully C, Laskaris G, Pindborg J, Porter SR, Reichart P. Oral manifestations of HIV infection and their management. 2. Less common lesions. *Oral Surg* 1991; **71**: 167–171.
25. Epstein JB, Scully C. Cytomegalovirus: a virus of increasing relevance to oral medicine and pathology. *J Oral Pathol Med* 1993; **22**: 348–353.
26. Scully C, Epstein JB, Porter SR. Oral hairy leukoplakia. *Lancet* 1989; **ii**: 1194.
27. Levy D, Ferro F, Greenspan D, Lennette E. Frequent isolation of HHV-6 from saliva and high seroprevalence of the virus in the population. *Lancet* 1990; **335**: 1047–1050.
28. Steeper TA, Ablashi DV, Salahuddin SZ, Saxinger C, Saltzman R, Schwartz B. The spectrum of clinical and laboratory findings resulting from human herpesvirus-6 (HHV-6) in patients with mononucleosis-like illness not resulting from Epstein–Barr virus or cytomegalovirus. *Am J Pathol* 1990; **93**: 776–783.
29. Chang Y, Cesarman F, Persin MS. Identification of new human herpesvirus-like DNA sequence in AIDS-associated Kaposi's sarcoma. *Science* 1994; **266**: 1865–1869.
30. Scully C, Cox M, Prime SS, Maitland NJ. Papillomaviruses: the current status in relation to oral disease. *Oral Surg* 1988; **65**: 526–532.
31. Scully C, Prime SS, Cox M, Maitland NJ. Infectious agents in the aetiology of oral cancer. In: Johnson NW (ed) *Oral Cancer: Detection of Patients and Lesions at Risk*. Cambridge: Cambridge University Press, 1991.
32. Ficarra G, Gaglioti D. Facial molluscum contagiosum in HIV-related patients. *Int J Oral Maxillofac Surg* 1989; **18**: 200–201.
33. Sugihara K, Reichart PA, Gelderblom HR. Molluscum contagiosum associated with AIDS: a case report with ultra-structural study. *J Oral Pathol Med* 1990; **19**: 235–239.
34. Brown LR, Mackler BF, Levy BM. Comparison of the plaque microflora in immunodeficient and immunocompetent dental patients. *J Dent Res* 1979; **58**: 2344–2352.
35. Scully C, Peterson DE. Oral infections in immunocompromised hosts. In: Millard D, Mason DK (eds) *Second World Workshop on Oral Medicine*. Chicago: Year Book (in press), 1997.
36. Hoecker JL, Pickering LK, Groschel D, Kohl S. *Streptococcus salivarius* sepsis in children with malignancies. *J Pediatr* 1978; **92**: 337–338.
37. Pizzo PA, Ladisch S, Witebsky FG. Alpha-haemolytic streptococci: clinical significance in the cancer patient. *Med Paediatr Oncol* 1978; **4**: 367–370.
38. Kern W, Kurrle E, Vanek E. High risk of streptococcal septicaemia after high dose cytosine arabinoside treatment for acute myelogenous leukaemia. *Klin Wochenschr* 1987; **65**: 773–780.
39. Cohen J, Worsley AM, Goldman JM, Donelly JP, Catvosky D, Galton DAG. Septicaemia caused by viridans streptococci in neutropenic patients with leukaemia. *Lancet* 1983; **ii**: 1452–1454.
40. Henslee J, Bostran B, Weisdorf D, Ramsay N, McGlave P, Kersey J. Streptococcal sepsis in bone marrow transplant patients. *Lancet* 1984; **i**: 393.
41. Leblanc T, Leverger G, Arlet G, Siguret V, Shaison G. Sepsis caused by *Streptococcus mitis* and *sanguis* II in neutropenic children. *Pathol Biol* 1989; **37**: 459–464.

42. Van de Leur JJJPM, Clasener HAL, Vollaard EJ, Van Turnhout JM. Infection prevention in neutropenia. In: Muller NF, Hekster YA (eds) *Progress in Clinical Pharmacy, Rational Use of Drugs*, pp. 329–330. The Hague: SDU 1989.
43. Guiot HFL, Van der Meer JWM, Van de Broek PJ. Prevention of viridans group streptococcal septicaemia in oncohematologic patient: a controlled comparative study on the effect of penicillin G and co-trimoxazole. *Ann Hematol* 1992; **64**: 260–265.
44. Burden AD, Oppenhaim BA, Crowther D *et al.* Viridans streptococcal bacteraemia in patients with haematological and solid malignancies. *Eur J Cancer* 1991; **27**: 409–411.
45. van de Leur JJJPM, Dofferhoff ASM, van Turnhout JM, Vollaard EJ, Clasener HAL. Colonization of oropharynx with staphylococci after penicillin in neutropenic patients. *Lancet* 1992; **340**: 861–862.
46. Dahlin YB, Holm AK. Changes in the oral microflora in patients with acute leukaemia and related disorders during the period of induction therapy. *Oral Surg* 1988; **65**: 411–417.
47. Galili D, Donitza A, Garfunkel A, Sela MN. Gram-negative enteric bacteria in the oral cavity of leukemia patients. *Oral Surg* 1992; **74**: 459–462.
48. Indrisana JP, Simon GL. Facial samonella abscess. *Ann Intern Med* 1989; **110**: 170.
49. Schiodt M, Pindborg JJ. AIDS and the oral cavity: epidemiology and clinical oral manifestations of human immune deficiency virus infection – a review. *Int J Oral Maxillofac Surg* 1987; **16**: 1–14.
50. Schmidt-Westhausen A, Fehrenbach FJ, Reichart PA. Oral Enterobacteriaceae in patients with HIV infection. *J Oral Pathol Med* 1990; **19**: 229–231.
51. Van Saene HKF, Martin MV. Do micro-organisms play a role in irradiation mucositis? *Eur J Clin Microbiol Infect Dis* 1990; **9**: 861–863.
52. Martin MV. Irradiation mucositis: a reappraisal. *Oral Oncol Eur J Cancer part B* 1993; **29B**: 1–2.
53. Zakowski P, Fligel S, Berlin OG. Disseminated *Mycobacterium avium-intracellulare* infection in homosexual men dying of acquired immunodeficiency. *J Am Med Assoc* 1982; **248**: 2980–2982.
54. Volpe F, Schwimmer A, Barr C. Oral manifestations of disseminated *Mycobacterium avium-intracellulare* infection in a patient with AIDS. *Oral Surg* 1985; **60**: 567–570.
55. du Moulin GC, Stottmeier KD. Waterborne mycobacteria: an increasing threat to health. *Am Soc Microbiol News* 1986; **52**: 525–529.
56. Cockerell CJ, Whitlaw MA, Webster GF, Friedman-Kien AE. Epithelioid angiomatosis: a distinct vascular disorder in patients with the acquired immunodeficiency syndrome or AIDS-related complex. *Lancet* 1987; **ii**: 654–656.
57. Walford N, Van der Wouw PA, Das PK, Ten Velden JJAM, Hulsebosch HJ. Epithelioid angiomatosis in the acquired immunodeficiency syndrome: morphology and differential diagnosis. *Histopathology* 1990; **16**: 83–88.
58. Speight PM, Zakrzewska J, Fletcher CDM. Epithelioid angiomatosis affecting the oral cavity as a first sign of HIV infection. *Br Dent J* 1991; **171**: 367–370.
59. Leboit PE, Berger TG, Egbert BM *et al.* Epithelioid haemangioma-like vascular proliferation in AIDS: manifestation of cat scratch disease bacillus infection. *Lancet* 1988; **i**: 960–963.
60. Relman DA, Loutit JS, Schmidt TM, Falkow S, Tompkins LS. The agent of bacillary angiomatosis – an approach to the identification of uncultured pathogens. *N Engl J Med* 1990; **323**: 1573–1580.
61. Perkocha LA, Geaghan SM, Yen TSB *et al.* Clinical and pathological features of bacillary peliosis hepatis in association with human immunodeficiency virus infection. *N Engl J Med* 1990; **323**: 1581–1586.
62. Slater LN, Welch DF, Hensel D, Coody DW. A newly recognized fastidious gram-negative pathogen as a cause of fever and bacteremia. *N Engl J Med* 1990; **323**: 1587–1593.
63. Relman DA, Falkow S, Le Boitt PE *et al.* The organism causing bacillary angiomatosis peliosis hepatis and fever and bacteremia in immunocompromised patients. *N Engl J Med* 1991; **324**: 1514.
64. Cockerell CJ, Tierno P, Friedman-Kien AE, Kim KS. The agent of bacillary angiomatosis. *N Engl J Med* 1991; **324**: 1511–1512.
65. Wilton JMA, Grifiths GS, Curtis MA *et al.* Detection of high-risk groups and individuals for periodontal diseases. *J Clin Perio* 1988; **15**: 339–346.
66. Johnson NW. Detection of high-risk groups and individuals for periodontal diseases. *Int Dent J* 1989; **39**: 33–47.
67. Porter SR. Immunological aspects of rapidly progressive periodontitis. PhD thesis, University of Bristol, UK 1987.
68. Ranney RR, Ruddy S, Tew JG, Welshimer HJ, Palcanis KG, Segreti A. Immunological studies of young adults with severe periodontitis. *J Perio Res* 1981; **16**: 390–402.
69. Porter SR, Scully C. Primary immunodeficiency. In: Jones JH, Mason DK (eds) *Oral Manifestations of Systemic Disease*, 2nd edn, pp. 112–161. London: Baillière Tindall, 1990.
70. Scully C, Mutlu S, Porter SR. Markers of disease susceptibility and activity for periodontal disease. In: Johnson NW (ed) *Periodontal Disease Markers of Disease Susceptibility and Activity*, pp. 139–178. Cambridge: Cambridge University Press, 1991.
71. Kinane DF, Davies RM. Periodontal manifestations of systemic disease. In: Jones JH, Mason DK (eds) *Oral Manifestations of Systemic Disease*, 2nd edn, pp. 112–161. London: Baillière Tindall, 1990.
72. Cianciola LJ, Genco RJ, Patters MR, McKenna J, van Oss CJ. Defective polymorhonuclear leukocyte function in a human periodontal disease. *Nature* 1977; **265**: 445–447.

73. Lavine WS, Maderaco EG, Stolman J *et al.* (1979) Impaired neutrophil chemotaxis in patients with juvenile and rapidly progressive periodontitis. *J Perio Res* 1979; **14**: 10–19.
74. Altman LC, Page RC, Vandesteen GE, Dixon LI, Bradford C. Abnormalities of leukocyte chemotaxis in patients with various forms of periodontitis. *J Perio Res* 1985; **20**: 553–563.
75. Kinane DF, Cullen CF, Johnston FA, Evans CW. Neutrophil chemotactic behaviour in patients with early-onset forms of periodontitis. I. Leading front analysis in Boyden chambers. *J Clin Perio* 1989; **16**: 242–246.
76. Kinane DF, Cullen CF, Johnston FA, Evans CW. Neutrophil chemotactic behaviour in patients with early-onset forms of periodontitis. II. Assessment using the under agarose technique. *J Clin Perio* 1989; **16**: 247–251.
77. Porter SR, Scully C. Periodontal aspects of systemic disease. In: Lang NP, Karring T (eds) *Proceedings of 1st European Workshop on Periodontology 1994.* London: Quintessence, pp. 375–438.
78. Scully C. Orofacial manifestations in chronic granulomatous disease of childhood. *Oral Surg Oral Med Oral Pathol* 1981; **51**: 148–151.
79. Bauer WH. The supporting tissues of the tooth in acute secondary agranulocytosis (arsphenamine neutropenia). *J Dent Res* 1946; **25**: 501–508.
80. Swenson HM, Redish CH, Manne M. Agranulocytosis: two case reports. *J Perio* 1965; **36**: 466–470.
81. Mishkin DJ, Akers JO, Darby CP. Congenital neutropenia. Report of a case and a biorationale for dental management. *Oral Surg Oral Med Oral Pathol* 1976; **42**: 738–745.
82. Gilman PA, Jackson DP, Guild HG. Congenital agranulocytosis: prolonged survival and terminal acute leukaemia. *Blood* 1970; **36**: 576–586.
83. Gilmour G, Scully C. Neutropenia and dental patients. *Br Dent J* 1986; **160**: 43–46.
84. Peterson DE, Minah GE, Overholser CD *et al.* Microbiology of acute periodontal infection in myelosuppressed cancer patients. *J Clin Oncol* 1987; **5**: 1461–1468.
85. Reynolds MA, Minah GE, Peterson DE *et al.* Periodontal disease and oral microbial successions during myelosuppressive cancer chemotherapy. *J Clin Perio* 1989; **16**: 185–189.
86. Deasy MJ, Vogel RI, Annes IK, Simon BI. Periodontal disease associated with preleukemic syndrome. *J Perio* 1976; **47**: 41–45.
87. Curtis AB. Childhood leukaemias: osseous changes in jaws on panoramic dental radiographs. *JADA* 1971; **83**: 844–847.
88. Lynch MA, Ship II. Initial oral manifestations of leukaemia. *JADA* 1967; **75**: 932–940.
89. Browne RM. Periodontal ligament features in blood and lymphoreticular disorders. In: Berkovitz BKB, Moxham BJ, Newman HN (eds) *The Periodontal Ligament in Health and Disease*, pp. 373–398. Oxford: Pergamon Press, 1982.
90. Porter SR, Luker J, Scully C, Glover S, Griffiths MJ. Oral manifestations of a group of British patients infected with HIV-1. *J Oral Pathol Med* 1989; **18**: 47–48.
91. Scully C, Porter SR. Leading article: orofacial manifestations of HIV infection. *Lancet* 1988; **i**: 987–989.
92. Gornitsky M, Pekovic DD. Involvement of human immunodeficiency virus (HIV) in gingiva of patients with AIDS. In: Mestecky J, McGhee JR, Bienenstock J, Ogra PL (eds) *Recent Advances in Mucosal Immunology*, Part A. pp. 553–62. New York, Plenum, 1987.
93. Winkler JR, Grassi M, Murray PA. Clinical description and etiology of HIV-associated periodontal diseases. In: Robertson PB, Greenspan JS (eds) *Perspectives on Oral Manifestations of AIDS*, pp. 49–70. Littleton MA: PSG 1988.
94. Winkler JR, Murray PA. Periodontal disease – a potential intraoral expression of AIDS may be a rapidly progressive periodontitis. *Calif Dent Assoc J* 1987; **15**: 20–24.
95. Pindborg JJ, Holmstrup PA. Necrotising gingivitis related to human immunodeficiency virus (HIV) infection. *Afr Dent J* 1987; **1**: 5–8.
96. Pindborg JJ, Thorn JJ, Schiodt M, Gaub J, Black FT. Acute necrotising gingivitis in an AIDS patient. *Danish Dentl J* 1986; **90**: 450–453.
97. Murray PA, Holt SC. Microbiology of HIV-associated gingivitis and periodontitis. In: Robertson PB, Greenspan JS (eds) *Oral Manifestations of AIDS*, pp. 105–18. Littleton MA: PSG, 1988.
98. Murray PA, Hoover CH, Greenspan D, Greenspan JS, Winkler JR. Microbiologic evaluation of AIDS virus associated periodontitis. *J Dent Res* 1987; **66**: 226.
99. Grassi M, Murray PA, Winker JR. Orale manifestationen von HIV-infektionen. Gegenwart und Zukunft. *Schweiz Monatsschr Zahnmed* 1987; **97**: 1537–1544.
100. Grieve WG, Murray PA, Winkler JR. The humoral response in AIDS-virus associated periodontitis. *J Dent Res* 1988; **66**: 256.
101. Murray PA, Grassi M, Winkler JR. The microbiology of HIV-associated periodontal lesions. *J Clin Perio* 1989; **16**: 636–642.
102. Akula SK, Creticos CM, Weldon-Linne CM. Gangrenous stomatitis in AIDS. *Lancet* 1989; **1**: 955.
103. Winkler JR, Murray PA, Hammerle C. Gangrenous stomatitis in AIDS. *Lancet* 1989; **2**: 108.
104. Giovannini M, Zuccotti GV, Fiocchi A. Gangrenous stomatitis in a child with AIDS. *Lancet* 1989; **2**: 1400.
105. Rotbart HA, Levin MJ, Jones JF *et al.* Noma in children with severe combined immunodeficiency. *J Pediatr* 1986; **109**: 596–600.
106. Ivanyi L, Lehner T. The effect of levamisole on gingival inflammation in man. *Scand J Immunol* 1977; **6**: 219–226.
107. Krohn S. Effect of the administration of steroid hormones on the gingival tissues. *J Periodontol* 1958; **29**: 300–306.

108. Safkan B, Knuuttila M. Corticosteroid therapy and periodontal disease. *J Clin Periodontol* 1984; **11**: 515–522.
109. Schuller PD, Freedman HL, Lewis DW. Periodontal status of renal transplant patients receiving immunosuppressive therapy. *J Periodontol* 1973; **44**: 166–170.
110. Rosenstein DI, Eigner TL, Levin MP, Chiodo GT. Rapidly progressive periodontal disease associated with HIV infection: report of a case. *JADA* 1989; **118**: 313–314.
111. Kardachi BJR, Newcomb GM. A clinical study of gingival inflammation in renal transplant recipients taking immunosuppressive drugs. *J Periodontol* 1978; **49**: 307–309.
112. Oshrain HI, Mender S, Mandel ID. Periodontal status of patients with reduced immunocapacity. *J Periodontol* 1979; **50**: 185–188.
113. Been V, Engel D. The effects of immunosuppressive drugs on periodontal inflammation in human renal allograft patients. *J Periodontol* 1982; **53**: 245–248.
114. Tollefsen T, Koppang HS, Messelt E. Immunosuppression and periodontal disease in man. Histological and ultrastructural observations. *J Perio Res* 1982; **17**: 329–344.
115. Tollefsen T, Saltvedt E, Koppang HS. The effect of immunosuppressive agents on periodontal disease in man. *J Perio Res* 1978; **13**: 240–250.
116. Sutton RBO, Smales FC. Cross-sectional study of the effects of immunosuppressive drugs on chronic periodontal disease in man. *J Clin Perio* 1983; **10**: 317–326.
117. Yeager BA, Hozie J, Weisman RA, Greenberg MS, Bilanik LT. Actinomycosis in the acquired immune deficiency syndrome complex. *Arch Otolaryngol Head Neck Surg* 1986; **112**: 1293–1295.
118. Felix DH, Wray D, Smith GLF, Jones GA. Oro-antral fistula: an unusual complication of HIV-associated periodontal disease. *Br Dent J* 1991; **171**: 61–62.
119. Watkins KV, Richmond AS, Langstein IM. Nonhealing extraction site due to *Actinomyces naesndii* in a patient with AIDS. *Oral Surg* 1991; **71**: 675–677.
120. Porter SR, Scully C. Orofacial manifestations in primary immunodeficiencies: polymorphonuclear defects. *J Oral Pathol. Med* 1993; **22**: 310–311.
121. Porter SR, Scully C. Orofacial manifestations in primary immunodeficiencies: T lymphocyte defects. *J Oral Pathol Med* 1993; **22**: 308–309.
122. Scully C, Porter SR. Orofacial manifestations in primary immunodeficiencies: common variable immunodeficiencies. *J Oral Pathol Med* 1993; **22**: 157–158.
123. Porter SR, Scully C. Orofacial manifestations in primary immunodeficiencies involving IgA deficiency. *J Oral Pathol Med* 1993; **22**: 117–119.
124. Porter SR, Scully C. Orofacial manifestations in the primary immunodeficiency disorders. *Oral Surg Oral Med Oral Pathol* 1994; **78**: 4–13.
125. Kirstila V, Tenovuo J, Ruuskanen O, Nikoskelainen J, Irjala K, Vilja P. Salivary defense factors and oral health in patients with common variable immunodeficiency. *J Clin Immunol* 1994; **14**: 229–235.
126. Norhagen G, Engstrom PE, Hammarstrom L. Immunoglobulin levels in saliva in individuals with selective IgA deficiency: compensatory IgM secretion and its correlation with HLA and susceptibility to infections. *J Clin Immunol* 1989; **9**: 279–286.
127. Norhagen G, Engstrom PE, Hammarstrom L, Smith CIE Nord CE. The microbial flora of saliva and faeces in individuals with selective IgA deficiency and common variable immunodeficiency. *Microbiol Ecol Health Dis* 1990; **3**: 269–275.
128. Engstrom GN, Engstrom PE, Hammarstrom L, Smith CIE. Oral conditions in individuals with selective immunoglobulin A deficiency and common variable immunodeficiency. *J Clin Periodontol* 1992; **63**: 984–989.
129. Dahlen G, Bjorklander J, Galinberg L, Slots J, Hanson LA. Periodontal disease and dental caries in relation to primary IgG subclass and other humoral immunodeficiencies. *J Clin Periodontol* 1993; **20**: 7–13.
130. Liese JG, Jendrossek V, Jansson A *et al.* Chronic granulomatous disease in adults. *Lancet* 1995; **346**: 220–223.

19

Hypersensitivity and anaphylaxis

Stephen R. Porter

Hypersensitivity represents an overreaction by appropriate immune responses. The immunological mechanisms that underly hypersensitivity can generally be classified according to their mediators and are summarized in Table 19.1. There is some overlap of these immunological mechanisms but outside the Gell and Coombs classification are other mechanisms sometimes, designated type IIa or V, that reflect antibody-mediated control of thyroid disease, control of lymphocyte function or cytokine-mediated vascular damage.

The present chapter will mainly detail aspects of hypersensitivity of relevance to oral disease and thus type-I mediated disease.

Type I (immediate) hypersensitivity

Type I hypersensitivity, sometimes termed immediate or atopic hypersensitivity, can affect up to 15% of the population and is clinically characterized by asthma, eczema, allergic rhinitis and urticaria often in patients with a family history of these or similar disorders. The type I hypersensitivity disorders may be genetically determined, for example in individuals who express human leukocyte antigen (HLA) B8 and DR3 antigens. The reaction depends upon the production of specific immunoglobulin E (IgE) antibodies to the foreign antigen that bind to mast cells and basophils. The binding of the foreign antigen to this cell-bound IgE causes degranulation of mast cells or basophils and the release of mediators (Table 19.2; Fig. 19.1).

There are at least two main types of mast cells – connective tissue (CTMC) and mucosal mast cells (MMC), differing in location, regulation and associated immunological mediators. The MMCs have a greater association with type I hypersensitivity than CTMCs. For example, there is increased MMC infiltration of the nasal mucosa of patients with allergic rhinitis during the pollen season and increased numbers of such cells in the bronchoalveolar lavage fluid of asthmatic individuals.

All immunoglobulins are made up of long and short polypeptide chains bound in a characteristic form for that immunoglobulin by disulphide bonds. The longer chains are termed heavy chains and are twice the molecular weight of the shorter light chains. The five classes of immunoglobulin, IgG, IgM, IgA, IgD and IgE, have heavy chains appropriately named γ, μ, α, δ and ϵ. The light chains are either χ or λ. Figure 19.2 shows the IgE structure. The C end of the heavy chains is called the Fc piece and is seen attached to the mast cell high-affinity Fc binding site. The N-terminal ends of the linked light and heavy chains are the specific antigen-binding sites called the Fab site or the idiotype, which are cross-linked by the antigen.

Degranulation of the mast cell is triggered when antigen binds to the IgE Fab receptors thereby cross-linking the two membrane-based Fc receptors. Degranulation can also occur via other immunological reactions, e.g. with anti-IgE autoantibodies or even high-molecular-weight carbohydrates such as lectins. Mast cells can be induced to degranulate via non-Fc

Table 19.1 Summary of type I to IV hypersensitivity reactions

	I: Immediate	*II: Cytotoxic*	*III: Immune complex*	*IV: Delayed*
Antigens	Pollens, moulds, mites, drugs, food and parasites	Cell surface or tissue-bound	Exogenous (bacteria, fungi, parasites) Autoantigens	Cell/tissue-bound
Mediators	IgE and mast cells	IgG, IgM and complement	IgG, IgM, IgA and complement	T_{DH} T_c-activated macrophages and lymphokines
Diagnostic tests	Skin-prick tests – wheal and flare RAST	Coombs test Indirect immuno-fluorescence (antibodies) Red-cell agglutination Precipitating antibodies	Skin test – oedema, erythema (Arthus reaction) Immune complexes	Skin test – erythema, induration (e.g. tuberculin test)
Time taken for reaction to develop	15-30 min	Rapid	4–12 h	12–48 h
Diseases and conditions produced	Asthma (extrinsic) Eczema (atopic) Urticaria Allergic rhinitis Anaphylaxis	Autoimmune haemolytic anaemia Transfusion reactions Haemolytic disease of newborn Goodpasture's syndrome Autoimmune pernicious anaemia Myasthenia gravis	Low-grade persistent infections, e.g. infective endocarditis Autoimmune, e.g. SLE, glomerulonephritis, rheumatoid arthritis Disease caused by environmental antigens, e.g. farmer's lung, pigeon fancier's lung	Contact dermatitis Pulmonary TB Graft-versus-host disease Insect bites Leprosy

IgE = Immunoglobulin E; T_{DH} = delayed hypersensitivity T cells; T_c = cytotoxic T cells; RAST = radioallergosorbent test; TB = tuberculosis; SLE = systemic lupus erythematosus.

Table 19.2 Main mediators generated by activation of the mast cell

Mediator	*Action*
Histamine	Vasodilation Increased vascular permeability Chemokinesis (increased random movement of cells) Bronchoconstriction
Heparin	Anticoagulant action
Tryptase	C_3 convertase action
β-Glucosaminidase	Cleaves glucosamine residues
Various chemotactic agents	Direct neutrophils, eosinophils, basophils and monocytes to site of activation
Leukotrienes (e.g. leukotriene B_4, SRS-A)	Vasodilation Increased vascular permeability Bronchoconstriction Chemotaxis and/or chemokinesis
Prostaglandins	Bronchoconstriction
Thromboxane	Platelet aggregation Vasodilation
Platelet-activating factor	Platelet activation

SRS-A = Slow-reacting substance of anaphylaxis.

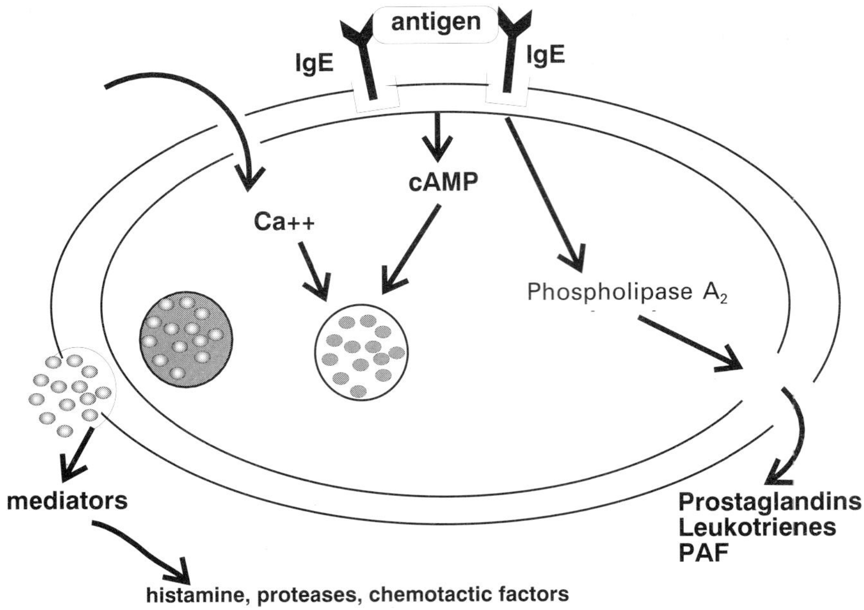

Fig. 19.1 Cross-linkage of the antigen to two mast-cell-bound immunoglobulin E (IgE) molecules induces a transient rise in cyclic adenosine monophosphate (cAMP) with influx of Ca ions. This causes degranulation and release of inflammatory mediators and activation of phospholipase A_2, which produces additional mediators. PAF = Platelet-activating factor.

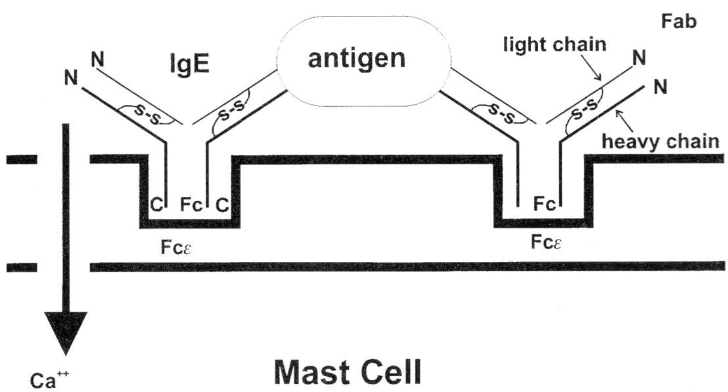

Fig. 19.2 The immunoglobulin E (IgE) molecule with its heavy-chain C-terminal end called the Fc piece, attached to the Fcε receptor site. Binding of the antigen to the N-terminal Fab end cross-linking two IgE molecules activates the mast cell.

receptor mechanisms, including the binding of complement components C3a or C5a, and drugs such as codeine and morphine. Whatever the mechanism, degranulation is initiated by a transient elevation of cyclic adenosine monophosphate (cAMP) levels and activation of phospholipase A_2 (Fig. 19.1). This involves an influx of calcium that initiates the migration of granules to the cell membrane and then exocytosis of the preformed granular contents. In addition there is synthesis of newly formed inflammatory mediators resulting from phospholipase A_2, acting on the cell membrane with the release of arachidonic acid. This is a substrate for the cyclooxygenase pathway giving rise to prostaglandins and thromboxanes, and via the lipoxygenase pathway to the leukotrienes (slow reacting substance of anaphylaxis; SRS-A). The main mediators derived from Fc -induced activation of the mast cells are indicated in Table 19.2. The outcome of the release of these mediators is vasodilation, increased vascular permeability and tissue influx of eosinophils, basophils, neutrophils and monocytes, tissue damage (via microthrombi formation), oedema, mucus secretion and possibly smooth-muscle contraction.

Thus, depending upon the site of the above reactions, there can be variable clinical outcomes – usually allergic rhinitis, asthma, urticaria and anaphylaxis.

Clinical manifestations of type I hypersensitivity

Allergic rhinitis

Rhinitis manifests as sneezing attacks, nasal discharge or nasal blockage occurring for more than 1 h for several days. Hayfever (seasonal rhinitis) affects 2–10% of the population, although up to 20% of young adults can be affected. Symptoms include nasal irritation, sneezing, nasal blockage and rhinorrhoea, occasional ocular discomfort and even an itching of the ears due to the common innervation of the pharynx and ear. Common allergens of hayfever include tree pollens from April to June, grass pollens from June to August and mould spores from July to September. *Perennial* allergic rhinitis is not seasonally associated but is mainly due to faecal particles of the house dust mite *Dermatophagoides pteronyssinus*, although other allergens include agents from urine, saliva or skin from domestic pets. Patients with perennial rhinitis can develop symptoms with non-specific stimuli such as cigarette smoke, washing powders, household detergents, perfumes, traffic fumes and emotional stress, all of which cause a non-allergic response.

Asthma

Asthma is clinically characterized by cough, wheeze, chest tightness and shortness of breath, often worse at night. Asthma has three main characteristics:

1. Limited airflow – usually reversible.
2. Hyperresponsiveness of the airway to a wide range of agents.
3. Inflammation of the bronchi with infiltration by eosinophils, T lymphocytes and plasma cells, with oedema, smooth-muscle hypertrophy, mucus plugging and epithelial changes.

The prevalence of asthma is increasing, particularly in persons in their second decade, indeed 10–15% of children in this age group can be affected.

Asthma can be classified as *extrinsic*, in which there is an identifiable external cause, and *intrinsic* (or cryptogenic) in which no causative agent can be identified. Extrinsic asthma is a feature of atopic individuals. These persons show positive prick-test reactions to common inhaled allergens, may have eczema in early childhood, can develop asthma-like symptoms in response to aspirin and other non-steroidal anti-inflammatory agents, and may be liable to other type I hypersensitivity disorders.

The pathogenesis of asthma includes both type I hypersensitivity and hyperresponsiveness of the airways. The allergens of extrinsic asthma are similar to those of allergic rhinitis; however, the most important allergen of this type of asthma is the faecal particles of house dust mites. The hyperresponsiveness of the airways in asthmatic patients is reflected by rapid and profound bronchoconstriction. This smooth-muscle contraction is also seen in response to agents such as histamine and methacholine (bronchial provocation tests) and also results in asthma-like features with exercise, wheezing and prolonged coughing after viral infections and problematic rhinitis or asthma. The precise pathogenic mechanisms of the bronchial hyperresponsiveness in asthma are unknown.

The investigation of asthma can be complex (Table 19.3) and the general management of asthma is outlined in Table 19.4.

Acute severe asthma

Acute severe asthma (asthmatic attacks, status asthmaticus) is a severe, life-threatening disorder characterized by: inability to complete a sentence in one breath, tachycardia (>110 beats/min), pulsus paradoxus (if very severe,

Table: 19.3 Investigation of asthma

Lung function studies	Improved FEV or PEFR following inhalation of bronchodilator
Peak flow charts	Variable PEFR throughout the day
Exercise tests	Exercise may induce asthmatic episode
Histamine or methacholine bronchial provocation	Histamine or methacholine induces a transient limitation of airflow in susceptible individuals
Trail of systemic corticosteroids	Prednisolone causes 15%+ improvement in airflow
Peripheral blood	Raised eosinophil count
Sputum	Eosinophils present in sputum in large numbers and/or clumps
Skin tests	Skin-prick testing may help determine allergens

FEV = Forced expiratory volume; PEFR = peak expiratory flow rate.

Table 19.4 Management of asthma

Control of extrinsic factors – allergens or other agents
Drug therapy
β Adrenergic agonists (salbutamol, terbutaline)
Anticholinergic bronchodilators (ipratropium bromide, oxitropium bromide)
Anti-inflammatories (sodium cromoglycate)
Inhaled corticosteroids (beclomethasone dipropionate, fluticasone propionate)
Systemic corticosteroids (prednisolone)
Other immunosuppressives (methotrexate, azathioprine, cyclosporin (rarely))

there is no paradoxus), silent chest, or little wheeze, due to inadequate airflow, possible cyanosis, partially disturbed consciousness, and electrocardiogram changes. Acute severe asthma is a medical emergency, the management of which is outlined in Table 19.5.

Urticaria and angioedema

Urticaria is clinically characterized by circumscribed, raised, erythematous, pruritic areas of oedema that involve the superficial portion of the dermis. When the oedematous process extends into the deep dermis and/or subcutaneous and submucosal layers, it is known as angioedema. Urticaria and angioedema may occur in any location together or individually.

The clinical features of urticaria can be variable and unpredictable. Typical lesions comprise circumscribed areas of oedema with a variable halo of erythema; others have only erythema, and some are bullous. The lesions can vary from pinprick size to 5–10 cm diameter. Angioedematous areas usually arise suddenly, rarely persist longer than 24–48 h, and may continue to recur for indefinite periods. Episodes of lesions of less than 6–8 weeks' duration are considered acute, whereas those persisting longer are termed chronic. Headache, dizziness, the sensation of a lump in the throat, hoarseness, wheezing, shortness of breath, nausea, vomiting, abdominal pain, diarrhoea and arthralgias may occur with or without urticaria.

Acute urticaria and angioedema often occur in individuals with a personal or family history of asthma, rhinitis or eczema and are presumed to be IgE-dependent. Interestingly however, these disorders do not commonly accompany an exacerbation of asthma, rhinitis or eczema and the prevalence of chronic urticaria or angioedema is not notably increased in atopic individuals.

Urticaria and angioedema do not always have an atopic basis. IgE-associated release of vasoactive mediators can arise in response to specific antigens or a variety of physical or emotional stimuli. Specific allergens that provoke urticaria and angioedema include foods such as shellfish, nuts and chocolate, drugs – notably penicillin – aeroallergens and *Hymenoptera* venom. Urticaria commonly occurs after direct contact with a variety of substances such as stinging nettles, animal hairs and chemicals. A classification of urticaria and angioedema is outlined in Table 19.6.

Table 19.5 Management of acute severe asthma in general practice

Uncontrolled asthma in adults
Speech normal
Pulse <110 beats/min
Respiration <25 breaths/min
Peak flow >50% of predicted or best

Treatment
Nebulized salbutamol 5 mg or nebulized terbutaline 10 mg
Monitor response 15–30 min after nebulization
If peak flow 50–75% of predicted or best give:
Oral prednisolone 30–60 mg and step up usual treatment

Alternatively, if peak flow >75% of predicted or best:
Step up usual treatment

Follow-up
Monitor symptoms and peak flow
Set up self-management plan
Review in surgery within 48 h
Modify treatment at review

Acute severe asthma in adults
Cannot complete sentences
Pulse ≥ 110 beats/min
Respiration ≥ 25 beats/min
Peak flow ≤ 50% of predicted or best

Treatment
Oxygen 40–60% if available
Nebulized salbutamol 5 mg or nebulized terbutaline 10 mg
Oral prednisolone 30–60 mg or intravenous hydrocortisone 200 mg
Monitor response 15–30 min after nebulization
If any signs of acute asthma persist:
Arrange hospital admission
While awaiting ambulance, repeat nebulized β_2-stimulant and give with nebulized ipratropium 500 μg or give subcutaneous terbutaline
or give slow intravenous aminophylline 250 mg (**important:** *not* if taking oral theophylline)
Alternatively, if symptoms have improved, respiration and pulse are settling, and peak flow >50% of predicted or best:
Step up usual treatment and continue prednisolone

Follow-up
Monitor symptoms and peak flow
Set up self-management plan
Review in surgery within 24 h
Modify treatment at review

Life-threatening asthma in adults
Silent chest
Cyanosis
Bradycardia or exhaustion

ARRANGE IMMEDIATE HOSPITAL ADMISSION

Treatment
Oral prednisolone 30–60 mg or intravenous hydrocortisone 200 mg (immediately)
Oxygen-driven nebulizer in ambulance
Nebulized* β_2-stimulant with nebulized ipratropium *or* subcutaneous terbutaline *or* slow intravenous aminophylline 250 mg (**important:** *not* if taking oral theophylline)

STAY WITH PATIENT UNTIL AMBULANCE ARRIVES

*If no nebulizer is available, give two puffs of β_2-stimulant using large-volume spacer and repeat 10–20 times.

Table 19.6 Classification of urticaria/angioedema

IMMUNOLOGICAL URTICARIA/ANGIOEDEMA
IgE-dependent
Atopic diathesis
Specific antigen sensitivity (foods, drugs, therapeutic agents, aeroallergens, animal danders, *Hymenoptera* venom, helminths)
Physical
Dermographism
Vibratory
Cold
Light
Cholinergic
Exercise-induced anaphylaxis
Contact
Complement-mediated
Hereditary angioedema
Acquired angioedema with malignant disorders or autoantibody
Necrotizing venulitis
Serum sickness
Reactions to blood products
NON-IMMUNOLOGICAL URTICARIA/ANGIOEDEMA
Direct mast cell-releasing agents
Opiates
Antibiotics
Curare, *d*-tubocurarine
Radiocontrast media
Agents that presumably alter arachidonic acid metabolism
Aspirin and non-steroidal anti-inflammatory agents
Azo dyes and benzoates
IDIOPATHIC URTICARIA/ANGIOEDEMA

Table 19.7 Investigation of urticaria/angioedema

In all patients
History and physical examination
Provocative tests for physical urticarias
Complete blood count and differential analysis
Erythrocyte sedimentation rate
Urinalysis
In selected patients
Stool examination for ova and parasites
Blood chemistry profile
Antinuclear factor
Hepatitis B virus surface antigen and antibody
Skin tests for IgE-mediated reactions
Radioallergosorbent test (RAST) for specific IgE
CH_{50}
Cryoproteins
Circulating immune complexes
Thyroid microsomal antibody
Skin biopsy

IgE = Immunoglobulin E; CH_{50} = Haemolytic complement level

Investigation and management of urticaria and angioedema

The investigation of urticaria and angioedema is outlined in Table 19.7. Provocation studies by skin-prick tests may help identify potential allergens but, as indicated above, urticaria and angioedema need not have an immune basis and it is often not possible to identify the provoking agent. The majority of other investigations are only indicated if there is some social or medical factor likely to be inducing the urticarial or angioedematous reactions. In general, antihistamines (anti-H_1) are the mainstay of therapy, although clearly avoidance of any identifiable precipitants is important. Some clinicians favour salicylate-free and food-additive-free diets.

Anaphylaxis

Anaphylaxis represents the most profound type I hypersensitivity reaction. There can be premonitory dizziness or faintness, skin tingling and reddening of the bulbar conjunctiva followed by urticaria, angioedema, bronchospasm (i.e. asthma-like features), abdominal pain and circulatory collapse. Anaphylaxis develops within the first hour of exposure to an allergen, is often severe and may be fatal.

Anaphylaxis usually develops on second exposure to the allergen; however, it may occur on first exposure if the agent is given over a period of days. It is more likely with the administration of drugs, particularly when given parenterally.

Penicillin allergy

Hypersensitivity to penicillin is probably the most clinically significant cause of anaphylaxis. Nevertheless, 90% percent of patients with a so-called penicillin allergy do not have a genuine allergic response to penicillin and have negative responses to skin-prick tests.

Skin tests to determine likely penicillin-allergy are carried out using major (penicilloyl polylysine; PLL) and minor (benzyl penicillin, benzyl penicillinolate and benzyl penilloate)

determinants. These agents are initially given as an epicutaneous scratch, then intradermally, provided there is no notable cutaneous or systemic reaction. Positive (e.g. histamine) and negative (e.g. diluent) controls are included.

Only 8–19% of patients with a history of penicillin allergy have a positive skin reaction. One per cent of patients with a history of penicillin allergy and a negative skin test develop an accelerated urticarial reaction, and 3% develop other mild symptoms. By contrast, the risk of acute allergic reactions, including anaphylaxis, with a positive history of penicillin allergy and a positive skin test is 50–70%. In addition, patients with a positive skin test to penicillin may have positive reactions to other β-lactam antibiotics such as ampicillin and cephalothin.

Procedures to desensitize penicillin-allergic individuals to penicillin have been described. The technique induces an immunotolerance by the administration of small doses of the antigen. Hypersensitivity to penicillin persists but the reaction is subclinical. The procedure is similar to that of skin testing and very occasionally induces an anaphylactic reaction.

About 10% of persons allergic to penicillin are also allergic to cephalosporins, which should not be given unless there is a specific microbiological indication in routine dental practice.

Aspirin allergy

Aspirin may precipitate an allergic reaction, e.g. urticaria or angioedema, or even anaphylaxis. It has been estimated that 10% of patients with asthma (particularly adults) may have an increased sensitivity to aspirin which manifests as flushing, rhinorrhoea and asthmatic episodes. Asthmatic patients who are sensitive to aspirin may be sensitive to other non-steroidal anti-inflammatory drugs (NSAIDs), such as ibuprofen, and diclofenac sodium. It must, however, be appreciated that hypersensitivity to analgesics is generally very rare, particularly in view of the vast consumption of these agents.

Local analgesic agents

Hypersensitivity to local analgesic agents is uncommon. The majority of the earlier reported cases have been in relation to procaine, whereas the number of detailed reports of lignocaine hypersensitivity seems to be very small. With the withdrawal of preservative-containing local analgesic agents, most complications of local analgesics are due to the accompanying patient anxiety and possible effects of the vasoconstrictor agents.

Other drugs

Allergic reactions to anxiolytics are rare, although the benzodiazepines and barbiturates may occasionally cause photosensitivity. The induction agents propanidid, Althesin, methohexitone and thiopentone can cause anaphylactoid reactions, such that Althesin and propanidid have been withdrawn. The neuromuscular blocker suxamethonium can induce anaphylactoid reactions and bronchospasm, particularly when given in combination with thiopentone. This risk may be increased in patients with a known history of atopic disease, a known history of drug allergy or those who have repeated general anaesthetics over a short period. Alcuranium, tubacurine and other muscle relaxants may occasionally cause hypersensitivity reactions.

Management of anaphylaxis

Anaphylaxis is a medical emergency and thus requires prompt effective treatment of laryngeal oedema, bronchospasm and hypotension. As anaphylaxis is more likely after parenteral administration, resuscitation facilities must always be available when such procedures are undertaken.

First-line treatment includes establishing the airway, restoration of blood pressure (laying the patient flat, raising the feet) and administration of adrenaline by injection. Adrenaline can be given subcutaneously in mild cases and can also be given intramuscularly, repeated every 5 min according to blood pressure and pulse, until improvement occurs. It should be noted that at least 10% of patients developing anaphylaxis outside hospital will require a repeat injection of adrenaline. Oxygen administration is also of primary importance.

Table 19.8 Adrenaline dosage in anaphylaxis

Adults
0.5 ml of a 1:1000 solution intramuscularly or 3–5 ml of a 1:10 000 solution intramuscularly or slowly intravenously
Children
0.01 ml of a 1:1000 solution per kg intramuscularly or 0.1 ml of a 1:10 000 solution per kg intravenously

Adrenaline should only be given intravenously in severe anaphylaxis and to patients who are being monitored appropriately, as ventricular fibrillation can develop. The appropriate dosages of adrenaline are indicated in Table 19.8.

An antihistamine (e.g. chlorpheniramine, given by slow intravenous injection in a dose of 10–20 mg) is a useful adjunctive treatment, given after adrenaline injection and continued for 24–48 h to prevent relapse. In patients on non-cardioselective β-blockers, severe anaphylaxis may not respond to adrenaline; hence the addition of β_2-adrenoreceptor stimulants such as salbutamol by intravenous injection should be considered.

Continuing deterioration requires further treatment, including intravenous fluids, intravenous aminophylline or a nebulized β_2-adrenoceptor stimulant (such as salbutamol or terbutaline) in addition to oxygen. Assisted respiration and possibly emergency tracheotomy may be necessary.

An intravenous corticosteroid, e.g. hydrocortisone (as sodium succinate) in a dose of 100–300 mg is of *secondary* value in the initial management of anaphylaxis as the onset of action is delayed for several hours, but should be given to prevent further deterioration in severely affected patients.

When a patient is so ill that there is no doubt as to adequacy of the circulation, the initial injection of adrenaline may need to be given *intravenously* (Table 19.8). When intravenous access is not possible, the adrenaline should be given intramuscularly. In adults, once an intravenous line is established, 1–2 l of colloid should be given rapidly. Colloid is more useful than crystalloid as capillaries remain leaky for longer to crystalloid than from colloid. Adrenaline can be repeated and a second bolus of colloid given.

Over 90% of patients with severe anaphylaxis will respond to this combination of adrenaline and colloid. If response remains poor, adrenaline should be infused. It is essential to ensure that the correct strength of adrenaline solution is used; anaphylactic shock kits need to make a very clear distinction between the 1 in 10 000 and 1 in 1000 strengths. It is also important that, where intramuscular injection might still succeed, time should not be wasted seeking intravenous access. For infants and children tibial injection may be necessary.

Some patients with severe allergy to insect stings or foods are encouraged to carry prefilled adrenaline syringes for self-administration during periods of risk. Adrenaline inhalations (Medihaler-epi) are much less effective, but may be useful for the individual without other symptoms who is beginning to develop angioedema and laryngeal oedema. Nevertheless, adrenaline injection is always the first line of treatment for patients with previous, very serious anaphylactic reactions.

Type II hypersensitivity

Type II hypersensitivity is IgG- or IgM-mediated. IgG or IgM class antibodies bind to a cell surface and activate the classical complement pathway, resulting in the components C5 to C9 forming the membrane attack complex (MAC) on the target cell surface. In addition C3b can bind to the target cell surface and act as an opsonin (agent that enhances phagocytosis) for neutrophils, eosinophils and monocytes/macrophages.

A second immunological mechanism of type II hypersensitivity is IgG-mediated. In this IgG antibodies bind via Fc receptors on macrophages, neutrophils, eosinophils and killer (K) cells. These IgG antibodies act as opsonin activators of phagocytosis by neutrophils and monocytes which take up the opsonized target cells or particles. This increased activation not only enhances phagocytes and killing of the target cell, but also causes increased release of immunological mediators such as superoxide and arachidonic acid from which prostaglandins and leukotrienes are synthesized.

The binding of IgG antibodies also enhances the binding of K cells to, and hence the death of, the target cell.

Type II hypersensitivity has no direct association with oral disease but does account for adverse transfusion reactions (e.g. inappropriate cross-matching of erythrocytes, or rarely platelets), haemolytic disease of the newborn, autoimmune haemolytic anaemias (e.g. Coombs-positive (IgG) in systemic lupus erythematosus; Coombs-negative (IgM) in *Mycoplasma pneumoniae* infection and some drug-induced haemolytic anaemias). Renal glomerular damage in Goodpasture's syndrome, blockage of postsynaptic acetylcholine receptors in myasthenia gravis and parietal cell damage in autoimmune pernicious anaemia are also due to type II hypersensitivity mechanisms.

Type III hypersensitivity (immune-complex disease)

Type III hypersensitivity disorders are due to the formation and deposition of complexes of antibody and antigen (immune complexes). These immune complexes can be generated in at least three main clinical circumstances:

1. Persistent infection, in which a weak immune response, coupled with a low-grade persistent infection, leads to the formation of complexes of antibody and invading microbe. This mechanism accounts for much of the damage associated with infective endocarditis.
2. In autoimmune disease, when autoantibodies bind to host antigens. The site of the antigen and hence deposition of immune complexes will influence the resultant tissue damage and clinical disease. This immunological mechanism underlies many autoimmune diseases, particularly rheumatoid arthritis, systemic lupus erythematosus, dermatomyositis and cryoglobulinaemia.
3. Low-grade, intermittent exposure to extrinsic agents can lead to immune complex function in the lungs, for example farmer's lung or pigeon-fancier's lung.

Deposition of the immune complexes triggers complement activation causing the generation of vasoactive and chemotactic agents (e.g. C3a and C5a), opsonins (e.g. C3b), release of inflammatory agents from adjacent mast cells and basophils, and thrombus formation. Immune complexes deposited in the tissues are unlikely to be effectively phagocytosed by neutrophils or monocytes, but give rise to tissue-damaging agents such as superoxides.

Serum sickness and the Arthus reaction are two useful demonstrations of type III hypersensitivity.

In serum sickness circulating immune complexes are deposited at sites of high vascularity, giving rise to glomerulonephritis and arthritis. Serum sickness was previously a consequence of injection of large amounts of horse-derived antidiphtheria serum into affected humans and is thus now only demonstrated by animal studies.

The Arthus reaction demonstrates the effects of local deposition of immune complexes and occurs when animals with high levels of specific IgG antibodies are injected subcutaneously or intradermally with antigen. After 4–10 h an area of oedema and haemorrhage develops at the site of injection induced by local immune complex formation. The reaction subsides after 48 h with complement and phagocyte activation.

Type IV hypersensitivity (delayed hypersensitivity)

Type IV or delayed hypersensitivity is a cell-mediated immune response and becomes clinically manifest over a period of 24–48 h after becoming exposed to the precipitant agent. The clinical disorders with such a basis are listed in Table 19.1 and are characterized by a heavy infiltration of T cells and macrophages. Although the biological role of the reaction is to eliminate persistent infections, especially microbes that can replicate within the lysosomes of the macrophages, the response to these antigens evokes a marked cellular inflammatory response and cytokine-induced tissue damage.

The foreign antigen, which may be a bacterium or a metallic molecule such as nickel bound to albumin, enters the host cell where it binds to a groove in the so-called HLA antigen molecule in the endoplasmic reticulum compartment of the cell. These HLA protein molecules are an essential part of the body's defence mechanism and are encoded by a series of genes on the short arm of chromosome 6 of each cell called the major histocompatibility complex (MHC; Fig. 19.3). The MHC genes are divided into three series – class I, class II and class III. Class I and class II antigens have different functions which are determined by the binding affinity of the MHC/HLA molecule to

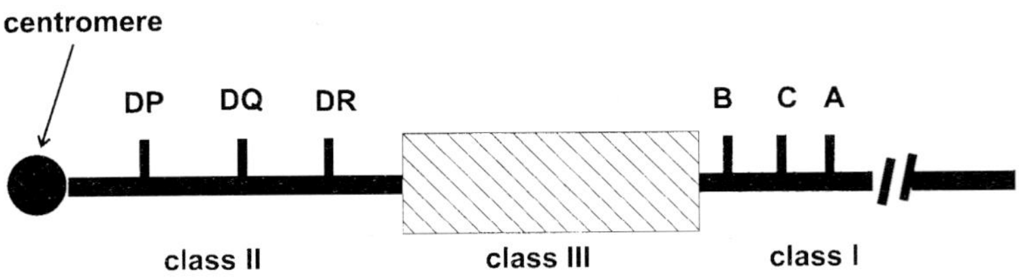

Fig. 19.3 The human leukocyte antigen–major histocompatibility complex (HLA–MHC) gene complex on the short arm of chromosome 6. HLA class 1 gene proteins A–C, when they present foreign antigen, are recognized by T-killer cells. Class II, including the HLA DR antigens, are recognized by the T-helper cells, and the class II genes encode the complement proteins.

a specific type of T cell. HLA class I proteins A, B and C in association with foreign antigens are recognized by cytotoxic (killer) T cells. The class II or DR antigens are recognized by helper T cells. The class III genes encode the complement system proteins. This specific or so-called MHC class-restricted T-cell binding is enhanced by the presence of the foreign antigenic peptide in the groove. Humans have a wide range of identifiable HLA molecules, some of which can be associated with certain diseases, such as HLA B27 in ankylosing spondylitis and A10, B7, DR3 in oral submucous fibrosis and other fibrotic diseases.

The HLA molecule and its bound foreign antigen travel to the surface of the cell where the antigen is presented to the appropriate T cells. Dendritic cells (Langerhan's cells) can also present foreign antigen in this way.

The CD4 receptor of a helper T cell links with class II HLA/antigen complexes and triggers the release of T-cell cytokines, including macrophage-activating factor (MAF) and macrophage migration inhibition factor (MIF) as well as attracting eosinophils, basophils and mast cells. One of the principal cytokines is interferon-γ, which not only activates macrophages but also increases the expression of the class II MHC HLA molecules so that more foreign antigen may be presented to the T cell. It also stimulates the production of other inflammatory cytokines such as tumour necrosis factor (TNF)-α and β, interferon-α and -β and interleukin-1 (IL-1) (Fig. 19.4). An

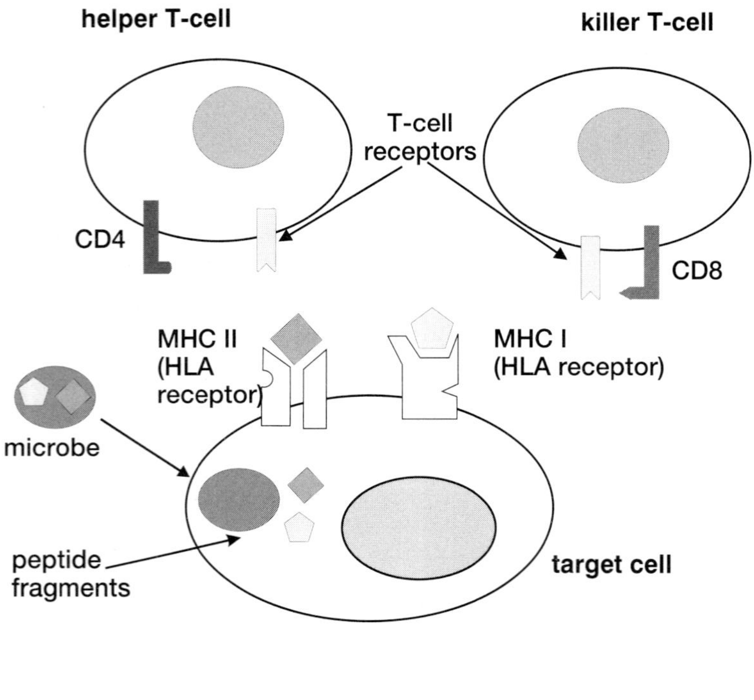

Fig. 19.4 The major histocompatibility complex I-human leukocyte antigen (MHC I–HLA) receptor protein presents antigen to killer T cells where it is recognized by the CD8 receptor, whereas the MHC II HLA receptor–antigen complex is recognized by the helper T cell CD4 receptor.

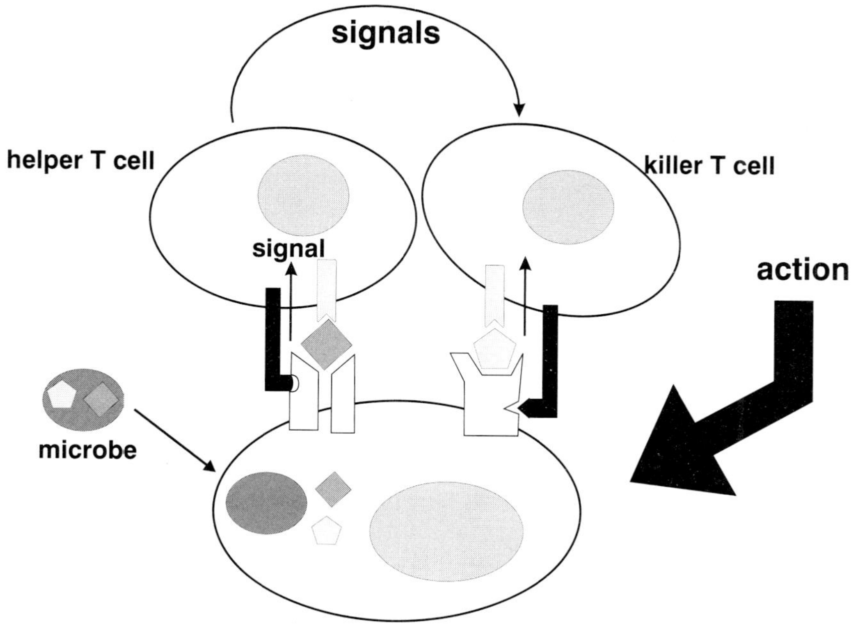

Fig. 19.5 Helper T cell activates killer T cell.

important part of this reaction is the activation of the killer T cell (Fig. 19.5). This process helps to kill the bacterium and the host presenting cell, and the MIF also prevents the macrophages from leaving the area, all of which produce the local raised erythematous irritant lesion seen in cutaneous examples of delayed hypersensitivity (see also Chapter 16).

It is possible to demonstrate previous exposure and thus possible delayed sensitivity to antigens *in vitro* by lymphocyte transformation testing (LTT). Exposure of lymphocytes of a patient with hypersensitivity to the implicated antigen causes DNA synthesis, which can be measured by determining the uptake of radioactive thymidine. Patients hypersensitive to the antigen have a rapid and high response (i.e. LTT), while the lymphocytes of non-hypersensitive patients do not respond. It is also possible to estimate possible delayed hypersensitivity by measuring the production of MIF by lymphocytes exposed to potential allergens.

Allergic contact dermatitis

Allergic contact dermatitis is probably the most relevant of the delayed hypersensitivity reactions to dental surgery, although both

Table 19.9 Type of delayed hypersensitivity reactions

Type	*Jones–Mate*	*Contact*	*Tuberculin*	*Granulomatous*
Antigen	Some proteins	Nickel, rubber	Mycobacterial and leishmaniasis antigens	Macrophages, e.g. persistent antigen or immune complexes or non-immunological antigens
Reaction tissue	24 h	48 h	48 h	4 weeks
Histology	Basophils, lymphocytes, mononuclear cells	Lymphocytes, macrophages with later oedema	Lymphocytes, monocytes, macrophages	Epithelioid cell granuloma, giant cells, macrophages, fibrosis ± necrosis
Clinical features	Skin sweating	Eczema-like	Local induction, swelling ± fever	Skin induration

acute and chronic graft-versus-host disease can give rise to oral manifestations.

Allergic contact dermatitis usually manifests as erythema, swelling, papules and papulovesicles. With prolonged exposure the skin can become dry, scaly and thickened.

Most allergens in contact dermatitis are of low molecular weight and act as haptens, binding to proteins to generate an appropriate allergen. Contact sensitivity is frequently directed towards this carrier-protein component, the hapten having induced antigenic changes in the carrier protein, e.g. albumin.

About 2–4% of populations may have allergic atopic dermatitis, the incidence being high in the chemical and metal industries. Frequencies and patterns of disease vary between countries and communities, reflecting patterns of exposure to different reagents.

Management of allergic contact dermatitis may include skin patch-testing in which a small amount of the allergen to which the patient is possibly sensitized is applied to a small area of the skin of the upper back. A positive test, i.e. the subsequent development of redness and/or wheal, indicates that the patient has an allergic contact sensitivity but this does not necessarily indicate that this agent is the cause of the patient's allergic contact dermatitis. Aside from avoiding the precipitating agents, treatment of allergic contact dermatitis mainly entails the use of topical corticosteroids, which may also be applied to reduce any inflammation.

Relevance of allergic contact dermatitis to dental surgery

A wide range of agents used in dentistry may cause allergic contact dermatitis in dental health care workers (Table 19.10).

Table 19.10 Some agents used in dentistry that may cause allergic contact dermatitis

Penicillin
Streptomycin
Formalin
Cetrimide
p-aminobenzoic acid
Lanolin
Benzocaine
Neomycin
Methylmethacrylate
Amethocaine
Latex
Mercury
Chromic acid
Chlorhexidine
Gluteraldehyde

Contact allergy only rarely affects the oral mucosa or the lips. The mucosa becomes red and oedematous and sometimes small vesicles develop, only to rupture and leave painful erosions. Allergens responsible for contact stomatitis include antibiotics such as streptomycin, neomycin and bacitracin, oils of casia and cloves, mercury, gold, vulcanite, flavouring agents such as cinnamon in toothpaste, epoxy resins, acrylic, eugenol, walnuts, polyether impression material and karaya gum. Some cases of lichen planus may have a similar pathogenesis. Both nickel-containing orthodontic wire and stainless-steel wire used in maxillofacial surgery can give rise to contact allergies. A type IV hypersensitivity in response to the nickel of non-precious alloy crowns was implicated in local periodontal destruction – albeit in one patient.

Contact cheilitis has occurred with the fluorescein stains in some lipsticks, carmine, oleyl alcohol, methyl heptine carbamate and other lipstick constituents. Peppermint, carvone, spearmint, citrus fruits, artichokes, nuts, pineapple, mangoes, asparagus and cinnamon oil can give rise to similar reactions.

Further reading

Assem ESK, Punnia-Moorthy A. Allergy to local anaesthetics: an approach to definitive diagnosis. A review with an illustrative study. *Br Dent J* 1988; **164**: 44–47.

Breathnach SM. Drug reactions. In: Champion RH, Burton JL, Ebling FJG (eds) *Textbook of Dermatology*, 5th edn, pp. 253–304. Oxford: Blackwell Scientific Publications, 1993.

Cascale TB, Sampson HA, Hanifin J *et al.* Guide to physical urticarias. *J Allergy Clin Immunol* 1988; **82**: 758.

Cawson RA, Curson I, Whittington DR. The hazards of dental local anaesthetics. *Br Dent J* 1983; **154**: 253–258.

Eichmann AR. Syphilis. In: Fitzpatrick T, Eisen AZ, Wolff K, Freeberg IM, Austen KF (eds) *Dermatology in General Medicine*, 4th edn. pp. 1483–1493. New York: McGraw-Hill, 1993.

Eley BM, Cox SW. The release, absorption and possible health effects of mercury from dental amalgam: a review of recent findings. *Br Dent J* 1993; **175**: 355–362.

Fisher M. Treatment of acute anaphylaxis. *Br Med J* 1995; **311**:731–733.

Gallagher GT. Oral mucous membrane reactions to drugs and chemicals. *Curr Opin in Dent* 1991; **1**: 777–782.

Gigli I, Rosen FS. Angioedema associated with complement abnormalities. In: Fitzpatrick T, Eisen AZ, Wolff K, Freeberg IM, Austen KF (eds) *Dermatology in General Medicine*, 4th edn. pp. 1494–1500. New York: McGraw-Hill, 1993.

Harper J. Genetics and genodermatoses. In: Champion RH, Burton JL, Ebling FJG (eds) *Textbook of Dermatology*, 5th edn, pp. 305–372. Oxford: Blackwell Scientific Publications, 1993.

Hodgson TA, Shirlaw PJ, Challacombe SJ. Skin testing after anaphylactoid reactions to dental local anaesthetics: a comparison with controls. *Oral Surg Oral Med Oral Pathol* 1993; **75**: 706–711.

Holmstrup P. Reactions of the oral mucosa related to silver amalgam: a review. *J Oral Pathol Med* 1991; **20**: 1–7.

Jacobsen KW, Branch LB, Nelson HS *et al.* Laboratory tests in chronic urticaria. *JAMA* 1980; **243**: 1644.

Kanerva L, Estlander T, Jolanki R. Occupational skin allergy in the dental profession. *Dermatol Clin* 1994; **12**: 517–532.

Leung DYM, Rodes AR, Geha RS, Scheider L, Ring J. Atopic dermatitis (atopic eczema). In: Fitzpatrick T, Eisen AZ, Wolff K, Freeberg IM, Austen KF (eds) *Dermatology in General Medicine*, 4th edn. pp. 1543–1564. New York: McGraw-Hill, 1993.

Mjor IA. Side-effects of dental materials (editorial). *Br Med J* 1994; **309**: 621–622.

Parish WE. Clinical immunology and allergy. In: Champion RH, Burton JL, Ebling FJG (eds) *Textbook of Dermatology*, 5th edn, pp. 253–304. Oxford: Blackwell Scientific Publications, 1993.

Porter SR, Scully C. Immunologically-mediated disease. In: Jones JH, Mason DK (eds) *Oral Manifestations of Systemic Disease*, 2nd edn. pp. 183–270. London: Baillière Tindall, 1990.

Roitt I, Brostoff J, Male D. *Immunology,* 2nd edn, pp. 125–130. Edinburgh: Churchill Livingstone, 1989.

Seymour RA, Walton JG. *Adverse Drug Reactions in Dentistry.* Oxford: Oxford University Press, 1988.

Soter N. Urticaria and Angioedema. In: Fitzpatrick T, Eisen AZ, Wolff K, Freeberg IM, Austen KF (eds) *Dermatology in General Medicine*, 4th edn. pp. 1483–1493. New York: McGraw-Hill, 1993.

Warfvinge G. Screening tests for sensitization potential of dental materials. *J Dent* 1994; **22** (suppl 2): S16–S20.

20

Autoimmunity and its oral manifestations

Andrew William Barrett and Mohammed F. Haque

Introduction

The breakdown of recognition of self and non-self cell and tissue antigens produces a variety of pathological entities which may affect the oral tissues. The exact incidence of these diseases is unknown, since they affect different populations in different ways. However, in western populations it is estimated that 1–2% of the population may be affected by one of the rheumatological autoimmune diseases. These include Sjögren's syndrome, one of the most common autoimmune diseases to affect the oral and perioral structures. To state categorically that a disease has an autoimmune aetiology, the immune response must be a primary event, not secondary to tissue injury by other cause. Many of the proposed schemes of autoimmunity remain hypothetical or are based on *in vitro* or animal model evidence, and the aim of this chapter is to discuss the phenomenon of autoimmunity in broad terms before focusing on oral manifestations of autoimmune disease.

Principles of autoimmunity

Self non-responsiveness

Physiologically, the host's immune system does not react destructively towards a tissue antigen present on its own cell membranes. Self antigens may be termed tolerogens, in contrast to immunogens, which induce a hostile response. Tolerance is thus the converse of immunity, and autoimmunity follows when the mechanisms governing self non-responsiveness and the ability of the immune system to distinguish tolerogens from immunogens are disrupted. A brief description of the normal mechanics of tolerance is therefore necessary. It is also worth reminding ourselves at this stage that specific immune responses are mediated by B and T lymphocytes, following an initial antigen presentation step.

B cells represent 5–15% of circulating lymphocytes and are produced in the bone marrow throughout life. The bone marrow appears to serve the same purpose in humans as the bursa of Fabricius (from which these cells derive their name) in chickens; that is, to prime the B cell to become an immunoglobulin (Ig), i.e. antibody, producing plasma cell. B lymphocytes are therefore involved in the humoral arm of the immune response. In addition, they can function as antigen-presenting cells (see below).

In contrast to B lymphocytes, T-cell precursors are released from the bone marrow and migrate to the thymus for priming – hence their name T lymphocyte. Within the thymus, the genes which determine the antigen-binding site of the T-cell receptor (see below) are activated, thus determining the range of antigens with which circulating T lymphocytes can interact. The factors which control the repertoire of antigens T cells can recognize are uncertain, but may be the result of interplay between developing T cells and thymic epithelium. The T lymphocyte does not produce antibody, but has a key role in orchestrating cell-mediated immune responses.

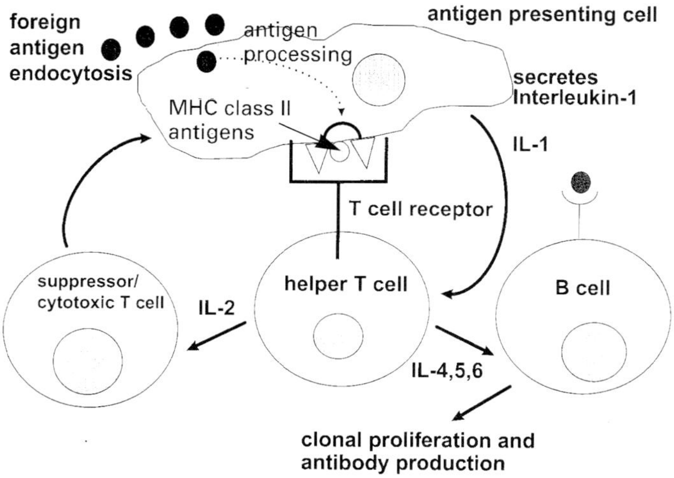

Fig. 20.1 The sequence of antigen presentation to a helper T lymphocyte, which then mediates the recruitment of T suppressor/cytotoxic cells and B lymphocytes. MHC = Major histocompatibility complex; IL-1 = interleukin-1.

Both B- and T-cell lymphocytes have, on their cell membranes, molecules responsible for recognition which are unique for a given clone of lymphocytes. In the case of B lymphocytes, this molecule is one of the five major classes of immunoglobulins – IgA, IgG, IgM, IgD or IgE. Hence Ig can exist freely after synthesis by the plasma cell or as membrane-bound receptors. The equivalent molecule on the T lymphocyte is the membrane-bound T-cell receptor which, though it shares some structural homology (similarity), is not an Ig. The T-cell receptor protein is composed of two chains with different amino acid sequences and molecular weights, and is thus referred to as a heterodimer (*hetero-* = different, *di-* = two, -*mer* =part or portion). Two types of T-cell receptor heterodimer have been identified and are termed αβ (alpha beta) and γδ (gamma delta). The majority of T cells express the former. These αβ T lymphocytes can also be subdivided in terms of expression of the two important cell surface molecules, CD4 and CD8 which, in mature cells, are mutually exclusive. The CD4 T cells supply helper function to B cells, whereas CD8 T cells are suppressor or cytotoxic in function. B cells require T-cell help before antibodies to many antigens can be produced. These are T-dependent antigens. Some antigens, however, can stimulate B cells directly – the T-independent antigens.

Whereas B cells may bind soluble antigen present in the fluid medium around them, T cells recognize and are activated by cell-bound antigens. Current evidence favours the view that protein antigens, such as viral or bacterial components, are processed into peptides suitable for display on special antigen-presenting cell membranes, where they are bound to the protein molecules of the major histocompatibility complex (MHC). The MHC is a set of genes located on the short arm of chromosome 6 which encodes molecules vital for effective immunity and whose importance became evident with the development of transplantation surgery. There are three groups of MHC genes; class I, the protein products of which are expressed by all nucleated cells; class II, which are expressed only by antigen-presenting cells and activated T lymphocytes; and class III, which are concerned with the components of the complement cascade.

These foreign antigen peptide–MHC complexes are recognized by specific T cells through their unique T-cell receptors, leading to the activation of the immune response (Fig. 20.1). The CD4 (helper) cells recognize antigenic peptides complexed with MHC class II molecules and CD8 (suppressor and cytotoxic) T cells recognize antigens associated with MHC class I molecules. These MHC molecules are also called human leukocyte antigens (HLA) and the MHC class I molecules, which include HLA-A, B and C, are, as mentioned above, expressed on the membranes of most nucleated cells. The immune system recognizes class I MHC molecules as self and does not normally induce an immune response against them. MHC class

II molecules, e.g. HLA-DR, DP and DQ, are normally expressed only by antigen-presenting cells or activated T lymphocytes. Three types of cell of bone marrow origin are now established as MHC class II-expressing antigen-presenting cells; these are B lymphocytes, macrophages and dendritic cells. There is also an association between the patient's inherited HLA profile and disease. For instance, HLA allotypes A10, B7 and DR3 are associated with a tendency to develop oral submucous fibrosis. The mechanisms by which the HLA profile predisposes to a disease are conjectural.

A further requirement for effective antigen presentation is the presence of certain costimulatory molecules. These molecules are not antigen-specific and do not, in isolation from the MHC class II molecules, induce T-cell proliferation, but they are none the less essential for full immune potency. They either take the form of soluble cytokines, for example interleukin (IL)-1, or are molecules bound to the antigen-presenting cell membrane, such as CD40, CD80 and CD86.

Tolerance may be partial, where there is a reduced antigen-induced responsiveness, or complete, where there is total antigen-induced unresponsiveness. This occurs within hours in T cells but may take days in B cells. T-cell tolerance also lasts longer and requires lower concentrations of antigen. It has been suggested that T-cell tolerance is of greater importance than B-cell tolerance because of the requirement of T-cell help for B-cell function, but the known antigen-presenting, as well as antibody-producing, function of B lymphocytes would imply a role for both.

With both T and B cells, the degree of tolerance is related to the persistence of the antigen. Polysaccharides or polymers of D-amino acids, which are antigens that are poorly degraded, tend to be better tolerogens. On the whole, large polymeric antigens are tolerated better than smaller molecules. In the case of the protein ovalbumin, for example, some degradation of the native protein is necessary before T cells are stimulated to respond to it. Thus, the peptides that are produced by the antigen-processing cell are immunogenic, whereas the whole protein is not. This rule is not universal, since some protein antigens require no modification to be immunogenic, and others become immunogenic by simple unfolding of the protein structure, before they are presented.

The concentration of antigen is another factor which affects T- and B-cell behaviour towards self tissues. Very low or high concentrations of antigen induce tolerance, whereas intermediate concentrations induce an immune response. Thus stimuli which, under some circumstances, favour tolerance will, under others, induce immunity.

Mechanisms of tolerance

The various means by which tolerance develops appear to be common to both T and B lymphocytes. The processes involved are termed:

1. Clonal abortion (synonymous with clonal deletion).
2. Clonal anergy (synonymous with clonal tolerance).
3. Antibody-forming cell blockade.
4. Clonal exhaustion or clonal paralysis.

Clonal abortion

Clonal abortion (deletion) was one of the earliest theories postulated to account for the absence of autoimmunity in normal individuals. As discussed above, within the thymus there is activation of the genes which give rise to the protein structure of the T-cell receptor. A single clone of T lymphocytes will have a specific T-cell receptor only expressed by that clone. Some T cells may develop which have a receptor which matches a self antigen and, if allowed to escape into the circulation, would have the potential to bind to, and mount an immune response against, that self antigen. It is therefore clearly beneficial for such clones to be deleted whilst still within the thymus. Whilst it is not the only means by which tolerance occurs, the deletion of potentially autoreactive precursor T-lymphocyte clones in the thymus is still accepted as contributory to the induction of tolerance. Clonal deletion may also be induced in B lymphocytes by exposure of precursors to concentrations of monomeric antigens too low to induce the formation of clones reactive to that antigen. This can also be demonstrated in adults, when it is termed 'low zone tolerance', and follows after multiple injections of subimmunogenic doses of antigen, to which the individual becomes tolerant.

Clonal anergy

Clonal anergy of T lymphocytes to a self peptide may also occur in the thymus, and there is *in vitro* evidence suggesting that, postthymically, T-helper cells become unresponsive to high concentrations of antigen even in a suitable form to be presented. Clonal anergy of B cells may develop with both T-dependent and T-independent antigens. In the case of T-dependent antigens, if CD4 T cells do not supply the necessary help, or if that help is suppressed, the B cells specific for that antigen cannot differentiate into Ig-producing plasma cells. In contrast, T-independent antigens present in very high concentrations seem to inactivate rather than stimulate B cells specific for that antigen, as mentioned above. Clonal anergy has been induced in either case.

Antibody-forming cell blockade

Antibody-forming cell blockade is similar to clonal anergy, and so high concentrations of antigen, especially multivalent T-independent antigens, can switch off plasma cells already actively synthesizing antibody.

Clonal exhaustion

Clonal exhaustion has been proposed to occur when B lymphocytes are stimulated with a T-independent antigen so that *all* the B cells of the clone differentiate into plasma cells, leaving none to react to the antigen if it is re-encountered. Likewise, strong stimulation of a T-cell clone both within and beyond the thymus leads to its rapid expansion, followed by rapid disappearance. This tolerance to the stimulating antigen is, in effect, a clonal deletion. Clonal paralysis applies to T cells and occurs where the T-cell receptor has bound its antigenic ligand in combination with the MHC molecule on the antigen presenting cell membrane, but the required costimulatory signals are absent and a stable anergic state develops.

The role of suppressor T cells in antigen-induced unresponsiveness is also unclear, but the immunosuppressive drug cyclophosphamide actually inhibits T suppressor induction. Tolerance in T-helper cells can be induced in the absence of T-suppressor cells, which therefore are not obligatory for tolerance to develop. T-suppressor cells do, however, mediate the phenomenon of low zone tolerance, referred to above.

The maintenance of tolerance to self antigens

Self non-reactivity may be maintained in additional ways, first by 'hiding' the antigen from the immune system, and second, by what is called idiotype regulation.

The first is illustrated by the so-called immunologically privileged sites. From the discussion on clonal deletion above, it is apparent that below a certain threshold concentration an antigen does not elicit an immune response. An antigen that is not 'seen' by the immune system at all will thus be a tolerogen. The cornea, which normally is a structure with neither a vascular nor a lymphatic supply, may be transplanted from one individual to another without danger of rejection. Rejection may occur, however, if the cornea was previously inflamed and, as a result, vascularized. Vascularization brings the foreign antigens of the donor cornea to the attention of the host immune system, which reacts accordingly. The cornea is therefore, physiologically, an immunologically privileged site. Similarly, the blood–brain barrier conceals central nervous system antigens from the immune system.

In the second, an antibody can itself act as an antigen. The antigenic site of the antibody molecule is called the *idiotype*. An idiotype may be defined as the antigenic characteristic of the variable (V) region of an immunoglobulin molecule and is made up of several *idiotopes* (Fig. 20.2). Since most antibodies are generated after maturation of the immune system, the idiotype of the antibody molecule is itself a non-self antigenic site. Any antigenic site which can generate the production of antibodies against itself is called an epitope. These anti-antibodies are referred to as *anti-idiotypes*. By binding to, and neutralizing, the idiotype autoantigens, anti-idiotypes may be one means of preventing autoimmunization. In the same way, a potentially autoreactive B-cell receptor, itself an immunoglobulin molecule possessing its own idiotype, may be bound by anti-idiotypes which block further interaction between the B-cell immunoglobulin receptor and its target self antigen, with the result that autoantibody production is switched off. A

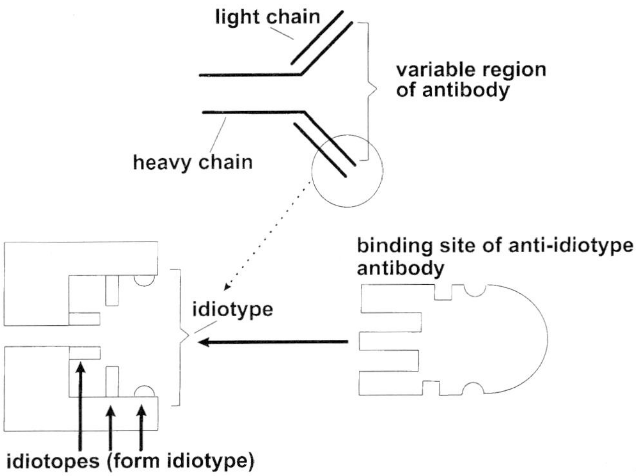

Fig. 20.2 The idiotype of an antibody molecule is located in the variable, light chain region where antigens are normally bound. The idio*type*, which is made up of several idio*topes*, has a distinct structure which can itself act as an antigenic determinant (or epitope), to which antibodies to the idiotype (anti-idiotypes) bind.

similar system may regulate T-lymphocyte activity, since the binding site of the T-cell receptor also acts as an idiotype.

Tolerance may also be maintained by inhibiting the presentation of self antigens, by interfering with antigen-processing mechanisms, by downgregulating the cell membrane expression of MHC class II molecules and/or costimulatory molecules, or by suppressing the synthesis of cytokines.

There are inevitably penalties for efficient self-tolerance. If self antigens 'avoid' an immune response, it is possible that a pathogen bearing an antigen similar enough to self will avoid it as well. Conversely, the immune system must have a 'repertoire' of antigens it responds to for immune competence, and so a self antigen resembling a foreign antigen that would normally elicit immunity may give rise to autoimmunization.

Natural autoantibodies and autoreactive lymphocytes

Autoantibodies are not invariably pathogenic and healthy individuals produce low titres of autoantibody without harm, possibly through the anti-idiotypic mechanism outlined above. Thus the production of non-pathogenic, or natural, autoantibodies is physiological and autoreactivity does not necessarily lead to autoimmunity. Titres of natural autoantibodies are raised in autoimmune diseases, but this may be the result of tissue damage following cell-mediated cytotoxicity, and so the rise is a consequence of the disease process rather than a primary factor. They are, however, very useful for diagnosis.

Natural autoantibodies are synthesized early in life and are of IgM isotype, but those which develop in older individuals are mainly IgG with some IgA, and tend to occur in females more than males. Most natural autoantibodies are produced by plasma cells which are differentiated from a subpopulation of B lymphocytes which express the antigen CD5. These B lymphocytes are not, however, able to generate autoantibodies to all antigens, possibly because of clonal abortion or clonal deletion.

The role of natural autoantibodies is uncertain. They tend to be directed against molecules which are highly conserved phylogenetically (i.e. by evolution) such as intranuclear components, hormones, cytokines or cell membrane constituents. They may, therefore, help remove normal byproducts of cell breakdown, or bind an exogenous antigen with an epitope which fits the autoantibody's idiotype closely enough. As a result, there is expansion of a B-lymphocyte clone which will synthesize new antibodies specific to that exogenous epitope. Another possible scenario is that circulating natural autoantibodies bind and neutralize foreign epitopes closely resembling self antigens, thus preventing the sort of cross-reactivity which causes infective endocarditis after a streptococcal infection. As with other B lymphocytes, the regulation of autoreactive B cells is a function of T lymphocytes.

Autoreactive T lymphocytes are also known to exist in normal individuals. This was proven by the *in vitro* observation that an individual's T lymphocytes will respond to autologous or syngeneic (i.e. from the same individual) non-T cells by clonal expansion. This phenomenon is termed the autologous mixed lymphocyte response. The precise role of autoreactive T lymphocytes *in vivo* is uncertain, but autoreactive T lymphocytes not dealt with by clonal deletion, clonal anergy and the other processes discussed above may provide inappropriate help to autoreactive B lymphocytes and consequent autoimmunity. Progress to disease, however, can only occur against a background of the correct genetic and environmental factors (see below).

Possible mechanisms of autoimmunity

The autoimmune diseases are organ-specific or non-organ-specific (Table 20.1). In an organ-specific autoimmune disease, the inappropriate response is directed against a single component of a single tissue. These can then be subdivided into those in which there is a specific lesion in a discrete target organ, the accompanying autoantibodies being directed against a specific component of that organ, and those where the lesions tend to be restricted to a single organ but the autoantibodies are not themselves organ-specific. An example is primary biliary cirrhosis, where the autoantibody reacts with all mitochondria but the only site affected is intrahepatic bile duct epithelium. Primary biliary cirrhosis is therefore designated as intermediate, as are several other autoimmune diseases (Table 20.1). In the non-organ-specific autoimmune diseases, the response targets a component present in many tissues and organs throughout the body; clinical signs and symptoms develop secondarily to the damage produced by the formation of immune complexes. These are composed of the autoantigen and autoantibody, an effect similar to type III hypersensitivity. In systemic lupus erythematosus, autoantibodies to double-stranded (native) DNA generate immune complexes which are deposited in blood vessels, glomerular capillaries, skin, joints, skeletal muscle and brain. The major impact this has on the vasculature and supporting tissues has led to the term connective tissue diseases being applied to the non-organ-specific autoimmune diseases.

High titres of autoantibodies, invariably of an IgG isotype, are usually associated with clinical disease. Pathogenic autoantibodies tend to be directed against crucial proteins. In systemic lupus erythematosus, there are autoantibodies to ribonucleoproteins essential for the correct splicing of RNA to form the functional messenger RNA capable of directing protein synthesis.

Normally, autoimmunization cannot occur because the necessary helper function is not available from host T lymphocytes, which are tolerant to self antigens. One can therefore hypothesize that autoimmunity might follow if this system is bypassed in some way. Several

Table 20.1 Classification of autoimmune diseases

Organ-specific	*Intermediate*	*Non-organ-specific*
Addison's disease	Autoimmune haemolytic disease	Dermatomyositis
Chronic atrophic gastritis	Autoimmune leukopenia	Polymyositis
Hashimoto's thyroiditis	Chronic active hepatitis	Progressive systemic sclerosis
Juvenile diabetes mellitus	Coeliac disease	Rheumatoid arthritis
Male infertility	Dermatitis herpetiformis	Systemic lupus erythematosus
Myasthenia gravis	Goodpasture's syndrome	
Pernicious anaemia	Idiopathic thrombocytopenia	
Primary myxoedema	?Linear IgA bullous dermatosis	
Premature ovarian failure	Pemphigoid	
Thyrotoxicosis (Graves' disease)	Pemphigus	
	Primary biliary cirrhosis	
	Sjögren's syndrome	
	Sympathetic ophthalmia	
	Ulcerative colitis	

IgA = Immunoglobulin A.

mechanisms have been proposed to explain how this might actually happen. These include: the exposure of antigens from normally immunologically privileged sites; antigenic modification; cross-reactivity; bypass of normal idiotype networks; polyclonal B-cell activation; and imbalance in the activity of T-helper and suppressor cells.

1. The immunologically privileged sites have been discussed above. Whilst trauma to most tissues does not usually elicit an autoimmune response against the damaged cells, trauma to the lens or male gonads, immunologically privileged sites containing antigens not normally exposed to the immune system, induces production of autoantibodies which, in the latter case, can result in sterility.
2. The immune system will recognize as foreign any self antigen that has undergone a structural alteration. An example of this is autoimmune haemolytic anaemia following methyldopa administration, where the methyldopa (or a metabolite) becomes a carrier for the rhesus e antigen. The new carrier acts as a hapten so that the rhesus e antigen is no longer recognized as self. Erythrocytes thus become the target of an autoimmune response
3. Exogenous antigenic determinants which are structurally similar to self antigens may induce an immune response which cannot distinguish host from foreign, and cross-react with both. The classic example of this phenomenon is infective endocarditis, where antibodies to the M protein of *Streptococcus* group A also bind to antigenic components of the endocardium, with severe consequences. There is also an element of this 'molecular mimicry' in Lyme disease and leprosy. The similarity between HLA-DR4 and HLA-DR1 with *Proteus mirabilis*, and that between mycobacterial antigens and heat shock protein 65, may be of importance in predisposing to rheumatoid arthritis. Heat shock proteins are the major antigens on many microbes, and since they are molecules which have been phylogenetically conserved (preserved through evolution), bacterial heat shock proteins can have a similar structure to those of humans. Heat shock protein 90 has been implicated as a specific causal factor in systemic lupus erythematosus.
4. Exogenous antigens resembling self may also interfere with protective idiotype networks and stimulate an autoimmune response as a consequence. A microbial antigen which resembles self and fits the anti-idiotype receptor on a T-helper cell will stimulate the T lymphocyte to activate all the B cells of that idiotype clone to produce autoantibodies. (Fig. 20.3). Alternatively, if antibodies are produced as a result of microbial infection which carry an idiotype which resembles the idiotype of a potentially autoreactive B cell closely enough, then T-helper lymphocytes carrying the anti-idiotype may again be activated inappropriately by the antimicrobial

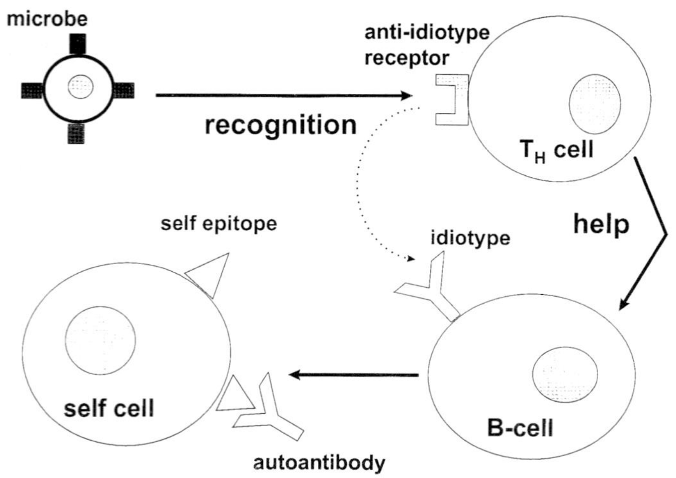

Fig. 20.3 By virtue of structural mimicry a microbe antigen is able to bind the anti-idiotype receptor of a T-helper cell. This anti-idiotype also recognizes the idiotype of a B lymphocyte and its immunoglobulins which can be synthesized and released as autoantibodies. As a consequence, when the T lymphocyte is stimulated by the microbe, it transmits helper signals to the B lymphocyte, which releases autoantibodies, and tissue destruction follows.

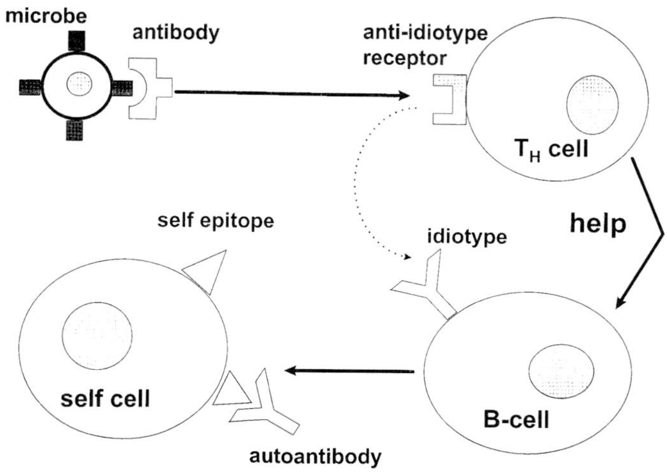

Fig. 20.4 A microbe has induced an antibody response. The antimicrobial antibodies bear an idiotype resembling the idiotype of a potentially autoreactive B lymphocyte. A T-helper cell with a receptor containing the anti-idiotype is stimulated when it recognizes the idiotypic structure on the antimicrobial antibody, and activates the autoreactive B cell, leading to autoantibody production and tissue damage.

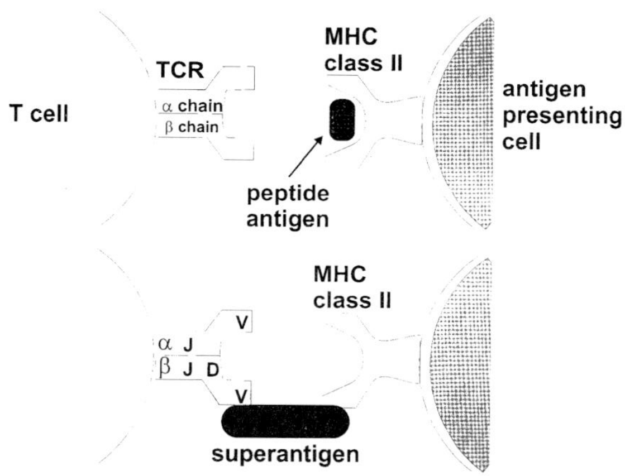

Fig. 20.5 Superantigens bypass the normal route of intracellular processing and bind directly as intact proteins to most class II major histocompatibility complex (MHC) molecules away from the peptide-binding groove. They react with the V segment of the β chain (Vβ) of the T-cell receptor (TCR) rather than the normal α and β antigen-binding site. Superantigens can react with all T cells with the appropriate Vβ gene, which is about 1 in 50 T cells, as opposed to 1 in 10^4 to 1 in 10^6 T cells. TCR has α and β chains, each with a joining segment, J, and a variable segment, V. The β chain also has a diversity segment, D.

antibody to stimulate the autoreactive B cell to release its autoantibodies (Fig. 20.4). Cross-reacting idiotypes have been suggested to play a role in the aetiology of rheumatoid arthritis and systemic lupus erythematosus, but it should be added that the role and significance of idiotype and anti-idiotype networks are ill-understood.

5. Some microbial antigens capable of inducing polyclonal (i.e. non-specific) T- and B-lymphocyte activation have recently attracted attention as potential factors in autoimmunity. These antigens have been named superantigens (Fig. 20.5). Most superantigens are bacterial exotoxins, including those produced by staphylococci, that cause food poisoning and toxic shock syndrome. By avoiding attachment to the cleft of a specific MHC class II molecule, and with an equally non-specific attachment to the T-cell receptor, the antigen-presenting cell is able to stimulate clonal expansion of many T lymphocytes 1 in 50 T cells as opposed to 1 in 10^4 to 10^6 with normal antigens (i.e. non-specifically). The bound T cells can then, in turn, activate many B-cell clones, resulting in the production of polyclonal autoantibodies. Staphylococcal superantigens have been implicated in the aetiology of animal models of multiple sclerosis. Superantigens on the Epstein–Barr virus and lipopolysaccharides in the wall of Gram-negative bacteria are able to interact directly with B lymphocytes, including those with the potential to synthesize autoantibodies.
6. The failure of T-cell suppression and increased T-helper activity have been

proposed to occur in systemic lupus erythematosus. This correlates with the histological finding of a predominance of CD4 T-helper cells in the perivascular lymphocytic aggregates of autoimmune diseases. Microbial factors, as well as 'confusing' the immune system by their resemblance to self antigens, induce inflammation which may release inflammatory mediators and cytokines which cause autoimmunity by another process. As discussed above, MHC class II molecule expression is normally restricted to the antigen-presenting cell and activated T cells. However, if there is loss of normal repression of MHC class II genes in other cells, these cells can then communicate with CD4 T cells and activate immune effector mechanisms. Such inappropriate HLA-D region expression has been observed in thyroid epithelium in patients with Graves' thyrotoxicosis. Similarly, the majority of cells in a joint with active rheumatoid arthritis are HLA-DR-positive, and in insulin-dependent diabetes mellitus, the β islets of the pancreas express MHC class II molecules.

The association of autoimmune disease with certain HLA-D region genes supports an active role for CD4 helper-inducer T cells, because of the interaction of CD4 T cells and MHC class II molecules during antigen presentation. The cytokine interferon-γ (IFN-γ), secreted by T cells, is a costimulatory molecule and IL-1, tumour necrosis factor-α (TNF-α) and TNF-β are other cytokines produced by local T lymphocytes which can act synergistically with IFN-γ. With the production of IL-1, antigen presentation can proceed. IL-1 also induces inflammation via the release of prostaglandin E_2 (PGE_2) and other acute-phase proteins. Other mediators may also induce IL-1 production, as illustrated by therapy with IL-2, which sometimes precipitates a Hashimoto-type thyroid autoimmunity; IL-6 may also have this ability.

The final means by which infective agents have been hypothesized to play a role in the tissue damage seen in autoimmune diseases, particularly those which are organ-specific, is by their physical presence at the site of the disease. This initiates a normal, local T-cell dependent inflammatory response directed specifically against the infective agent (rather than against self). Mycobacteria are again suspected as a cause of tissue destruction in this way.

Inevitably perhaps, a role for apoptosis (programmed cell death) has also been proposed in the development of autoimmunity. It is now accepted that apoptosis has a crucial role in the development of the normal immune system, since this is how clones are deleted in the thymus. Work in animal models has shown that overexpression of *bcl*-2, one of the genes that prevents a cell entering programmed cell death, produces the clinical features of autoimmunity. There is complementary suppression of the genes which promote apoptosis. Whether these findings will translate to human autoimmunity remains to be seen.

It is not easy to explain how an immunoglobulin molecule, reactive to a host intracellular component, penetrates the cell membrane and remains intact to bind to its target in the cytoplasm or nucleus. Even if this occurs, it is still difficult to explain how these autoantibodies to intracellular components cause the manifestations of disease seen clinically. The target antigen must therefore be accessibly located. This is most likely to be on the target cell membrane, where it is easier to understand how autoantibody binding would cause patholological changes. This has been shown to be the case with some thyroid autoantigens. In myasthenia gravis, autoantibodies to acetylcholine receptors cause their aggregation, or diminish receptor half-life and block transmitter function. Alternatively, autoantibody binding might result in complement-mediated lysis or antibody-dependent cell-mediated cytotoxicity through the action of natural killer cells or macrophages.

Genetic and environmental factors involved in the initiation of autoimmunity

Although defects in immune regulation suggest a genetic explanation, the numerous ways in which exogenous agents also appear to be involved show that environmental factors must also be of significance. This conclusion is further supported by the fact that, in an identical twin with autoimmune disease, the chance of the sibling also being affected is less than 100%. In systemic lupus erythematosus, it is of the order of 65%. In rheumatoid arthritis it is at most 30–40% and may be as low as 15%. It remains uncertain, therefore, how a genetic trait develops into clinical disease.

HLA typing has shown that all autoimmune diseases have an HLA association, either with an MHC class I or class II gene or, in the case of systemic lupus erythematosus, with MHC class III (complement) genes. The HLA association is important as MHC genes influence the repertoire of T lymphocytes emerging from the thymus, and the range of idiotypes within the T-cell receptor. It would also be reasonable to expect that genes regulating immunoglobulin structure, antigen processing and intracellular transport also influence the development of autoreactive T lymphocytes.

Other genes not directly associated with immune responsiveness can also be involved, and an example is the ability to acetylate, and thus inactivate, certain drugs. Patients who are slow acetylators are at risk of developing an iatrogenic systemic lupus erythematosus if treated with some drugs.

Females are more commonly affected by autoimmune disease than males, though the ratio varies between diseases. In insulin-dependent diabetes mellitus it is 2:1, but in systemic lupus erythematosus it rises to 8:1. The reasons for this are unclear, but presumably relate to the fact that females produce higher natural autoantibody titres to a greater variety of autoantigens, thus increasing the liklihood that autoimmunization will occur. Clearly the processes involved are complex, as pregnancy and the use of the contraceptive pill affect the severity of autoimmune disease differently.

There is also an age effect which varies between autoimmune diseases. Insulin-dependent diabetes mellitus characteristically affects young patients, whilst rheumatoid arthritis has a later onset.

The role of methyldopa in autoimmune haemolytic anaemia has already been alluded to, but several drugs and toxic chemicals are known to cause autoimmune reactions. Polyvinyl chloride (PVC) has been implicated in scleroderma, and more mundane factors such as diet and stress may have a role too. The net result of all these factors, and the degree of influence they have exerted, probably determines which disease develops.

Oral manifestations of autoimmune disease

Sjögren's syndrome

Sjögren's syndrome is also included amongst the autoimmune diseases intermediate between organ-specific and non-organ-specific (Table 20.1) since exocrine glands throughout the body may be affected. Primary Sjögren's syndrome involves only the eyes and mouth, whereas secondary Sjögren's syndrome develops against a background of one of the connective tissue autoimmune disorders, most commonly rheumatoid arthritis or systemic lupus erythematosus. The disease has a 9:1 (or higher) female preponderance. There is a wide variation in age at presentation, though most patients fall in the range from the fourth to seventh decades, the disease running a chronic course. The incidence is thought to be 3–5% amongst geriatric populations. There is also a significantly higher incidence (2–3 times that of the general population) of the allotype HLA-DR3 amongst sufferers, although HLA associations do show racial variation. HLA-B8, HLA-DR2 and HLA-DR4 have also been reported to be abnormally frequent amongst patients with Sjögren's syndrome.

Because the salivary glands are often the site of latent viruses, it is perhaps not surprising that environmental factors have been implicated in Sjögren's syndrome. The MHC class II expression observed in ductal epithelium in affected salivary glands is probably modulated by IFN-γ, the presence of which could itself be a response to viral infection. Raised antibody titres to herpesviruses, including Epstein–Barr virus, human herpesvirus-6 and cytomegalovirus, have been reported but the results are inconsistent between studies; indeed normal titres to these agents have also been demonstrated. Associating the onset of Sjögren's syndrome with an acute infection with these, or any other agent, is difficult because the exact point of onset of disease is difficult to determine accurately.

The retroviruses have also attracted attention as possible aetiological factors in Sjögren's syndrome because of the lymphocyte abnormalities, lymphoma predilection and reported cases of acquired immunodeficiency syndrome (AIDS) where the signs and symptoms included parotitis and keratoconjunctivitis sicca. One of the autoantibodies present in high titres in patients with Sjögren's syndrome, the La (SS-B) autoantigen, shares amino acid sequences with retroviruses, raising the possibility that this autoantibody is raised as a result of molecular mimicry. It should be remembered, however, that viral RNAs are often not immunogenic.

All exocrine glands, including the major and minor salivary glands, may be replaced by a lymphocytic infiltrate, about three-quarters of which are T cells. The vast majority of these express αβ T-cell receptors, with CD4 and CD8 T lymphocytes in a ratio of 3:1. T lymphocytes with γδ receptors are sparse within the salivary T-cell infiltrate and apparently play an insignificant role in Sjögren's syndrome, though this is not the case in other rheumatoid autoimmune diseases. Fifty per cent of the infiltrating lymphocytes (T and B) show upregulation of activation markers, such as the IL-2 receptor, and reduced numbers and activity of natural killer lymphocytes. Although the ductal epithelial cells express MHC class II molecules, HLA-DR expression may also be seen in non-specific sialadenitis.

Plasma cells differentiated from hyperactive B lymphocytes produce a hypergammaglobulinaemia, and serological investigations reveal high titres of rheumatoid factor and a variety of extractable antinuclear autoantibodies, including those named Ro (SS-A) and La, in 50–90% of Sjögren's sufferers, but no autoantibody is absolutely specific for Sjögren's syndrome. Antisalivary duct antibodies (i.e. an organ-specific autoantibody) may also be present, but these appear to be a consequence of glandular destruction rather than the cause of it. The autoantibodies are detected by indirect immunofluorescence on frozen sections of rat, mouse or monkey tissue, often liver, to which the patient's serum has been applied.

Although Sjögren's syndrome generally follows a benign course, these patients have a 20–44 times greater likelihood of developing lymphoma, in most cases a low-grade B-cell lymphoma of mucosa-associated lymphoid tissue (MALT). Genetic studies using Southern blotting, the polymerase chain reaction and *in situ* hybridization demonstrate heavy-chain gene rearrangements and that light-chain restriction (κ more commonly than λ) may be present in 15–20% of labial gland biopsies from patients with no clinical evidence of lymphoma. Approximately 40% of these patients will go on to develop lymphoma, sometimes many years later. In some instances, however, it is clear that monoclonality is a later event. By contrast, in parotid lymphoepithelial lesions, not all of which are associated with overt Sjögren's syndrome, there may be light-chain restriction in almost 80% of patients.

Vesiculobullous lesions

Several mucocutaneous diseases which are immunologically mediated affect the oral mucosa. Whilst some of the conditions described below, such as pemphigus, pemphigoid and dermatitis herpetiformis, are undoubtedly autoimmune in nature, some of the others are idiopathic. In these cases some of the observations which have raised the possibility of an autoimmune aetiology are discussed. Although restricted to skin and mucosae, the fact that lesions are often anatomically dispersed has led them to be classified, as with Sjögren's syndrome, as autoimmune diseases intermediate between organ-specific and non-organ-specific (Table 20.1).

Pemphigus

Two varieties of pemphigus affect the oral mucosa – the far commoner pemphigus vulgaris and the rare pemphigus foliaceus. Pemphigus vegetans appears to be a variant of the former, and pemphigus erythematosus of the latter. Fogo selvagem, or Brazilian pemphigus, is also a form of pemphigus foliaceus. There are other types of pemphigus, but they are restricted to the epidermis and oral involvement is virtually unheard of. All forms of pemphigus are autoimmune diseases, the autoantibodies of which are directed against intercellular components of stratified squamous epithelium. The autoantigen is situated in the immediately suprabasal layers in pemphigus vulgaris, but is located more superficially in the stratum spinosum in pemphigus foliaceus. This difference manifests in the level at which the characteristic intra-epithelial separation seen histologically occurs.

Oral blisters or vesicles are invariably ulcerated at presentation, though it is usually possible to elicit a positive Nikolsky sign. The ulcers are irregular, often ragged and, though shallow, painful with a tendency not to heal. The incidence is estimated at between 0.5 and 3.2 per 100 000 per annum, with an equal sex distribution and inclination to occur in the fifth and sixth decades. Children and adolescents are only exceptionally affected. Oral signs and symptoms occur in 70% of patients, and 50% will only develop overt disease in the mouth.

Genetic factors appear to have a strong influence and patients with HLA-DR4 or HLA-DR6 genes are at 24 and 1.5 times respectively higher relative risk of contracting pemphigus vulgaris. There are racial variations in HLA allotypes predisposing to pemphigus. The first to be identified was HLA-A10 in Japanese and Jewish patients. Over 90% of patients of Jewish origin have been reported to express the HLA-DR4 allotype, and the combination of HLA-A26, B38 and DR4 has an especially high frequency in sufferers. Given the importance of HLA-DR4 in Sjögren's syndrome (see above), it is interesting that pemphigus has been reported to occur in conjunction with other autoimmune diseases, including rheumatoid arthritis, Sjögren's syndrome and mucous membrane pemphigoid.

Both bound and circulating autoantibodies are detectable in pemphigus, mainly of an IgG isotype, notably IgG4. IgG4 does not fix complement and the extent to which complement mediates pemphigus is unclear. However, IgM and IgA isotypes may be present in up to 50% of cases. High titres are often, but not always, associated with active disease. In pemphigus vulgaris, the autoantigen is an E-cadherin, a transmembrane glycoprotein and member of one of the four groups of adhesion molecules. The autoantigen shows some homology with the 160-kDa E-cadherin often referred to as desmoglein 1, which is the antibody-binding site in pemphigus foliaceus. However, the pemphigus vulgaris autoantigen is thought to be specific to the immediately suprabasal desmosomes, whereas desmoglein 1 is a core component of all desmosomes. Presumably there is also an element of site-specificity to the targeted desmoglein 1 in pemphigus foliaceus and these variations give some indication to the heterogeneity of desmosomal structure. Clearly these proteins are of importance in cell–cell adhesion and an autoimmune response against them, amplified by complement and proteolytic processes (the latter attributable to plasminogen activator release by keratinocytes) produces the typical acantholysis.

Pemphigoid

Of the two main forms of pemphigoid, mucous membrane pemphigoid affects the oral mucosa much more frequently than does bullous pemphigoid, which is principally a disease of skin. The term cicatricial pemphigoid is generally used interchangeably with mucous membrane pemphigoid, and though the two may be the same disease, some authorities believe purely ocular cicatricial pemphigoid to be a separate entity. In mucous membrane pemphigoid the mucosal surfaces of the mouth, larynx, nose, oesophagus, genitals and conjunctiva are involved much more commonly than skin. The mouth is often the only affected site. Despite the alternative term, mucous membrane pemphigoid rarely causes scarring anywhere but the eye, and blindness is thus a serious complication of the condition. It is not, however, fatal, in contrast to untreated pemphigus. Oral vesicles rarely last long, though blood-filled blisters may sometimes be seen and there may be a positive Nikolsky sign. Ulceration is therefore generally the presenting feature, the ulcers being painful, often with a well-defined margin, typically persisting for weeks before healing. All manifestations of pemphigoid produce an autoimmune response to components of the basement membrane zone proteins, though the precise target epitope in mucous membrane pemphigoid remains unidentified (see below). The result is cleavage of the epithelium from the underlying lamina propria.

About twice as many women as men contract the disease, which affects elderly individuals. The age range of onset is 40–80 years, with most patients in the seventh decade.

In contrast to pemphigus, there is no racial predilection and no consistent finding of an HLA allotype which predisposes to disease.

Both mucous membrane and bullous pemphigoid show a linear pattern of IgG (generally IgG4 and IgG1) and complement fraction C3 in the basement membrane zone with direct immunofluorescence of perilesional mucosa, with IgM and IgA positive in about a quarter of cases. Direct immunofluorescence is positive in skin in about 40% of patients with mucous membrane pemphigoid. Light and electron microscopic studies of mucous membrane and bullous pemphigoid show very similar features, and the main distinction between the two (other than anatomical location) is the absence in the former of any circulating autoantibodies, at least using conventional methods, with consequently negative indirect immunofluorescence. This is inconsistent with an autoimmune disease, but techniques such as immunoblotting have suggested that a circulating autoantibody is indeed present in mucous membrane pemphigoid. The circulating titre of autoantibody in bullous pemphigoid does not reflect the severity of disease, and it remains to be seen whether this is the case in mucous membrane pemphigoid.

Two autoantigens have been identified in bullous pemphigoid; both are hemidesmosomal proteins located in the upper lamina lucida of the basement membrane zone. The major autoantigen is a polypeptide of 230 kDa, situated intracellularly at the point where the integrin adhesion molecule $\alpha_6\beta_4$ links with the keratin filaments in hemidesmosomes. The minor autoantigen has a molecular weight of 180 kDa and forms the vital link between the basal cell and the basement membrane zone. It is a transmembrane polypeptide which also contains extracellular domains and has recently been designated as type XVII collagen.

The autoantigen in mucous membrane pemphigoid is located in the lower lamina lucida, and though it cross-reacts with, and has a similar molecular weight to, the 180 kDa minor bullous pemphigoid antigen, its nature has not been pinpointed for certain. The integrin $\alpha_3\beta_1$ attracted interest in this context, since it mediates adhesion of basal keratinocytes to the basement membrane zone. However, its distribution is unchanged in mucous membrane pemphigoid, though expression is weaker. Expression of the integrin α_6 subunit becomes patchy in mucous membrane pemphigoid, and what remains is located on the epithelial aspect of the bulla at the same site as the autoantibody binds, thus rendering it a strong candidate as the elusive autoantigen in mucous membrane pemphigoid.

As might be expected, increased numbers of antigen-presenting cells, in the form of Langerhans cells, have been reported in skin lesions of bullous and ocular lesions of mucous membrane, with most of the infiltrating lymphocytes helper T cells.

Dermatitis herpetiformis

Although also generally held to be principally a skin disease, oral lesions may occur in 70% of patients who develop dermatitis herpetiformis, even if they are not the presenting feature. All patients have a gluten-sensitive enteropathy, but often without any overt manifestations of coeliac disease. The condition has a 2:1 male preponderance and predisposing allotypes cited are HLA-B8, HLA-DR3, which are common to coeliac disease, and HLA-DR2, which is not. HLA-DR7 and HLA-DQ2 are also reported as highly frequent in coeliac disease. Direct immunofluorescence usually shows a focal, granular IgA and fibrinogen deposition adjacent to the basement membrane zone at the tips of the dermal papillae, where microabscesses are also found on routine staining, though linear IgA staining may be seen in 10–15% of cases. The IgA is polyclonal and, though it lacks the secretory component, probably originates in the gut mucosa in response to gluten.

Circulating autoantibodies to gliadin have traditionally been the marker of dermatitis herpetiformis with indirect immunofluorescence, but some studies have shown this to be present in only two-thirds of cases and sometimes may be found in patients with other vesiculobullous diseases. Gliadin has therefore been superseded in this respect and autoantibodies to endomysial and reticulin connective tissue are now accepted as being more specific features of dermatitis herpetiformis and coeliac disease.

Epidermolysis bullosa acquisita

Epidermolysis bullosa is a complex of approximately 20 conditions, of which only epidermolysis bullosa acquisita is non-hereditary, or at least clinically absent at birth. All produce subepithelial bullae similar in appearance histologically to those in the other lesions described above. However, the bullae in epidermolysis bullosa acquisita contain few cells, or contain a predominance of erythrocytes. Although cell-poor bullae may also be seen in pemphigoid, leukocytes, notably eosinophils, are more commonly present in this condition. Linear IgG and C3 deposition is seen just below the basement membrane on direct immunofluorescence, and electron microscopy reveals the cleavage to occur below the lamina densa, with amorphous material seen at the same site. Indirect immunofluorescence is negative, but there is evidence that the autoantigen in epidermolysis bullosa acquisita is a component of type VII collagen, and whereas $\alpha_6\beta_4$ staining is diminished in pemphigoid, it is normal in epidermolysis bullosa acquisita.

Erythema multiforme

Erythema multiforme is an acute mucocutaneous disease which usually affects young adults, either as a single attack or as recurrent episodes. Some authorities designate the more common form minor, when oral signs and symptoms may be absent, and the systemic form affecting multiple skin and mucosal sites major. The latter is equivalent to Stevens–Johnson syndrome.

The lesions of erythema multiforme are believed by some authorities to develop as a result of vasculitis which follows immune complex deposition in blood vessel walls. In superficial blood vessels of the dermis, IgM and C3 may indeed be identified by direct, and circulating immune complexes by indirect immunofluorescence. However, other sources specifically comment on the absence of vasculitis and there is now some evidence that a cell-mediated immune response is mounted against keratinocytes. There are also changes in Langerhans cell morphology and location. An explanation for this remains to be ascertained, but herpes simplex virus has been implicated as the stimulus. As there is an influx of both T helper and suppressor cells, it can be speculated that either a viral antigen is presented by Langerhans cells in combination with MHC class I molecules to CD8 T suppressor cells, or that viral antigens mimicking or altering keratinocyte phenotypes are causing an autoimmune response mediated by CD4-T helper lymphocytes in association with class II MHC molecules. An increased likelihood of developing erythema multiforme associated with herpes simplex virus has been observed in patients with the HLA-DQ3 allotype.

Lichen planus

Lichen planus is a chronic mucocutaneous condition which affects the oral mucosa more commonly than any of the diseases so far described. Although not usually included amongst the vesiculobullous diseases, the rarity of vesicles and bullae in patients with oral lichen planus may merely be a reflection of the trauma that also explains why intact oral blisters are uncommon in pemphigus and pemphigoid. The bullous variant of lichen planus may therefore be more frequent than is believed, but manifest clinically as erosive lichen planus. An autoimmune aetiology has yet to be determined, however, though some features hint at such a pathogenesis.

Lichen planus is characterized by sub- and intraepithelial T-lymphocyte infiltration and degeneration of the basal layer. The appearances are thus suggestive of an inappropriate T-cell-mediated immune response directed against an as yet unknown antigen. As in other oral inflammatory and ulcerative situations, there is induced HLA-DR expression by keratinocytes which may be focal or extensive.

Direct and indirect immunofluorescence has failed, to date, to identify a lichen planus-specific autoantigen. Indirect immunofluorescence has been reported as showing IgG, IgA and IgM deposition in the stratum spinosum and granulosum of epidermis, if serum is applied to autologous tissue sections, or if serum from a patient with oral lichen planus is applied to an allogeneic section of skin from a patient with cutaneous lichen planus. Drug-induced lichenoid reactions, but not lichen planus, may sometimes give a positive reaction to the basal keratinocyte membrane with indirect immunofluorescence. Direct immunofluorescence, however, is only exceptionally positive for immunoglobulins in oral mucosa, and then only with a weak, granular distribution. In contrast, there is often strong linear deposition of fibrinogen and C3 along the basement membrane zone, a non-specific feature.

Lupus erythematosus

Lupus erythematosus is an uncommon autoimmune disease presenting as two main forms, systemic and discoid. The allotypes HLA-DR2 and DR3 are believed to predispose to systemic lupus erythematosus. Either may give rise to oral lesions which resemble lichen planus both clinically and histologically. Systemic lupus erythematosus produces oral lesions in approximately 20% of cases, but there are few data on the figure for discoid lupus erythematosus, and in neither are oral lesions commonly the presenting feature. Whereas systemic lupus erythematosus may give rise to multisystem pathology, discoid lupus erythematosus tends to be a mucocutaneous disease producing localized rashes, sometimes of a photosensitive nature, which rarely produces arthralgia or significant autoantibody production. Mild systemic lupus erythematosus can be difficult to distinguish from discoid lupus erythematosus and occasionally there may be transition between the two. Sjögren's syndrome is a complication in approximately 30% of cases of systemic lupus erythematosus.

Direct immunofluorescence of frozen sections shows granular deposition of complement fractions, usually C3, and immunoglobulins at the basement membrane zone. Normal epithelium distant from the lesion is positive in systemic lupus erythematosus, whereas only the lesion is positive in discoid lupus erythematosus. Serologically, systemic lupus erythematosus is characterized by high titres to double-stranded (native) DNA in 40–60% and antinuclear antibodies in about 95% of cases.

Miscellaneous

Lupus erythematosus has also been reported in acquired immunodeficiency syndrome (AIDS), though the most common autoimmune disease associated with human immunodeficiency virus (HIV) infection is thrombocytopenic purpura, which can cause purple patches in the oral mucosa resembling Kapsosi's sarcoma and a haemorrhagic diathesis. The other connective tissue diseases, polymyositis, dermatomyositis and progressive systemic sclerosis (scleroderma), may occasionally affect the oral tissues.

Further reading

Ackerman AB, Penneys NS, Clark WH. Erythema multiforme exudativum: distinctive pathological process. *Brit J Dermatol* 1971; **84**: 554–556.

Camisa C, Allen CM, Bowen B, Olsen RG. Indirect immunofluorescence of oral lichen planus. *J Oral Pathol* 1986; **15**: 218–220.

Feldman M. Immunological tolerance and self non-responsiveness. In: McGee JO'D, Isaacson PG, Wright NA (eds) *Oxford Textbook of Pathology*, vol. 1, pp. 293–306. Oxford: Oxford University Press, 1992.

Fry L. Dermatitis herpetiformis. *Bailliere's Clin Gastroenterol* 1995; **9**: 371–393.

Isenberg DA, Horsfall AC (eds). *Autoimmune Diseases – Focus on Sjögren's Syndrome*. Oxford: βIOS Scientific Publishers, 1994.

Jones J, Downer CS, Speight PM (1995). Changes in the expression of integrins and basement membrane proteins in benign mucous membrane pemphigoid. *Oral Dis* 1995; **1**: 159–165.

Karjalainen TK, Tomich CF. A histopathologic study of oral mucosal lupus erythematosus. *Oral Surg Oral Med Oral Pathol* 1989; **67**: 547–554.

Lamey P-J, McCartan BE, MacDonald DG, Mackie RM. Basal cell cytoplasmic autoantibodies in oral lichenoid reactions. *Oral Surg Oral Med Oral Pathol* 1995; **79**: 44–49.

Roitt I. *Essential Immunology*, 7th edn. London: Blackwell Scientific Publications, 1991.

Williams DM. Vesiculobullous mucocutaneous disease: pemphigus vulgaris. *J Oral Pathol Med* 1989; **18**: 544–553.

Williams DM. Vesiculo-bullous mucocutaneous disease: benign mucous membrane pemphigoid and bullous pemphigoid. *J Oral Pathol Med* 1990; **19**: 16–23.

Williams DM. Non-infectious diseases of the oral soft tissue: a new approach. *Adv Dent Res* 1993; **7**: 213–219.

21

The pathophysiology of cardiorespiratory arrest and the principles of post-resuscitation intensive care

Susan J. Wright

Oxygen supply to the tissues is dependent on both cardiac output (which is determined by blood volume and myocardial function) and the oxygen tension of arterial blood (which reflects respiratory status). Disturbances of these parameters may occur individually or together, and may progress to combined cardiorespiratory collapse. Life support measures are then required to restore the oxygen supply to vital organs, such as the brain, heart, kidneys and liver, while attempts to restore normal cardiorespiratory function are made. Survival following cardiorespiratory arrest is enhanced if resuscitation is promptly instituted by skilled resuscitators, and a clear understanding of the mechanisms of cardiorespiratory collapse is essential to the efficient management of these patients.

Causes of cardiorespiratory arrest

The factors which may precipitate cardiorespiratory arrest may be primarily cardiac or non-cardiac.[1]

Primary cardiac cause ('sudden cardiac death')

Although atherosclerosis is the commonest underlying cause of sudden cardiac death, myocardial infarction itself is by no means assumed to have occurred prior to cardiac arrest. For example, rupture of an atheromatous plaque may cause a focal area of ischaemia, which triggers a life-threatening dysrhythmia. Cobb *et al.*[2] reported that 25% of patients who had been successfully resuscitated from ventricular fibrillation were found to have no electrocardiogram (ECG) changes indicative of myocardial infarction in the days following cardiac arrest. Nevertheless, many patients with underlying coronary obstructive disease do have a previous history of angina, myocardial infarction or heart failure and, in the clinical setting, such patients must be recognized to be at increased risk of sudden cardiac death. Other primary cardiac causes of cardiac arrest include coronary artery spasm, valvular heart disease (including acute valve prolapse and disintegration or obstruction of a prosthetic heart valve), conduction defects (such as atrioventricular block), cardiomyopathy, myocarditis and infective endocarditis.

Primarily non-cardiac cause

Cardiac arrest occurs in these patients when the heart is deprived of nutrients, is subjected to an abnormal chemical environment or is impeded by physical forces which impair cardiac function. These conditions may arise in a number of ways.

Respiratory failure

If arterial blood is inadequately oxygenated by the lungs, the resulting myocardial hypoxia will lead, ultimately, to cardiac arrest. Children and pregnant women, in particular, may develop hypoxaemia with alarming rapidity as their basal oxygen requirements are high. Failure of the respiratory system to provide adequate arterial oxygen content may arise as a result of:

1. Airway obstruction from the presence of a foreign body, blood or secretions in the airway, postoperative swelling, laryngospasm or reduced pharyngeal muscle tone (see below).
2. Respiratory depression or paralysis of respiratory muscle activity. This may be secondary to the injudicious use of sedative drugs or general anaesthetic agents and neuromuscular blocking drugs, or may be precipitated by obesity, neuromuscular disease and chest wall deformities or injury.
3. Pulmonary gas diffusion defect. Normal diffusion of gases between the alveolus and pulmonary capillaries may be impaired in any of a large number of chronic lung diseases, and in the presence of pulmonary oedema.
4. Inadequate inspired oxygen concentration. In clinical practice, this is only likely to be encountered as a complication of mismanaged anaesthesia, or as a result of inadequate mixing of oxygen and nitrous oxide during rewarming of Entonox cylinders which have been exposed to temperatures lower than 7°C. Hypoxia-induced myocardial dysfunction is exacerbated by the acidosis and hypercapnia that accompany respiratory failure and accelerate progression toward cardiac arrest.

Hypovolaemia

Major blood loss or extravasation of fluid from the intravascular compartment (for example, during anaphylaxis, or following burn injuries) causes hypotension and reduced tissue perfusion. Coronary blood flow is dependent on the systemic diastolic pressure which, if inadequate to ensure adequate myocardial perfusion, will cause ischaemia and cardiac arrest.

Metabolic disturbances

Radical changes in the chemical environment can lead to myocardial fibre dysfunction. Normal heart function can be maintained only within narrow limits of levels of:

1. Potassium (which may be abnormal as a result of liver disease, potassium supplementation, gastrointestinal losses or diuretic therapy).
2. pH. Myocardial function is particularly sensitive to acidosis, which may be caused by tissue hypoperfusion, sepsis, renal disease, diabetic ketoacidosis or drugs such as metformin.
3. Calcium.

Temperature

Cardiac rate and force of contraction are impaired by progressive hypothermia to the point of cardiac arrest at approximately 28–30°C. In some individuals, and especially in children, organized cardiac contraction may continue down to a temperature of 15–20°C. The cerebral protection conferred by reduced metabolic requirements of the brain at these temperatures has led to the successful resuscitation of some patients after prolonged immersion in cold water.

Drug therapy and toxins

Most sedative and general anaesthetic drugs are both cardiac and respiratory depressants. If given in overdose they may lead to cardiac arrest, either as a result of direct myocardial depression or as a result of the hypoxia caused by respiratory insufficiency. The toxic effects of local anaesthetic agents include both generalized central nervous system depression, which may result in respiratory arrest (with subsequent cardiac hypoxia) and dose-dependent depression of myocardial contraction and conduction pathways. Inadvertent intravascular injection of adrenaline-containing solutions may lead to ventricular tachyarrhythmias and cardiac arrest, particularly in a patient whose myocardium has been sensitized to the effects of catecholamines by the prior administration of the anaesthetic halothane. For this reason the recommended maximum dosages of both local anaesthetic drugs and adrenaline (100 μg, or 8 ml of 1:80 000 adrenaline over a 10-min period) should be adhered to. Felypressin, a potent vasoconstrictor which has no effects on the myocardium, is preferable to adrenaline in this regard. Anaphylactoid reactions to administered drugs can lead to profound cardiovascular collapse and respiratory embarrassment from bronchospasm. Severe reactions may culminate in cardiorespiratory arrest.

Mechanical impairment of cardiac function

Extracardiac physical forces which may prevent normal cardiac output include tension pneumothorax, haemorrhagic cardiac tamponade, pneumopericardium, ruptured diaphragm, and massive pulmonary air or thromboembolism.

Diagnostic and therapeutic procedures

Reflex brady- and tachyarrhythmias may result from surgical manipulation, for example dental extraction, cardiac catheterization or bronchoscopy.

Cardiac rhythms associated with cardiac arrest

The victim of a cardiorespiratory arrest may be found to have one of three cardiac dysrhythmias:

1. Ventricular fibrillation (VF) or pulseless ventricular tachycardia (VT).
2. Asystole.
3. Electromechanical dissociation (EMD).

Ventricular fibrillation/pulseless ventricular tachycardia

VT may cause a catastrophic fall in cardiac output (and thus a pulseless, collapsed patient) if myocardial function is severely compromised, particularly if the ventricular rate is very rapid. ECG monitoring reveals broad QRS complexes which are regular (Fig. 21.1). Without treatment, VT frequently progresses to VF, in which coordination of action of the myocardial fibres is lost and electrical depolarization and contraction become apparently random (Fig. 21.1). On direct observation, the ventricles would be seen to be quivering rather than beating. Initially, the force of fibre contraction is strong (coarse VF), but as ischaemia persists, the movement becomes weaker (fine VF, which may be mistaken for asystole on an ECG monitor) and eventually there is a deterioration to the point of asystole. VF is the underlying rhythm in 75% of patients suffering sudden cardiac death and is most commonly associated with pre-existing heart disease, hypothermia or high levels of circulating catecholamines, whether endogenous or exogenous in origin. Whatever the precipitating cause, consciousness is lost within 10–20 s of the onset of VF, but this rhythm carries the best prognosis for successful resuscitation.

Asystole

Asystole constitutes complete standstill of the myocardial fibres (Fig 21.1), and is the underlying rhythm in 25% of cardiac arrests. It may be preceded by VF and other dysrhythmias. Asystole may be precipitated by massive myocardial ischaemia, or by selective ischaemia involving the cardiac conducting tissues. It is also associated with non-cardiac causes of cardiac arrest such as hypoxia, hypovolaemia and biochemical derangement. A patient is predisposed to asystole in the presence of β-blockade or in conditions of high parasympathetic activity (which depress the sinoatrial and atrioventricular nodes), such as reflex responses to traction on the extraocular muscles or surgical manipulation of the bowel.

Electromechanical dissociation

Electromechanical dissociation (EMD) is a form of cardiac arrest characterized by profound pump failure, with the absence of cardiac output despite normal or near-normal ECG activity (Fig. 21.1). EMD is relatively rare. It may be primary (due to failure of excitation-contraction coupling, precipitated by myocardial infarction, for example) or secondary to mechanical forces which prevent the heart from functioning as a pump (such as tension pneumothorax).

The mechanism of EMD is unclear, but is thought to be related to intracellular acidosis and autonomic effects.

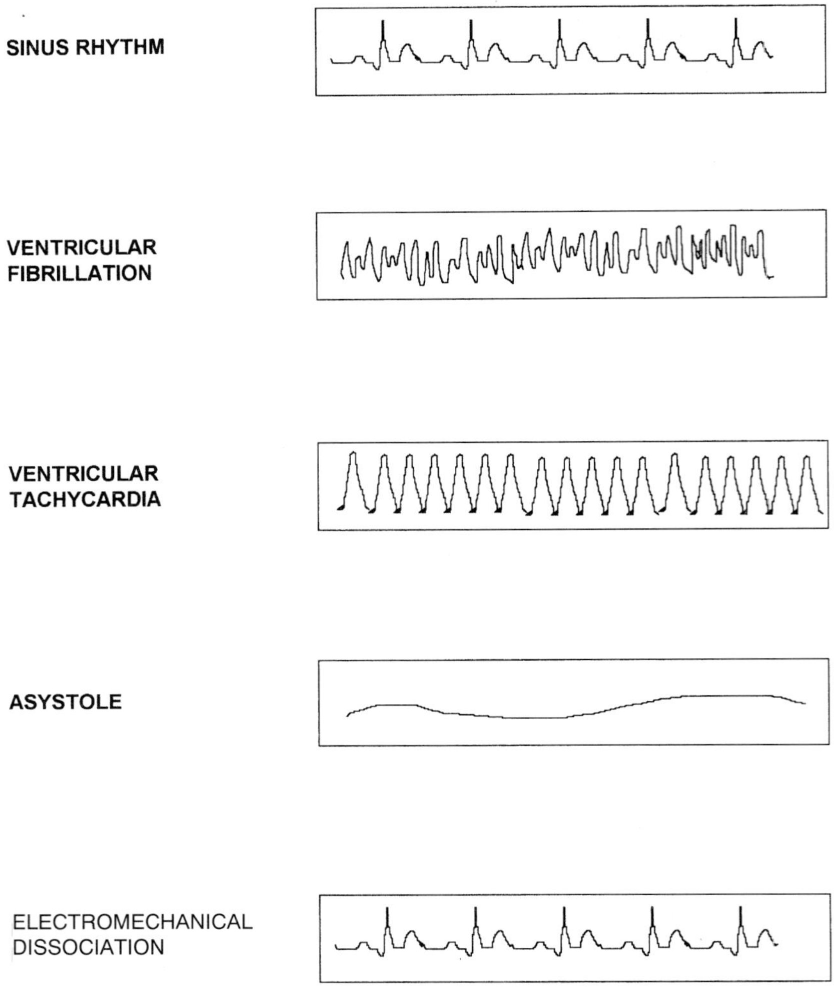

Fig. 21.1 The ECG appearances of cardiac rhythms associated with cardiorespiratory arrest.

The recognition and management of cardiorespiratory arrest

The patient suddenly falls deeply unconscious, pale and cyanosed. The carotid and femoral pulses are absent and respiration is gasping or absent. The pupils may be dilated and unresponsive (although this is an unreliable sign).

The object of cardiopulmonary resuscitation (CPR) is the restoration of tissue perfusion, and particularly that of the brain. Until a spontaneous circulation (in other words, the patient's own cardiac output) and normal respiration are restored, oxygenation must be supported by artificial ventilation and a cardiac output must be achieved by external cardiac massage. Basic life support (Fig. 21.2) and advanced life support (Figs 21.3–21.5), which together constitute CPR, are summarized in the UK Resuscitation Council protocols shown.

Basic life support (Fig. 21.2)

Basic life support incorporates airway maintenance and basic ventilation techniques, which are performed with chest compressions to generate a cardiac output (albeit only approximately 30% of the normal cardiac output at best). Recent research[3] has examined the

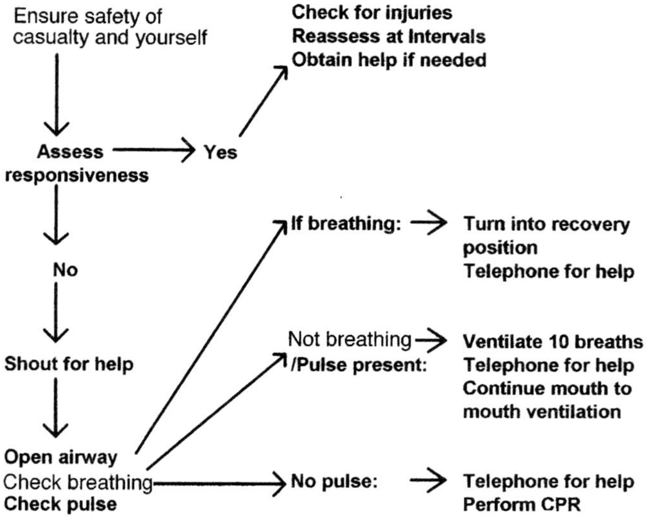

Fig. 21.2 Basic life support: sequence of resuscitation[7].

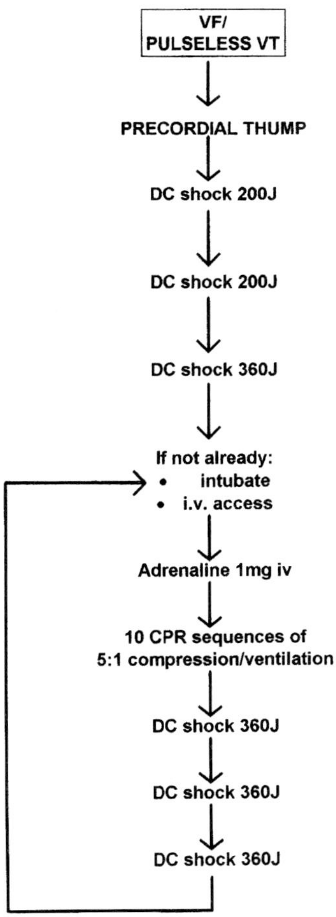

Fig. 21.3 Advanced life support: management of ventricular fibrillation (VF)/pulseless ventricular tachycardia (VT). CPR = Cardiopulmonary resuscitation; DC = direct current.

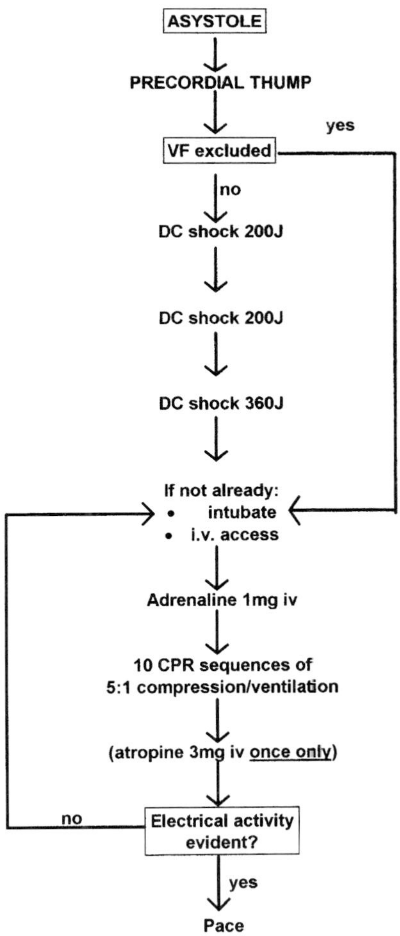

Fig. 21.4 Advanced life support: management of asystole. VF = Ventricular fibrillation; DC = direct current.

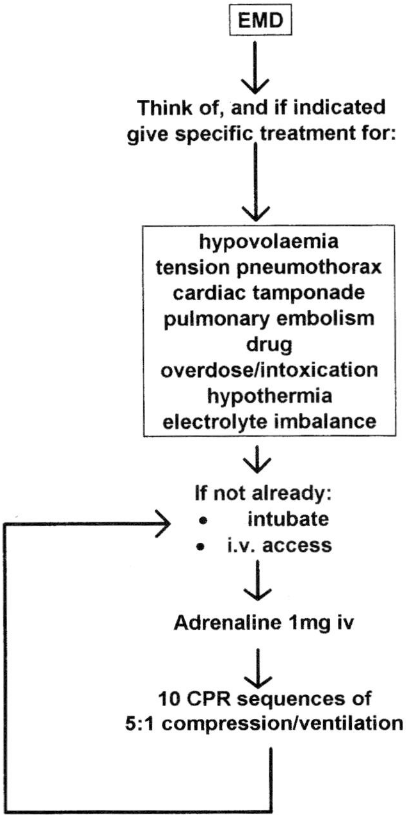

Fig. 21.5 Advanced life support: management of electromechanical dissociation (EMD). CPR = Cardiopulmonary resuscitation.

effect of interposed abdominal compression performed at the same time as conventional chest compression CPR and found significant haemodynamic augmentation, although this technique has yet to be adopted widely.

Recognition of the compromised airway is vital to those whose work involves maxillofacial procedures. The patient with upper airway obstruction will have laboured breathing, with paradoxical movement of the abdomen and thorax (i.e. the chest wall moves inwards and the abdominal wall outwards during inspiration) and reduced air movement at the nose or mouth. Frequently, breathing is noisy with gurgling, inspiratory stridor or the crowing sound typical of laryngospasm. As the obstruction and hypoxia worsen, the patient becomes increasingly distressed, eventually becoming cyanosed and losing consciousness as a result of hypoxia. If the problem is unrecognized, secondary cardiac arrest will ensue. The causes of upper-airway obstruction, and their management, are outlined below:

1. Reduced pharyngeal muscle tone in a semiconscious patient, with the tongue falling back into the pharynx. This may compound other causes of upper-airway compromise in the immediate postoperative period, and is a particular problem in obese patients. The basic techniques of airway maintenance comprise:
   (a) Chin lift (by placing one's fingers at the tip of the chin and elevating the mandible).
   (b) Jaw thrust (by placing one's fingers behind the angle of the mandible on each side and displacing the mandible anteriorly).
   (c) Head tilt (by extending the head on the neck to elevate the hyoid bone and therefore lift the tongue away from the posterior pharyngeal wall). This manoeuvre should not be performed on any patient with existing or suspected cervical spine injury as it may cause spinal cord damage.

   If available, adjuncts to basic airway maintenance such as the Guedel oropharyngeal airway or a nasopharyngeal airway may help relieve obstruction until the return of consciousness.

2. The presence of a foreign body in the mouth or pharynx, for example dentures, mouth or throat packs or inhaled objects. In adults the finger may be swept around the mouth to exclude the presence of a foreign body, but an object firmly lodged in the pharynx or larynx which cannot be moved by either thumping the choking patient's back between the scapulae or by performing abdominal thrusts will require laryngoscopy and removal by Magill forceps. If the airway obstruction is recognized early and the patient is still conscious, this procedure is likely to be difficult, and careful general anaesthesia (usually induced by inhalation of anaesthetic agents in this situation) may be required.
3. The presence of fresh blood, clot, or vomitus in the pharynx or larynx. It is usually possible to remove these liquids and semisolids with the use of a Yankauer sucker or suction catheter placed gently

Notes on cardiopulmonary resuscitation (CPR)

Ventilation	Aim for 800–1200 ml tidal volume (the amount normally required to achieve visible expansion of the chest) over approximately 2 s Allow the chest to fall fully during expiration (normally 2–4 s)
Chest compression	Aim to depress the sternum 4–5 cm, spending equal periods of time in the compressed and released phases Perform compressions at a rate of approximately 80/min, without waiting for expiration to occur after each breath
One rescuer present	Deliver 2 breaths of expired air after every 15 chest compressions
Two rescuers present	Deliver 1 breath of expired air after every 5 chest compressions

into the mouth, with care taken not to stimulate the larynx to the point of precipitating laryngospam in the conscious or semiconscious patient. Patients whose jaws have been wired intraoperatively may require urgent removal of the wires to relieve obstruction by semisolid matter in the upper airway. For this reason wire cutters are kept by the bedside of such patients as a matter of routine. The potential for aspiration of semisolid or liquid material by an unconscious or semiconscious patient should be borne in mind; the resulting lung contamination may develop into life-threatening aspiration pneumonia.

4. Oedema. Patients are frequently given steroids perioperatively in an attempt to reduce the extent of oedema formation in tissue which has been manipulated. However, pharyngeal and laryngeal oedema may be severe enough (and, in the case of anaphylaxis, may progress very rapidly) to precipitate complete upper-airway obstruction. If the problem is diagnosed early enough, the airway may be secured by orotracheal intubation after careful inhalational general anaesthesia, but when the situation is acute and critical hypoxia threatens, the obstruction has to be relieved by performing needle cricothyroidotomy (followed by jet insufflation of oxygen into the trachea), surgical cricothyroidotomy (with insertion of a tracheostomy tube) or emergency tracheostomy. The choice of procedure will be governed both by the urgency of the situation and the experience of the operator. The presence of oedema and altered anatomical landmarks in the postoperative patient may make the procedure practically difficult.
5. Laryngospasm. Stimulation of the larynx, for example by insertion of an oropharyngeal airway or the presence of laryngeal blood or secretions in a semiconscious patient, may precipitate spasm of the laryngeal muscles and airway obstruction. Laryngospasm is usually self-limiting, but may progress to the point of severe hypoxia. Treatment may be effected with the use of continuous positive airway pressure (CPAP) or by the administration of a muscle relaxant, such as suxamethonium, following which the patient will require sedation and ventilation by hand until the drug action wears off (typically 5 min).
6. Facial trauma. Both soft-tissue disruption and bone fractures may precipitate upper-airway obstruction. The management principles follow the progression of intervention from insertion of an oropharyngeal airway to provision of a surgical airway as above, depending on the severity of the injury. Nasopharyngeal airways should not be inserted into patients with suspected basal skull fractures because of the possibility that the airway will pass upwards into the brain. Similarly, the risk of cord injury precludes the use of head tilt to maintain a patent airway in patients with suspected cervical spine injury.

All patients with airway obstruction should be given oxygen in as high a concentration as possible. In certain situations, a helium–oxygen mixture, heliox, may be given via a face mask to improve gas movement across the site of obstruction (helium is more dense than nitrogen and therefore produces a smaller pressure gradient across a narrow orifice under conditions of turbulent flow).

Advanced life support

Figures 21.3–21.5 outline the advanced life support management of the underlying heart rhythms in cardiac arrest. If the patient's heart rhythm changes, the new treatment algorithm is commenced from the beginning, even if that rhythm has been treated at a previous point in the resuscitation. Tracheal intubation and obtaining intravenous access should not be allowed to interrupt basic life support for longer than 30 s; if intravenous access is difficult to secure, most drugs may be given via the tracheal tube, in a dosage double that normally given intravenously (with the exception of sodium bicarbonate and calcium salts, which are not suitable for endotracheal administration).

Management of ventricular fibrillation/pulseless ventricular tachycardia

The management of these rhythms is identical. VF is the most important rhythm to recognize and manage correctly, first because it is the most common rhythm underlying cardiac arrest and second because it carries the greatest likelihood of successful resuscitation. If the cardiac arrest is witnessed, particularly if ECG monitoring is already in progress and the rhythm is seen to change to VF or VT, a sharp precordial thump (over the lower half of the sternum) may terminate the dysrhythmia and restore a cardiac output. This procedure, which is rapidly and easily performed, therefore heads the treatment algorithm for VF, before the administration of three sequential DC shocks. The chance of restoring a spontaneous cardiac output in a patient in VF is highest if defibrillation is carried out within 90 s of cardiac arrest, and diminishes thereafter; the likelihood of successful resuscitation is minimal if defibrillation is first attempted longer than 8 min after the cardiac arrest. Rapid defibrillation therefore constitutes the overwhelming priority in the management of VF; basic life support techniques do not improve the situation (but slow the deterioration in the patient's status until defibrillation can be carried out) and therefore should not be allowed to delay defibrillation.

A 200 J shock is usually effective in the cardioversion of treatable VF and is associated with less myocardial damage than 360 J, which is used if two initial shocks of 200 J are unsuccessful. (The first 200 J shock causes a reduction in thoracic impedance which leads to a greater amount of energy being delivered to the myocardium during the subsequent 200 J shock.) The sequence of three shocks is delivered without pause for chest compression or ventilation. Adrenaline is administered during each loop of the treatment algorithm (which correlates to approximately every 2 min) *not* to enhance the likelihood of successful defibrillation but to increase vital organ perfusion during basic life support.[4]

After three loops of the algorithm have been performed, additional drug therapy may be considered, such as sodium bicarbonate and antiarrhythmic drugs (lignocaine, bretylium, amiodarone). However, none of these agents have been shown to alter the outcome from cardiac arrest and defibrillation remains the mainstay of treatment for VF or pulseless VT.

Management of asystole

The likelihood of successful resuscitation from asystole is very low (rate of survival to hospital discharge, <2%[5]). However, as VF may be confused for asystole on an ECG monitor (for example, if a lead has become detached, or if the monitor gain is not maximal), the initial management is the same as that for VF if the latter, more easily treatable rhythm, cannot be excluded. Once asystole is positively identified, the treatment algorithm pursues a pattern of repeated loops of chest compression and ventilation, with adrenaline administration during each loop. Atropine is administered only once during resuscitation from asystole; one 3 mg dose is large enough to effect total vagal blockade and interrupt any parasympathetic influences that may be contributing to asystole or a profound bradycardia. If, having completed three loops of the treatment algorithm, the patient remains asystolic, high-dose adrenaline (5 mg) should be considered. After 15 min of unresponsive asystole, however, successful resuscitation is highly unlikely except in patients with hypothermia, poisoning or near-drowning, and unless these situations apply, consideration should be given to abandoning resuscitation attempts.

Management of electromechanical dissociation

The treatment algorithm, which is shown in Figure 21.5, is dominated by the need to find the cause of the EMD so that appropriate therapy, for example needle thoracostomy in the case of a tension pneomothorax, may be instituted immediately. Mechanical causes carry the highest chance of successful treatment.

Principles of post-resuscitation intensive care

Cardiac arrest in the hospital environment carries a survival rate of 15–20%. Immediate resuscitation to full cardiorespiratory and neurological recovery occurs in a minority of cases; most successfully resuscitated patients have temporary or permanent complications which require careful management in the intensive therapy unit (ITU) setting.

Tissue injury during cardiac arrest may be a consequence of:

1. Ischaemia, causing oedema which further impairs tissue perfusion. Tissue death follows the rapid depletion of energy sources, such as glucose and adenosine triphosphate.
2. Multiple organ failure. Failure of one vital organ system is frequently associated with impairment of function of others.
3. Reperfusion injury. The hyperaemia which follows periods of tissue hypoperfusion is associated with the release of oxygen-derived free radicals and other toxic mediators of tissue damage.

Thus the successfully resuscitated patient is, initially, frequently unconscious and hypotensive, with inadequate respiration. Continued care on the ITU is aimed at restoration of normal cardiorespiratory status with preservation of vital organ function, particularly that of the brain and kidneys.

The cardiovascular system

Restoration of normal blood pressure and vital organ perfusion is a critical factor in the prevention of permanent neurological deficit and other vital organ dysfunction. Augmentation of the cardiac output with the use of inotropes, treatment of persistent dysrhythmias or restoration of blood volume by fluid administration may be required. In cases of profound cardiac pump failure, intra-aortic balloon counterpulsation may be employed.

The respiratory system

The patient should remain intubated and ventilated until the return of consciousness, with adequate cough and gag reflexes to protect the airway from aspiration of foreign matter. Pulmonary damage may have occurred during resuscitation, from aspiration of vomit, rib fractures, lung contusion or pneumothorax. Combined with residual respiratory depression of central origin, these factors usually necessitate the use of continued mechanical ventilation with increased inspired concentrations of oxygen. In the past it was usual to hyperventilate the patient to reduce carbon dioxide levels and thus reduce intracranial pressure (ICP), but current practice aims to maintain normocapnia, with avoidance of any rises in ICP which may result from coughing or straining, hypercapnia or cerebral oedema, with the aim of minimizing neurological damage. Mechanical ventilation usually necessitates the use of sedative infusions with or without neuromuscular blockade.

The central nervous system (CNS)

The organ most sensitive to hypoxia is the brain. Following cessation of cerebral blood flow, electroencephalogram (EEG) activity is minimal after 10 s and cerebral glucose stores are exhausted in one minute. Irreversible damage occurs after ischaemia of greater than 3–4 min duration. If resuscitation attempts fail to restore cerebral oxygen delivery within this period, although the patient may survive the circulatory arrest, permanent neurological damage may result. However, the brain can be protected from permanent damage by maintenance of a cerebral blood flow as low as one-seventh of normal.[6] Correctly performed CPR will result in cerebral blood flow adequate for the prevention of permanent cerebral dysfunction, although it invariably causes depression of function. Patients who at the time of cardiorespiratory arrest are unconscious with fixed, dilated pupils, may still regain normal cerebral function. Neurological well-being after cardiorespiratory arrest is best ensured by immediate resuscitation with:

1. Rapid re-establishment of spontaneous cardiac output.
2. Scrupulous maintenance of normal pH, blood gas and electrolyte levels in the post-resuscitation period.
3. Ventilation to achieve a normal arterial carbon dioxide tension to avoid rises in ICP that may be associated with hypercapnia.

The following measures, which aim to improve neurological outcome, have all been used but none have been shown conclusively to be effective:

1. Hypothermia to 35°C. Hypothermia is used primarily in patients who are hyperthermic on presentation.
2. Barbiturate coma reduces cerebral activity and therefore metabolic requirements, and protects against the adverse effects of fitting. Its value after arrest is unclear.
3. Steroids – although used primarily in the prevention of intracranial hypertension in patients with slow-growing brain tumours, steroids may lessen free radical damage in ischaemic brain. They have no proven effect on neurological outcome in this setting.
4. Calcium antagonists such as nimodipine are believed to improve outcome but do not as yet enjoy widespread use.
5. Anticoagulants and diuretics have been employed in the past, but there is little evidence to support their use.

Renal function

Maintenance of urine output may be aided by the correction of hypovolaemia and diuretics such as mannitol or frusemide. The infusion of dopamine to increase renal blood flow does produce a diuresis but has not been shown to improve renal outcome, and may in fact be detrimental to the patient. Its popularity in critical care is therefore diminishing. Short-term haemofiltration or long-term renal dialysis may be required.

Metabolic control

Strict control of blood biochemistry, in particular pH, blood gases, potassium and calcium levels, is essential for optimal function and recovery of the heart and brain.

Thus, restoration of ECG activity alone does not constitute successful resuscitation; the aim of life support techniques during and after cardiopulmonary arrest is the restoration of stable, spontaneous cardiorespiratory function in a patient free from neurological deficit or renal impairment. The likelihood of achieving such success is greatest if:

1. The response times to basic and advanced life support by well-trained personnel are short.
2. The underlying rhythm is VF.
3. Successful cardioversion is achieved within 3 min (and not longer then 8 min).
4. In a situation where defibrillation is delayed for more than 3 min, CPR is instituted promptly and maintained.

Scott[7] reported a 28-day survival rate of 24% in patients who had suffered VF cardiac arrests, and 11.5% in patients with asystole. With the factors favourable for good outcome listed above, a discharge recovery rate of 50% for patients developing VF in a coronary care unit can be expected.[8] The resuscitation skills of attending personnel are critical to patient outcome; understanding of the underlying pathophysiology is vital to appropriate management.[9]

References

1. Baskett PJ. Cardiopulmonary resuscitation. In: Nimmo WS, Smith G (eds) *Anaesthesia*, pp. 951–974. Oxford: Blackwell, 1989.
2. Cobb LA, Werner J, Trobough G. Sudden cardiac death – a decade's experience without hospital resuscitation. *Mod Con Cardiovasc Dis* 1980; **49**: 31–36.

3. Babbs CF. The evolution of abdominal compression in cardiopulmonary resuscitation. *Acad Emerg Med* 1994; **1**: 469–477.
4. Ornato JP. Use of adrenergic agonists during CPR in adults. *Ann Emerg Med* 1993; **22**: 411–416.
5. Niemann JT. Current concepts: cardiopulmonary resuscitation. *N Engl J Med* 1992; **327**: 1075–1180.
6. Gilston A, Resnekov L. *Cardiorespiratory Resuscitation*. London: Heinemann Medical, 1971.
7. Scott RPF. Cardiac resuscitation in a teaching hospital – a survey of cardiac arrests occurring outside intensive care units and emergency rooms. *Anaesthesia* 1981; **36**: 526–530.
8. Mackintosh AF, Crabb ME, Brennan H, Williams JH, Chamberlain DA. Hospital resuscitation from ventricular fibrillation in Brighton. *Br Med J* 1979; **1**: 511–513.
9. Handley AJ, Swain A (eds). *Advanced Life Support Manual*, 2nd edn. London: Resuscitation Council (UK), 1994.

22

Peripheral nerve damage and repair

G. Rex Holland and Peter P. Robinson

Introduction

The orofacial region is more densely supplied with a greater variety of nerves than any other region of the body. The face, the lips and the oral mucosa have precise tactile, proprioceptive, chemosensitive, nociceptive and thermal sensory mechanisms associated with monitoring the local external environment, inspired air and the composition and physical properties of ingested food and liquids. The finely controlled motor activities involved in facial expression, mastication and speech require exact neuromuscular control. An extensive autonomic efferent innervation controls regional blood flow and secretions from the many exocrine glands in the area. Injury to the nerves in this region can lead to significant functional disturbances.

Peripheral nerve structure

A peripheral nerve, such as the lingual or inferior alveolar nerve, consists of a number of elements. The axon is the peripheral extension of the neuron and its cell body will lie, in the case of most sensory axons, in the sensory ganglion. In the case of autonomic nerves the cell bodies will lie in the cervical chain or peripheral autonomic ganglion, and in motor axons they will be in the motor nucleus. Larger, faster conducting axons (A fibres) are surrounded by a myelin sheath – a multilayered insulation formed by a Schwann cell spiralling around the axon during development. Narrower, slower axons lack this sheath but several are protected within a Schwann cell, tucked into infoldings or pockets. The combination of multiple non-myelinated axons and their protecting Schwann cell is known as a Remak bundle or non-myelinated nerve fibre. A peripheral nerve consists of a large number of myelinated axons and non-myelinated nerve fibres surrounded by a specialized arrangement of connective tissue (Fig. 22.1).

The nerve fibres lie within a loose matrix, the endoneurium, containing collagen fibres, fibroblasts and capillaries and characterized by large extracellular spaces. The collagen fibres are arranged to support the nerve fibre as endoneurial sheaths. Groups of nerve fibres and their surrounding endoneurium are bundled together into fascicles surrounded by a dense, strong connective tissue sheath, the perineurium, that provides both mechanical and chemical protection. The perineurium consists of up to 15 layers of flattened cells, the number of layers being related to the size of the fascicle. The cells are very tightly apposed but between the layers are capillaries and both collagen and elastic fibres. Septa of perineurium subdivide large fascicles. The outer layer of the perineurium merges with the surrounding looser connective tissue, the epineurium, which provides cushioning protection outside and between the fascicles. It varies in extent but is largest near joints and at other sites

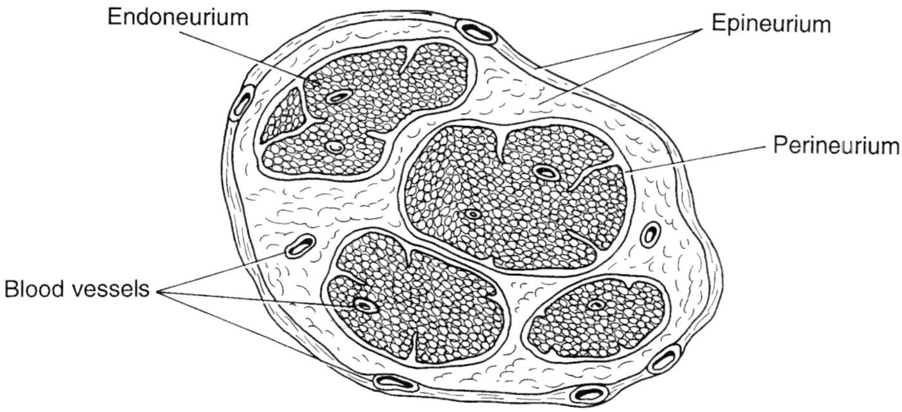

Fig. 22.1 The basic anatomy of a peripheral nerve as seen in cross-section. It consists of several (in this example, four) fascicles. Each fascicle consists of a variable number of myelinated and non-myelinated axons surrounded by a connective tissue sheath, the perineurium. Within the fascicle a loose connective tissue, the endoneurium, supports the axons, occasionally condensing into septa that incompletely subdivide the fascicle. The fascicles are themselves supported in a loose connective tissue, the epineurium, the outer part of which is organized into multiple layers of dense cells and collagen fibres to form a protective sheath. Blood vessels travel in all compartments of the neural connective tissue. When a nerve is transected, both connective tissue and axons are separated. When a nerve is crushed, the connective tissue elements stay in continuity. The denser outer layers of the epineurial sheath provide a material through which sutures can be passed to allow reapposition of transected nerves. A very precise approach calls for the suturing together of individual fascicles via the perineurium, but there is little evidence to suggest that this improves recovery.

where nerves undergo movement. The epineurium contains a vascular plexus from which branches supply the perineurium and endoneurium. The outer layer of the epineurium is denser, delimiting the nerve from the surrounding structures. A superficial adventitial layer, sometimes called the paraneurium, attaches the nerve loosely to the surrounding tissues.

This complex connective tissue ensheathment of the axons is what provides them with protection. The outcome of a given injury is related much more to its effect on the connective tissue sheath than its effect on the axon itself. Following all but the lightest of trauma (which merely disturbs the axon without disrupting it), the distal component of the axon undergoes Wallerian degeneration and must be replaced during recovery by regenerating sprouts. When the axon is thus damaged but the ensheathments remain intact, recovery is good. When the connective tissue elements are damaged, the guidance they provide for regenerating sprouts is lost and the prognosis for recovery is much worse.

Normal nerve function

Effective neural function requires that the special patterns and arrangements of innervation be maintained. When these are disturbed by injury, normal function is not possible. The features of the peripheral nervous system that are most likely to be affected by injury include the following.

Target specificity

Sensory axons are specialized to respond to a limited range of stimuli. That specialization is often conferred by a modification of the axon at its peripheral termination or by an arrangement with a unique receptor such as the taste bud. Motor nerves supply muscle fibres in specific groupings that vary in size (numbers of muscle fibres per motor unit) or in location, allowing for a particular effect in terms of force and direction when the unit is activated. Autonomic nerves form several different groups with varying vasomotor and/or secretomotor functions. When a nerve is injured these special targets and patterns are lost and may not be restored. Reinnervation may occur by collateral branches of other nerves[1,2] but the targets innervated and the pattern created may be inappropriate.

Differential density

Touch discrimination varies in precision, the lips and the tip of the tongue being particularly sensitive. Fine discrimination calls for a high density of innervation that may be lost or reduced following injury.

Characteristic conduction velocity

Nerves of different sensory types vary in conduction velocity. Fine touch, for example, is carried by fast conducting fibres and pain by slow fibres. After damage, recovered nerves have reduced conduction velocities.

Central support

In addition to the metabolic support from the vascular system, every axon is supported and supplied with neurotransmitters by its cell body, agents passing along the nerve by axonal transport. Injury may disturb or disrupt this supply. Temporary disturbances may be reversible but in the majority of situations nerve injury separates the axon distal to the injury site from its central support and it will undergo Wallerian degeneration.

Central connections

The neurons of the peripheral nervous system interact with each other and other neurons via their central connections within the central nervous system. Damage to the peripheral extension of a neuron results in changes in these central elements. If neurons die, for example, their input into the central integration is lost and there may be secondary effects in addition to the loss of specific peripheral or sensory activities. It has been shown, for example, that the neural damage caused by pulpectomy (small fibres) results in changes in the threshold and receptive fields of facial mechanoreceptors (large fibres).[3] Similarly, it is possible that the loss of large-fibre sensory input could result in changes in the perception of small, nociceptive fibre input.

Axon reflexes

It has been suggested that an underestimated function of peripheral afferents is to control blood flow and perhaps other functions by axon reflexes.[4] This mechanism would consist of activity generated in one branch of an axon being carried down another branch of the same axon, resulting in the release of a neuroactive agent that may, for example, result in vasodilatation. While the basic mechanism can be demonstrated experimentally, the physiological extent and importance is not clear. This action would, however, be disrupted by injury.

A classification of nerve injuries

The most widely accepted classifications of nerve injury take into account the importance of the connective tissue elements. A series of definitions originally described by Seddon[5] has been expanded by Sunderland[6] and is shown in Table 22.1.

Nerves may be damaged in a number of ways. Infections directly affecting peripheral nerve include leprosy, diphtheria, herpes zoster and poliomyelitis, and other viruses such as herpes simplex may lie latent within neural tissue, becoming intermittently active. Autoimmune mechanisms are thought to be responsible for Guillain–Barré syndrome and a proportion of facial nerve palsies. Idiopathic degenerative diseases such as inflammatory polyradiculoneuropathy[7] have a peripheral component. Peripheral nerves can also be involved in the pathological changes of more generalized disorders. For example, the small-vessel changes seen in diabetes will produce a peripheral neuropathy, as can other conditions which cause a vasculitis. Severe infections which result in tissue necrosis (e.g. osteomyelitis) will also affect any peripheral nerves in the region. Benign and malignant neoplasms can impinge on peripheral nerves and produce neurological symptoms.

However, the description in this chapter is limited to injuries of traumatic origin that may

Table 22.1 Classification and consequences of nerve injury

Sunderland (1951)[11]	*Sedden (1943)*[5]	*Injury*	*Result*	*Effect*	*Recovery*
First-degree	Neuropraxia	Minor compression	No axonal degeneration or connective tissue disruption Local ischaemia and intraneural oedema. In some cases, local narrowing and segmental demyelination	Temporary conduction block	Full recovery – days if only conduction block, longer if there is segmental demyelination
Second-degree	Axonotmesis	More severe crush	Wallerian degeneration distal to injury site (disintegration and phagocytosis of myelin and axons); endoneurial sheaths intact	Longer loss of sensation	Slow but good recovery. Regenerating axons guided to correct targets by intact endoneurial sheaths. Time course dependent on distance regenerating axons must travel.
Third-degree	Axonotmesis	More severe crush or stretch	Wallerian degeneration distal to injury site; endoneurial sheaths disrupted, perineurium intact	Permanently altered sensation	Endoneurial guidance lost. Appropriate peripheral reconnection incomplete. Limited recovery of sensation
Fourth-degree	Axonotmesis	Very severe crush or stretch	Axonal continuity lost; endoneurium and perineurium disrupted; epineurium intact	Permanently altered sensation	Poor prognosis without surgical intervention
Fifth-degree	Neurotmesis	Transection of entire nerve trunk	Axonal continuity lost; endoneurium, perineurium and epineurium disrupted	Permanently altered sensation	Very poor prognosis without reapposition. Surgery complicated by scarring and separation of cut ends

be encountered in dental practice, and most of which may arise as a complication of oral surgical procedures. As examples, compression injuries to the inferior alveolar nerve may occur when third molars that lie in close proximity to the mandibular canal are being elevated. Transection injuries are likely when the nerve passes between the roots of a third molar that is being extracted. Stretch injuries (usually third- or fourth-degree injuries) may occur to the mental nerves during surgical flap retraction.

This classification does not cover all possibilities, such as partial division combined with stretching, that may occur if a nerve comes into contact with a rotary instrument. Similarly, minor injuries caused by a needle stab during an inferior alveolar nerve block injection[8] or toxic chemical insults that may be induced by local anaesthetic solutions[9] or extruded root canal filling materials[10] are also not included.

Degeneration and regeneration following injury

The events following nerve section have been examined in great detail (see reviews[11,12]). As well as the degeneration that occurs distal to the injury and which was first characterized by Waller,[13] degeneration usually extends a short distance proximally. There are, in addition, responses in the neuron cell body which range from chromatolysis (swelling of the nucleus and condensation of basophilic material) to cell death.[14] The connective tissue elements distal to the injury survive but undergo changes. Schwann cells within the endoneurial sheath proliferate and form the bands of Büngner within a fragmented chain of connective tissue islands that formerly supported axons. If axons reinnervate the area, these connective tissue elements reorganize to fulfil their supporting role (Figs 22.2 and 22.3).

After injury there is a delay before regeneration occurs, during which the neuronal cell body changes its role from maintenance to synthesis. Axonal sprouts then appear at the cut end of the damaged axons, several per axon.[15] The fate of these sprouts and their ability to reinnervate target organs are determined by conditions in the periphery. Neurotrophic substances are produced by the connective tissue elements that formerly supported the axons and the sprouts are attracted towards these.[16] Target tissues also produce neurotrophic substances.[17] When a functional connection is made with a target organ the regenerative process declines. Ideally, one sprout per injured axon would re-establish its connection with an appropriate target and the remaining sprouts die back, but studies have shown that a single axon centrally can support two or more axons in the periphery.[18] Clearly following those injuries in which the connective tissue elements survive, regeneration is more successful as an accurate guiding pathway is in place.

After complete nerve section, regenerating axons enter the endoneurial sheaths of the distal stump at random and may be led to inappropriate targets. A number of consequences may follow. Innervation may not be restored and areas may remain anaesthetic or paralysed. Two sprouts from one axon may survive and innervate separate receptive fields,[18] leading to sensory abnormalities. The obstruction of regenerating axons can cause multiple sprouts to develop and give rise to a neuroma – a disorganized mass of axons and connective tissue. Neuromas may be highly sensitive to mechanical stimuli and circulating catecholamines, and may discharge spontaneously. This is one possible aetiology for the development of dysaesthesia.[19]

Symptoms following injury

Disruption of a sensory nerve will produce anaesthesia or hypoaesthesia (reduced sensation) of the supplied area. This may lead to self-inflicted damage to the affected area. As recovery progresses, paraesthesia (abnormal sensation) occurs and can include tingling, itchiness, coldness, wetness, pins and needles and apparent swelling. These sensations may arise spontaneously or in response to stimulation. As neural activity can originate from the injury site the sensations do not necessarily indicate impending recovery. Misdirected regeneration, in which nerves follow the wrong endoneurial tubes will result in false localization due to misinterpretation at the cortical level. Rarely, nerve injury is followed by long-term pain or

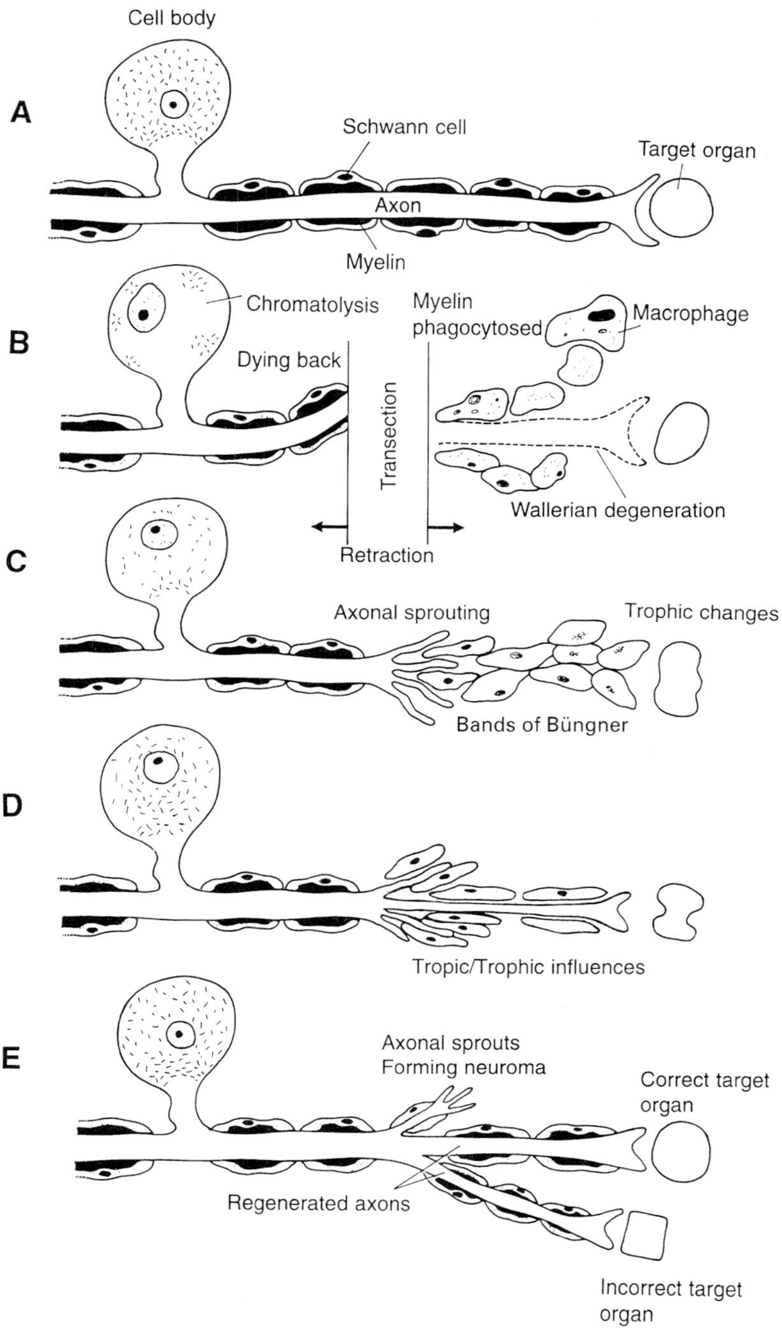

Fig. 22.2 A diagrammatic representation of the fate of a transected axon. (A) An intact myelinated axon with a series of Schwann cells producing the insulating myelin. Transection of the axon (B) results in Wallerian degeneration of the axon distal to the injury. Myelin in the distal Schwann cells breaks down and is phagocytosed by macrophages. The Schwann cells themselves survive but, in the absence of an axon, form groups of cells surrounded by a basement membrane, the bands of Büngner. The target organ may undergo degenerative trophic changes or disappear (e.g. taste buds). Proximally, the axon dies back to the next node of Ranvier. Regeneration begins shortly after injury (C) with changes in the cell body, particularly the nucleus, associated with increased protein synthesis. Multiple sprouts appear from the cut end of the axon and grow towards the distal stump, attracted by neurotrophic substances produced by the cells in the bands of Büngner and/or the target organ. If there is good approximation of the nerve ends, the sprouts will rapidly become reassociated with the isolated Schwann cells and be guided to the target organ (D). The Schwann cells reorganize and form new myelin, and the relationship of the axon terminal and the target organ can be re-established (E). If the cut ends of the nerve trunk are widely separated, it is more unlikely that good recovery will occur and abnormalities may persist. Target organs may be left denervated and may atrophy. Sprouts may locate and innervate inappropriate targets or, if no target organ is located, axonal sprouts may persist as a neuroma (E).

discomfort and this may present in several possible ways. Hyperaesthesia is an increased sensitivity in the affected area, and hyperalgesia is an increase in pain sensation evoked by painful stimuli. Allodynia, which is a painful response to an innocuous stimulus, may also occur. Together these unpleasant disturbed sensory patterns should be termed dysaesthesias. Clinically there is a spectrum of changes which are often difficult to categorize. Symptoms resulting from injury to specific nerves will be described below.

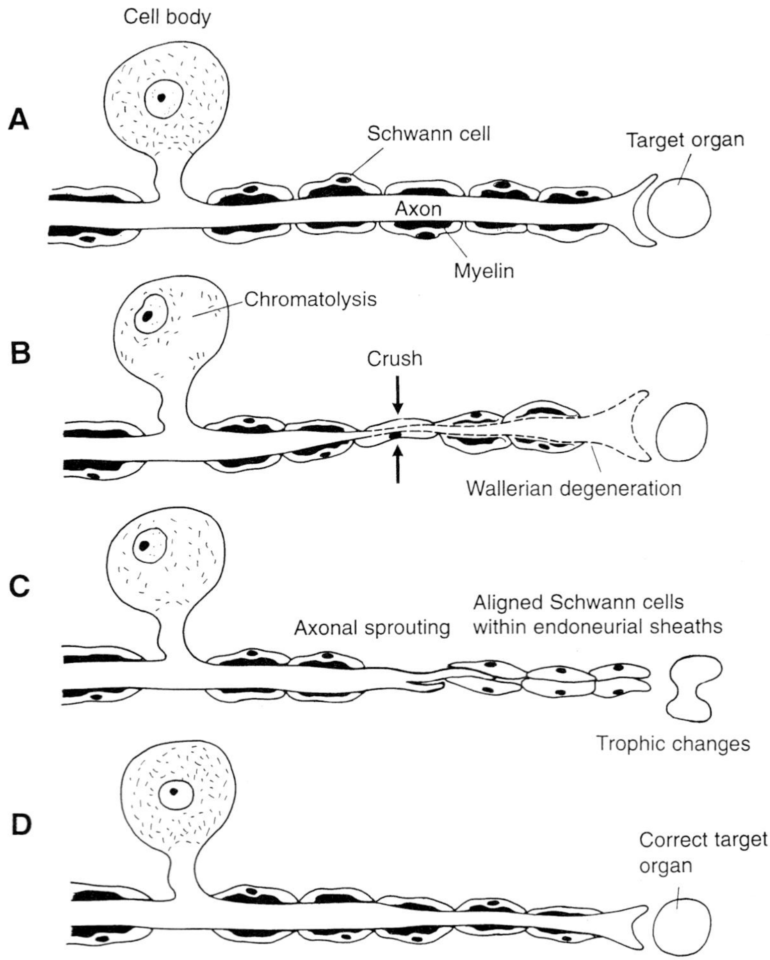

Fig. 22.3 The fate of a crushed axon. (A) The intact axon. After a crush injury the distal axon undergoes Wallerian degeneration but, in contrast with a transected axon, continuity of the supporting Schwann cells and endoneurial sheaths is not lost (B). These tissues remain in alignment and, when the damaged axon sprouts, the guidance they provide returns the growing axon terminal to the target organ (C). Normal relationships (and usually function) are restored with little inappropriate reinnervation (D).

Prevalence and consequences of nerve injuries following dental procedures

Tooth extraction and pulpectomy

When teeth are extracted or the pulp removed as part of a root canal procedure, several hundred axons are severed and their target organ removed. Such loss of sensory input has been described as deafferentation and some chronic pain syndromes have been linked to this process.[20] In experimental animals changes in the activity and morphology of central neurons have been reported in response to pulpectomy and tooth extraction[3,21,22] and one report of behavioural changes, possibly indicating pain, has been published.[23] However, symptoms are rare following these routine clinical procedures unless a whole nerve trunk is also traumatized. Histological animal studies suggest that after tooth extraction[24,25] and pulpectomy,[26] pulpal and periodontal fibres reorganize into nerve bundles and innervate new targets. As indicated above, obstruction of regenerating axons could give rise to a neuroma and it has been suggested that activity in neuromas formed at extraction sites may be responsible for some examples of chronic orofacial pain.[27] Conclusive evidence for this aetiology is lacking.

Removal of impacted teeth

One of the most common causes of nerve injury in the orofacial region is surgical removal of impacted mandibular third molars, because of the proximity of these teeth to the inferior alveolar and lingual nerves.

Inferior aveolar nerve

Reported incidences of inferior alveolar nerve injury range from 1.3%[28] to 7.8%.[29] The average incidence reported in a series of 17 studies published since 1940 (taking into account the number of cases in each study) is approximately 4%.[30–32] Some anatomical arrangements predispose to injury, including proximity of the molar roots to the mandibular canal,[31,33–35] the presence of complete bone coverage[32] and the angulation of the impacted tooth; the incidence is higher with mesioangular[31] or horizontal[31,34] teeth. The incidence has also been shown to rise with the age of the patient, from 1.2% in a 14–24-year-old group, through 2.4% in the 25–34-year-old group, to 9.7% in patients over 35.[36]

Injury to the inferior alveolar nerve causes ipsilateral sensory disturbance from the skin on the lower lip and chin, the oral mucosa of the lower lip, the buccal gingivae and mucosa from the midline to the premolar region, as well as the pulps and periodontal ligaments of the mandibular teeth. Autonomic changes, though occasionally detectable, are rarely reported.[37] Fortunately, in most instances, complete anaesthesia is only temporary and in one study the ability to detect light touch stimuli had recovered in all areas by 4 months after nerve compression and by 8 months after nerve section.[37] However, some sensory abnormalities persist and reports suggest that permanent changes following inferior alveolar nerve injury occur in up to 2.2% of cases with an average incidence of 0.7%.[28,29,32,34,38] Persistence of sensory abnormalities also relates to the type of initial injury, as long-term sensory change occurs in all patients who have experienced inferior alveolar nerve transection and in about half of those who have suffered compression.[37] There is also little evidence of improvement beyond 9 months following compression and after 12 months following nerve section.[37]

There seem to be two patterns of recovery following inferior alveolar nerve injury: either uniform improvement over the entire anaesthetic area (presumably due to recovery or regeneration of nerves that previously supplied the area) or shrinkage in size of the affected area (by collateral ingrowth of sprouts from adjacent nerves).[37,39]

Lingual nerve

In the third molar area the lingual nerve lies between 2 mm above and 7 mm below the alveolar crest in the vertical plane, and 0–3 mm from the lingual plate in the horizontal plane, lying directly against the bone in 62% of cases.[40] Reports of the incidence of lingual nerve injury following third molar removal vary over a wide range, from 0.2%[41] to 22%.[42] The average incidence reported in a series of 14 studies published since 1970 (taking into account the number of cases in each study) is approximately 7%.[30,31,43,44] On average, 0.7% of cases show permanent sensory loss.[29,32,43,44]

The variability in incidence of nerve damage may be attributed to a number of factors, including differences in time interval following surgery before testing, differences in the tests used, and variations in the surgical technique. Elevation of a lingual mucoperiosteal flap, as is common practice in the UK, raises the chances of injury considerably.[45] Injury is also more likely when the tooth is deeply impacted and the surgery long and difficult.[43,44]

The lingual nerve in the third molar region contains mechanosensitive, thermosensitive and nociceptive afferents, and vasomotor fibres. In addition it has at this point acquired taste fibres from the facial nerve via the chorda tympani, and autonomic fibres controlling secretion in the submandibular and sublingual salivary glands. Injury to the nerve results in ipsilateral sensory loss from the dorsal and ventral surfaces of the tongue anterior to the circumvallate papillae, and from the mucosa and gingiva lingual to the mandibular teeth. Taste sensation will be lost from this region of the tongue and taste buds and fungiform papillae will disappear but will redifferentiate after reinnervation.[46] Patients do not report changes attributable to the loss of secretomotor or vasomotor fibres and often do not notice the loss of taste. Interestingly, the recovery of tongue sensation appears to begin in the anterior region[47] but this may merely reflect the higher density of nerve fibres in this region.[48]

Other nerves

The surgical removal of impacted lower premolars can result in injury to the mental nerve, usually during retraction of the mucoperiosteal flap.[49,50] The mylohyoid nerve may be injured during the removal of lower third molars, most commonly when using the lingual split technique, with a reported incidence of 1.4%.[32] This causes sensory loss from a small area of skin on the point of the chin.[51] Overextension of a relieving incision up the external oblique ridge during third molar surgery may damage the buccal nerve,[52] resulting in loss of sensation from part of the buccal mucosa.[53] The incidence of this complication is not known. The nasopalatine nerve may be severed during the elevation of a palatal flap to permit extraction of impacted upper canines but the presence of a second innervation from the greater (anterior) palatine nerves prevents sensory loss.[54]

Facial fractures

Displacement of the bone fragments can lead to significant damage to the inferior alveolar nerve after mandibular fractures;[55] to the infraorbital nerve after fractures of the zygomatic complex;[56] and to the facial nerve after temporal bone fractures,[57] mandibular condyle fractures[58,59] and unfortunate dislocations.[60] The majority of injuries will be due to nerve compression, or stretching during displacement, and permanent sensory disturbance may follow both mandibular and zygomatic fractures.[61] It has been suggested that the techniques used to provide fixation of fractured mandibles may themselves contribute to the extent of nerve damage[55,62] and that rigid fixation of fractures of the zygomatic complex may reduce permanent disturbance;[56] there is no good evidence from controlled trials to confirm these suggestions.

Osteotomies

Osteotomies of both maxilla and mandible may result in nerve damage. Estimates of the proportion of patients experiencing sensory disturbance following a sagittal split osteotomy of the mandible vary, but not widely. Yoshida *et al.*[63] reported that shortly after surgery 67% of patients show sensory loss; Walter and Gregg[64] reported a similar incidence of 69.4% shortly after surgery. Permanent sensory disturbance has been reported to occur in 8%,[65] 15%[63] or 25%[66] of patients. The more recent the report, however, the lower the proportion of patients with long-term changes, presumably due to improved surgical technique. Facial nerve palsy has been reported as a very rare (0.26%) complication of sagittal split osteotomy.[67–69] Although vertical subsigmoid osteotomies should divide the ramus of the mandible proximal to the mandibular foramen, the incidence of inferior alveolar nerve disturbance can be quite high (acute 36%, long-term 8%[70]). With extensive maxillary osteotomies, sensory loss in the area of the infraorbital nerve is as high as 79%.[71] In two recent studies 6 months after Le Fort I osteotomies, the region supplied by the greater palatine and superior alveolar nerves showed incomplete recovery, while the infraorbital region showed full recovery at 6–12 weeks.[72,73]

Salivary gland surgery

Removal of the submandibular salivary gland can result in damage to the lingual nerve as it crosses the submandibular duct, or the hypoglossal nerve which lies deep to the gland. Parotid gland surgery places all branches of the facial nerve at risk and can also result in Frey's syndrome, which is gustatory sweating. This is thought to result from regeneration of the divided parasympathetic secretomotor fibres in the auriculotemporal nerve to sweat glands in the skin. This inappropriate reinnervation is possible because both types of terminal are cholinergic.

Experimental observations on injured trigeminal nerves

Orofacial nerves respond to injury in generally the same way as spinal nerves. However, studies on the trigeminal system have revealed some features of the response that are attributable to special local characteristics. The trigeminal nerves are shorter than their spinal counterparts and injuries often occur much closer to the central ganglia and nuclei than in the spinal system. Central responses tend to be greater the closer the injury is to the central nervous system.[74] In addition, some trigeminal branches, in particular the lingual nerve, contain a particularly wide variety of nerve fibre types, including those subserving general sensation, special sense, nociception, and vasomotor and secretomotor functions, which renders them highly susceptible to disorganization at the injury site. Some trigeminal branches, such as the inferior alveolar, follow an intra-bony course where mechanical protection and support are greater than in spinal nerves, but there is also the potential for compression due to oedema in the canal. The inferior alveolar and lingual nerves have been subjected to the most extensive experimental observations.

Inferior alveolar nerve

For much of its course the inferior alveolar nerve is within the mandibular canal and firmly supported by connective tissue. When transected the nerve will not retract and apposition is usually good. This leads to excellent recovery, which has been documented in a number of experimental studies.[75–79] Though excellent, the recovery is not perfect. Three months after transection, axon counts proximal to the injury show a reduction in the number of non-myelinated axons, whereas distally there is an increase in fibre number, due to branching.[78] Target organs do re-establish their connections. The dental pulp is reinnervated but with a reduced number of smaller fibres with thinner myelin sheaths.[77] The regenerated fibres have reduced conduction velocities, greater variation in mechanoreceptive fields and produce smaller compound action potentials in the teeth when stimulated.[75] Some functional links may be re-established better than others. Pulpal axons will reinnervate dentinal tubules and allow the dentine to regain its sensitivity to mechanical and thermal stimuli,[80] whereas reinnervated periodontal mechanoreceptors have significantly higher force thresholds, lower discharge frequencies and adapt more rapidly than normal.[79] During normal recovery the reinnervating axons develop from sprouts arising from the central end of the transected nerve. If regeneration of the nerve is impeded, sprouts from other ipsilateral and contralateral nerves form collateral branches that will reinnervate the tissue, though to a lesser extent than would occur in unimpeded recovery.[1,75] It appears that the stimulus which initiates this collateral ingrowth may be nerve growth factor.[81,82]

Lingual nerve

The lingual nerve differs from the inferior alveolar in that its vulnerable section lies within a thin layer of overlying soft tissue. When transected the cut ends of the nerve retract and may become misaligned and separated by scar tissue. Regeneration across a gap is much less successful than regeneration between closely apposed segments. The lingual nerve also differs in being composed of a broad range of distinct fibre types. This, combined with the separation of the proximal and distal components after transection, makes the regeneration of fibres along appropriate endoneurial tubes less likely. This is borne out experimentally by the poor level of recovery after unrepaired nerve section.[48,83] The mechanosensitive axons that do recover have smaller receptive fields and higher thresholds than normal. There is also a reduction in the proportion and sensitivity of gustatory and thermosensitive axons in the chorda tympani, and autonomic secretomotor and vasomotor responses are reduced.[48,83] Crush injuries do not result in separation of the nerve trunk and experimentally the innervation of the tongue following this type of injury differs little from normal.[48,83,84] In patients suffering from long-standing sensory loss following lingual nerve injury it is likely that the nerve has been partially or completely transected, although very occasionally an intact nerve constricted by scar tissue can result in this problem (Figs 22.4–22.7).

Techniques for diagnosis and assessment of recovery

Thorough reviews of the evaluation of trigeminal nerve injuries[85] and the monitoring of recovery[86] have recently been published. The subjective assessment given by the patient should be followed by a physical examination and sensory testing. The relatively small number of patients complaining of persistent pain/dysaesthesia may require additional assessments of their ability to cope with the condition. This would be similar to that applied to all

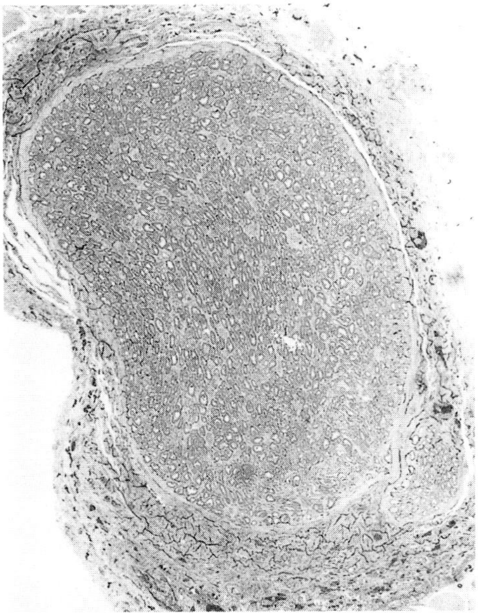

Fig. 22.4 A light micrograph of normal cat lingual nerve. It consists of two fascicles, one large (the lingual branch of the trigeminal nerve) and one small (the chorda tympani) surrounded by a common epineurium. Toluidine blue × 140.

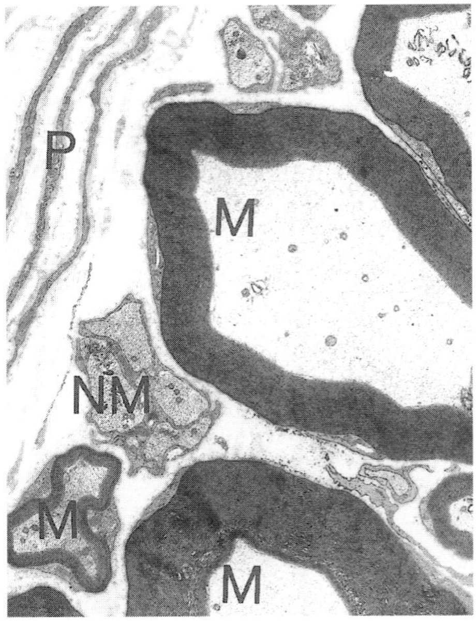

Fig. 22.6 An electron micrograph of a normal cat lingual nerve. Both large and small myelinated (M) and non-myelinated (NM) axons are present. Part of the perineurium (P) is also visible. × 8000.

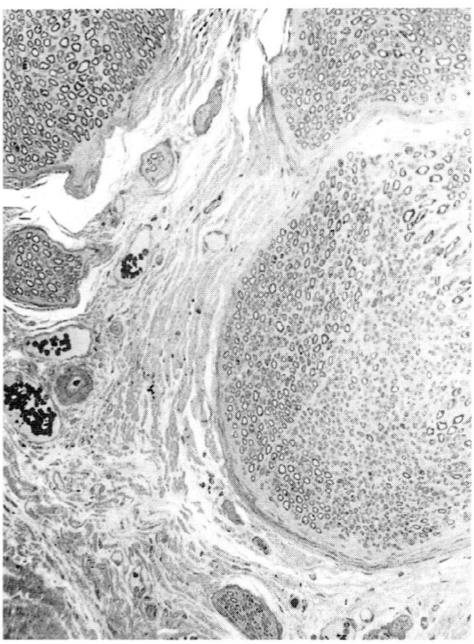

Fig. 22.5 A light micrograph of part of a lingual nerve that was transected 3 months earlier but not repaired. This section is taken distal to the injury and shows extensive regeneration. During recovery the nerve trunk has divided into multiple fascicles of varying size. Toluidine blue × 140.

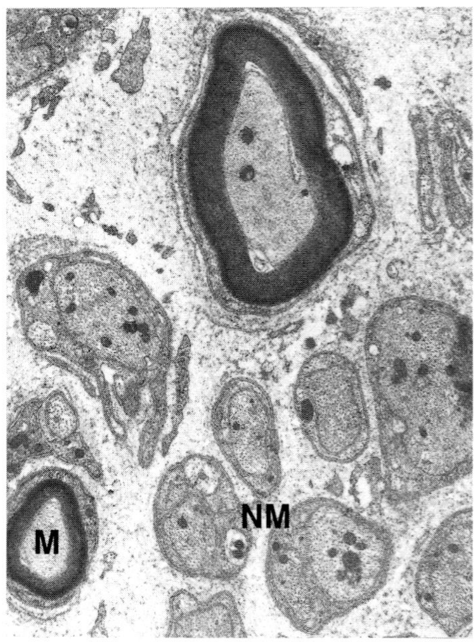

Fig. 22.7 An electron micrograph of part of a lingual nerve that was transected 3 months earlier but not repaired. This section is taken distal to the injury and shows regenerating fibres. There is a predominance of small myelinated (M) and non-myelinated (NM) axons. × 8000.

chronic pain patients and is beyond the scope of the present discussion. The much more common condition of reduced or absent sensation has been assessed with a number of tests which range from the simple perception of a wisp of cotton wool, a blunt probe and pinprick,[39] to include two-point discrimination,[87] thermal and electrical stimulation,[88] sharp/blunt differentiation,[43] brush stroke direction[64] or somatosensory evoked potentials.[44]

In one study the tests that were most likely to detect persistent sensory abnormalities were localization, pinprick sensation threshold and two-point discrimination,[37] although the most sensitive (and important) indicator is the patient's subjective report.

No accepted standard protocol for monitoring sensory changes exists but a series of simple tests may be recommended:[89]

1. Light touch sensation: a von Frey hair (a filament of nylon suture mounted on a rigid handle and adjusted in length to produce a known bending force of 20 mN) is applied randomly and the area in which this cannot be felt is mapped.
2. Pinprick (pain) sensation: a spring-mounted pin producing a variable force of up to 150 mN[6] is applied randomly and the area in which this cannot be felt is mapped.
3. Pinprick (pain) sensation threshold: the same instrument is applied with increasing force to normal and affected areas and the patient is asked to indicate the point at which the sensation becomes sharp rather than dull.
4. Two-point discrimination: pairs of blunt probes with separations ranging from 2 to 20 mm[6,89] are drawn across the surface and the minimum separation consistently reported as two is the discrimination threshold.

During the initial stages of recovery it is not possible to distinguish between anaesthesia resulting from nerve crush or that following nerve section. Eventual return to normal two-point discrimination and localization indicates that the injury is most likely to have resulted from nerve compression.

Tests must be performed at intervals which permit decisions on whether or not surgical intervention is indicated. Accordingly, we recommend that initial observations should be made within 2 weeks of the injury. For the inferior alveolar nerve, tests should be repeated at 1, 3, 6 and 12 months after the injury and for the lingual nerve should be repeated at monthly intervals until there is evidence of progressive recovery, and less frequently thereafter.

Treatment

Inferior alveolar nerve

A variety of surgical approaches have been advocated as follows:

1. Decompression.[90–92]
2. Approximation and suture of cut ends.[87,92,93]
3. Grafting.[94–98]
4. Neurolysis (release of constricting scar tissue at the site of injury).[93]

Although good overall success rates are reported (80%;[92] 73.7%[99]), there is little objective evidence to support this, and no clear comparisons between the outcome following different surgical techniques. The case for early or delayed repair has been discussed by Donoff[100] and Gregg.[101] At present, a realistic approach would be:

1. For patients presenting with paraesthesia in the early postoperative period, surgical intervention is not indicated but their progress should be monitored to ensure adequate functional recovery.
2. For patients with anaesthesia, radiographs should be taken to ensure that bone has not been dislodged into the mandibular canal, creating an obstruction to regeneration.[87] Any obstruction present should be removed. Otherwise, immediate repair of the nerve is indicated only if the nerve has been surgically divided and the nerve ends have not remained in apposition in the mandibular canal. The only other positive indication for microreconstructive surgery is in patients with persistent traumatic pain or dysaesthesia suspected to be arising from a neuroma.[102] Excision of the damaged segment of nerve sometimes relieves or reduces the dysaesthesia but it may recur and without repair the excision may also leave permanent anaesthesia.

Lingual nerve

If accidental transection of the lingual nerve is detected at operation, it should be repaired immediately using epineurial sutures. Usually, however, injury is only discovered as impaired sensation following surgery. At that stage it is not possible to distinguish between anaesthesia caused by a crush injury and that caused by nerve section, and as the prognosis from a crush injury is good without intervention, no treatment is indicated initially. Surgical repair is, however, indicated if there is no clear evidence of progressive sensory recovery by 3–4 months after the injury.[47] This short delay does not appear to worsen the outcome significantly.[103,104] If at exploration the nerve is intact and appears normal but is constricted by scar tissue, treatment should be limited to freeing of the nerve (neurolysis). This is rare and much more commonly there is a clear area of nerve damage.

A neuroma may be visible as a substantial expansion at the injury site. The neuroma and damaged area should be removed and if, after mobilization of the central and distal stumps, the gap is less than 1 cm, the cut ends of the nerve can be approximated directly using epineurial sutures.[105,106] For gaps greater than 1 cm, grafts may be necessary. Donor tissue from the sural or great auricular nerves has been used but the results are often poor.[107,108] Frozen muscle autografts are effective experimentally[109,110] and may provide an alternative which avoids donor site morbidity.

Success is variable,[107] but can be acceptable, even after late repair.[111] LaBanc and Gregg[99] report an overall success rate of 80%.

Acknowledgement

We would like to thank Mr P. Elliott for drawing Figures 22.1–22.3.

References

1. Holland GR, Robinson PP. A morphological study of the collateral reinnervation of the cat's canine tooth. *Exp Neurol* 1987; **98**: 489–498.
2. Kinnman E, Aldskogius H. Collateral reinnervation of taste buds after chronic sensory denervation: a morphological study. *J Comp Neurol* 1988; **270**: 569–574.
3. Hu JW, Dostrovsky JO, Lenz YE, Ball GJ, Sessle BJ. Tooth pulp deafferentation is associated with functional alterations in the properties of neurons in the trigeminal spinal tract nucleus *J Neurophysiol* 1986; **56**: 1650–1668.
4. Olgart L, Edwall L, Gazelius B. Involvement of afferent nerves in pulpal blood-flow reactions in response to clinical and experimental procedures in the cat. *Arch Oral Biol* 1991; **36**: 575–581.
5. Seddon HJ. Three types of nerve injury. *Brain* 1943; **66**: 237–288.
6. Sunderland S. *Nerves and Nerve Injuries*, 2nd edn. Edinburgh: Churchill Livingstone, 1978.
7. Dyck PJ, Lais, AC, Ohta M, Bastron, JA, Okazaki H, Groover RV. Chronic inflammatory polyradiculoneuropathy. *Mayo Clin Proc* 1975; **50**: 621–637.
8. Stacy GC, Hajjar G. Barbed needle and inexplicable paresthesias and trismus after dental regional anaesthesia. *Oral Surg Oral Med Oral Pathol* 1994; **77**: 585–588.
9. Nickel AA. A retrospective study of paresthesia of the dental alveolar nerves. *Anesth Prog* 1990; **37**: 42–45.
10. Brodin P. Neurotoxic and analgesic effects of root canal cements and pulp-protecting dental materials. *Endodont Dent Traumatol* 1988; **4**: 1–11.
11. Sunderland S. A classification of peripheral nerve injuries producing loss of function. *Brain* 1951; **74**: 491–516.
12. Lundborg G. *Nerve Injury and Repair*. Edinburgh: Churchill Livingstone, 1988.
13. Waller AV. Experiments on the section of the glossopharyngeal and hypoglossal nerves of the frog, and observations of the alterations produced thereby in the structure of their primitive fibres. *Phil Trans Roy Soc* 1850; **5**: 924–925.
14. Holland GR, Robinson PP. Cell counts in the trigeminal ganglion of the cat after inferior alveolar nerve injuries. *J Anat* 1990; **171**: 179–186.
15. Bray GM, Aguayo AJ. Regeneration of peripheral unmyelinated nerves. Fate of the axonal sprouts which develop after injury. *J Anat* 1974; **117**: 517–529.
16. Kuffler DP. Promoting and directing axon outgrowth. *Mol Neurobiol* 1994; **9**: 233–243.
17. Lundborg G, Dahlin L, Danielsen N, Zhao Q. Trophism, tropism, and specificity in nerve regeneration. *J Reconstr Microsurg* 1994; **10**: 345–354.
18. Horch KW, Lisney SJW. On the number and nature of regenerating myelinated axons after lesions of cutaneous nerves in the cat. *J Physiol* 1981; **313**: 275–286.
19. Devor M. Neuropathic pain and injured nerve: peripheral mechanisms. In: Wells JCD, Woolf CJ (eds) *Pain Mechanisms and Management*, pp. 619–630. Edinburgh: Churchill Livingstone, 1991.
20. Tasker RR, Organ LW, Hawrylyshyn P. Deafferentation and causalgia. *Res Publ Assoc Res Nerv Ment Dis* 1980; **58**: 305–329.

21. Aldskogius H, Arvidsson J, Grant G. The reaction of primary sensory neurons to peripheral nerve injury with particular emphasis on transganglionic changes. *Brain Res* 1985; **357**: 27–46.
22. Johnson LR, Westrum LE, Canfield RC. Ultrastructural study of transganglionic degeneration following dental lesions. *Exp Brain Res* 1983; **52**: 226–234.
23. Black RG. A laboratory model for trigeminal neuralgia. In: Bonica JJ (ed) *Advances in Neurology* vol. 4. pp. 651–658. Raven Press, New York, 1974
24. Fried K, Arvidsson J, Robertson B, Pfaller K. Anterograde horseradish peroxidase tracing and immunohistochemistry of trigeminal ganglion tooth pulp neurons after dental nerve lesions in the rat. *Neuroscience* 1991; **43**: 269–278.
25. Mason AG, Holland GR. The reinnervation of healing extraction sockets in the ferret. *J Dent Res* 1993; **72**: 1215–1221.
26. Holland GR. A histological comparison of periapical inflammatory and neural responses to two endodontic sealers in the ferret. *Arch Oral Biol* 1994; **39**: 539–544.
27. Ratner EJ, Person P, Kleinman DJ, Shklar G, Socransky SS. Jawbone cavities and trigeminal and atypical facial neuralgias. *Oral Surg Oral Med Oral Pathol* 1979; **48**: 3–20.
28. Schultze-Mosgau S, Reich RH. Assessment of inferior alveolar and lingual nerve disturbances after dentoalveolar surgery, and of recovery of sensitivity. *Int J Oral Maxillofac Surg* 1993; **22**: 214–217.
29. Rood JP. Permanent damage to inferior alveolar and lingual nerves during the removal of impacted mandibular third molars. Comparison of two methods of bone removal *Brit Dent J* 1992; **172**: 108–110.
30. Goldberg MH, Nemarich AN, Marco WP. Complications after mandibular third molar surgery: a statistical analysis of 500 consecutive procedures in private practice. *J Am Dent Assoc* 1985; **111**: 277–279.
31. Wofford, DT, Miller, RI. Prospective study of dysesthesia following odontectomy of impacted mandibular third molars. *J Oral Maxillofac Surg* 1987; **45**: 15–19.
32. Carmichael FA, McGowan DA. Incidence of nerve damage following third molar removal: a West of Scotland oral surgery research group study. *Br J Oral Maxillofac Surg* 1992; **30**: 78–82.
33. Howe GL, Poynton HG. Prevention of damage to the inferior dental nerve during the extraction of mandibular third molars. *Br Dent J* 1960; **109**: 355–563.
34. Kipp DP, Goldstein BH, Weiss WW. Dysesthesia after mandibular third molar surgery: a retrospective study. *J Am Dent Assoc* 1980; **100**: 185–192.
35. Rood JP, Shehab BA. The radiological prediction of inferior alveolar nerve injury during third molar surgery. *Br J Oral Maxillofac Surg* 1990; **28**: 20–25.
36. Bruce RA, Fredrickson GC, Small GS. Age of patients and morbidity associated with mandibular third molar surgery. *J Amer Dent Ass* 1980; **101**: 240–245.
37. Robinson PP. Observations on the recovery of sensation following inferior alveolar nerve injuries. *Br J Oral Maxillofac Surg* 1988; **26**: 177–189.
38. Rood JP. Degrees of injury to the inferior alveolar nerve sustained during the removal of impacted mandibular third molars by the lingual split technique. *Br J Oral Surg* 1983; **21**: 103–116.
39. Rood JP. Lingual split technique. Damage to inferior alveolar and lingual nerves during removal of impacted mandibular third molars. *Br Dent J* 1983; **154**: 402–403.
40. Kiesselbach JE, Chamberlain JG. Clinical and anatomic observations on the relationship of the lingual nerve to the mandibular third molar region. *J Oral Maxillofac Surg* 1984; **42**: 565–567.
41. Van Gool AV, Ten Bosch JJ, Boering, G. Clinical consequences of complaints and complications after removal of the mandibular third molar. *Int J Oral Surg* 1977; **6**: 29–37.
42. Von Arx DP, Simpson MT. The effect of dexamethasone on neuropraxia following third molar surgery. *Br J Oral Maxillofac Surg* 1989; **27**: 477–480.
43. Mason DA. Lingual nerve damage following lower third molar surgery. *Int J Oral Maxillofac Surg* 1988; **17**: 290–294.
44. Blackburn CW, Bramley PA. Lingual nerve damage associated with the removal of lower third molars. *Br Dent J* 1989; **167**: 103–107.
45. Robinson PP, Smith KG. Lingual nerve damage during lower third molar removal: a comparison of two surgical methods. *Br Dent J* 1996; **180**: 456–461.
46. Robinson PP, Winkles P. The number and distribution of fungiform papillae and taste buds after lingual nerve injuries in cats. *Arch Oral Biol* 1991; **36**: 885–891.
47. Blackburn CW. A method of assessment in cases of lingual nerve injury. *Br J Oral Maxillofac Surg* 1990; **28**: 238–245.
48. Robinson PP. The effect of injury on the properties of afferent fibres in the lingual nerve. *Br J Oral Maxillofac Surg* 1992; **30**: 39–45.
49. Simpson HE. Injuries to the inferior dental and mental nerves. *J Oral Surg* 1958; **16**: 300–305.
50. Bodner L, Oberman M, Shteyer A. Mental nerve neuropathy associated with compound odontoma. *Oral Surg Oral Med Oral Pathol* 1987; **63**: 658–660.
51. Roberts GDD, Harris M. Neuropraxia of the mylohyoid nerve and submental analgesia. *Br J Oral Surg* 1973; **11**: 110–113.
52. Hendy CW, Smith KG, Robinson PP. The surgical anatomy of the buccal nerve. *Br J Oral Maxillofac Surg* 1995; **34**: 457–460.
53. Hendy CW, Robinson, PP. The sensory distribution of the buccal nerve. *Br J Oral Maxillofac Surg* 1994; **32**: 384–386.

54. Langford RJ. The contribution of the nasopalatine nerve to sensation of the hard palate. *Br J Oral Maxillofac Surg* 1989; **27**: 379–386.
55. Iizuka T, Lindqvist C. Sensory disturbances associated with rigid internal fixation of mandibular fractures. *J Oral Maxillofac Surg* 1991; **49**: 1264–1268.
56. De Man K, Bax W. The influence of the mode of treatment of zygomatic bone fractures on the healing process of the infraorbital nerve. *Br J Oral Maxillofac Surg* 1988; **26**: 419–425.
57. Grobman LR, Pollak A, Fisch U. Entrapment injury of the facial nerve resulting from longitudinal fracture of the temporal bone. *Otolaryngol Head Neck Surg* 1989; **101**: 404–408.
58. Goin DW. Facial nerve paralysis secondary to mandibular fracture. *Laryngoscope* 1980; **90**: 1777–1785.
59. Brookes CN. Facial nerve paralysis complicating bilateral fractures of the mandible: a case report and review of the literature. *Br J Oral Maxillofac Surg* 1988; **26**: 149–154.
60. Ferguson JW, Stewart IA, Whitley BD. Lateral displacement of the intact mandibular condyle. Review of literature and report of case with associated facial nerve palsy. *J Craniomaxillofac Surg* 1989; **17**: 125–127.
61. Larsen OD, Nielsen A. Mandibular fractures. II. A follow-up study of 229 patients. *Scand J Plast Reconstr Surg* 1976; **10**: 219–226.
62. Blakey GH, Zuniga JR. Lingual nerve injury associated with superior border wire fixation. *Int J Adult Orthodont Orthognath Surg* 1992; **7**: 115–117.
63. Yoshida T, Nagamine T, Kobayashi T *et al.* Impairment of the inferior alveolar nerve after sagittal split osteotomy. *J Craniomaxillofac Surg* 1989; **17**: 271–217.
64. Walter TM, Gregg JM. Analysis of postsurgical neurologic alteration in the trigeminal nerve. *J Oral Surg* 1979; **37**: 410–414.
65. Leira JI, Gilhuis-Moe OT. Sensory impairment following sagittal split osteotomy for correction of mandibular retrognathism. *Int J Adult Orthodon Orthognath Surg* 1991; **6**: 161–167.
66. Rittersma J. Total mandibular alveolar osteotomy. *J Oral Surg* 1981; **39**: 903–906.
67. De Vries K, Devriese PP, Hovinga J, Van Den Akker HP. Facial palsy after sagittal split osteotomies. A survey of 1747 sagittal split osteotomies. *J Craniomaxillofac Surg* 1993; **21**: 50–53
68. Zafarulla MY. Iatrogenic facial nerve injury. *Int J Oral Surg* 1985; **14**: 544–546.
69. Dendy RA. Facial nerve paralysis following sagittal split mandibular osteotomy: A case report. *Br J Oral Surg* 1973; **11**: 101–105.
70. Hall HD, Mckenna SJ. Further refinement and evaluation of intraoral vertical ramus osteotomy. *J Oral Maxillofac Surg* 1987; **45**: 684–688.
71. Brouns JJ, Freihofer HP. Long-term results on the quadrangular osteotomy. *Int J Oral Maxillofac Surg* 1992; **21**: 192–198.
72. Rosenberg A, Sailer HF. A prospective study on changes in the sensibility of the oral mucosa and the mucosa of the upper lip after Le Fort I osteotomy. *J Craniomaxillofac Surg* 1994; **22**: 286–293.
73. Shehab Al-Din OF, Coghlan KM, Magennis P. Sensory nerve disturbance following Le Fort I osteotomy. *Int J Oral Maxillofac Surg* 1996; **25**: 13–19.
74. Lieberman HR. Some factors affecting retrograde neuronal responses to axonal lesions. In: Bellairs R, Gray EG (eds) *Essays on the Nervous System*, pp. 71–105. Oxford: Clarendon Press, 1974.
75. Robinson PP. Reinnervation of teeth, mucous membrane and skin following section of the inferior alveolar nerve in the cat. *Brain Res* 1981; **220**: 241–253.
76. Fried K, Erdelyi G. Inferior alveolar nerve regeneration and incisor pulpal reinnervation following intramandibular neurotomy in the cat. *Brain Res* 1982; **244**: 239–268.
77. Holland GR, Robinson PP. Reinnervation of the canine tooth pulp after section of the inferior alveolar nerve in the cat. *Brain Res* 1985; **329**: 300–303.
78. Holland GR, Robinson PP. The number and size of axons central and peripheral to inferior alveolar nerve injuries in the cat. *J Anat* 1990; **173**: 129–137.
79. Loescher AR, Robinson PP. Properties of reinnervated periodontal mechanoreceptors after inferior alveolar nerve injuries in cats. *J Neurophysiol* 1989; **62**: 979–983.
80. Holland GR, Matthews B, Robinson PP. An electrophysiological and morphological study of the innervation and reinnervation of cat dentine. *J Physiol* 1987; **386**: 31–43.
81. Doubleday B, Robinson PP. The role of nerve growth factor in collateral reinnervation by cutaneous C-fibres in the rat. *Brain Res* 1992; **593**: 179–184.
82. Doubleday B, Robinson PP. Nerve growth factor depletion reduces collateral sprouting of cutaneous mechanoreceptive and tooth-pulp axons in ferrets. *J Physiol* 1994; **481**: 709–718.
83. Robinson PP. The reinnervation of the tongue and salivary glands after lingual nerve injuries in cats. *Brain Res* 1989; **483**: 259–271.
84. Holland GR, Robinson PP. A quantitative morphological study of the recovery of cat lingual nerves after transection or crushing. *J Anat* 1995; **188**: 289–297.
85. Zuniga JR, Essick GK. A contemporary approach to the clinical evaluation of trigeminal nerve injuries. In: Labanc JP, Gregg JM (eds) *Oral and Maxillofacial Surgery Clinics of North America*, vol. 4. pp. 353–368. Philadelphia: WB Saunders, 1992.
86. Essick, G. K. Comprehensive clinical evaluation of perioral sensory function. In: Labanc JP, Gregg JM (eds) *Oral and Maxillofacial Surgery Clinics of North America: Trigeminal Nerve Injury: Diagnosis and Management*, vol. 4. pp. 503–526. Philadelphia: WB Saunders, 1992.

87. Merrill RG. Prevention, treatment and prognosis for nerve injury related to the difficult impaction. *Dent Clin North Am* 1979; **23**: 471–488.
88. Ferdousi AM, Macgregor AJ. The response of peripheral branches of the trigeminal nerve to trauma. *Int J Oral Surg* 1985; **14**: 41–46.
89. Robinson PP, Smith KG, Johnson FP, Coppins DA. Equipment and methods for simple sensory testing. *Br J Oral Maxillofac Surg* 1992; **30**: 387–389.
90. Merrill RG. Decompression for inferior alveolar nerve injury. *J Oral Surg* 1964; **22**: 291–330.
91. Merrill RG. Further studies in decompression for inferior alveolar nerve injury. *J Oral Surg* 1966; **24**: 233–238.
92. Mozsary PG, Syers CS. Microsurgical correction of the injured inferior alveolar nerve. *J Oral Maxillofac Surg* 1985; **43**: 353–358.
93. Donoff RB, Guralnick W. The application of microneurosurgery to oral–neurological problems. *J Oral Maxillofac Surg* 1982; **40**: 156–159.
94. Hausamen JE, Samii M, Schmidseder R. Repair of the mandibular nerve by means of autologous nerve grafting after resection of the lower jaw. *J Maxillofac Surg* 1973; **1**: 77–78.
95. Haschemi A. Partial anastomosis between the lingual and mandibular nerves for restoration of sensibility in the mental nerve area after injury to the mandibular nerve. *J Maxillofac Surg* 1981; **9**: 225–227.
96. Wessberg GA, Wolford LM, Epker BN. Simultaneous inferior alveolar nerve graft and osseous reconstruction of the mandible. *J Oral Maxillofac Surg* 1982; **40**: 384–390.
97. Kaban LB, Upton J. Cross mental nerve graft for restoration of lip sensation after inferior alveolar nerve damage: report of a case. *J Oral Maxillofac Surg* 1986; **44**: 649–651.
98. Pogrel MA, Kaban LB. Injuries to the inferior alveolar and lingual nerves. *J Cal Dent Assoc* 1993; **21**: 50–54.
99. Labanc JP, Gregg J. Trigeminal nerve injuries. Basic problems, historical perspectives, early successes and remaining challenges. In: Labanc JP, Gregg JM (eds) *Oral and Maxillofacial Surgery Clinics of North America: Trigeminal Nerve Injury: Diagnosis and Management*, vol. 4. pp. 277–283. Philadelphia: WB Saunders, 1992.
100. Donoff RB. Surgical management of inferior alveolar nerve injuries (part I). The case for early repair. *J Oral Maxillofac Surg* 1955; **53**: 1327–1329.
101. Gregg JM. Surgical management of inferior alveolar nerve injuries (part II). The case for delayed management. *J Oral Maxillofac Surg* 1995; **53**: 1330–1333.
102. Labanc JP, Van Boven RW. Surgical management of inferior alveolar nerve injuries. In: Labanc JP, Gregg JM (eds) *Oral and Maxillofacial Surgery Clinics of North America: Trigeminal Nerve Injury: Diagnosis and Management*, vol. 4. pp. 425–437. Philadelphia: WB Saunders, 1992.
103. Smith KG, Robinson PP. The effect of delayed nerve repair on the properties of regenerated afferent fibres in the chorda tympani. *Brain Res* 1995; **691**: 142–152.
104. Smith KG, Robinson PP. An experimental study on the recovery of the lingual nerve after injury with or without repair. *Int J Oral Maxillofac Surg* 1995; **24**: 372–379.
105. Smith KG, Robinson PP. The reinnervation of the tongue and salivary glands after two methods of lingual nerve repair in the cat. *Arch Oral Biol* 1995; **40**: 373–383.
106. Smith KG, Robinson PP. An experimental study of lingual nerve repair using epineurial sutures or entubulation. *Br J Oral Maxillofac Surg*1995; **33**: 211–219.
107. Mozsary PG, Middleton RA. Microsurgical reconstruction of the lingual nerve. *J Oral Maxillofac Surg* 1984; **42**: 415–420.
108. Riediger D, Ehrenfeld M, Cornelius CP. Micronerve surgery on the inferior alveolar and lingual nerve with special consideration for nerve replacement. In: Riediger, D, Ehrenfeld M (eds) *Microsurgical Tissue Transplantation*, pp. 189–194. Illinois: Quintessence, 1989.
109. Smith KG, Robinson PP. The reinnervation of the tongue and salivary glands after lingual nerve repair by stretch, sural nerve graft or frozen muscle graft. *J Dent Res* 1995; **74**: 1850–1860.
110. Smith KG, Robinson PP. An experimental study of three methods of lingual nerve defect repair. *J Oral Maxillofac Surg* 1995; **53**: 1052–1062.
111. Robinson PP, Smith KG. A study on the efficacy of late lingual nerve repair. *Br J Oral Maxillofac Surg* 1995; **34**: 96–103.

23

Orofacial pain – pathophysiology and clinical presentation

Behnam Aghabeigi

Introduction

Pain is the most common symptom that compels patients to seek medical and dental therapy and constitutes a serious health and economic problem. It has been estimated that in the industrialized countries 15–20% of the population have acute pain and between 25 and 30% suffer from chronic pain. This costs American society 79 billion dollars annually.[1]

Dentists and dental specialists are concerned with two of the most common pains. The first is acute orofacial pain arising from the teeth and associated structures and the second is chronic craniofacial pain, which is believed to account for 40% of all chronic pain problems.[2] An understanding of the pathophysiology of pain is needed by all those involved in pain relief. The aim of this chapter is to present some pathophysiological concepts, particularly those which may have an important effect on patient management.

Definitions

Traditional views of pain are reflected in definitions such as that of *Butterworths Medical Dictionary*:[3] 'the distressing sensation excited by noxious stimuli of sufficient intensity acting on nerve endings'. It goes on to define psychogenic pain as 'pain which occurs without any organic cause and is due to a disorder of mind'.

Although much pain results from noxious stimulation, it can also occur from non-noxious stimuli, as well as spontaneously when there is no stimulus at all. Wall and Devor[4] have shown that sensory impulses from the dorsal root ganglia (the site where sensory neurons make their first synapse) are constantly being transmitted into the central nervous system (CNS) even under normal conditions. This means that we have a potential source of neural impulses present at all times which can reach a conscious level of pain as a result of any decrease in central inhibitory control. Thus, newer concepts regard pain as a subjective psychological state rather than an unpleasant sensory activity that is induced solely by noxious stimulation. The definition of pain adopted by the International Association for the Study of Pain (IASP)[5] defines pain as 'an unpleasant sensory and emotional experience associated with actual or potential tissue damage or described in terms of such damage'. This definition avoids linking pain to a stimulus and regards pain always as an affective state, that is, an emotional experience and not merely the perception of a pure sensation. However, the affective state of pain differs from other affective states in that it is always referred or projected to some part of the body with varying degrees of precision.[6] Unlike elation or sorrow, pain is always 'felt' in some part of the body, even when that part is no longer present, as in the case when pain is felt in a 'phantom limb' after its amputation.

Pathophysiology

Chemical basis of nociception

Pain is provoked when a variety of substances are released or injected into the tissues. These pain-producing substances can be released by trauma, infection, allergenic reaction, neurogenic reflexes and central emotional changes from cell membranes, mast cells and nerve endings. This leads to the excitation of free nerve endings which act as nociceptors or peripheral sense organs that respond to the noxious stimulus. This group of substances includes histamine, bradykinin, potassium, acetylcholine, prostaglandins, leukotrienes and the neuropeptides.

Among these noxious substances prostaglandins have attracted much attention in the recent past. Their biosynthesis involves the free radical peroxidation of arachidonic acid by cyclooxygenase or lipoxygenase enzymes (Fig. 23.1). Prostaglandin E_2 (PGE_2) has hyperalgesic properties and sensitizes the nerve endings and lowers their threshold to all kinds of stimulation. The analgesic action of aspirin and the other non-steroidal anti-inflammatory analgesic drugs (NSAIDs) is believed to be due to inhibition of cyclooxygenase. In addition to their peripheral action, NSAIDs seem to possess a central analgesic action as well.[7]

Arachidonic acid can also be metabolized via the lipoxygenase pathway. This is not inhibited by NSAIDs (Fig. 23.1). Leukotriene B_4 (LTB_4) is a hyperalgesic substance[8] which is derived from the 5–lipoxygenation of arachidonic acid. This is the result of the action of the lipoxygenase enzyme on the fifth carbon atom bond of arachidonic acid. LTB_4 has been identified in the saline aspirates of the painful temporomandibular joint (TMJ),[9] as has been 15-hydroxyeicosatetraenoic acid (15-HETE), which is the breakdown product of 15-hydroperoxyeicosatetraenoic acid (15-HPETE), another known hyperalgesic agent produced via the lipoxygenase pathway. This may explain why the NSAIDs are not fully successful in the relief of chronic TMJ pain. However, in an unpublished open trial the lipoxygenase inhibitor Novalgin (dipyrone, Hoechst) was superior to ibuprofen (Boots). However, compliance was poor and may have been attributable to the patients' reluctance to seek transient relief for a mild to moderate pain. Furthermore, preliminary studies of therapeutic use of a free radical scavenger, the enzyme superoxide dismutase, in painful TMJs seem promising.[10]

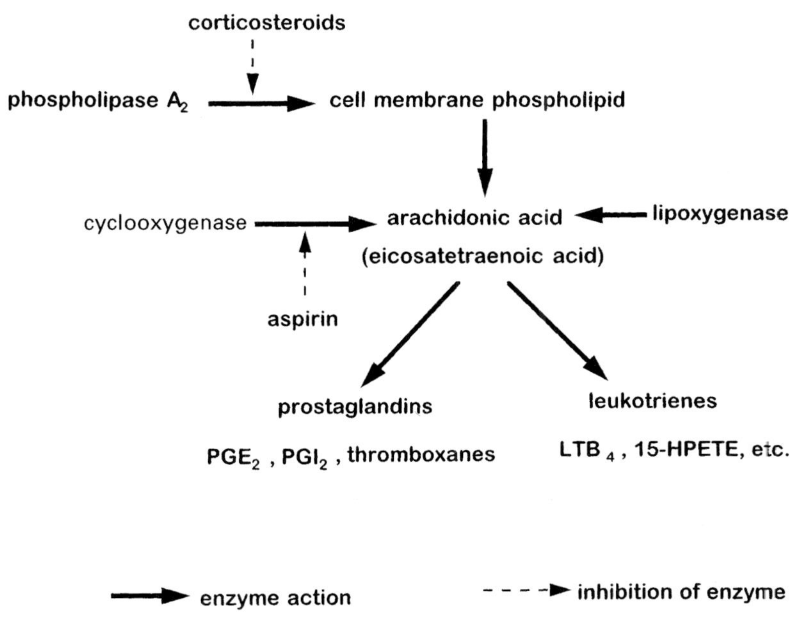

Fig. 23.1 Pathways of arachidonic acid metabolism. PG = Prostaglandin; LTB_4 = leukotriene B_4; 15-HPETE = 15-hydroperoxyeicosatetraenoic acid.

Although acute and some types of chronic hyperalgesia are due to a continuous generation of pain mediators by damaged tissue, there is evidence that certain mediators such as the neuropeptide substance P[11] and PGE_2[12] as well as 15-HPETE[13] can induce a state of prolonged hyperalgesia which is not due to continuous tissue destruction, by sensitizing the peripheral nociceptors (peripheral sensitization).[14] Furthermore, there is evidence that activation of peripheral nociceptors as a consequence of tissue damage can lead to hyperexcitability of central neurons at the spinal dorsal horn, also resulting in unexpected prolonged hyperalgesia (central sensitization).[15] Wall and Devor[4] have shown that repeat surgery on experimental animals enhanced pain – a phenomenon now called wind-up. The genetic basis for this appears to be upregulation, i.e. increased concentration and activity of two regulatory genes called c-*fos* and c-*jun* in the spinal nucleus nerve cells. This would place one of the causes of persistent pain well out of the reach of surgery.[16] Central sensitization may be avoided in clinical practice by a nerve block infiltration of a local analgesic prior to surgery, even when carried out under a general anaesthetic, i.e. pre-emptive analgesia.[17] These observations may also be relevant in explaining other chronic painful conditions without evident structural changes.

It has also been suggested that stress can lead to the peripheral release of neuropeptides such as substance P (SP).[18] SP plays an important role in neurogenic inflammation.[19] It leads to the production of oxygen free radicals, release of interleukins from macrophages and PGE_2 from synoviocytes. The TMJ capsule and disc are innervated by many SP-containing fibres[20] and Holmlund *et al.*[21] have also found these neuropeptides in painful joints.

Pain transmission

Free nerve endings which act as nociceptors are present in all orofacial tissues including the skin, oral mucosa, the temporomandibular joint, periodontium, tooth pulp, periosteum and muscles.[22] Bone itself has SP and calcitonin gene-related peptide (CGRP)-containing nerve endings.[23] These become excited by noxious stimuli and the impulses are transmitted via three major classes of nociceptive afferents:[24]

1. C-polymodal fibres. These have a diameter of 0.3–3 µm and are unmyelinated with a conduction velocity (cv) of 0.5–2 m/s. They respond to strong mechanical, thermal and chemical stimuli.
2. Aδ fibres. These are 2–5 µm in diameter and thinly myelinated with a cv of 5–30 m/s.
3. Aβ fibres. These are 6–22 µm in diameter and heavily myelinated with a cv of 33–75 m/s. In one study almost half the myelinated dental axons in the trigeminal nerve conducted at Aβ velocities.[25]

Studies of electrically stimulated teeth have found that the most sensitive fibres are activated by low-stimulus intensities and evoke 'prepain' sensations, whereas higher intensities cause sharp pain, and the highest cause an unpleasant ache.[26] As single-fibre studies in animals show that Aβ fibres are more sensitive than Aδ fibres and that C-fibres are least sensitive, it is probable that prepain, sharp pain and dull ache correspond to Aβ, Aδ and C-fibre activation.[27]

Abnormal conducting patterns may occur in nerves after experimentally induced demyelination and this has been suggested as a pathogenesis of trigeminal neuralgia,[22] a paroxysmal pain which is characteristically provoked by the stimulation of myelinated fibres by light touch. Plaques of demyelination are frequently found in the descending trigeminal tract and in the lemniscal systems, but it is not possible to argue that such plaques are either necessary or sufficient to cause tic douloureux. Nevertheless, trigeminal neuralgia is associated with plaques of demyelination in multiple sclerosis and sites of nerve compression by cerebral arteries.

Although teeth are extensively innervated by Aβ, Aδ and C-fibre axons, it is not possible to prove that all these fibres are nociceptive afferents. It is likely that some are autonomic efferents. Although nerve fibres enter the dentinal tubules, the actual mechanism of dentinal sensitivity is unclear. Three major theories are:

1. Activation of the intradentinal extensions of pulpal nerves.
2. A transduction mechanism involving the odontoblast or its dentinal process.
3. A hydrodynamic mechanism within the dentinal tubules and pulp.

The first theory has largely been abandoned as there is no satisfactory evidence to show

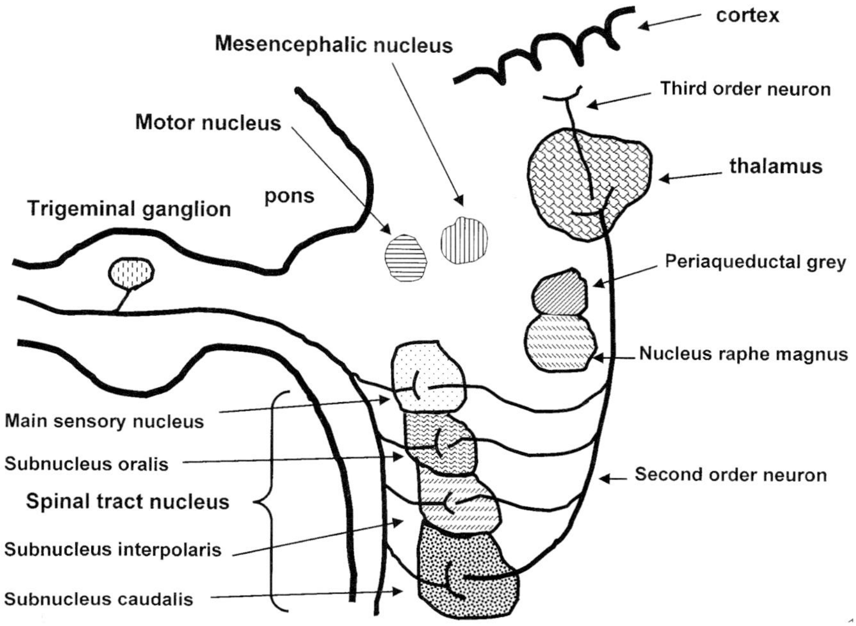

Fig. 23.2 Sensory transmission from trigeminal nerve endings to cerebral cortex. The unipolar cell bodies of primary neurons are located in the trigeminal (Gasserian) ganglion. Other cranial nerves supplying the orofacial region follow a similar course. For clarity connections from the midbrain periaqueductal grey (PAG) and medullary nucleus raphe magnus (NRM) to the trigeminal sensory complex are not shown.

that there are nerves in the outer highly sensitive dentine. Furthermore, agents that cause pain, when applied to the skin, do not do so when applied to dentine.[28] It has also been shown experimentally that the existence of nerve fibres in dentine is not a necessary prerequisite for its sensitivity.[29]

The second theory considers the odontoblast to be a receptor coupled to the nerves in the pulp. It used to be argued that because the odontoblast was of neural crest origin it could have retained an ability to transduce and propagate an impulse. However, dentine remains sensitive despite the destruction of not only the intradentinal nerve fibres but also the odontoblast layer.[29] This gives support to the concept that transmission of external irritation from the dentine surface to the pulp nerves must be indirect. The hydrodynamic theory of dentine sensitivity fits much of the experimental and morphological data. It proposes that the fluid movement through the tubules distorts the adjacent pulp and is sensed by its free nerve endings. This theory explains why topical anaesthetics fail to block dentine sensitivity and why pain is produced by dehydration, hypertonic solutions, thermal change and mechanical probing. The increased sensitivy at the dentinoenamel junction is explained by the profuse branching of the tubules in this region.

Once generated, the impulse in the orofacial nerves travels mainly via the trigeminal nerve but also by the sensory roots of the facial, glossopharyngeal, vagus and upper cervical nerves. SP is the neurotransmitter at the primary sensory synapse. This neuropeptide is synthesized by the nerve cell body and can be released antidromically. In fact, it is interesting to note that approximately four times as much SP is transported peripherally as centrally.[30] SP has been measured in dentine and dental pulp[31] and is believed to play a role in the reception and transmission of pain in dentine.[32] Another receptor system that transmits and modulates nociceptive information is the *N*-methyl-D-aspartate (NMDA) receptor system. Its activation by excitatory amino acids released from the nerve terminals lead to the synthesis of nitric oxide. This molecule might play an important role as an intracellular and intercellular mediator in the CNS.[33] The central processes of the primary neurons enter the brainstem and synapse on second-order neurons at various levels of the trigeminal brainstem sensory nuclear complex (Fig. 23.2), which consists of:

1. The main sensory trigeminal nucleus, which is rostrally located and receives periodontal and some pulpal afferents.

2. The spinal tract of the trigeminal nucleus, which is more caudally located. The spinal tract is divided into the subnucleus oralis, subnucleus interpolaris and subnucleus caudalis.

The subnucleus caudalis extends into the cervical spinal cord and merges with the spinal dorsal horn. It serves as the principal relay site of orofacial nociceptive information and is similar in structure and projection to the spinal dorsal horn, which is the principal component of the spinal nociceptive mechanism. Evidence suggests that the subnucleus caudalis is homologous to the substantia gelatinosa of the spinal dorsal horn and acts as a 'gating' mechanism capable of modulating sensory information.[34] From the brainstem, sensory information may then be relayed directly to third-order neurons in the thalamus and from there to cerebral cortex.

There is reason to believe that the sensory and affective aspects of pain are subserved in part by separate neural mechanisms.[35] The spinothalamic projection to ventrobasal thalamus and its projection to the somatosensory cortex are required for the discriminative sensory aspect of pain. This is the means whereby the nature and source of pain are determined. However, projections to the medial thalamus and from the medial thalamus to the frontal cortex seem to be concerned with the affective aspect of pain. This view is supported by observation of patients who have undergone frontal lobotomy.[36] Interestingly, these patients usually obtained striking relief of their pain problem but with no impairment in their ability to detect and identify noxious stimuli as painful. The suffering was thus eliminated with no effect on the purely sensory aspect of their pain. Increased prefrontal brain activity is also detected by positron emission tomography in patients with chronic facial pain suggesting that this area may enhance pain perception.[37]

Pain modulation

The concept of pain modulation is based on the evidence that neural impulses are altered as they travel up to the higher centres. It has been traditional to divide pain into organic and psychogenic, organic being pain which has resulted from an identifiable structural lesion, while psychogenic not only labelled those pains without such a lesion but also implied a supratentorial psychiatric disturbance. This view is no longer held. The emphasis is now on the many factors that influence the excitation and inhibition of the painful experience. Whether pain is generated by a noxious stimulation of the tissues or occurs as a result of a central affective disturbance is no longer of great concern. Pain is now regarded as a sensory and emotional experience that always involves structural and biochemical changes somewhere in the body.

Melzack and Wall[38] proposed their gate-control theory to explain the variability of the painful experience. Later, they modified this theory based on new information.[39] These theories have proven to be among the most important developments in the field of pain research and therapy. As a result, psychological variables such as past experience, attention and other cognitive activities have been integrated into current research and therapy on pain processes. The gate-control theory, however, is not able to explain several chronic pain problems, such as phantom limb pain.[40] A substantial number of children who are born without a limb feel a phantom of the missing part, suggesting that the neural network, or neuromatrix, that subserves body sensation has a genetically determined substrate and is modified by sensory experience.[41]

The pain modulating network

There appears to be a specific central nervous system network for pain control. Analgesia may be demonstrated by the stimulation of brain sites such as the periaqueductal grey (PAG) and nucleus raphe magnus (NRM; Fig. 23.2) in animals and humans. This has provided powerful evidence for a highly selective brainstem control of nociceptive transmission.[42] This system is also involved in emotional and motivational functions and other complex behaviour.

Although there has been much emphasis on the pain-suppressing effect of the modulation system, the brainstem-modulating neurons have a bidirectional control of transmission in that the network has both excitatory and inhibitory actions on pain conduction.[43] These concepts are incorporated in the new model of the gate-control theory (Fig. 23.3). Therefore pain can result from either the loss of

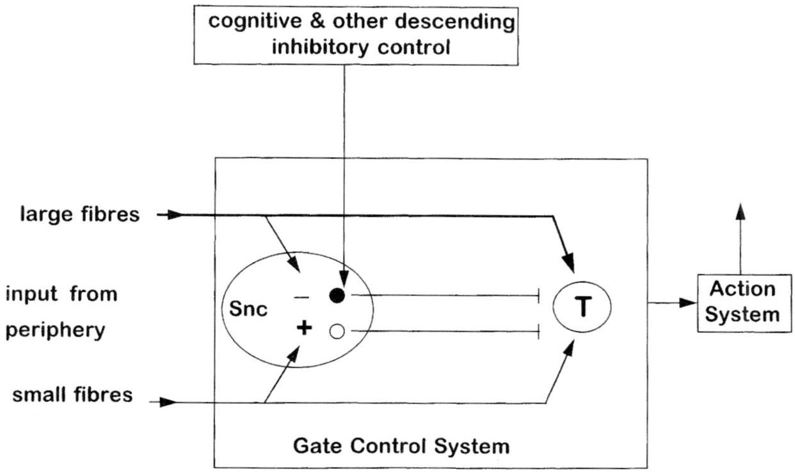

Fig. 23.3 The gate-control theory. The transmission of nerve impulses from the afferent fibres to the central transmission cell (T) of the medullary trigeminal sensory complex is modulated by a gate-control system. An inhibitory effect exerted by subnucleus caudalis (Snc) on the afferent fibre terminals is increased by large-diameter fibre input and decreased by activity in small diameter fibres. This model includes excitatory (white circle) and inhibitory (black circle) links from the Snc to T as well as descending inhibitory control from the brainstem system. Cognitive (conscious) influences are also possible.

inhibitory control or the activation of excitatory modulating neurons.

The anatomical, chemical and physiological bases of pain modulation are progressively being unravelled. Analgesia produced by the pain-modulating network is believed to be mediated by endogenous opioid substances which are synthesized by nerve cells and have pharmacological properties nearly identical to those of narcotic analgesic drugs. The first endogenous opioid peptides discovered were leucine enkephalin and methionine enkephalin.[44] Since their discovery, other opioid peptides have been identified throughout the body. One of the most potent of these is β-endorphin (endogenous morphine). Its precursor, pro-opiomelanocortin, which originates in the infundibular nucleus of the basal hypothalamus, also gives rise to the adrenocorticotrophic hormone (ACTH). However, it is interesting that ACTH antagonizes the analgesic effects of β-endorphin.[45] This may also be of some relevance to chronic pain conditions, as patients with chronic idiopathic pain syndromes are reported to have higher levels of cortisol in their blood.[46]

It has been a widely held view that the endogenous opioids are involved in anaesthesia or analgesia produced by hypnosis and acupuncture.[47] However, recent controlled studies question this view.[48]

Cytochemical studies of the pain-modulating networks have also revealed that, in addition to the endogenous opioid peptides, a variety of other neurotransmitters are involved in the control of pain transmission. The monoamines serotonin and noradrenaline are present in the brainstem neurons and both inhibit spinal cord pain transmission cells.[49,50]

The endogenous opioid system and the monoaminergic network interact and recent studies have shown that morphine may activate the descending serotoninergic pathway and so modulate dental pain transmission.[51]

Monoamines have also been implicated in the pathogenesis of chronic pain and are of particular importance as they can be manipulated by a variety of pharmacological agents, thus raising the possibility of new centrally acting analgesic agents. In fact, there is evidence that the well-established value of tricyclic antidepressants in chronic pain management[52] relates to their potency as blockers of the reuptake of both noradrenaline and serotonin.[53,54] The use of antidepressants as analgesics opens up an entirely new approach to drug treatment for chronic pain. These drugs do not produce tolerance and dependence and their side-effects have been considerably diminished with the development of novel agents such as the specific serotonin reuptake inhibitors, e.g. fluoxetine.

Chronic and recurrent idiopathic orofacial pain

Psychological and biochemical aspects

The basis of chronic pain that is persistent or recurrent pain differs from acute pain. The initiating mechanisms in cases of chronic nociceptive pain such as rheumatoid arthritis or uncontrolled malignancy are readily recognizable. However, many pains have no recognizable aetiology, and these include migraine, tension headache, facial migraneous neuralgia and the specific orofacial problems of facial arthromyalgia (FAM), atypical (idiopathic) facial pain, atypical odontalgia and oral dysaesthesia. These common idiopathic chronic orofacial pain problems that may present individually, sequentially or simultaneously in any patient (see section on clinical presentation below). Despite popular belief, there is no controlled evidence that they arise from malocclusion.[55,56] There is a substantial body of work to show that many chronic pains are stress-related.[57,58] However, it is not clear how stress leads to pain or any other psychosomatic illness. There is increasing evidence that points to an organic basis for all such disturbances. Thus receptors, neurons and neurochemical changes are involved in all pain disorders, both psychological (functional) and structural (organic).

It has recently been revealed by positron emission tomography that patients with atypical facial pain had increased contralateral cingulate cortex activity in response to both heat and pain.[37] This area is concerned with attention which suggests an enhanced alerting mechanism in response to peripheral stimuli which could therefore be processed as pain in some patients.

There have been several reports of a higher level of stressful life events in idiopathic facial pain patients,[57,58] although Marbach *et al.*[59] did not find any difference between TMJ patients and controls with regard to their desirable and undesirable life events. However, it was found that these patients had fewer sources of emotional support, thus indicating stress as an imbalance between the demand on the individual and coping ability. It would therefore seem that whether or not the amount of stress endured is higher than normal, chronic pain patients have personalities that are in some way more vulnerable.[60] The psychological features of importance include an unstable or inadequate parental background, poor adaptation to school or work, marital and financial difficulties, chronic illness in the family and bereavement.[61] Whereas chronic pain does not imply psychopathology, a proportion of patients may experience diagnosable and important psychiatric conditions. Using a structured clinical interview to diagnose mental disorders according to the criteria set by the *Diagnostic and Statistical Manual of Mental Disorders*, third edition, revised (DSM-III-R) we found that the lifetime prevalence of depression and posttraumatic stress disorder (PTSD) is higher than in the general population.[62] Despite this, almost half of the patients had a clear lifetime history of psychiatric illness and 75% had no current psychiatric problems and remained purely idiopathic.

Whether pain arises from depression or depression is reactive to pain has been argued extensively in the literature. This suggests that a common metabolic vulnerability may predispose to both idiopathic pain and depression even if both do not occur in the same individual, and is supported by the high incidence of depression in chronic pain patients and the pain relief achieved by tricyclic antidepressants in non-depressed psychiatrically normal patients.[61]

The concept of pain vulnerability is underlined by the clinical observation of different pains occurring in some patients at different stages of life.[58,63] In childhood such patients suffer from abdominal or ear pain, in adolescence TMJ pain or dysmenorrhoea, and later abdominal pain (usually the irritable bowel syndrome), neck and back pain and pruritus. There is also an association with PTSD.[62] If this concept is not recognized, the differential diagnosis of each pain episode may be misleading and clinically unhelpful, with the tendency to attribute the disorder to purely local abnormalities rather than a generalized problem. This vulnerability may be genetically transmitted as children of TMJ pain patients seem to suffer from a higher incidence of illness and injury.[64]

One of the promising fields of study to explain this phenomenon seems to be the CNS serotonin system, which is believed to be involved in the pathogenesis of both pain and depression. Drugs such as reserpine, which deplete CNS monoamines, produce not only depression but also spontaneous pain, including atypical odontalgia (Harris, personal communication). Patients with idiopathic pain syndromes have low concentrations of serotonin metabolites in their cerebrospinal fluid,[65] but it has

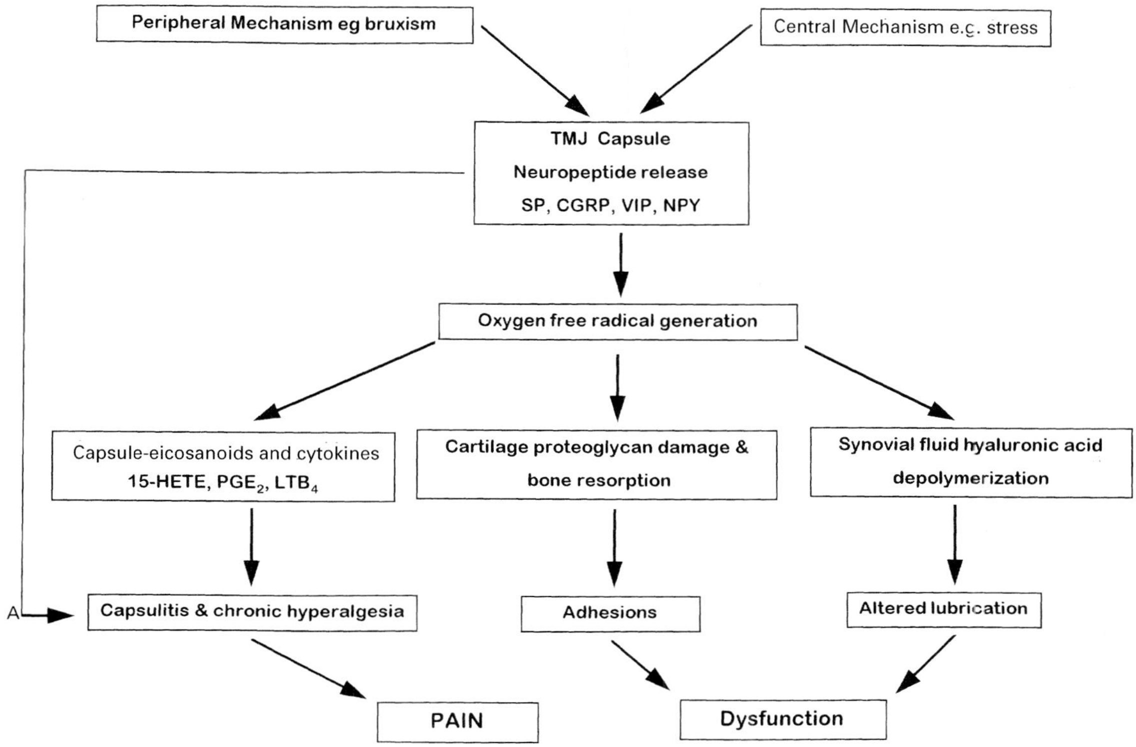

Fig. 23.4 Diagrammatic hypothesis of temporomandibular joint (TMJ) pain and dysfunction. SP = Substance P; CGRP = calcitonin gene-related peptide; VIP = vasoactive intestinal peptide; NPY = neuropeptide Y; 15-HETE = 15-hydroxyeicosatetraenoic acid; PGE_2 = prostaglandin E_2; LTB_4 = leukotriene B_4. A = Neuropeptides and eicosanoids interact to produce chronic algesiae.

been suggested that this abnormality does not alter during the course of the illness and may be a marker of an increased risk of developing a chronic pain syndrome.[66] Besides central serotonin system markers, chronic pain and depression share a number of other biological abnormalities, such as: hypercortisolaemia, an abnormal dexamethasone suppression test, and low serum and urine melatonin levels.[67] However, these are state markers, i.e. they reflect the current state of the patient and the studies did not establish whether or not they are permanent traits of the patients. Impaired conjugation of tyramine sulphate is a trait (unchanging) marker of endogenous depression. It has been shown that following a standard dose of tyramine the chronic facial pain patient has an impaired urinary excretion of tyramine sulphate.[68] Furthermore, although half of the patients had a history of depression and 10% were currently depressed, the lowest tyramine sulphate conjugation levels occurred in those who had never been depressed. These findings, together with the finding that both tricyclic and monoamine oxidase inhibitor antidepressants are highly effective in the treatment of chronic pain syndromes, provide further support that a common biological abnormality may underlie the pathogenesis of both chronic pain and depression.

Harris[69] has put forward a credible hypothesis for idiopathic facial pain (Fig. 23.4). Emotional strain, together with local physical stress (such as bruxism), in a biochemically and psychologically vulnerable subject promotes the release of neuropeptides in the target tissues such as the joint capsule, muscles and periodontal membrane or dental pulp. SP and other neuropeptides can cause vasodilatation and inflammation generating free radicals from leukocytes. This would account for the painful but reversible capsulitis and synovitis in facial arthromyalgia. Localized free radical damage of cell membranes also produces algesic eicosanoids such as PGE_2 and 15-HPETE which, with the neuropeptides, could produce chronic pain.[11,13] Thus, in FAM, stress in a psychologically and biochemically vulnerable subject produces capsulitis and myofascial pain. The synovitis impairs lubrication and movement, giving rise to the classic clicking and sticking with trismus. With free radical-induced damage to the fibrocartilage, movement becomes increasingly impaired with adhesion formation which can readily be seen on arthroscopy. This may ultimately lead to an anteriorly displaced disc without reduction. However, the same peripheral pain mechanism could apply to other related pains. The intensity of such pains, their duration and response to reassurance, placebo and active therapy is undoubtedly determined by central psychological factors which modulate pain.

In summary, pain is multifactorial and when interpreting the results of animal research models one must consider psychophysiological phenomena associated with pain perception. The significance of, and concern for, the consequences of the painful experience in humans makes it different from that experienced by animals. Many consider that clinical pain as we know it is a unique experience peculiar to human beings.

Clinical presentation

For clinical purposes orofacial pain may be classified as follows:

1. Nociceptive.
2. Idiopathic and psychogenic.
3. Neuropathic.
4. Vascular.

Nociceptive implies a known cause of tissue damage, and neuropathic pain arises from a primary disorder affecting a nerve cell or its neuron. The relationship of psychological factors to the group of common idiopathic pains has been discussed in the previous section.

General considerations

As pain is a totally subjective experience which cannot be simultaneously shared and reported by another individual, it is clinically important to accept the subject's description of the pain experience. Conversely, it is unhelpful to question or reject it. As defined earlier pain is an unpleasant psychological experience due to either, physical or emotional trauma, or a combination of both. The intensity of this experience is strongly influenced by the patient's emotional make-up and cultural background. It is equally important for the clinician to realize that his or her diagnosis and management of the condition will be influenced by professional training, and emotional and cultural attitudes to the patient's problem. In clinical practice it is essential to assume that, even in the absence of clinical features, the pain process represents both central and peripheral end-organ changes.

Diagnosis

The most important aid to the diagnosis of pain is the history, which must be followed by a careful clinical examination and appropriate investigations, including radiographs and where appropriate, a computerized or magnetic resonance scan. The history should establish the nature of the pain, including:

1. Its character, e.g. sharp, dull, throbbing, burning or stabbing.
2. The site or sites from which it arises, and to which it travels. This is best recorded as a simple line drawing (Fig. 23.5).
3. Its timing. When did the first attack occur? Occasionally previous attacks are withheld by the patient as being irrelevent. Note the frequency, duration of subsequent episodes, the time of day, in particular whether the pain is worse in the morning, afternoon, evening or night, and if it prevents or disturbs sleep.
4. The provoking factors, especially hot, cold, sweet and sour food or drink, biting, chewing, yawning or talking. Also the effect of anxiety, anger or alcohol.
5. The relieving factors, such as heat, analgesics or alcohol.
6. Associated phenomena, e.g. swelling, unpleasant taste, discharge, bruxism, trismus, nasal obstruction, altered sensation, epiphora.
7. Any current or previous episodes of pain in the head, neck, back, chest, abdomen (especially irritable bowel syndrome), pelvis or pruritus.

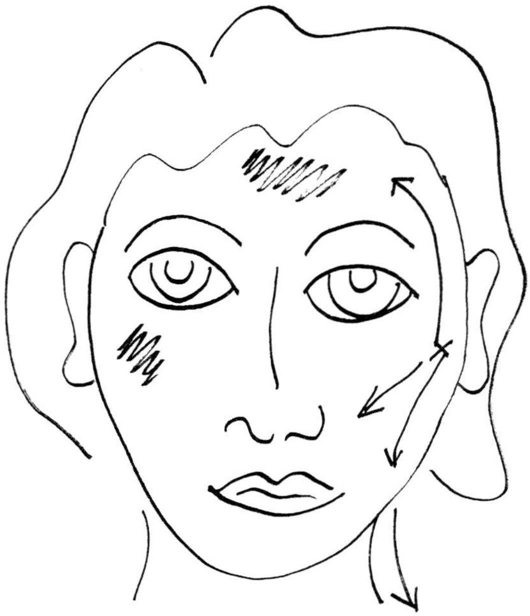

Fig. 23.5 A line drawing in the patient's notes is the simplest means of recording the site and distribution of pain.

8. Does the patient suffer from anxiety or depression? Has he or she been treated for depression? Emotional factors such as anxiety or depression associated with occupational and family problems are of crucial importance.
9. The current and previous general medical history and drug therapy.
10. Family problems, including parental separation, ill health or bereavement.A simple family tree provides the best record (Fig. 23.6).

Nociceptive

The teeth and supporting structures

Pulpal pain

In the early stages of pulpitis pain may present as a transient response of the exposed dentinal tubules to acid, sweet and thermal changes. Later an inflamed pulp causes an intense throbbing pain which is characteristically worse at night. It may be poorly localized or referred to the opposite jaw on the same side, or even obscured by painful ipsilateral reflex muscle spasm.

The dentition must be carefully examined with a mirror and probe for cavities, loose restorations and the occasionally overlooked split tooth crown. Systematic percussion to detect periapical inflammation and electric pulp testing for vitality are valuable diagnostic aids. When subjective localization is difficult, local analgesia may help; a successful infiltration over the site will confirm the diagnosis. However, with chronic idiopathic or psychogenic pain such as atypical odontalgia or atypical facial neuralgia the response to local analgesia is variable and therefore unreliable as a diagnostic aid.

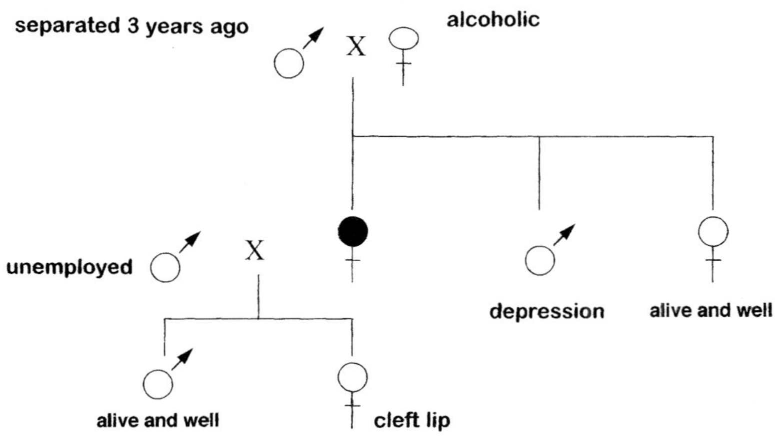

Fig. 23.6 An example of a family tree which provides a simple record of family history. ♀ is pain patient.

Radiographs must include a full mouth survey. Where periapical films are required these should be long cone projections to eliminate distortion of multirooted tooth anatomy. An occipitomental view of the antra may be invaluable.

Treatment will vary from desensitization of the exposed dentine, sedative dressings over the irritated pulp to pulp extirpation, abscess drainage or extraction.

Periodontal pain

This tends to be dull and continuous and, though relieved initially by clenching the teeth, this later aggravates it. The periodontitis may be a primary inflammation of a periodontal pocket or secondary to pulpitis or split tooth.

The underlying cause must be established and this will determine the treatment which may include the drainage of pus, and the application of a counterirritant antiseptic, such as tincture of iodine, to the inflamed periodontal tissues or antibiotics. Spot-grinding gives immediate relief from occlusal trauma. Definitive care is by periodontal surgery, root canal therapy or extraction.

Bone pain

This varies from a dull to a severe throbbing, and may arise from an alveolar osteitis, infected cysts, fractures or osteomyelitis. Inflammation of the inferior dental nerve gives rise to the pathognomonic mental analgesia. However, an accumulation of subperiosteal pus from one of the mandibular premolars may produce this sign and simulate an osteomyelitis.

Treatment of infection is antibiotic therapy and the appropriate surgery to drain the exudate and remove any sequestra. Rarely, such pains become chronic if the condition is not adequately controlled.

The tongue

Lingual pain may be sharp or burning and is often referred to the ear. It is provoked by spiced food or drink and by swallowing. The benign mucosal causes include aphthous and viral ulceration, erosive lichen planus, pemphigoid and the atrophic glossitis of vitamin B_{12} deficiency due to primary or postgastrectomy pernicious anaemia. Occasionally geographical tongue and severe iron deficiency give rise to discomfort. The exclusion of malignant ulceration, especially at the lateral border or posterior third of tongue, is always important and for this reason examination must include these areas which can only be seen when the tongue is drawn forwards by holding it with a dry gauze swab. Any suspicious lesion must be biopsied.

Carcinoma of the posterior third of the tongue may give rise to pain even when the lesion is palpable but not visible. When persistent due to an inoperable lesion, relief may be achieved by dividing the glossopharyngeal nerve in the tonsillar fossa.

Probably the most common lingual pain is idiopathic glossodynia or glossopyrosis. This is a burning discomfort, usually of emotional origin, constantly present during waking hours and often of long standing. Unlike lingual mucosal pain, it is relieved by eating and drinking. The tongue is normal in its appearance but may present with a bright red surface with an indented scalloped margin due to a combination of vasodilatation and bruxism. This condition is discussed under oral dysaesthesia in the section on chronic idiopathic pain.

The temporomandibular joint and masticatory muscles

Acute

This may follow damage to the meniscus or capsule due to excessive uncoordinated jaw movements or direct trauma. The pain is moderate to severe, well-localized and aggravated by chewing, talking and yawning. Movements are markedly restricted and the jaw deviates to the painful side on attempted opening. A tender effusion may be palpable. In older patients clinical and radiological evidence of osteoarthritis should be sought after. Treatment consists of resting the joint by a soft diet and the provision of adequate analgesia, such as ibuprofen 400 mg 4-hourly after food.

Other acute inflammatory lesions are rare and include in children, juvenile rheumatoid arthritis (Still's disease), a panarthritis following rubella immunization. In adults acute rheumatoid arthritis of the TMJ is uncommon and again part of the systemic disease.

Treatment is essentially anti-inflammatory analgesics. Steroids may be required for severe exacerbation of the rheumatoid conditions. Most cases become chronic pain with acute exacerbations.

Chronic dysfunction – facial arthromyalgia (the TMJ dysfunction syndrome, myofascial pain dysfunction syndrome)

This is discussed under chronic idiopathic pain, above.

Osteoarthrosis

Although primarily a degenerative condition, Toller[70] has observed the clinical and radiological manifestations in young patients, which he suggests are a direct consequence of untreated facial arthromyalgia. This transition from a functional to a structural disturbance may be quite prevalent as many older patients are aware that emotional tension and bruxism are related to episodes of joint pain. The bouts of pain are well-localized to the affected joint and provoked by movement, especially chewing. The joint is tender and crepitus may be audible or apparent on palpation. Occasionally there is a painful effusion. When the pain is sharp and severe, the differentiation from a trigeminal neuralgia in an old person can be difficult. Furthermore, in some patients a temporomandibular osteoarthrosis would appear to be the trigger site for a true paroxysmal neuralgia.

There is often a lack of occlusal support due to either unreplaced teeth or old ill-fitting dentures. Many of these patients appear to wear such dentures continually both day and night for many years.

Radiographic changes are best seen on the transpharyngeal and panoramic views of the joint. They will include a loss of cortical definition, flattening or erosions of the condylar head, subarticular cyst formation and calcification in the insertion of the lateral pterygoid tendon.

Treatment

Treatment consists of a course of an anti-inflammatory analgesic such as ibuprofen 400 mg three times daily, or diclofenac sodium 150 mg a day in divided doses or 100 mg of the slow-release preparation, especially if there is a painful effusion. These are best taken with food to prevent gastric irritation.

Persistent pain should be investigated by arthroscopy. Smoothing of the condylar head by open surgery, repair of a perforated meniscus or its replacemant with a temporalis myofascial flap are occasionally required. The atrophic joint, especially resulting from iatrogenic damage, may require an allopastic relacement.

Correction of the occlusion with adequate dentures is of primary importance in those patients with missing teeth.

The maxillary antrum

Acute sinusitis presents as a dull severe maxillary ache on one or both sides which is worse on bending. The premolar and molar teeth are often periostitic, which gives a false impression of pulpitis. The patient has usually had a recent upper respiratory tract infection and is aware of nasal obstruction and discharge; however, this is not invariable. Clinically the antra are tender to pressure and an occipitomental radiograph will show an opaque sinus, often with a fluid level.

Acute sinusitus responds to antibiotics and steam inhalations.

Chronic sinusitis rarely gives rise to facial or dental pain, but all too frequently an antral opacity due to polyps or mucosal thickening attracts unnecessary medical or surgical treatment, especially where the pain is chronic idiopathic or psychogenic in nature.

Antral tumours, especially carcinoma, are unfortunately painless unless they give rise to obstruction and secondary infection. However, these lesions must be excluded during any examination for facial pain by careful scrutiny of the occipitomental radiograph. The panoral tomograph may not reveal lesions in the medial part of the antrum and a computed tomographic (CT) scan may be necessary for the diagnosis.

The ears

Occasionally a painful otitis externa due to a furuncle, fungal infection or impacted wax can be referred to the mandibular area. The pain is elicited on rotating the concha, in which case the external auditory meatus should be examined. Treatment is by antibiotics or removal of the wax.

The salivary glands

The pain is usually dull and well-localized and is characteristically provoked by eating and associated with a swollen gland. Pus may be expressed from the duct, the opening of which is inflamed.

Where these features are acute and persistent one must consider the possibility of mumps, in which case the swelling may become bilateral and the patient is not only febrile but occasionally develops testicular, pancreatic or mammary inflammation. The serum may be screened for mumps S and V antibodies when the patient is first seen and 10 days later.

Calculi should be sought by plain radiographs and duct obstruction may be confirmed by sialography after the inflammatory phase has subsided. A persistent tender nodule in the parotid may be an adenoid cystic carcinoma and therefore requires surgical exploration. An ultrasound or CT scan will help to identify a space-occupying lesion.

Tonsils

A peritonsillar abscess (quinsy) not uncommonly presents as maxillary pain with trismus. A swelling of the palate between tonsillar fossa and uvula will be apparent. Treatment is with antibiotics, incision and drainage of the abscess. This can be done with a short-acting intravenous anaesthetic with the head of the supine patient well-extended to prevent inhalation of the pus.

Eyes

Acute glaucoma has been described as presenting with acute facial pain. However, the associated disturbance of vision and a palpably hard eye should establish the diagnosis. Pilocarpine and surgery are both used as treatment.

Elongated styloid process (Eagle's syndrome)

This questionable condition has been reported as being the cause of painful dysphagia. The elongated process is said to be palpable in the tonsillar fossa or evident on radiography and the recommended treatment is by surgical excision of the styloid process. However, in these patients serious consideration should be given to an alternative diagnosis of psychogenic atypical facial neuralgia or glossopharyngeal neuralgia. Rarely, a fractured styloid process can be the cause of acute pain, but surgical intervention is infrequently required.

Cardiac angina

On rare occasions the first presentation of ischaemic heart disease is angina related to exercise but referred to the angle of the left mandible. The explanation of this phenomenon may be a common autonomic sensory innervation.

The investigation will include an electrocardiogram.

Cancer

Chronic pain due to uncontrolled cancer in the orofacial region is treated with increasing doses of opioids such as morphine or heroin together with antidepressants. However, the elimination of underlying infection, palliative surgery or debulking with laser therapy are essential adjuncts.

Idiopathic and psychogenic pain

This is the most common cause of facial pain after toothache. Although severe attacks of recent onset do present for treatment, most are of sufficient duration to be classified as a chronic facial pain.

Four symptom complexes present either separately or together suggesting a common aetiology: facial arthromyalgia (TMJ dysfunction syndrome, myofascial pain dysfunction syndrome), atypical facial pain (atypical facial neuralgia), atypical odontalgia and the oral dysaesthesias.

The underlying mechanisms of these pains are unknown; many appear to be precipitated by or maintained by adverse life events, hence the description of psychogenic pain. However it is important to reassure the patient that the pain experience is real and that it represents 'chemical changes in the nerves and blood vessels comparable to migraines and tension headaches'.

Psychogenic pain may arise as:

1. A result of stress in a previously normal individual.
2. A feature of an emotional disturbance such as anxiety or depression.

3. An abnormal personality trait, e.g. obsessional or 'hysterical', now described as somatization.
4. Rarely, as a manifestation of psychosis.

The first two appear to be the most common causes and are readily amenable to treatment, even when the pain is of long standing. There is a wide age range, extending from the first decade upwards. The characteristic FAM patient is difficult to define and includes individuals with obsessional perfectionist traits.[71] Lefer[72] and Lupton[73] have both noted a tendency to self-denial and repression in these patients in relation to their personal problems, which accounts for their somatic manifestation. Feinmann and Harris[61] showed that, although these conditions are stress-related, 60% were psychiatrically normal with a third showing features of depression, and there was a small group of patients with personality disorders or psychosis. This may be compared with 20% with psychatric symptoms in a control group of other pain patients.

The common underlying problems related to the onset or perpetuation of the pain include, in young patients, parental separation, school examinations or sibling rivalry, whereas with older patients a history of family illness or bereavement, marital disharmony or professional stress is common. Even positive events such as promotion, marriage or moving house may be important related factors. It is therefore important in taking the history discreetly to explore both personal and family problems. The condition may present in an acute form but is often part of a long series of intermittent episodes. A small number of patients present with a personality disorder, or a psychiatric illness such as depression.

As stated, pain of emotional origin is common, especially in the orofacial region and it is clinically fallacious to assume that these complaints are imaginary. Indeed in most pain conditions the same peripheral structural and biochemical disturbances are responsible for the symptoms, whether of psychogenic or organic origin, and therefore the quality and intensity of the pain in both groups are indistinguishable.[74]

The key to the diagnosis of psychogenic pain, probably more than any other pain, is the history, i.e. general medical, family and social history. In many cases this appears to have been overlooked. Unfortunately, some patients often manifest a lack of psychological insight. They are reluctant to accept an emotional explanation for their pain, but insist that an organic cause must be found. This is of considerable clinical importance as they may decline drug therapy or psychiatric help but will readily submit to surgery. The clinician must recognize that a long-standing severe pain with no characteristic provoking or relieving factors, and no neurological or radiological signs, is unlikely to have a simple structural cause. However, the patient's precise definition of the site, descriptions of swelling, ulceration, discharge or haemorrhage, though all unsubstantiated, may persuade the surgeon to operate. This can range from the denervation or extraction of a tooth, exploration of the TMJ or antrum, to the excision of a salivary gland or sectioning of a division of the trigeminal or glossopharyngeal nerves. These procedures give relief for a short period, often no more than 10 days, and then the pain returns. Invariably the surgeon justifies the intervention by calling it an exploratory procedure, whereas often there has been failure to recognize a psychogenic pain syndrome and its appropriate therapy.

A paroxysmal trigeminal neuralgia sometimes can provoke a more continuous atypical facial neuralgia component. This latter may be due to reactionary depression caused by the primary neuralgia. Where both are present together the clinician may assume erroneously that the tic douloureux has become uncontrollable, whereas the therapy should be adjusted to include an antidepressant drug in addition to carbamazepine. Contrariwise, trigeminal neuralgia may suddenly change its character from intermittent paroxysmal attacks controlled by carbamazepine to a more continuous pain responding only to antidepressant drugs. Again, these patients have a background of significant emotional stress.

Facial arthromyalgia

Symptoms vary from a clicking uncomfortable jaw joint on chewing, talking and yawning, to a continuous dull ache with severe exacerbations, often described as earache. The pain radiates widely to the masseteric, temporal, occipital and mastoid areas or down into the neck. The patient on questioning may also give a history of headaches, disturbed hearing and tinnitus, cervical, lumbar or pelvic pain. The condition has also a strong association with pruritic skin conditions, vasomotor rhinitis,[75] peptic ulceration and irritable bowel and has therefore the characteristics of a generalized pain syndrome.

Bruxism and other tension-relieving habits are commonly found, although it seems that these habits do not have a causal relationship but are merely features of the condition.

Patients tend to fall into two groups: those who wake in the morning with pain and trismus which gradually subsides – the nocturnal grinders – and those who develop a dull ache during the day, especially towards evening when tired – the diurnal clenchers. The pain rarely seems to prevent or disturb sleep, and has often troubled the patient for many weeks or even intermittently for many years. Tenderness is most commonly present in the temporalis and masseter muscles and beneath the condylar head adjacent to the lobe of the ear, described as earache, but may also be detected over the mastoid process and the anterior border of sternomastoid, which the patient describes as swollen glands. Trismus is usual, with deviation of the mandible towards the affected side on opening. Ridging of the buccal mucosa and tongue margins due to bruxism, and worn facets on the teeth, are helpful diagnostic features. The dentition must be examined for pulpitic teeth.

Dysfunction may progress from minor limitation of opening with clicking or sticking to a marked lock prior to opening – a closed lock – or on attempted closure – an open lock. Both represent impaired translation of the meniscus due to disturbed synovial lubrication and are descibed as an anterior displacement with reduction. If this progresses to an anteriorly displaced adherent meniscus without reduction, opening is limited to less than 30 mm. In both these situations fibrillar adhesions may be seen on arthroscopy.

Atypical facial pain (idiopathic facial pain)

This is a common form of facial pain, usually described as a continuous dull ache, with intermittent excruciating throbbing episodes which are localized to a non-muscular site, such as the teeth and alveolus or over the maxillary antrum. It may be bilateral and is not provoked by jaw movement and rarely relieved by analgesics. Occasionally there is a strong resemblance to facial migrainous neuralgia, attacks being associated with nasal stuffiness or obstruction, and waking the patient in the early hours of the morning. Bouts may last for hours or days and the patient may give a history of intermittent episodes over a period of many years. A common feature is that the pain may be provoked or potentiated by dental treatment. Apart from occasional marked hyperaemia of the oral mucosa or slight oedema of the face, there are no clinical signs. Infiltrating the pain site with local anaesthetic often gives temporary relief but has no diagnostic significance.

Atypical odontalgia

Odontalgia, i.e. toothache is usually due to infective or traumatic inflammation of the pulp or periodontal membrane, but patients may present with identical clinical features without any obvious cause. The pain is severe and throbbing in character and the teeth are hypersensitive to any stimulus, be it pressure or thermal. It is often widespread and bilateral but occasionally may be precisely localized. Some appear to have been precipitated by a dental procedure such as the fitting of a bridge or an extraction, but they are invariably made worse by any further active treatment.

Typically, there is a history of pain accelerated by unnecessary pulp extirpations and extractions. The remaining teeth, even when sound and vital, are tender to percussion. The problem appears to be a state of hyperalgesia of the pulp and periodontal pain receptors due to persistent vasodilatation.[76] Careful investigation will reveal significant emotional problems in some. Others may not have any of the features of a primary psychogenic disorder and attempts to force one on them does not produce any therapeutic advantage.

These patients are best considered to have a variant of atypical facial neuralgia and can be treated in the same manner. The temptation to devitalize or extract teeth must be strenuously resisted.

Oral dysaesthesia

The most common presentation of this condition is the burning tongue, which has been called glossopyrosis or glossodynia. Occasionally the gingiva and lips are also involved, or the denture-bearing areas of the hard palate and lower alveolus, making the wearing of a denture impossible.

The patient is often middle-aged and female but can be any age or either sex. The picture is invariably one of a burning sensation that gradually increases in severity and frequency until it is present for the greater part of every day. It is not felt on waking but very quickly builds up to its maximum intensity. It may be unilateral or bilateral. The most striking feature is the relief usually obtained by eating or drinking. This leads to chewing of gum or other food as a palliative. Mucosal pains of the tongue are made worse by food and drink and this distinction is crucial in making the diagnosis.

The fear of cancer is the patient's greatest concern, and occasionally a bright-red tongue with scalloped margins, due to compression against the adjacent teeth, all too readily supports this suspicion. Additional minor worries, such as that of iron and vitamin deficiency or of pernicious anaemia, may have been created by indiscriminate prescribing. It is essential to establish that such a deficiency exists before trying empirical therapy. Similarly, antifungal treatment should be reserved for the clinically obvious candidosis or that confirmed by a microbiological smear and culture.

Variants of this condition are the persistent nasty taste, descibed as salty or purulent or halitosis, and the dry-mouth sensation. This last may present with either adequate or overtly inadequate salivary flow, but sialography and labial gland biopsies to eliminate Sjögren's disease should be normal.

As stated, these complaints would appear to be common reactive manifestations to stress, although in elderly patients this is not always evident and the symptoms may persist despite all therapy.

Those with insight and a short history often respond dramatically to explanation and reassurance, or to an antidepressant drug or a phenothiazine, such as trifluoperazine 2 mg twice a day.

Psychosis and facial pain

Rarely these pains may present as a feature of a psychotic illness.without any special qualitative characteristics. The distinguishing clinical features are to be detected in the behaviour of the patient whose story, which is often followed later by a long letter, invariably contains unusually vivid or bizarre details. Paranoid accusations seem to be an essential element: dentists, doctors, relations or religious and racial groups have all contributed to the patient's suffering. Occasionally the incongruous emotional reactions of schizophrenia are manifest and discreet questioning usually reveals previous psychiatric treatment and a family history of instability. Care must be taken in examining putative lesions which are usually factitious, that is, self-inflicted with a finger nail, needles or a corrosive agent such as aspirin, an undiluted antiseptic or household cleansing agents.

Rarely, one encounters the more florid Münchausen syndrome where the patient skilfully and repeatedly induces unwary surgeons to carry out operations for delusional symptoms which may include pain.[77] Psychiatric treatment is essential.

Somatopsychic problems

These vary from the recognizable simple overreaction to a dental procedure to more aggressive conditions. Anxious, obsessional and depressed states of mind will amplify pain and create agitation after what appears to be a normal surgical operation. Strong compassionate reassurance is essential and antipsychotic sedation with the usual analgesic will generally bring the problem under control.

However, unstable patients with a history of psychiatric illness may be thrown into a state of agitated paranoia by dental or surgical treatment. The procedure may have been relatively benign, such as the fitting of a new and therefore unfamiliar denture, or have involved an anaesthetic and surgery for the removal of teeth. The common factor appears to be intraoral disturbance which triggers off an aggressive vociferous attack on the dentist's competence and reputation. With the inevitable discomfort, bleeding and swelling following surgery, the patient may complain violently of facial mutilation, the destruction of hearing and balance and the retention of multiple foreign bodies in the throat.

These psychotic reactions, however, appear to be an exaggerated response to real discomfort, and rather than abandon the patient one should bravely attempt to restore the *status quo ante*. New dentures must be carefully adjusted replicas of the previous set, or if possible, of the natural teeth. Firm reassurance and appropriate relief for surgical sequelae are important. Antipsychotic sedation, such as trifluoperazine or flupenthixol, is invaluable, but when the disturbance or delusions are marked, specialist psychiatric advice is mandatory.

Idiopathic pain management

For successful management it is important to identify:

1. Not only the features of the facial pain but also chronic pain disorders elsewhere, e.g. the head, neck, back, irritable bowel and the pelvis (often endometriosis) and pruritus.
2. Predisposing adverse life events, especially in the family history, and any emotional or psychiatric disturbance.
3. Sensitive carious cavities and pulpal inflammation must be excluded. Major restorative dental procedures should be avoided as they can create intractable problems which tend to obscure the aetiology and complicate treatment.
4. Reassurance is important; many patients respond well to the explanation that the pain is real, not imaginary, arising in cramped muscle and dilated blood vessels as a response to emotional stress.
5. A bite guard worn either at night or during the day between meals discourages bruxism and may be effective in relieving joint pain and trismus. It is useful in young patients and those who are reluctant either to take psychotropic drugs, even when they are used as muscle relaxants. However, such physical therapy should be limited to 3 months if unsuccessful.
6. Patients unresponsive to physical therapy, those with an obvious psychogenic background or with marked pain respond well to a tricyclic antidepressant such as nortriptyline 10–75 mg or lofepramine 70–210 mg taken at night and increased slowly over 6 weeks, maintaining this regime until the patient has been symptom-free for at least 3 months. Side-effects such as dry mouth, drowsiness and constipation may be a problem but often diminish with treatment. The serotonin-specific uptake inhibitors such as fluoxetine 20–40 mg may also be effective with fewer muscarinic side-effects, that is, less drowsiness,dry mouth and constipation. The antidepressant drugs have been shown to be highly effective in non-depressed patients in many chronic pain conditions and may act by enhancing 5-hydroxytryptamine central pain suppressor activity as well as elevating mood. It is equally important to emphasize that the drug therapy is not being used to treat depression, but has a direct effect in relieving the painful muscles and blood vessels.

   Medication must be combined with regular reviews to provide reassurance and to achieve drug compliance. With psychotic or agitated patients additional medication such as small doses of a phenothiazine, for example, trifluoperazine 2–4 mg b.d. or flupenthixol 0.5–1.5 mg b.d. as a supplement to the tricyclics, may be required. These are best taken at breakfast and lunch.

   Occasionally the response is better to a monoamine oxidase inhibitor such as phenelzine 15 mg three times daily taken at 08.00, 12.00 and 16.00 h each day. Parstelin (tranylcypromine 10 mg, trifluoperazine 1 mg) three times daily, should be tried if these regimes fail. Reluctance to take medication and placebo side-effects are common problems which are usually overcome with firm reassurance.
7. With joint pains which have not responded to physical or medical therapy, arthroscopy provides a means of establishing the presence of intra-articular adhesions and eliminating them by lysis and lavage. A normal joint or hyperaemic synovium are indications for continued medical therapy with antidepressant medication. A rigid adherent or perforated meniscus is an indication for arthrotomy. It is often possible to mobilize the meniscus from its anteromedial displacement and carry out a meniscopexy. The grossly degenerate meniscus may be replaced with a temporalis

myofascial finger flap. Surgery carried out for intractable pain without obvious indications not only provides limited pain relief but may intensify the condition. Further surgery then will often make the pain intractable and create further dysfunction and deformity.

Once the condition is cured, it is important to warn patients that they may relapse from time to time should the provoking factors recur. This enables the patients to accept minor degrees of recurrent discomfort and helps to protect them from unnecessary and inappropriate treatment.

Persistent pain or a marked emotional disturbance are indications for referral to a liaison psychiatrist. However, where possible the patient should be kept under review to exclude any latent structural pathology. It is also important where the symptoms are severe to exclude any suicidal intent and in particular never to prescribe sedatives alone, as they tend to intensify rather than relieve depression. Frequent assessment at the outset is not only reassuring to the patient but also provides a clearer picture of the underlying personal and social background. Curiously enough, those with refractory pain are often relatively uncomplaining and appear to be satisfied with continued consultations and support, even though the same unchanging symptoms are discussed and treatment is prescribed. A regular regimen of simple analgesics supplemented with an antidepressant drug appears to be the most effective therapy. Rarely, vigorous attempts to deprive some of these intractable pain patients of their symptoms may precipitate a crisis such as dramatic syncopal attacks, urinary retention, whole-body analgesia, ataxia or a frank psychotic state.[72,78] All may occur without detectable neurological cause and cease as suddenly as they arise.

Neuropathic pain

Primary neuralgias

These may affect the trigeminal, glossopharyngeal nerves and the superior laryngeal branch of the vagus. Their aetiology is unknown, although viral damage to the ganglia, compression of the intracranial nerve roots by small vascular loops[79] or by dural bands, and narrowing of the foramina, have all been proposed, but the evidence is questionable. Paroxysmal neuralgia may also be an early feature of demyelinating disease. In addition ill-defined foci of chronic osteitis within the jaws have also been incriminated.[80]

Paroxysmal trigeminal neuralgia (tic douloureux)

This is the most common form of the condition. It usually presents in the elderly as a severe stabbing pain lasting seconds, provoked by talking, chewing or swallowing, or by touching a specific area, the so-called trigger zone. This is often found to be insensitive immediately after an attack. The most common sites of pain are the mandibular–mental and maxillary–canine areas. The ophthalmic distribution of the trigeminal nerve is usually spared. Attacks may be repeated throughout the day but rarely occur at night. Though periods of remission can be expected, the condition tends to persist throughout life. There are no objective neurological signs.

Occasionally the patient describes a persistent ache or burning sensation between paroxysmal attacks. This has the characteristics of an atypical facial neuralgia (see below) and is probably a depressive vascular pain arising as a secondary reaction to the paroxysmal neuralgia.

Treatment

The anticonvulsant carbamazepine (Tegretol) 100–400 mg three times daily controls the condition in over two-thirds of patients. It is important to introduce the drug gradually to avoid nausea and ataxia. The slow-release preparation produces fewer side-effects and may be taken 12-hourly. These symptoms or an allergic dermatitis may necessitate its withdrawal and replacement with phenytoin 100 mg four times a day. Unfortunately, this drug is not as effective and may need to be supplemented with clonazepam. Contrary to early reports, agranulocytosis due to carbamazepine is uncommon.

Where drug therapy is inadequate or immediate relief is essential, good control can be achieved by injecting 2 ml of 90% alcohol or 2 ml of 5% phenol in glycerine into the mental or infraorbital foramina, taking care to avoid entering a blood vessel by aspirating before injecting. The alcohol can also be infiltrated in the region of the mandibular foramen at the lingula. In all cases, give 1 ml of 2% lignocaine 5 min before the alcohol to avoid unnecessary pain. The relief may last 6–12 months but occasionally adjacent areas develop trigger zones. Peripheral neurectomy and cryotherapy at these sites has comparable results.

Where these local measures fail, intraganglionic radiofrequency thermocoagulation may be performed through the foremen ovale under radiographic control. The advantage of the latter technique is that the thermal damage may be modulated to destroy only unmedullated pain fibres, preserving sensation and reducing paraesthesia. The last resort is an intracranial preganglionic section of the mandibular and/or maxillary nerves or, where necessary, a total postganglionic nerve section, that is, between the ganglion and the brainstem.[81] Where the ophthalmic division is sectioned, a tarsorrhaphy is required to protect the insensitive cornea. Illingworth[82] has described a posterior fossa operation dividing the main sensory root near to the pons and sparing the more medially placed light touch and corneal reflex fibres as well as the motor root. Jannetta[79] proposes that intracranial vascular loops compressing the trigeminal nerve are responsible for the problem and advocates exploration and decompression of the nerve.

Glossopharyngeal neuralgia is brought on by swallowing and is felt in the ear and faucial area. Analogous treatment, where applicable, is used for glossopharyngeal and superior laryngeal neuralgia.

Secondary neuralgias

Secondary neuralgias are caused by lesions irritating the trigeminal nerve or ganglion. They may initially mimic a primary neuralgia but later present as a more persistent pain with local sensory, reflex or motor disturbances. For this reason they will be discussed as chronic nociceptive pain. They can be classified into extracranial, cranial base and intracranial lesions.

Extracranial lesions

The mental nerve produces two causes of neuralgia in the elderly patient. The first arises from the continued use of an old lower denture where there is marked alveolar resorption, leading to compression of the mental nerve by the buccal flange. The pain can be elicited by digital compression and there is usually radiographic evidence of a superficial mental foremen. Treatment is by relieving the denture over the site of the nerve or, where this is ineffective, the latter may be set down surgically below the alveolar surface.

In the second presentation, bony compression of the mental nerve may give rise to intermittent severe paroxysmal pain indistinguishable from a true tic douloureux and which can be bilateral. Usually there is radiological evidence of a narrowed mental foramen. Again, this is a problem of old age, although the patient may have a well-preserved alveolar ridge. Treatment consists of decompression of the mental nerve by carefully removing a ring of bone from around the margin of the foramen.

Causalgia

Causalgia is rare in the jaws and is a difficult diagnosis to make with certainty. It presents as a well-localized persistent burning or throbbing pain, usually at the site of a traumatic surgical procedure which preceded the onset of symptoms. The commonest site is the lower third molar or mental region, and may follow a history of a difficult extraction or occasionally a local anaesthetic injection into the inferior alveolar nerve. Relief can only be obtained by a complete local analgesic blockage of all sensory pathways from the area which may be diagnostic. Some causalgias have been attributed to traumatic neuromas, but unfortunately localization of the neuroma for excision may be difficult.

It is important to distinguish causalgia from atypical facial pain, which is achronic idiopathic pain relieved by antidepressant drug therapy. The differential diagnosis may be difficult, especially as an atypical facial pain can be converted into a causalgia by repeated irrelevant surgery. Here a careful study of the patient and an attempt to relieve the pain initially with a course of antidepressants are essential. Nerve blocks tend to have a variable initial effect on atypical facial pain, but do not give the long-term relief they provide for a true causalgia.

Where the pain is repeatedly abolished by a simple inferior dental nerve block, avulsion of the damaged portion of the nerve or exploration by means of a sagittal split osteotomy and excision of a traumatic neuroma is indicated.

The only alternative to these procedures is the continued use of analgesics. Opioids such as tramadol require continued supervision and should be substituted for sedation and minor analgesics at intervals to reduce the problems of addiction.

Frey's syndrome, facial gustatory sweating and flushing

Frey's syndrome is a burning pain in the temporal area associated with flushing and sweating on eating. Occasionally there is a persistent hyperalgesia between attacks. It occurs after damage to the parotid by inflammation, surgery or occasionally a condylar fracture, and has been reported after cervical sympathectomy, and the ingestion of certain foods, including cheese, especially in diabetic neuropathy.[83] The syndrome has been attributed to aberrant parasympathetic secretomotor fibres reinnervating the cut ends of the sympathetic vaso- and sudomotor cholinergic nerves. However, recovery in the postsurgical group suggests that the cause may be a lack of inhibitory sympathetic tone.

Avulsion of the auriculotemporal nerve, intracranial section of Jacobson's nerve, which conveys the parasympathetic fibres to the area, has been recommended, but the effectiveness of these procedures is questionable. Relief is possible: the application of a 1% glycopyrronium bromide roll-on lotion provides an average 3–day control of symptoms;[84] a possible contraindication is narrow-angle glaucoma. An aluminium hexachloride antiperspirant applied before meals may control the gustatory sweating.

Herpes zoster

This presents initially as pain followed by a vesicular eruption of the skin overlying the branch of the trigeminal nerve, along which the activated varicella virus has spread. The pain may precede the rash by up to 48 h and, if localized to a tooth, this may be extracted unnecessarily. To abolish the pain and aid rapid recovery, acyclovir 800 mg 5 times daily is taken immediately for 7 days by mouth. The dose may be doubled and also given intravenously in the immunocompromised.

Postherpetic neuralgia

This has been attributed to destruction of the large myelinated sensory fibres by the zoster virus, so abolishing their modulating effect on the substantia gelatinosa gate mechanism. It is however a rare complication which takes the form of attacks of pain of varying severity localized to scarred areas of increased or diminished sensation – the so-called anaesthesia dolorosa. The pain usually diminishes in 6 months to 2 years. Where the virus has infected the geniculate ganglion, the patient will also have facial palsy – the Ramsay Hunt syndrome.

As treatment the minor analgesics should always be used initially, supplemented with a tricyclic antidepressant. The application of capsiacin (0.075% cream) 3–4 times a day may help by depleting the peripheral sensory neurons (C fibres) of SP. If severe, a low-addictive opioid such as tramadol may be necessary. The condition is not amenable to surgery.

Nasopharyngeal carcinoma (Trotter's syndrome)

This may occur in young people, especially in Asia, and is due to the oncogenic Epstein–Barr virus. It classically arises in the fossa of Rosenmüller behind the opening of the eustachian tube and obstructs its aperture, producing conductive deafness. The tumour infiltrates laterally the mandibular division of the trigeminal nerve, giving rise to the important combination of facial pain, cutaneous analgesia and wasting of the masseter muscle. Direct invasion of the soft palate and the medial pterygoid produces ipsilateral elevation of the uvula, dysphagia and trismus. Further extension towards the base of the skull eventually involves other cranial nerves.

The lesion may be demonstrated by CT. Treatment is by radiotherapy and cytotoxic drugs.

Cranial base lesions

Pyogenic inflammation (Gradenigo's syndrome)

Rarely, middle-ear infection may spread to the apex of the petrous temporal bone, where the osteitis involves both the abducent nerve and the trigeminal ganglion. This presents as a lateral rectus palsy and facial pain with or without cutaneous analgesia. Other painful lesions of the cranial base include meningeal sarcoid, nasopharyngeal tumours extending upwards, intracranial lesions extending downwards and secondary carcinoma from elsewhere. These may give cranial nerve neuropathies with disturbed facial sensation rather than pain. Rarely, Paget's disease may lead to platybasia (indentation of the posterior cranial fossa) with neurological disturbance.

Intracranial lesions

Disseminated sclerosis

This may present as a tic douloureux but should be considered if the neuralgia is accompanied by other neurological features such as a loss of taste, disturbance in facial sensation and neurological changes elsewhere. This presentation tends to occur more frequently in younger patients. The diagnosis may be confirmed by magnetic resonance imaging scan.

Tabes dorsalis

This is now an exceedingly rare cause of severe paroxysmal facial pain. It is associated with Argyll Robertson pupils and positive serological tests for syphilis. Treatment with carbamazepine is effective.

Tumours of the posterior cranial fossa

The classical example is the schwannoma (acoustic neurinoma) arising on the eighth cranial nerve in the cerebellopontine angle. The trigeminal, facial and the vestibuloacoustic cranial nerves are enclosed in the narrow triangular space between the pons, cerebellum and medial surface of the petrous bone. Thus, the enlarging neuroma produces trigeminal pain and sensory loss, deafness and ataxia. These, together with nystagmus and a reduced corneal reflex, may be observed clinically. Further investigations should include CT.

Although this is a benign lesion, early removal is essential to reduce operative and postoperative complications.

Middle cranial fossa lesions

These include pituitary tumours and aneurysms of the internal carotid artery. The latter enlarge within the cavernous sinus. Both ultimately exert pressure on the optic track and nerves contained in the cavernous sinus, which include the ophthalmic and maxillary and the third, fourth and sixth cranial nerves. Thus tumours in this region produce facial pain and cutaneous analgesia together with disturbances in vision and in extraocular movements. Investigations will include angiography and CT.

Vascular pains

Migraine

This is a recurrent unilateral throbbing headache associated with visual disturbances, nausea and ataxia. The pain is intensified by sneezing, coughing and movements of the head. It appears to be due to painful pulsatile extracranial vasodilatation associated with intracranial vasoconstriction. There are a multitude of precipitating factors, which include hormonal and emotional disturbances, hypoglycaemia, alcohol and foods containing vasoactive amines such as cheese (tyramine) and chocolate (β-phenylethylamine) but many cases remain idiopathic.

Some patients achieve relief with simple analgesics, which include aspirin 1 g or ibuprofen 400 mg. A combination of analgesic and a continuous course of a tricyclic antidepressant such as nortriptyline 10–25 mg can be highly effective in preventing frequent attacks.

The vasoconstrictor ergotamine tartrate is widely used – 2 mg sublingually, 0.36–0.72 mg by inhaler or 0.25–0.5 mg intramuscularly or subcutaneously. However, ergot preparations have to be given as early as possible in the attack for satisfactory relief, and can add to the malaise and nausea of the attack if repeated too frequently. The drug should be avoided in pregnancy and in patients with vascular disease.

Sumatriptan 100 mg orally as soon as possible after the onset of the attack and repeated no more than 300 mg in 24 h, or 6 mg may be taken subcutaneously and repeated once in 24 h.

Facial migrainous neuralgia (also known as Horton's syndrome, Sluder's syndrome, cluster headaches, histamine cephalalgia, sphenopalatine neuralgia, vidian nerve neuralgia, alarm clock headache, etc.)

The many names for this condition reflect the problems associated with its diagnosis and treatment.[85] As with other types of migraine, the pain is attributed to spastic dilatation of blood vessels, which in this condition are the maxillary branches of the external carotid artery. It affects principally men and classically occurs at night, waking the patient in the early hours – hence the name alarm clock headache. It is an intense throbbing pain, usually lasting about half an hour, and the patient may notice that the eye is red and the nose feels congested on that side. The attacks occur at regular intervals and are sometimes repeated as a series over a period of a week or more before they subside. Occasionally, alcohol or coffee are precipitating factors.

The attacks may be prevented with ergotamine suppositories used nightly before going to sleep, until a phase of remission occurs. However, pizotifen is much more acceptable and may be taken in range of 500 µg to 3 mg nocte. As with simple migraine, tricyclic antidepressant drugs are also a valuable prophylactic. However, there appears to be a strong clinical association between facial arthromyalgia, migraine,[81] facial migrainous neuralgia and atypical facial neuralgia, suggesting that they all represent related vascular pain mechanisms.

Giant cell arteritis

Although classically occurring in the temporal region, these inflammatory foci within an artery wall may affect other branches of the external carotid, producing severe facial pain. It is usually a condition of old age and may be associated with diabetes mellitus. An arteritis may also be a presenting feature of polymyalgia rheumatica, when the patient will complain of widespread stiffness and joint pain. Where a superficial vessel such as the facial artery is involved, a tender nodule may be palpable; on exploration it will prove to be a firm, pale and tortuous section of blood vessel. This should be excised for histology. The erythrocyte sedimentation rate will be high and the rheumatoid serological tests positive.

When the maxillary artery is involved, the pain presents as intermittent claudication in the muscles of mastication and of the tongue brought on by eating.

Systemic steroids commencing with prednisone 60 mg a day are essential to prevent involvement of the ophthalmic artery, leading to blindness. The dose will be maintained for 10 days and then reduced as the condition comes under control.

References

1. Bonica JJ. General considerations of chronic pain. In: Bonica JJ (ed) *The Management of Pain*, pp. 180–183. Philadelphia: Lea & Febiger, 1990.
2. Schiffman E, Fricton JR. Epidemiology of TMJ and craniofacial pain. In: Friction JR, Kroening RJ and Hathaway KM (eds) *TMJ and Craniofacial Pain. Diagnosis and Management*, p. 1–10. St Louis: EuroAmerica, 1989.
3. *Butterworths Medical Dictionary*, 2nd edn, p. 1230. London: Butterworths, 1978.
4. Wall PD, Devor M. Sensory afferent impulses originate from dorsal root ganglia as well as from periphery in normal and nerve injured rats. *Pain* 1983; **17**: 321–339.
5. Merskey H (ed). Classification of chronic pain: description of chronic pain syndromes and definition of pain terms. *Pain* 1986; suppl 3: S1.
6. Wyke BD. The surgical physiology of facial pain. *Br Dent J* 1958; **104**: 153–168.
7. Brune K, Menzel-Soglowek S, Zeihofer HU. Differential analgesic effects of aspirin like drugs. *Drugs* 1992; **44**: 52–58.
8. Levine JD, Gooding J, Donatoni P, Borden L, Goetzl EJ. The role of the polymorphonuclear leucocyte in hyperalgesia. *J Neurosci* 1985; **5**: 3625–3629.
9. Quinn JH, Bazan NG. Identification of prostaglandin E_2 and leukotriene B_4 in the synovial fluid of painful, dysfunctional temporomandibular joints. *J Oral Maxillofac Surg* 1990; **48**: 968–971.
10. Lin Y, Pape HD, Friedrich R. Use of superoxide dismutase (SOD) in patients with temporomandibular

joint dysfunction. A preliminary study. *Int J Oral Maxillofac Surg* 1994; **23**: 428–429.
11. Nakamura-Craig M, Smith TH. Substance P and peripheral inflammatory hyperalgesia. *Pain* 1988; **38**: 91–98.
12. Ferreira SH, Lorenzetti BB. Prostaglandins hyperalgesia. A metabolic process. *Prostaglandins* 1981; **21**: 789–792.
13. Follenfant RL, Nakamura-Craig M, Garland LG. Sustained hyperalgesia in rats evoked by 15-hydroxy-tetraenoic acid is attenuated by the protein kinase inhibitor H-7. p. 133. *J Br Pharm Soc* 1990; **99**: (abstracts published as supplement to this volume).
14. Perreira SH, Lorenzetti BB, De Campos DI. Induction, blockade and restoration of a persistent hypersensitive state. *Pain* 1990; **42**: 365–371.
15. Dubner R. Pain and hyperalgesia following tissue injury; new mechanisms and new treatments. *Pain* 1991; **44**: 213–214.
16. Cousins MJ. Prevention of postoperative pain. In: Bond MR, Charlton JE, Woolf CJ (eds) *Proceedings of the VI World Congress on Pain*. Oxford: Elsevier Science, 1991.
17. Tverskoy M, Cozacov, Ayache M, Bradley EL, Kinssin I. Postoperative pain after inguinal herniorrhaphy with different types of anaesthesia. *Anesth Analg* 1990; **70**: 29–35.
18. Matis WL, Lavker RM, Murphy GF. Substance P induces the expression of an endothelial-leukocyte adhesion molecule by microvascular endothelium. *J Invest Dermatol* 1990; **94**: 492–495.
19. Levine JD, Goetzl EJ, Basbaum AI. Contribution of the nervous system to the pathophysiology of rheumatoid arthritis and other polyarthrides. *Rheum Dis Clin North Am* 1987; **13**: 360–383.
20. Johansson AS, Isacsson G, Isberg A, Granholm AC. Distribution of substance P like immunoreactive nerve fibers in temporomandibular joint soft tissues of monkey. *Scand J Dent Res* 1986; **94**: 225–230.
21. Holmlund A, Ekblom A, Hansson P, Lind J, Lundberg T, Theodorsson E. Concentrations of neuropeptide substance P, neurokinin A, calcitonin gene related peptide, neuropeptide Y and vasoactive intestinal polypeptide in synovial fluid of the human temporomandibular joint. *Int J Oral Maxillofac Surg* 1991; **20**: 228–231.
22. Sessle BJ. The neurobiology of facial and dental pain: present knowledge, future directions. *J Dent Res* 1987; **66**: 962–981.
23. Hukanen M, Konttinen YT, Rees RG, Gibson SJ, Fatavirpa F, Polak JM. Innervation of bone from normal and arthritic rats by SP and CGRP containing fibres. *J Rheumatol* 1992; **19**: 1252–1259.
24. Fields HL. *Pain Syndromes in Neurology*, p. 2. London: Butterworths, 1990.
25. Cadden SW, Lisney S, Matthews B. Thresholds to electrical stimulation of nerves in cat canine tooth pulp with A beta, A delta and C fiber conduction velocities. *Brain Res* 1983; **261**: 31–41.
26. Azerad J, Woda A. Sensations evoked by bipolar intrapulpal stimulation. *Pain* 1977; **4**: 145–152.
27. Narhi M. The characteristics of intradental sensory units and their response to stimulation. *J Dent Res* 1985; **64**: 564–571.
28. Torneck CD. Dentine-pulp complex. In: Ten Cate AR (ed) *Oral Histology, Development, Structure and Function*. p. 188. St Louis: CV Mosby, 1989.
29. Narhi MVO. Intradental sensory units. In: Inoki R (ed) *Dynamic Aspects of Dental Pulp. Molecular Biology, Pharmacology and Pathophysiology*. pp. 144–145. London: Chapman & Hall, 1990.
30. Brimijoin S, Lundberg JM, Brodin E, Hokfelt T, Nilsson G. Axonal transport of SP in the vagus and sciatic nerves of the guinea pig. *Brain Res* 1980; **191**: 443.
31. Gores M, Oehme P, Zuhrt R. The significance of endogenous peptides for dental pulp pain. *Zahn Mund Kisferhgilkd* 1989; **77**: 531–536.
32. Akai M, Wakisaka S. Neuroregulators-neuropeptides. Distribution of peptidergic nerves. In Inoki R (ed) *Dynamic Aspects of Dental Pulp. Molecular Biology, Pharmacology and Pathophysiology*, p. 346. London: Chapman and Hall, 1990.
33. Zochodne DW, Murray M, Nag S, Riopelle RJ. A segmental chronic pain syndrome in rats associated with intrathecal infusion of NMDA: evidence for selective action in the dorsal horn. *Canad J Neur Sci* 1994; **21**: 24–28.
34. Shigenaga Y, Nakatani J. Distribution of trigemino-thalamic projection cells in the caudal medulla of the cat. In: Matthew B, Hill RG (eds) *Anatomical, Physiological and Pharmacological Aspects of Ttrigeminal Pain*, pp. 163–174. Amsterdam: Elsvier Biomedical, 1982.
35. Fields HL. In: Fields HL (ed) *Pain Syndromes in Neurology*. London: Butterworths, 1990.
36. Barber TX. Toward a theory of pain: relief of chronic pain by prefrontal leucotomy, opiates, placebo and hypnosis. *Psychol Bull* 1959; **36**: 436–460.
37. Derbyshire SW, Jones AK, Devani P, Watson JD, Frackowiak RS. Cerebral responses to pain in patients with atypical facial pain measured by positron emission tomography. *J Neurol Neurosurg Psychiatry* 1994; **57**: 1166–1177.
38. Melzack R, Wall PD. Pain mechanisms: a new theory. *Science* 1965; **150**: 971–979.
39. Melzack R, Wall PD. *The Challenge of Pain*. London: Pelican, 1988.
40. Melzack R. Pain: past, present and future. *Can J Exp Psychiatry*1993; **47**: 615–629.
41. Melzack R. Phantom limbs and the concept of a neuromatrix. *Trends Neurosci* 1990; **13**: 88–92.
42. Basbaum AI, Fields HL. Endogenous pain control mechanisms, review and hypothesis. *Ann Neurol* 1978; **4**: 451–462.
43. Fields HL, Heimricher MM. Anatomy and physiology of a nociceptive modulatory system. *Phil Trans R Soc Lond (Biol)* 1985; **308**: 361–374.
44. Hughes J, Smith TW, Kosterlitz HW, Fothergill LA, Morgan BA, Morris HR. Identification of two related

pentapeptides from the brain with potent opiate activity. *Nature* 1975; **256**: 577–579.
45. Smoke T, Fields HL. ACTH blocks opiate-induced analgesia in the rat. *Brain Res* 1980; **212**: 202–206.
46. Blumer D, Zorick F, Heilbronn M, Roth T. Biological markers for depression in chronic pain. *J Nerv Ment Dis* 1982; **170**: 425–428.
47. Hirst M. The changing nature of pain control: clinical aspects of endorphin and enkephalins. *J Can Dent Assoc* 1985; **7**: 493–497.
48. Morget V, Foster A, Laverriere MC *et al.* Mechanism of analgesia induced by hypnosis and acupuncture. Is there a difference? *Pain* 1991; **45**: 135–140.
49. Yaksh TL. Direct evidence that spinal serotonin and noradrenalin terminals mediate the spinal antinociceptive effects of morphine in periaqueductal gray. *Brain Res* 1979; **160**: 180–185.
50. Basbaum AI, Moss MS, Glazer EJ. Opiate and stimulation produced analgesia: the contribution of the monoamines. *Adv Pain Res Ther* 1983; **5**: 323–339.
51. Yonehara N, Shibutani T, Imai Y, Inoki R. Involvement of descending monoaminergic systems in the transmission of dental pain in the trigeminal nucleus caudalis of the rabbit. *Brain Res* 1990; **508**: 234–240.
52. Feinmann C, Harris M. Psychogenic facial pain: management and prognosis. *Br Dent J* 1984; **156**: 205–208.
53. Botney M, Fields HL. Amitriptyline potentiates morphine analgesia by a direct action on the central nervous system. *Ann Neurol* 1983; **13**: 160–164.
54. Taiwo U, Fabian A, Pazoles C, Fields HL. Further studies on the mechanism of the potentiation of morphine antinociception of monoamine uptake inhibitors. *Pain* 1985; **21**: 329–338.
55. Takenoshita Y, Ikebe T, Yamamoto M, Oka M. Occlusal contact area and temporomandibular joint symptoms. *Oral Surg Oral Med Oral Pathol* 1991; **72**: 388–394.
56. Pullinger AG, Seligman DA, Gombein JA. A multiple logistic regression analysis of the risk and relative odds of temporomandibular disorders as a function of common occlusal features. *J Dent Res* 1993; **72**: 968–979.
57. Speculand B, Hughes AO, Gross AN. Role of stressful life experiences in the onset of TMJ pain dysfunction. *Commun Dent Oral Epidemiol* 1984; **12**: 197–202.
58. Feinmann C, Harris M, Cawley R. Psychogenic facial pain: presentation and management. *Br Med J* 1984; **228**: 436–438.
59. Marbach JJ, Lennon MC, Dohrenwend BP. Candidate risk factors for temporomandibular pain and dysfunction syndrome: psychosocial, health behaviour, physical illness and injury. *Pain* 1988; **34**: 139–151.
60. Southwell J, Deary IJ, Geissler P. Personality and anxiety in temporomandibular joint syndrome patients. *J Oral Rehabil* 1990; **17**: 239–243.
61. Feinmann C, Harris M. Psychogenic facial pain. The clinical presentation. *Br Dent J* 1984; **156**: 165.
62. Aghabeigi B, Feinmann C, Harris M. Prevalence of post-traumatic stress disorder in patients with chronic idiopathic facial pain. *Br J Oral Maxillofac Surg* 1992; **30**: 360–364.
63. Engel GL. Psychogenic pain and the pain-prone patient. *Am J Med* 1959; **196**: 129–136.
64. Raphael KG, Dohrenwend BP, Marbach JJ. Illness and injury among children of temporomandibular pain and dysfunction syndrome (TMPDS) patients. *Pain* 1990; **40**: 61–64.
65. Almay BGL, Haggendal J, von Knorring L, Oreland L. 5-HIAA and HVA in CSF in patients with idiopathic pain disorders. *Biol Psychiatry* 1987; **22**: 403–412.
66. von Knorring L. Affect and pain: neurochemical mediators and therapeutic approaches. In: Dubner R, Gebhart GF, Bond MR (eds) *Proceedings of the Vth Congress on Pain* pp. 243–253. Amsterdam: Elsvier Science, 1988.
67. von Knorring L. The pathogenesis of chronic pain syndromes. *Nord Psykiatr Tidsskr* 1989; **43** (suppl 20): 35–43.
68. Aghabeigi B, Feinmann C, Glover V *et al.* Tyramine conjugation deficit in patients with chronic idiopathic temporomandibular joint and orofacial pain. *Pain* 1993; **54**: 159–163.
69. Harris M. The surgical management of idiopathic facial pain produces intractable iatrogenic pain? *Br J Oral Maxillofac Surg* 1996; **34**: 1–3.
70. Toller PA. Temporomandibular joint arthropathy. *Proc R Soc Med* 1974; **67**: 153–159.
71. Moulton RE. Emotional factors in non-organic temporomandibular joint pain. *Dent Clin North Am* 1966; 609–620.
72. Lefer L. A psychoanalytic view of a dental phenomenon psychosomatics of the temporomandibular joint pain–dysfunction syndrome. *Contemp Psychiatry* 1966; **2**: 135–150.
73. Lupton DE. Psychological aspects of temporomandibular joint dysfunction. *J Am Dent Assoc* 1969; **79**: 131–136.
74. Woodforde JM, Merskey H. Personality traits of patients with chronic pain. *J Psychosom Res* 1972; **16**: 167–172.
75. Berry DC. Mandibular dysfunction pain and chronic minor illness. *Br Dent J* 1969; **127**: 170–175.
76. Rees RT, Harris M. Atypical odontalgia. *Br J Oral Surg* 1979; **16**: 212–218.
77. Oldham L. Facial pain as a presentation in Von Munchausen's syndrome: a case report. *Br J Oral Surg* 1974; **12**: 86–90.
78. Delaney JF. Atypical facial pain as a defense against psychosis. *Am J Psychiatry* 1976; **133**: 1151–1154.
79. Jannetta PJ. Trigeminal neuralgia and hemifacial spasm – etiology and definitive treatment. *Trans Am Neurol Assoc* 1975; **100**: 89–91.
80. Ratner EJ, Persch P, Kleinman DJ, Shklar G, Sokranoky SS. Jawbone cavities and trigeminal and atypical facial neuralgias. *Oral Surg Oral Med Oral Pathol* 1979; **48**: 3–20.
81. Henderson WR. Trigeminal neuralgia – the pain and its treatment. *Br Med J* 1967; **1**: 7–15.

82. Illingworth RD. Selective posterior fossa trigeminal nerve section for treatment of trigeminal neuralgia. *Proc R Soc Med* 1974; **67**: 770.
83. Watkins PJ. Facial sweating after food: a new sign of diabetic autonomic neuropathy. *Br Med J* 1973; **1**: 583–587.
84. Hays LL, Novack AJ, Worsham JC. The Frey syndrome: a simple effective treatment. *Otolaryng Head Neck Surg* 1982; **90**: 419–425.
85. Ball JI, Walton JN. Periodic migrainous neuralgia. *Br Med J* 1964; **1**: 219–221.

24

Orofacial neuropathies and their clinical manifestations

Malcolm Harris

Introduction

The relatively small anatomical area of the mouth and face is subject to a great variety of neurological disturbances, some of which are of little concern to the oral specialist. Only those relevant to our clinical practice will be discusssed here.

Examination of the cranial nerves is a simple procedure and where appropriate must be followed by a full neurological examination of all systems. Computerized tomographic (CT) scans and magnetic resonance imaging (MRI) are invaluable when appropriately applied to the diagnosis of these lesions.

Classification

Where a clinical presentation such as a cranial nerve disorder is unfamiliar, the diagnostic problem should be considered using the 'surgical sieve'. One of the most effective forms of this classification is the subdivision into congenital or acquired, remembering that certain disorders such as drug or viral defects may be acquired *in utero*. The acquired disorders may then be subdivided into traumatic: inflammatory, which includes physical, chemical, radiation, and the all-important infective group.

Infective inflammatory agents include viruses, prions, bacteria, fungi and parasites. Autoimmune disorders also belong here in inflammation. This leaves cysts, neoplasms, both benign and malignant, endocrine, nutritional deficiency and idiopathic conditions.

The olfactory nerve (I cranial nerve)

The sense of smell can be readily tested with small bottles containing aromatic substances such as oil of cloves, peppermint, acetic acid, ground coffee, etc. With the eyes closed and each nostril occluded in turn, the patient is asked to detect and if possible identify the substances.

Anosmia is invariably associated with loss of taste, as flavour is dependent on the sense of smell. The most common cause of anosmia is an upper respiratory tract viral infection; however, the sense of smell may also be lost following anterior cranial fossa fractures or neurosurgery involving the cribriform plate, and in frontal lobe tumours. Smell is usually normal in psychogenic disturbances of taste.

The optic nerve (II cranial nerve)

A simple assessment of the visual fields may be obtained by asking the patient to sit opposite the examiner and gaze at the examiner's nose whilst the latter waves his or her outstretched forefinger at the four points of the compass in a vertical plane.

Maxillofacial trauma is the principal cause of visual disturbance in our clinical practice. Acute and permanent amaurosis (blindness) may follow a retrobulbar haemorrhage within the orbital fascial cone due to a zygomatic or maxillary fracture (Fig. 24.1) and has also been reported as a consequence of elevating a

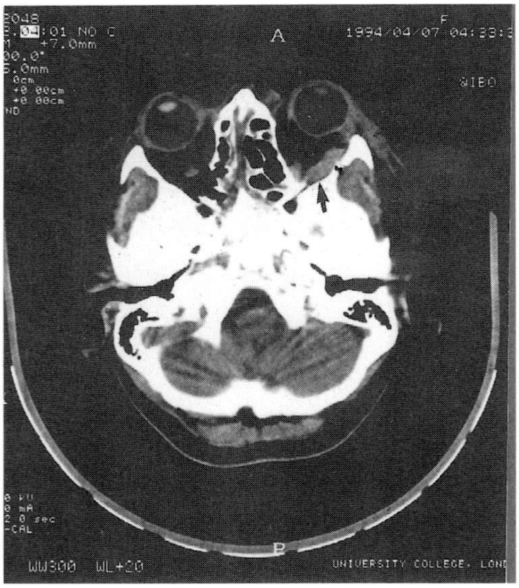

Fig. 24.1 Axial computed tomographic scan showing a left sided retrobulbar haemorrhage producing proptosis. Note the minimum displacement of the adjacent zygomatic fracture.

depressed zygoma. This has been attributed to the sudden proptosis caused by the haematoma creating retinal artery vasospasm.[1] There is however evidence that stretching of the nerve produces ischaemia and impaired conduction due to spasm of the external vasa nervorum, whilst the retinal artery remains patent.[2]

Immediate decompression of the haematoma through a wide subciliary or frontonasal incision is essential to evacuate the haematoma, together with megadose steroids (see below) until the vision is stable. However, blindness may also follow blunt trauma to the forehead, even without any evident orbital fracture or haematoma. This has been attributed to distortion of the nerve within the canal, or more proximally at the chiasma, where it will produce bilateral field defects. The eye shows a sluggish or absent pupillary reflex and loss of vision.

A CT or MRI scan is essential to localize any fracture or haematoma. Mega-dose steroids such as dexamethasone 3 mg/kg initially followed by 1–3 mg/kg 6-hourly for 24 h reducing to 1 mg/kg/per day may restore sight. If there is no response after 12 h the optic nerve should be decompressed via a transethmoid sphenoidotomy with removal of the medial wall of the canal. Similarly, traumatic displacement of the orbital plate of the greater wing of the sphenoid which makes up part of the posterior lateral wall of the orbit may also be rotated medially against the optic nerve and requires a lateral or temporal approach to reduce the fracture and restore vision.[3] Iatrogenic damage may follow the innappropriate insertion of bone grafts to repair the orbital floor.

Transient amaurosis (blindness) is also a rare but dramatic complication of an inferior dental nerve block.[4] The mechanism is thought to be the intra-arterial injection of the local anaesthetic and vasoconstrictor. The local anaesthetic bolus refluxes from the inferior dental into the adjacent middle meningeal artery. It reaches the orbit through an uncommon anomaly of the maxillary artery circulation in which its middle meningeal branch supplies the retina through the superior orbital fissure. This produces both angiospasm of the central retinal artery with ischaemia and perhaps anaesthesia of the retina. There may be additional extraocular palsies, including the abducent nerve[5] The condition appears to be reversible within an hour without treatment, though the patient must be carefully examined to exclude any latent impairment of the visual field. Rarely, ischaemia due to unrecognized giant cell (temporal) arteris may lead to blindness; for this reason the immediate use of high-dose corticosteroids is essential where this condition is suspected.

Both benign and malignant tumours may affect sight. Insidious loss of the outer visual fields – bitemporal hemianopia – occurs when a pituitary tumour or meningioma compresses the medial retinal optic fibres where they decussate at the chiasma (Fig. 24.2). Aggressive uncontrolled maxillary antral carcinoma may invade the orbit, producing proptosis and blindness. Bilateral spread of the tumour through the ethmoid air cells may follow.

Papilloedema, that is, oedema of the optic disc (nerve), is usually associated with raised intracranial pressure, and conversely pallor of the optic disc may be a manifestation of multiple sclerosis.

In all cases a full ophthalmic examination, including a visual field chart (not Hess), is essential (Fig. 24.3).

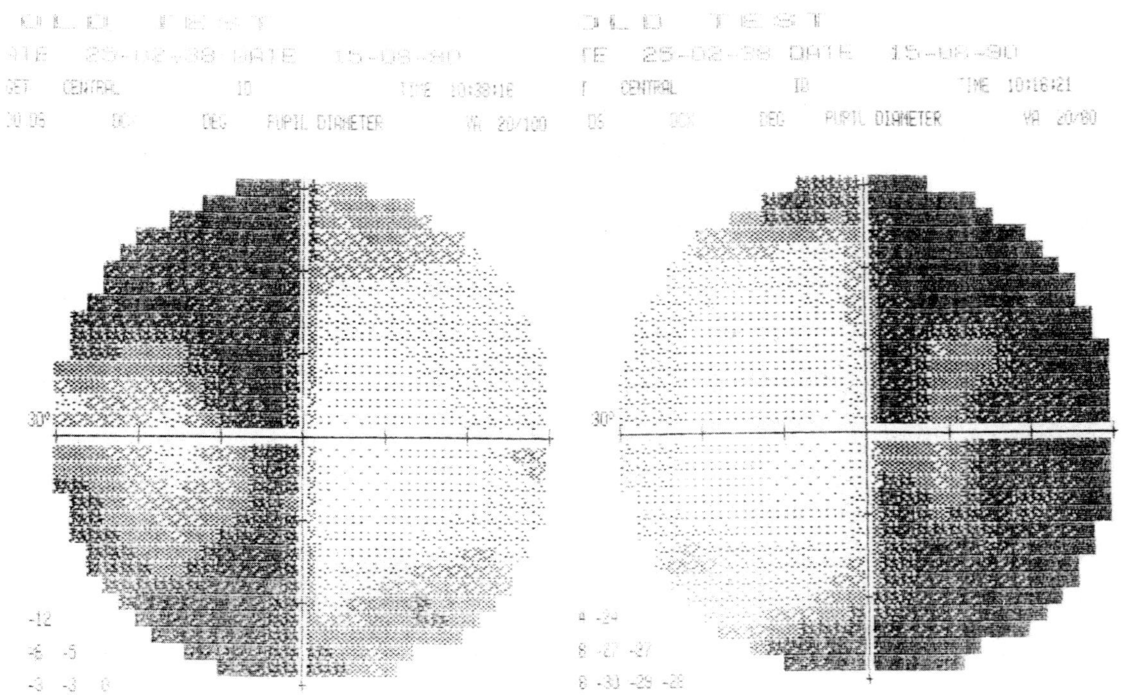

Fig. 24.2 Bitemporal hemianopia shown on a perimeter chart. This followed a fracture of the skull base. The peripheral dark area is loss of vision, leaving a central light area representing tunnel vision.

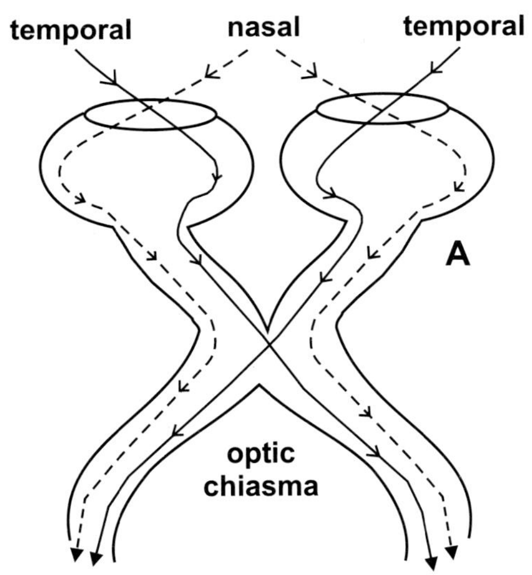

Fig. 24.3 Central visual pathways. Light from objects in the outer (temporal) visual fields passes through the lens to activate the nasal side of the retina, following which the sensory stimuli pass proximally to the occipital visual cortex after decussating at the optic chiasma.

Light from objects in the nasal visual field crosses through the lens to activate the outer retina and then the visual stimulus passes proximally without decussation.

Lesions at A produce total blindness in that eye, whereas those at the chiasma only affect the decussating medial retinal fibres and give rise to a bitemporal hemianopia.

The oculomotor, trochlear and abducent nerves (III, IV and VI cranial nerves)

Ophthalmoplegias

The external ocular movements of the eye can be tested by asking the patient to follow the examiner's finger to the four points of the compass with his or her eyes, whilst keeping the head fixed facing the examiner.

The third nerve innervates the rectus muscles, which elevate, depress and adduct the globe of the eye, and also the elevator of the upper eyelid – the levator palpabrae superioris. Damage to this branch will produce complete ptosis, that is, paralysis of the upper eyelid movement. This important nerve also conveys the parasympathetic sphincter nerve fibres to the iris which constrict the pupil (see below).

The trochlear nerve contributes a downwards and outwards movement of the globe through the superior oblique muscle. The abducent nerve innervates the lateral rectus muscle.

Disturbances in coordinated movement, the ophthalmoplegias, will give rise to double

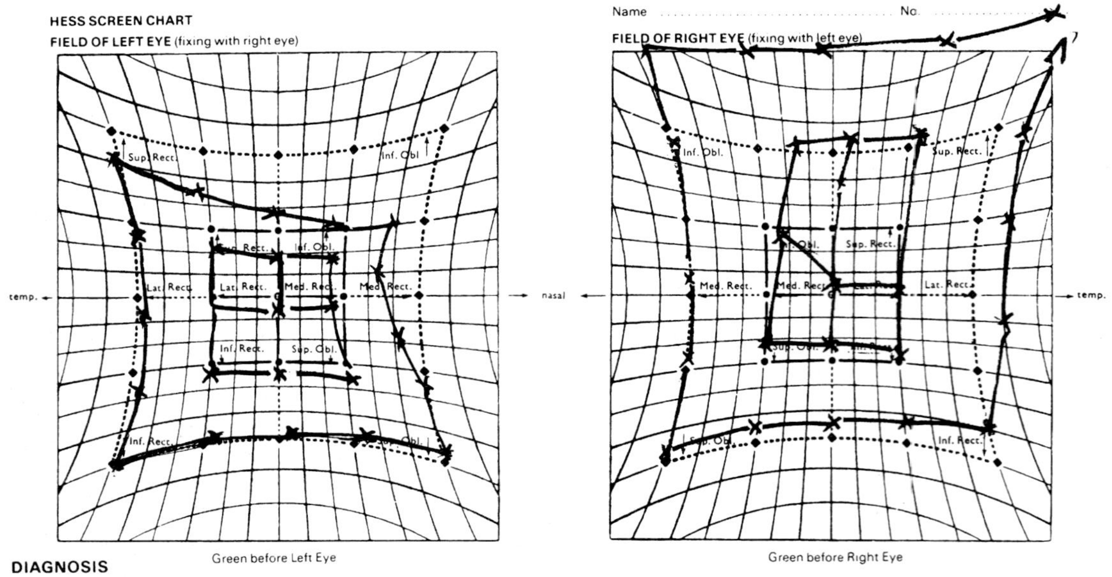

Fig. 24.4 Hess chart showing limitation of upward gaze due to entrapment of the orbital fascia by a greenstick blowout fracture.

vision. This diplopia is most marked in the direction of the disturbed muscle function.

Trauma is the most relevant cause of ophthalmoplegia. All eye injuries should have a full orthoptic examination with a Hess chart to provide a detailed baseline for management (Fig. 24.4).

The fractured zygoma is often associated with a transient ipsilateral neuropraxia of the abducent nerve with impaired movement and diplopia on lateral gaze. Early resolution suggests the cause to be oedema and haematoma, although occasionally the CT scan reveals direct muscle involvement by medially displaced bone fragments. Gross disturbances in suspension of the eye, especially due to fractures above Whitnall's tubercle inside the lateral orbital rim, will also give rise to diplopia if the external ocular muscles cannot compensate.

Impaired eye movement is also found in blowout injuries. Blowout fractures of the orbital floor are usually the result of a buckling stress fracture created by trauma to the intact inferior orbital margin or zygoma, rather than an acute rise in orbital hydraulic pressure.[6] The hydraulic explanation for blowout fractures is unlikely in the absence of gross injury to the globe.

Most ophthalmoplegias in many blowout injuries are likely to be the consequence of oedema and haematoma producing local muscle guarding, as they often resolve spontaneously within 10 days. The rare trapping of the inferior orbital fascia (not the inferior rectus muscle) in the fracture margin is usually seen in children and adolescents and can be detected by noting retraction of the globe and increased intraocular pressure when upward gaze is attempted.[7] Retraction of the globe is seen from side-holding a pencil or vertical margin of a card in front of the eye as a reference point. Severe ophthalmoplegias also arise from medial wall and roof blowouts.These lesions are readily visualized by an axial CT scan.

Maxillary fractures through the superior orbital fissure containing the III, IV, VI nerves and the ophthalmic division of V produce varying degrees of ptosis, mydriasis (dilated pupil) and impaired eye movements, together with a loss of supraorbital cutaneous sensation (Fig. 24.5.). Recovery is usually slow but complete. Rarely, the optic nerve or ophthalmic artery in the adjacent optic foramen are also damaged, leading to blindness. This has been called the orbital apex syndrome.

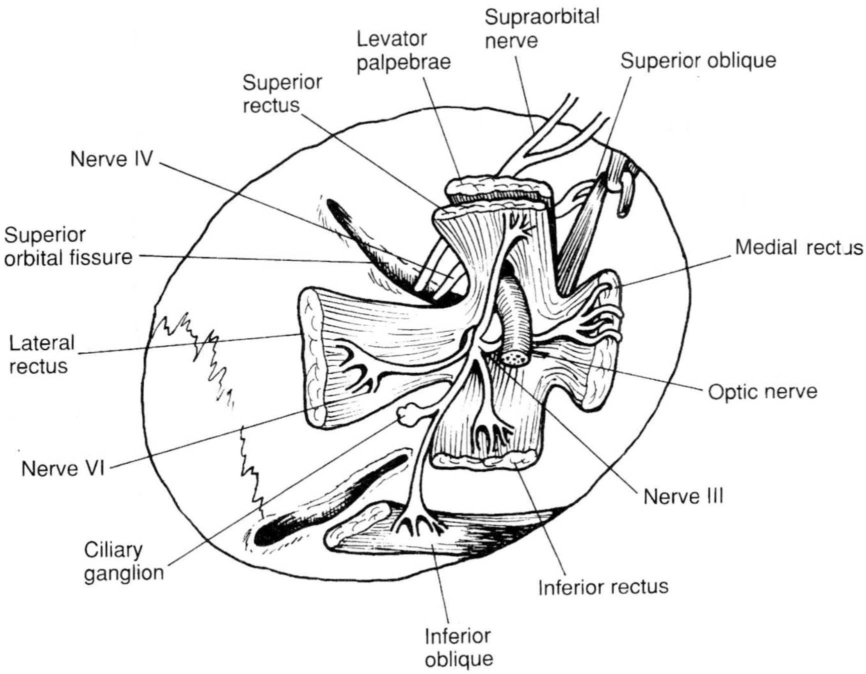

Fig. 24.5 Neuroanatomy of the superior orbital fissure and optic canal.

Bilateral compression injuries of the skull, especially in children, can produce a transverse fracture of the skull base with elevation of the apices of the petrous temporal bones damaging the overlying VI nerves. This neuropraxia gives rise to a bilateral abducens palsy which is also reversible.[8] With gross disruption of the sphenoid air sinus air may be drawn into the skull through the torn dura, producing a pneumocele. This will be seen as a radiolucent area on a lateral skull radiograph outlining the brain and ventricular system.

Transient abducent nerve palsy has also been described following a posterior superior alveolar nerve block.[5] The most likely explanation for this is penetration of the inferior orbital fissure by the needle, allowing infiltration of the anaesthetic around the lateral rectus muscle itself.

Ophthalmoplegias manifesting tumours and aneurysms of the middle cranial fossa are discussed in the section on the V nerve, below.

Head injuries affecting the midbrain area may disturb the supranuclear control of external ocular movement. Here there is a loss of conjugate eye movement, but with retained individual function of the III, IV and VI cranial nerves. Such patients may also suffer damage to adjacent structures such as the hypothalamus or pituitary.

Pupillary disturbances

The pupils should be of moderate and equal size and react briskly to light, directly and consensually. The consensual reflex depends on the light impulse from one retina passing to the other side through the optic chiasma, activating the contralateral light reflex. The size of the pupil is controlled by a balance between the parasympathetic sphincter action, which is mediated by fibres travelling with the oculomotor nerve, and the sympathetic dilator fibres which accompany blood vessels and also partially activate levator palpebrae superioris.

Lesions of the III nerve will therefore produce a dilated pupil (mydriasis). Direct trauma to the globe may also give an isolated mydriasis, which is usually transient.

A small pupil (myosis) in a conscious patient, when associated with slight ptosis and dry anhidrotic skin on the ipsilateral face and palm of hand, constitutes Horner's syndrome.

This arises when there is damage to the sympathetic outflow from the spinal segments of T1 and T2. The most common cause is cervical node involvement by a thoracic tumour such as bronchial carcinoma, but cervical injuries and fractures of the necks of the upper ribs may also be responsible.

It is obvious that the pupillary light reflex requires intact optic nerves in addition to the parasympathetic component of III nerve. In the unconscious patient pupillary size and disturbances in this reflex are important signs of increased intracranial pressure due to haemorrhage or oedema. Initially there is irritation of the III nerve with a transient myosis but soon compression of the nerve impairs conduction, producing an ipsilateral dilation with impaired response to light. As the pressure is transmitted across the falx cerebri in the midline, the contralateral pupil also becomes dilated and unresponsive. Immediate decompression with burr holes is essential.

The rare bilateral irregular small Argyll Robertson pupils are unresponsive to light but retain a reaction to accommodation, due to syphilis, and must be distinguished from the idiopathic unilateral dilated Holmes–Adie pupil which reacts slowly to light and accommodation.

Papilloedema, that is, oedema of the retina due to increased intracranial pressure, is difficult to detect in acute cases and requires experience with the ophthalmoscope. Engorgement of the central retinal vein causes a filling of the central optic pit and blurs the margins of the optic disc.

The corneal reflex is discussed under the trigeminal nerve, below.

The trigeminal nerve (V cranial nerve)

The trigeminal nerve is the principal conductor of oral and facial sensation, apart from a small area at the angles of the mandible. The simplest means of testing its function is to use cotton wool or a Frey's hair (see Chapter 22) for light touch, and a pin or probe for pain. Two-point discrimination may be compared between affected and normal areas using a pair of dressing forceps and a ruler. Taste may be assessed with sweet, sour and bitter solutions, but it should be remembered that this sense is mostly flavour and is mediated by the olfactory nerve. More refined techniques are described in neurological textbooks.

The patient is instructed to close the eyes and say 'now' or raise a finger when touched. This attempts to measure an all-or-nothing response. Hesitation in response implies an area of impaired perception which can then be examined more carefully. Intraorally the probe and a fine blunt wooden stick may be used and in addition teeth should be tested for vitality with an electric pulp tester, heated gutta percha or ethyl chloride on a pledget of cotton wool.

The corneal reflex is a very sensitive test of the ophthalmic division. For this a fine-twist cotton wool is touched first on the white insensitive sclerotic area then on to the adjacent cornea, with the patient looking away from the examiner. Immediate closure of the eye signifies an intact reflex. It is repeated for the opposite side.

Motor function is assessed by palpating temporalis and masseter tone with the patient clenching and relaxing the jaw.

Disturbances in facial sensation

The loss of sensation in the mouth and face either alone or accompanied by pain or paraesthesia may represent a variety of lesions along the course of the trigeminal nerve and its intracranial pathways. For this reason an examination of the cranial nerves should always be carried out whenever non-odontogenic pathology is suspected. The causes of altered sensation may be classified as extracranial, intracranial and somatoform disturbances (psychogenic).

Extracranial (see also Chapter 22)

Trauma

A frequent cause of sensory disturbance is the extraction of the mandibular third molar due to its proximity to the inferior dental, lingual and mylohyoid nerves (Fig. 24.6). The inferior dental nerve lesion is usually considered to be a neuropraxia from direct compression, although infarction following thrombosis of its vascular supply cannot be excluded. The sensory loss is detectable in the ipsilateral

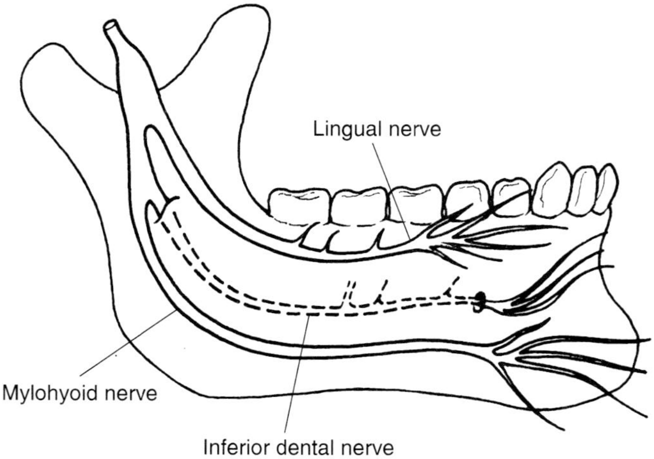

Fig. 24.6 Diagram showing the relationship of the inferior dental, lingual and mylohyoid nerves.

lower lip from the vermilion border extending downwards for a distance of 3–4 cm. The patient also complains of a dead sensation in the teeth because of sensory loss in the periodontal membranes. Recovery is usually slow but sure, varying from 1 to 6 months. Rarely, the apices of the third molar enclose the nerve and so elevation produces a permanent severance (neurotmesis), which may also occur as a result of fractures or osteotomies (see Chapter 22). Sensory impairment also occurs following accidental division of the nerve in the region of the mental foramen. A rare cause of mental anaesthesia is associated with condylar fractures. This has been attributed to nerve damage by the displaced condylar neck but if the sensory loss is widespread it probably results from a linear fracture of the skull base extending from the condylar fossa to the foramen ovale, producing a haematoma around the mandibular nerve at its origin (see also intracranial causes, below).

Sensory loss will arise from the inadvertent injection of root canal medicaments through the tooth apex into the inferior dental canal; this should be removed immediately. This may done by an apicectomy approach for premolars or a sagittal split for molars.

Lingual nerve neuropraxia commonly follows retraction of the lingual flap during the surgical removal of the lower third molar. At this site it lies immediately adjacent to the bone and is separated from it only by the periosteum. In some patients the nerve also appears to be very superficial. Common sensation and taste generally recover within 4 weeks, but a persistent disturbance beyond this time carries a poor prognosis without surgical intervention.

The mylohyoid nerve is a mixed sensory and motor nerve which branches off the inferior dental nerve above the lingula and then travels independently downwards and forwards on the lingual aspect of the mandible below the level of the lingual nerve. In some individuals it is included within a canal in the cortical plate. Thus it may be damaged during the removal of an impacted third molar, at mandibular osteotomy or when reducing a prominent mylohyoid ridge. The peripheral sensory loss consists of a circular area of anaesthesia 2–3 cm in diameter at the lower border of the chin. Recovery usually takes place in 4–8 weeks.

Fractures of the zygoma and maxilla involving the infraorbital canal commonly produce an area of infraorbital sensory loss with associated numbness of the maxillary premolar teeth. A similar lesion may follow a Caldwell–Luc operation.

Patients will need to be reassured about the uncomfortable paraesthesia associated with the recovering nerve. It is essential to warn of the possible occurrence of these lesions preoperatively. This reduces both postoperative concern and litigation.

Inflammation (see also intracranial causes of dysaesthesia)

One of the classic signs of acute osteomyelitis of the mandible is mental anaesthesia, though it is rare in the chronic forms of the disease, or in osteoradionecrosis. Occasionally infra-orbital anaesthesia occurs in acute maxillary sinusitis with empyema of the antrum. Again, drainage produces rapid relief, but radiographic follow-up to exclude a neoplasm is necessary.

Herpes zoster may damage branches of the trigeminal nerve and leave a permanent sensory deficit. Viral sensory neuropathy may also be a manifestation of human immunodeficiency virus (HIV) infection. Benign cysts of the mandible rarely cause mental and labial anaesthesia, except where there has been resorption of the canal wall and acute infection involving the neurovascular bundle.

Benign tumours, including large ameloblastomas, do not cause facial anaesthesia. An uncommon exception is the neurofibroma of the mandibular nerve.

Malignant tumours which involve any part of the extracranial course of the trigeminal nerve invariably produce sensory loss which may be associated with pain. These include primary carcinomas of the antrum, invasive carcinomas of the alveolus, osteo-, chondro- and fibrosarcomas and lymphomas. Tumour metastases, including those from the bronchus, breast, kidney, prostate, thyroid and pancreas, may simulate these primary neoplasms, and should also be borne in mind. Investigations include biopsy, radiographs, calcium chemistry and plasma proteins, a CT scan and a technetium bone scan. Occasionally multiple myeloma and Burkitt's lymphoma may infiltrate the mandible, producing labial anaesthesia without any detectable radiographic or bone scan changes. This is thought to be due to resorption within the cortical plates, with inhibition of reactive bone formation, which is normally detected by the nuclide scan. Leukaemic cells may also infiltrate the inferior dental canal[9] or a haematoma due to a primary or secondary thrombocytopenia may follow an inferior dental injection and produce a transient mental anaesthesia.

The peculiar presentation of the nasopharyngeal carcinoma (Trotter's syndrome) involves sensory loss, pain, palatal dysfunction, deafness and trismus, due to the tumour involving the adjacent trigeminal nerve branches, eustachian tube and the muscles of mastication.

Intracranial

Trauma

Fractures of the base of skull may damage a variety of cranial nerves. Direct trauma to the skull or indirect stress transmitted upwards by the mandibular condyle can produce a fracture passing through the foramen ovale, or rarely the apex of the petrous temporal bone, damaging the trigeminal ganglion. The sensory loss is principally in the distribution of the mandibular division.

Anaesthesia in the supraorbital region, associated with varying degrees of ophthalmoplegia, may result from fractures involving the superior orbital fissure. Here the ophthalmic division of the trigeminal nerve is damaged, together with the oculomotor, abducent and trochlear nerves. The patient characteristically cannot elevate the eyelid and also has a dilated pupil owing to damage to the parasympathetic component of the oculomotor nerve.

Inflammation

Apart from viral infections, consider meningeal sarcoid. This idiopathic chronic granulomatous condition also involves the skin, eyes and hilar lymph nodes (as seen on chest X-ray), which may help to establish the diagnosis. The serum angiotensin-converting enzyme is now prefered to the Kveim test, which is usually but not invariably positive. A palatal mucosal biopsy may reveal characteristic giant cell granulomas.

However, in some areas of the world tuberculous basal meningitis, leprosy and meningovascular syphilis produce similar chronic disturbances. Therefore serological tests for syphilis should be carried out. Tabes dorsalis, which affects the dorsal sensory tracts of the spinal cord, may give rise to facial analgesia, or merely an interval between the stimulus and perception of a pinprick. Later, light touch and differentiation of heat and cold are also lost.

Trigeminal sensory neuropathy is an idiopathic disturbance of sensation in one or more divisions of the trigeminal nerve.[9] It is usually transient, lasting a few weeks to months, and rarely may be associated with motor loss and Horner's syndrome. There is slight evidence that it occurs in a mild epidemic form. As some patients insist that it follows a dental injection, the cause could be the activation of neurotrophic virus. The patient complains of a sudden awareness of a painless area of facial numbness which will include the associated intraoral mucosa and teeth. Where the mandibular division is involved, there is a disturbance or loss of taste. Apart from these peripheral neurological signs, there are no obvious diagnostic features. Although recovery usually takes place within 6 months, there may be persistent paraesthesia, and trigeminal neuralgia may be a late complication.[10]

The autoimmune diseases rheumatoid arthritis, systemic lupus erythematosus and scleroderma may involve the vasa nervorum of the trigeminal nerve and give rise to a transient facial anaesthesia. Occasionally an additional complication is a sore red tongue from an associated autoimmune pernicious anaemia. The diagnosis is difficult if the neurological disturbance precedes the systemic manifestations of these diseases. A full examination, the erythrocyte sedimentation rate, autoimmune antibody studies, serum electrophoresis and serum vitamin B_{12} estimations may be necessary to exclude these disorders.

Disseminated sclerosis is often a disease of adolescence and early adult life. A plaque of demyelination in the pons can give rise to facial anaesthesia and hemiageusia (taste loss). The numbness is often associated with formication or even paroxysmal trigeminal neuralgia and may be transient. Sensory, motor and reflex disturbances elsewhere characterize the condition. An MRI scan is required to reveal the lesions.

Drug neuropathies

Hydroxystilbamidine isethionate, which was used for the treatment of protozoal infections, produced a bilateral facial neuropathy in 50% of patients. The numbness and a painful paraesthesia could last for months or years. As all drugs may produce protean side-effects, the patient's medication should always be carefully excluded when diagnosing a baffling neuropathy.

Vascular

Intracranial aneurysms, by virtue of their increasing size within a limited space, compress nerves and so produce disturbances in facial sensation, indistinguishable from those of any intracranial tumour. The basilar–vertebral lesions in the posterior cranial fossa tend to involve the other lower cranial nerves in addition to the trigeminal, presenting like a cerebellopontine lesion. The fusiform aneurysm of the internal carotid within the cavernous sinus gives rise to early oculomotor signs as well as anaesthesia and pain in the ophthalmic and maxillary nerve areas.

The posterior inferior cerebellar branch of the vertebral artery divides into an internal and an external branch. The internal branch supplies the middle lobe of the cerebellum and the side of the medulla, and thrombosis within it will involve the spinal tract of the fifth nerve, the adjacent spinothalamic tract which conveys sensation from the opposite side of the body, and the cerebellar tracts. This produces ipsilateral analgesia of the face and contralateral analgesia of the trunk and limbs. The cerebellar damage gives rise to vertigo and vomiting, with nystagmus and incoordination of the arm and leg on the same side. A limited thrombosis may only cause sudden transitory cerebellar signs, leaving a residual facial anaesthesia. The sixth to the tenth cranial nuclei can also be infarcted. This presentation may also occur with sarcoid. MRI and angiography are required to investigate these lesions.

Tumours

Intracranial primary tumours include, in order of frequency of occurrence, acoustic neuroma (schwannoma), meningioma, pituitary adenoma, schwannoma of the fifth nerve, and the cholesteatoma or 'pearly tumour' arising in the middle ear. Involvement of the nerve roots by these tumours or by secondary carcinoma may give rise to symptoms in only one division.

The schwannoma (acoustic neurinoma) arises on the vestibular branch of the eighth cranial nerve or, more rarely, on the seventh nerve or the trigeminal nerve. As all three cranial nerves occupy the narrow triangular space between the lateral surface of the pons and the cerebellum, called the cerebellopontine angle, the expanding lesion produces a variety of related clinical features (Fig. 24.7). These vary in predominance, and include headache,

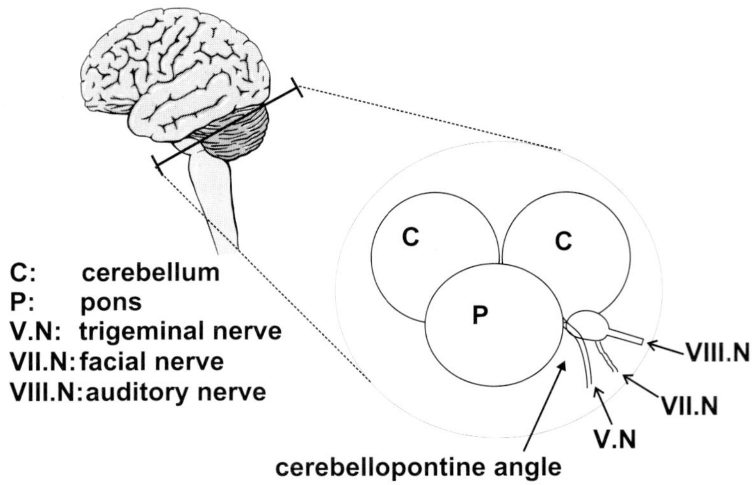

Fig. 24.7 Diagram showing the structures of the cerebellar angle, where an acoustic neuroma arising from the VIII nerve can compress the VII nerve and V nerve, giving rise to loss of hearing, ataxia, nystagmus, facial weakness, and facial sensory loss and/or pain.

unsteadiness of the feet, vomiting, facial numbness, vertiginous attacks and deafness.

Unfortunately, symptoms may precede signs by many years.Therefore a CT or MRI scan is essential with persistent symptoms, especially where there is any evidence of sensory loss.

Syringobulbia is thought to be a developmental defect in the closure of the spinal cord, which results in an expanding cavity lined with glia. It may arise in the medulla, or as a medullary, or even a pontine, extension of a syringomyelia. The cavitation often commences in the posterolateral part of the cord, but it can expand bilaterally from the midline near the spinal canal. Pressure atrophy of the spinal nucleus and its decussating fibres impairs the sensation of pain and temperature but the perception of light touch is unaffected, producing a so-called dissociated sensory loss.

Characteristically, the analgesia advances across the face, converging towards the nose, which is the last area to be affected. Extension into the pons gives rise to weakness of the muscles of mastication and paralysis of the palate, larynx and tongue. A Horner's syndrome results from involvement of the sympathetic fibres descending to their thoracolumbar outflow.

Involvement of the long spinal tracts will produce a variety of widespread motor and sensory changes in the trunk and limbs.

CT scan will reveal expansion of the internal auditory meatus. Early surgical removal is recommended to reduce both mortality and morbidity.

Somatiform (psychogenic, hysterical) sensory loss

Somatiform anaesthesia of the face represents a subconscious dissociation of facial sensation from perceptive awareness and is probably best considered to be a psychogenic anaesthesia. The patient cannot feel his or her face, despite the absence of any neurological disorder. The tendency towards somatiform disorders is not understood, but it is probably inborn. Depression is also capable of inducing similar delusional symptoms. It is essential not to overlook latent disease when making the diagnosis of both benign trigeminal neuropathy and somatiform sensory loss.

Three aspects of the somatiform symptom are recognized. First, it is a product of suggestion and may be derived from an organic disorder of the patient or a close relative, or may for instance follow the anaesthesia of a dental injection. The patient uncritically accepts this suggestion and thus becomes convinced that his or her face is 'numb'. However, as this notion of a numb face is unlikely to conform with the anatomical nerve supply, its margins may be sharply defined and include the cervical innervation of the angle of the jaw or fail to extend beyond the hairline. Where the anaesthesia is hemifacial, vibration will not be perceived, even though normally it would be transmitted through the bone to the unaffected side. Corneal, palatal and pharyngeal reflexes may also be lost.

Second, the functional loss is usually associated with a psychological gain. For example, responsibility is evaded, a mental conflict is resolved, or sympathy and attention are directed to the patient. The advantage, however, is not always evident. Finally there may be a symbolic element in the symptom, related to the face's important emotional significance which is seen, for example, in such phrases as 'to lose face', implying the loss of respect or prestige.

The condition usually responds to supportive psychiatric therapy but must be vigilantly followed up by the surgeon or neurologist to exclude a latent neoplasm.

Disturbance in taste (cachageusia or dysageusia) (see also Chapter 13)

Taste is a complex experience consisting of the appreciation by the tongue of the basic bitter, sweet, acid and salt stimuli and the more subtle flavours detected by olfaction. Common sensation within the mouth probably also enhances both. The chorda tympani branch of the facial nerve with the olfactory and the trigeminal nerves make up the principal taste pathways. The additional taste buds on the posterior third of tongue and fauces are supplied by the ninth and tenth cranial nerves.

Testing solutions should include quinine (bitter), sugar (sweet), dilute hydrochloric acid and saline. They can be applied in turn, asking first if the patient tastes anything and if he or she nods affirmatively, releasing the tongue for the answer.

However, it is important to distinguish between the loss of flavour due to anosmia, seen temporarily in a common cold or permanently following fractures of the anterior cranial fossa, and pure loss of taste. The latter occurs most commonly after traumatic lesions of the lingual nerve, or damage to the chorda tympani in Bell's palsy and in other lower motor neuron lesions of the facial nerve.

Most aberrations of taste met by the oral surgeon take the form of a bitter or salty taste in the absence of any obvious gross sepsis or salivary disorder. This symptom can be considered one of the so-called psychogenic oral dysaesthesias. It should be treated with sympathetic reassurance and antidepressant drug therapy. Occasionally the problem is best described as a monosymptomatic hypochondriacal psychosis which may respond to an antipsychotic drug such as flupenthixol or the tricyclic clomipramine.

Trigeminal neuropathy and occasionally alcohol injections of the gasserian ganglion also give rise to an ipsilateral loss of taste. Other intracranial disorders affecting taste include infarcts, tumours and demyelinating disease, all of which usually present with other symptoms and signs. Occasionally hallucinations of taste and smell may be a presenting feature of a temporal lobe abscess or tumour involving the uncinate gyrus. These so-called uncinate fits are usually associated with a strong sense of fear. Finally many patients suffer a disturbance of taste with drug therapy, especially antibiotics such as metronidazole and ampicillin.

The facial nerve (VII cranial nerve)

This nerve has three functions: maintaining muscular tone, without which the facial tissues droop; facial muscular activity, such as closing the eyes or labial movement; and emotional expression.

Its sensory component is principally concerned with taste.

Prior to testing function, one should compare facial expression and movement between the two sides of the face. Impaired blinking, a sagging cheek and flattening of the nasolabial crease are features of a facial palsy. The following basic actions are then examined:

1. Raising the eyebrows to test frontalis corrugator activity.
2. Tightly closing the eyes for obicularis oculi sphincter function.
3. Asking the patient to grin, to examine the retractor muscles acting on the angles of the mouth.
4. Taste may also be tested, as described earlier.

Facial palsy

The many causes of facial palsy are described in neurological textbooks. They may be classified as congenital or acquired, the former being associated with second branchial arch defects.

Lower motor neuron damage occasionally arises following head injuries involving the base of skull. Fractures of the petrous bone give rise to an immediate palsy due to a direct neurapraxia, or to a delayed paralysis. The latter has been attributed to either compression by oedema or ischaemia of the nerve. Injury within the medial part of the petrous temporal bone is usually associated with nerve deafness, which may be permanent. Such injuries may also produce ataxia and nystagmus due to vestibular damage. By contrast, fractures through the middle ear cause a combination of conductive deafness and loss of taste. The prognosis for traumatic palsies is good, especially in delayed cases and recovery is usually complete.

Surgical trauma to the main branches is associated with access to the temporomandibular joint and parotid salivary gland; occasionally a push-back sagittal split osteotomy and submandibular incisions may compromise the marginal mandibular branch. Intracapsular injections of local anaesthetic may also give a transient paresis.

Bell's palsy is the most common lower motor neuron lesion. Although the condition is held to be idiopathic, there is evidence that the lesion may be due to the herpes-zoster virus. It is often epidemic, and occasionally vesicles may be detected around the auricle or anterior fauces from which the virus has been recovered. The frequency and severity of this neuropathy compared to those affecting other cranial nerves are undoubtedly due to the seventh nerve's passage through a long narrow bone canal which leads to compression and ischaemia when it becomes swollen. The patient often wakes with a marked one-sided facial weakness which prevents wrinkling of the forehead and closure of the eyelids and allows an ugly traction of the lips over to the normal side on smiling.

Buccinator shows an obvious loss of tone which interferes with speech and leaves an accumulation of food in the buccal sulcus. Some patients may be aware of a disturbance in taste on the affected side. Hyperacusis due to paralysis of the stapedius muscle is not common. There is a contralateral deviation of the tongue on protrusion which is probably due to disturbance in the proprioceptive function of the chorda tympani, but this soon disappears as the tongue adapts to the altered shape of the mouth.[11] Eighty-five per cent make a good recovery, the majority in 2–4 weeks; the remainder are left with combinations of paralysis and inappropriate movement.

Early treatment with corticosteroids has been claimed to improve the rate and degree of recovery.[12] One regime is a course of dexamethasone 8 mg 12-hourly for a week, gradually reducing the dose over the following week.

Adhesive tape such as Sellotape or Blenderm (3M) gives simple immediate support to the face at rest.

If recovery is poor, alternative means of masking this socially debilitating condition must be considered. The oldest technique is the fascia lata sling which can give good static support, with additional movement provided by transferring the insertion of masseter to the angle of the mouth. Unfortunately, the fascial sling makes dental treatment difficult and the wearing of a full lower denture impossible.

A contoured gold weight inserted into the upper eyelid is also a simple way of facilitating closure.

Some surgeons favour an early facial–accessory or facial–hypoglossal nerve anastomosis. With the latter, tongue wasting on the affected side is not a great problem but to ensure satisfactory reinnervation, the operation should be done within 3 months of the nerve damage, otherwise both the peripheral part of the nerve and facial muscles will have undergone extensive atrophy. Very good movements are claimed for 80% of patients, with the advantage of developing good reflex movement of the eyelids.

Anderl[13] has had success with cross-facial nerve grafting from the sound to lame side using sural nerve grafts. After the cross-facial nerve graft has taken, an additional approach with long-standing cases is that of innervated muscle transplantation to animate the face. Pectoralis minor may be grafted by microvascular and microneural anastomosis into the affected side, gaining its innervation from the previously inserted cross-facial sural graft.[14]

A less complicated alternative is to graft a segment of the latissimus dorsi muscle with its thoracodorsalis nerve, which is long enough to reach across to the opposite active facial nerve.

Where there is a troublesome epiphora or where the cornea is insensitive following Ramsay Hunt syndrome (geniculate herpes involving the facial nerve), a lateral tarsorrhaphy is also essential and is readily performed under a local anaesthetic.

Facial weakness associated with a parotid swelling is highly suggestive of a malignant tumour, indicating a CT or ultrasound scan and fine-needle aspiration or open excisional biopsy.

Clonic facial spasm

The patient suffers from intermittent twitching of the facial muscles which may be brief and localized or involve the whole of one side of the face. The most commonly affected muscle is the sphincter of the eye and here there is often a history of emotional stress or chronic fatigue. Occasionally the problem arises after a Bell's palsy or Ramsay Hunt syndrome but many are idiopathic and hence termed cryptogenic. The condition may progress with increasing muscle weakness.

Treatment of the condition is difficult and unsatisfactory. Mild tics due to emotional stress will respond to counselling, rest and sedation or antidepressant drugs. Behavioural therapy may also be of value. Severe localized spasm may be eliminated by injections of botulinum toxin.

Ramsay Hunt syndrome

It is difficult to be sure whether this is a variant of Bell's palsy or a separate condition. The patient presents initially with pain in the ear, which is followed by a lower motor neuron paralysis. However, vesiculation in the external ear, loss of tears due to involvement of the greater superficial petrosol nerve and loss of ipsilateral taste are characteristic features. There may also be unilateral perceptive deafness, tinnitus and vertigo due to involvement of the VIII nerve.The treatment is the same as Bell's palsy.

Marcus Gunn or jaw-winking syndrome

This rare condition can be congenital or follows trauma or surgery in the facial area. The patient complains of ptosis or paradoxical oculopalpebral movements provoked by chewing and mandibular movement. The condition is not understood and the outcome appears to be variable. There is no known treatment.

The auditory nerve (VIII cranial nerve)

Loss of hearing may be conductive or perceptive.The assessment of deafness can be considered in three stages; simple tests, tuning-fork tests and audiometry.

A simple method is to whisper a number about 30–50 cm from the patient's nearer ear whilst occluding the far ear with a finger. Slight vibration of this finger will help to obscure any external sound. The examiner then moves to the opposite side and this is repeated.This is a crude test of conductive deafness.

The Rinne test is carried out with a heavy tuning fork which is struck and held close to the external auditory meatus. This tests the conduction of sound through the air and by the ossicles. As soon as the patient signals that he or she can no longer hear the vibrations, the base of the fork is applied firmly to the mastoid process; the vibrations are transmitted through the bone to be detected by the auditory nerve. If the patient finds that air conduction of sound is better than bone conduction, he or she has a normal or positive Rinne, which means that if there is deafness on that side it will be nerve deafness. However, if a deaf patient can hear the tuning fork when applied to the mastoid bone, so that bone conduction is better than air conduction, this is a negative Rinne, implying a conductive, (i.e. air-conductive) deafness.

Further examinations, including those of the vestibular apparatus, require an appropriate specialist.

It is important to examine the external ear and tympanic membrane with an auroscope. Blood may be seen behind or extruding through a torn tympanic membrane in fractures of the skull base, or adhering to the membrane where the canal has been breached in condylar surgery. It is worth remembering that immobilization of the mandible can lead

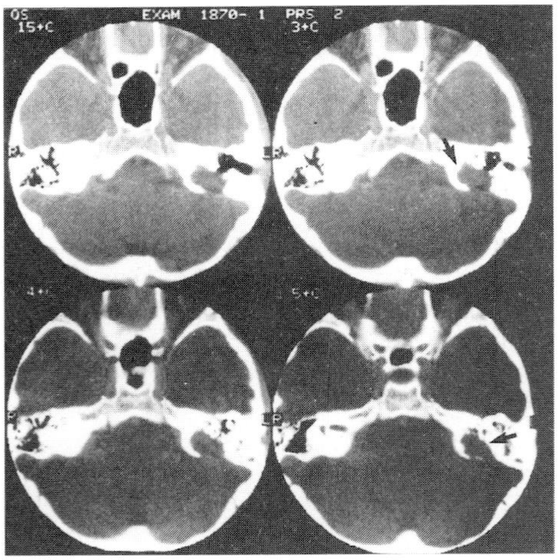

Fig. 24.8 Axial computed tomographic scan showing bone destruction and expansion by a cholesteatoma arising in the left middle ear cleft and presenting as facial pain and anaesthesia. This bone loss could be mistaken for a cerebellopontine angle neuroma.

to accumulation and impaction of wax which is normally cleared by condylar movements.

Causes of conductive deafness include wax or blood in the external auditory meatus as a result of trauma or infection of the middle ear, especially when the tympanic membrane is involved. Obstruction of the eustachian tube by a nasopharyngeal tumour will also produce a conductive deafness. Otosclerosis, in which new bone forms around the footplate of the stapes, is an insidious cause of conductive deafness in young people.

With perceptive deafness the pathology involves the labyrinth or cranial nerve itself and includes senile deafness (presbycusis), viral infections, drugs such as streptomycin, gentamicin, aspirin and quinine, Ménière's disease and intracranial tumours such as the acoustic neuroma (Fig. 24.7) or cholesteatoma (Fig 24.8). Rarely, perceptive deafness may be a feature of base-of-skull fractures involving the petrous temporal bone due to damage to the cochlea or auditory nerve.

The glossopharyngeal, vagus and accessory nerves (IX, X and XI cranial nerves)

These may be considered together, as isolated lesions of each are rare. The glossopharyngeal nerve (IX) supplies taste and common sensation to the posterior third of tongue and oropharynx. It therefore subserves the sensory component of the gag reflex, which can be evoked by touching the back of the pharynx with a dental mirror handle.

The vagus (X) supplies the motor side of this reflex with its fibres to the soft palate and larynx.

The accessory nerve (XI) supplies trapezius and sternomastoid and may be tested by elevating both shoulders. Any weakness may be confirmed by asking the patient to push his or her head laterally against the examiner's hand. The principal cause of accessory disturbance is infiltration by cervical lymph node carcinomatosis, which is invariably obvious, or following a block dissection of the neck.

Otherwise these three nerves are usually involved together by lesions in the posterior cranial fossa, where they cross to the jugular foramen or below the base of skull. The main cause is tumours such as the chemodectoma arising from the vagal or carotid body.

Hypoglossal nerve (XII cranial nerve)

The hypoglossal nerve provides motor fibres to the tongue. When disturbed, there is dysarthria and the tongue protrudes to the affected side. With upper motor neuron lesions the side of the tongue is small and spastic and with lower motor neuron lesions the tongue shows wasting.

Surgical trauma, usually when excising metastatic squamous cell carcinoma in the submandibular region, may damage the nerve. Other palsies are rare and are usually isolated cranial mononeuropathies, possibly of viral origin.

References

1. Varley EWB, Holt-Wilson AD, Watson PG. Acute retinal arterial occlusion following reduction of a fractured zygoma and its successful treatment. *Br J Oral Surg* 1968; **6**: 31–36.
2. Anderson RL, Panje WR, Gross CE. Optic nerve blindness following blunt forehead trauma. *Ophthalmology* 1982; **89**: 445–455.
3. Funk GF, Stanley RB, Becker TS. Reversible visual loss due to impacted lateral orbital wall fractures. *Head Neck* 1989; **11**: 295–300.
4. Blaxter PL, Britten MJA. Transient amaurosis after mandibular nerve block. *Br Med J* 1967; **1**: 681.

5. Marinho ROM. Abducent nerve palsy following dental local analgesia. *Br Dent J* 1995; **179**: 69–70.
6. Fujino TJ. Experimental 'blowout' fracture of the orbit. *J Plast Reconstr Surg* 1974; **54**: 81–82.
7. Fells P. Acute enophthalmos. *Trans Ophthalmol Soc UK* 1982; **102**: 88–89.
8. Goubran GF. Traumatic bilateral abducent nerve palsies. *Br J Oral Surg* 1978; **15**: 268–275.
9. Blau JN, Harris M, Kennett S. Trigeminal sensory neuropathy. *N Engl J Med* 1969; **281**: 873–876.
10. Harris W. Paroxysmal neuralgic tic as a sequel of trigeminal neuritis. *Br Med J* 1935; **1**: 1112–1114.
11. Harris M, Rood JP. Tongue deviation and Bell's palsy. *Br Med J* 1977; **2**: 20–21.
12. Taverner D, Cohen SB, Hutchinscn BC. Comparison of corticotrophin and prednisone in the treatment of idiopathic facial paralysis (Bell's palsy). *Br Med J* 1971; **4**: 20–22.
13. Anderl H. Cross-face nerve transplantation in facial palsy. *Proc R Soc Med* 1976; **69**: 781–783.
14. Harrison DH. Current trends in the treatment of established unilateral facial palsy. *Ann R Coll Surg Engl* 1990; **72** Suppl 2: 94–98.

Glossary

Adenine A nitrogenous base, one member of the base pair adenine–thymine (A–T)

Alleles Alternative forms of a genetic locus; a single allele for each locus is inherited separately from each parent (e.g. at a locus for eye colour the allele might result in blue or brown eyes)

Amino acid Any of a class of 20 molecules that are combined to form proteins in living things. The sequence of amino acids in a protein and hence protein function are determined by the genetic code

Amplification An increase in the number of copies of a specific DNA fragment; can be *in vivo* or *in vitro*. *See* cloning, polymerase chain reaction

Antioncogene Genes that repress uncontrolled cell division and differentiation

Arrayed library Individual primary recombinant clones (hosted in phage, cosmid, yeast artificial chromosome, or other vector) that are placed in two-dimensional arrays in microtitre dishes. Each primary clone can be identified by the identity of the plate and the clone location (row and column) on that plate. Arrayed libraries of clones can be used for many applications, including screening for a specific gene or genomic region of interest as well as for physical mapping. Information gathered on individual clones from various genetic linkage and physical map analyses is entered into a relational database and used to construct physical and genetic linkage maps simultaneously; clone identifiers serve to interrelate the multilevel maps. *Compare* library, genomic library

Autoradiography A technique that uses X-ray film to visualize radioactively labelled molecules or fragments of molecules; used in analysing length and number of DNA fragments after they are separated by gel electrophoresis

Autosome A chromosome not involved in sex determination. The diploid human genome consists of 46 chromosomes, 22 pairs of autosomes, and 1 pair of sex chromosomes (the X and Y chromosomes)

Bacteriophage Viruses that infect bacteria – often abbreviated to phage

Base DNA is synthesized from specific bases, namely, adenine, cytosine, guanine and thymine. In RNA molecules, thymine is replaced by uracil

Base pair (bp) Two nitrogenous bases (adenine and thymine or guanine and

	cytosine) held together by weak bonds. Two strands of DNA are held together in the shape of a double helix by the bonds between base pairs
Base sequence	The order of nucleotide bases in a DNA molecule
Base sequence analysis	A method, sometimes automated, for determining the base sequence
Biotechnology	A set of biological techniques developed through basic research and now applied to research and product development. In particular, the use by industry of recombinant DNA, cell fusion and new bioprocessing techniques
bp	*See* base pair
C chromosome banding	A technique for generating stained regions around centromeres
cDNA	*See* complementary DNA
cDNA library	A complete cDNA library for a given cell-type or biological organ (e.g. kidney, lung, etc.) will represent every gene sequence that is being actively transcribed in that particular cell/organ
cen	Abbreviation for chromosome centrometre
Centimorgan (cM)	A unit of measurement of recombination frequency. One centimorgan is equal to a 1% chance that a marker at one genetic locus will be separated from a marker at a second locus due to crossing over in a single generation. In human beings, 1 cM is equivalent, on average, to 1 million bp
Centromere	A specialized chromosome region to which spindle fibres attach during cell division
Chromosomes	The self-replicating genetic structures of cells containing the cellular DNA that bears in its nucleotide sequence the linear array of genes. In prokaryotes, chromosomal DNA is circular, and the entire genome is carried on one chromosome. Eukaryotic genomes consist of a number of chromosomes whose DNA is associated with different kinds of proteins
Chromosome walking	The process of moving linearly along a chromosome by the sequential isolation of overlapping DNA clones
Clones	A group of cells derived from a single ancestor
Cloning	The process of asexually producing a group of cells (clones), all genetically identical, from a single ancestor. In recombinant DNA technology, the use of DNA manipulation procedures to produce multiple copies of a single gene or segment of DNA is referred to as cloning DNA
Cloning vector	DNA molecule originating from a virus, a plasmid or the cell of a higher organism into which another DNA fragment of appropriate size can be integrated without loss of the vector's capacity for self-replication; vectors introduce foreign DNA into host cells, where it can be reproduced in large quantities. Examples are plasmids, cosmids and yeast artificial chromosome; vectors are often recombinant molecules containing DNA sequences from several sources
cM	*See* centimorgan
Code	*See* genetic code
Codon	*See* genetic code
Complementary DNA (cDNA)	DNA that is synthesized from a messenger RNA template; the single-stranded form is often used as a probe in physical mapping
Complementary sequences	Nucleic acid base sequences that can form a double-stranded structure by matching base pairs; the complementary sequence to G-T-A-C is C-A-T-G
Conserved sequence	A base sequence in a DNA molecule (or an amino acid sequence in a protein) that has remained essentially unchanged throughout evolution

Contig map — A map depicting the relative order of a linked library of small overlapping clones representing a complete chromosomal segment

Contigs — Groups of clones representing overlapping regions of a genome

***cos* site** — A specific DNA sequence occuring in bacteriophage DNA that is recognized by viral enzymes involved in the packaging of DNA into the bacteriophage head

Cosmid — Artificially constructed cloning vector containing the *cos* gene of phage λ. Cosmids can be packaged in λ-phage particles for infection into *Escherichia coli*; this permits cloning of larger DNA fragments (up to 45 kb) than can be introduced into bacterial hosts in plasmid vectors

Crossing over — The breaking during meiosis of one maternal and one paternal chromosome, the exchange of corresponding sections of DNA, and the rejoining of the chromosomes. This process can result in an exchange of alleles between chromosomes. *Compare* recombination

Cytosine (C) — A nitrogenous base, one member of the base pair G–C (guanine and cytosine)

Dalton — A unit of mass commonly used to describe biological molecules. Effectively equal to the mass of one hydrogen atom

Deletion — The removal of a sequence of DNA and joining together of the sequences on either side

***de novo* mutation** — A mutation occurring spontaneously in the genome that has not been inherited through the parental germline

Deoxyribonucleotide — *See* nucleotide

Diploid — A full set of genetic material, consisting of paired chromosomes, one chromosome from each parental set. Most animal cells except the gametes have a diploid set of chromosomes. The diploid human genome has 46 chromosomes. Compare haploid

DNA (deoxyribonucleic acid) — The molecule that encodes genetic information. DNA is a double-stranded molecule held together by weak bonds between base pairs of nucleotides. The four nucleotides in DNA contain the bases adenine (A), guanine (G), cytosine (C) and thymine (T). In nature, base pairs form only between A and T and between G and C; thus the base sequence of each single strand can be deduced from that of its partner

DNA probes — *See* probe

DNA replication — The use of existing DNA as a template for the synthesis of new DNA strands. In humans and other eukaryotes, replication occurs in the cell nucleus

DNA sequence — The relative order of base pairs, whether in a fragment of DNA, a gene, a chromosome, or an entire genome. *See* base sequence analysis

Domain — A discrete portion of a protein with its own function. The combination of domains in a single protein determines its overall function

Double helix — The shape that two linear strands of DNA assume when bonded together

Duplication — The copying and insertion of a DNA sequence usually adjacent to the original sequence

Electrophoresis — A method of separating large molecules (such as DNA fragments or proteins) from a mixture of similar molecules. An electric current is passed through a medium containing the mixture, and each kind of molecule travels through the medium at a different rate, depending on its electrical charge and size. Separation is based on these differences. Agarose and acrylamide gels are the media commonly used for electrophoresis of proteins and nucleic acids

Endonuclease — An enzyme that cleaves its nucleic acid substrate at internal sites in the nucleotide sequence

Enzyme — A protein that acts as a catalyst, speeding the rate at which a biochemical reaction proceeds but not altering the direction or nature of the reaction

Escherichia coli — Common bacterium that has been studied intensively by geneticists because of its small genome size, normal lack of pathogenicity and ease of growth in the laboratory

EST — Expressed sequence tag. *See* sequence tagged site

Eukaryote — Cell or organism with membrane-bound, structurally discrete nucleus and other well-developed subcellular compartments. Eukaryotes include all organisms except viruses, bacteria, and blue-green algae. *Compare* prokaryote. *See* chromosomes

Euchromatic — The region comprising all of the genome in the interphase nucleus except the heterochromatin

Evolutionarily conserved — *See* conserved sequence

Exogenous DNA — DNA originating outside an organism

Exons — The protein-coding DNA sequences of a gene. *Compare* introns

Exonuclease — An enzyme that cleaves nucleotides sequentially from free ends of a linear nucleic acid substrate

Expressed gene — *See* gene expression

FISH (fluorescence *in situ* hybridization) — A physical mapping approach that uses fluorescein tags to detect hybridization of probes with metaphase chromosomes and with the less condensed somatic interphase chromatin

Flow cytometry — Analysis of biological material by detection of the light-absorbing or fluorescing properties of cells or subcellular fractions (i.e. chromosomes) passing in a narrow stream through a laser beam. An absorbance or fluorescence profile of the sample is produced. Automated sorting devices, used to fractionate samples, sort successive droplets of the analysed stream into different fractions depending on the fluorescence emitted by each droplet

Flow karyotyping — Use of flow cytometry to analyse and/or separate chromosomes on the basis of their DNA content

Gamete — Mature male or female reproductive cell (sperm or ovum) with a haploid set of chromosomes (23 for humans)

Gene — The fundamental physical and functional unit of heredity. A gene is an ordered sequence of nucleotides located in a particular position on a particular chromosome that encodes a specific functional product (i.e. a protein or RNA molecule). *See* gene expression

Gene expression — The process by which a gene's coded information is converted into the structures present and operating in the cell. Expressed genes include those that are transcribed into messenger RNA and then translated into protein and those that are transcribed into RNA but not translated into protein (e.g. transfer and ribosomal RNAs)

Gene families — Groups of closely related genes that make similar products

Gene library — *See* genomic library

Gene locus — The physical location on a chromosome at which a gene resides

Gene mapping — Determination of the relative positions of genes on a DNA molecule (chromosome or plasmid) and of the distance, in linkage units or physical units, between them

Gene product — The biochemical material, either RNA or protein, resulting from expression of a gene. The amount of gene product is used to measure how active a gene is; abnormal amounts can be correlated with disease-causing alleles

Genetic code — The sequence of nucleotides, coded in triplets (codons) along the messenger RNA, that determines the sequence of amino acids in protein synthesis. The DNA sequence of a gene can be used to predict the messenger RNA sequence, and the genetic code can in turn be used to predict the amino acid sequence

Genetic cross-over During meiosis, homologous chromosomes pair together. Exchange of DNA can occur between the two chromosomes to produce a recombinant chromosome with a different genotype to either of the original parent chromosomes

Genetic engineering technologies *See* recombinant DNA technologies

Genetic linkage mapping The process used to identify regions of DNA that are physically close or linked to each other. During meiotic cell division, physically close DNA markers will nearly always be inherited together on the same daughter chromosome. Genetic linkage mapping analyses the cosegregation of different DNA marker loci in large numbers of genetic offspring

Genetic map *See* linkage map

Genetic material *See* genome

Genetics The study of the patterns of inheritance of specific traits

Genome All the genetic material in the chromosomes of a particular organism; its size is generally given as its total number of base pairs

Genome projects Research and technology development efforts aimed at mapping and sequencing some or all of the genome of human beings and other organisms

Genomic DNA DNA represented in the chromosomal DNA content of a cell

Genomic library A collection of clones made from a set of randomly generated overlapping DNA fragments representing the entire genome of an organism. *Compare* library, arrayed library

Genotype The genetic constitution of an organism

Guanine (G) A nitrogenous base, one member of the base pair G–C (guanine and cytosine)

Haploid A single set of chromosomes (half the full set of genetic material), present in the egg and sperm cells of animals and in the egg and pollen cells of plants. Human beings have 23 chromosomes in their reproductive cells. *Compare* diploid

Heterochromatin Regions of the genome that are maintained in a condensed state and are not expressed

Heteroduplex (hybrid) DNA A double-stranded DNA.DNA molecule formed by complementary base pairing of single-stranded DNA molecules. (NB: DNA.RNA heteroduplexes can also be formed by the same process)

Heterozygosity The presence of different alleles at one or more loci on homologous chromosomes

Heterozygote An individual with different alleles at the same genetic locus

Homeobox A short stretch of nucleotides whose base sequence is virtually identical in all the genes that contain it. It has been found in many organisms, from fruit flies to human beings. In the fruit fly, a homeobox appears to determine when particular groups of genes are expressed during development

Homologies Similarities in DNA or protein sequences between individuals of the same species or among different species

Homologous chromosomes A pair of chromosomes containing the same linear gene sequences, each derived from one parent

Homology A term used to describe the extent of similarity between DNA, RNA and protein sequences – totally identical DNA sequences are 100% homologous

Homozygote An individual with identical alleles at the same genetic locus

HTF-island	A region of the mammalian genome rich in the dinucleotide C_pG. So called because restriction enzyme digestion with H_{paII} produces a fraction of tiny DNA fragments (H_{paII} tiny fragments or HTF). These regions are often associated with gene sequences
Human gene therapy	Insertion of normal DNA directly into cells to correct a genetic defect
Hybridization	The process of joining two complementary strands of DNA or one each of DNA and RNA to form a double-stranded molecule
Hypervariable DNA	Regions of DNA that contain multiple copies of simple repeat DNA sequences. The number of copies can vary greatly between individuals of the same species
Informatics	The study of the application of computer and statistical techniques to the management of information. In genome projects, informatics includes the development of methods to search databases quickly, to analyse DNA sequence information and to predict protein sequence and structure from DNA sequence data
Informative DNA marker	Polymorphic DNA markers are informative in genetic matings when the parents are heterozygous for the marker in question. The chances of this occurring are increased when a marker displays multiple alleles. The mating is said to be fully informative when both parents are heterozygous and partially informative when only one parent is heterozygous for the DNA marker under investigation
***In situ* hybridization**	Use of a DNA or RNA probe to detect the presence of the complementary DNA sequence in cloned bacterial or cultured eukaryotic cells
Intergenic distance	The distance, genetic or physical, between different gene loci
Interphase	The period in the cell cycle when DNA is replicated in the nucleus, followed by mitosis
Introns	The DNA base sequences interrupting the protein-coding sequences of a gene; these sequences are transcribed into RNA but are cut out of the message before it is translated into protein. *Compare* exons
Inversion	The 180° rotation and reinsertion of a chromosomal DNA segment relative to the surrounding DNA sequences
In vitro	Outside a living organism
Karyotype	A photomicrograph of an individual's chromosomes arranged in a standard format showing the number, size and shape of each chromosome type; used in low-resolution physical mapping to correlate gross chromosomal abnormalities with the characteristics of specific diseases
kb	*See* kilobase
Kilobase (kb)	Unit of length for DNA fragments equal to 1000 nucleotides
Kilodaltons (kD)	Abbreviation for 1000 daltons
Library	An unordered collection of clones (i.e. cloned DNA from a particular organism) whose relationship to each other can be established by physical mapping. *Compare* genomic library, arrayed library
Linkage	The proximity of two or more markers (e.g. genes, restriction fragment length polymorphism markers) on a chromosome; the closer together the markers are, the lower the probability that they will be separated during DNA repair or replication processes (binary fission in prokaryotes, mitosis or meiosis in eukaryotes), and hence the greater the probability that they will be inherited together
Linkage map	A map of the relative positions of genetic loci on a chromosome, determined on the basis of how often the loci are inherited together. Distance is measured in centimorgans (cM)
Localize	Determination of the original position (locus) of a gene or other marker on a chromosome

Locus (plural loci) The position on a chromosome of a gene or other chromosome marker; also, the DNA at that position. The use of locus is sometimes restricted to mean regions of DNA that are expressed. *See* gene expression

Macrorestriction map Map depicting the order of and distance between sites at which restriction enzymes cleave chromosomes

Mapping *See* gene mapping, linkage map, physical map

Marker An identifiable physical location on a chromosome (e.g. restriction enzyme cutting site, gene) whose inheritance can be monitored. Markers can be expressed regions of DNA (genes) or some segment of DNA with no known coding function but whose pattern of inheritance can be determined. *See* restriction fragment length polymorphism

Mb *See* megabase

Megabase (Mb) Unit of length for DNA fragments equal to 1 million nucleotides and roughly equal to 1 cM

Meiosis The process of two consecutive cell divisions in the diploid progenitors of sex cells. Meiosis results in four rather than two daughter cells, each with a haploid set of chromosomes

Messenger RNA (mRNA) RNA that serves as a template for protein synthesis. *See* genetic code

Metaphase A stage in mitosis or meiosis during which the chromosomes are aligned along the equatorial plane of the cell

Mitosis The process of nuclear division in cells that produces daughter cells that are genetically identical to each other and to the parent cell

mRNA *See* messenger RNA

Multifactorial or multigenic disorders *See* polygenic disorders

Multiplexing A sequencing approach that uses several pooled samples simultaneously, greatly increasing sequencing speed

Mutation Any heritable change in DNA sequence. *Compare* polymorphism

Nitrogenous base A nitrogen-containing molecule having the chemical properties of a base

Nucleic acid A large molecule composed of nucleotide subunits

Nucleoside A purine or pyrimidine base linked to the pentose D-ribose or 2-deoxy-D-ribose

Nucleotide A subunit of DNA or RNA consisting of a nitrogenous base (adenine, guanine, thymine, or cytosine in DNA; adenine, guanine, uracil, or cytosine in RNA), a phosphate molecule and a sugar molecule (deoxyribose in DNA and ribose in RNA). Thousands of nucleotides are linked to form a DNA or RNA molecule. *See* DNA, base pair, RNA

Nucleus The cellular organelle in eukaryotes that contains the genetic material

Oncogene A gene, one or more forms of which is associated with cancer. Many oncogenes are involved, directly or indirectly, in controlling the rate of cell growth

Overlapping clones *See* genomic library

PCR *See* polymerase chain reaction

Penetrance A term used to describe the phenotypic effects of gene expression – a fully penetrant disease gene might cause a severe clinical phenotype, whereas when the gene is expressed at reduced penetrance, a milder clinical phenotype will be apparent

Phage A virus for which the natural host is a bacterial cell

Phenotype The outward appearance or characteristics of an organism as determined by the interaction of the genotype and environment

Physical map A map of the locations of identifiable landmarks on DNA (e.g. restriction enzyme cutting sites, genes) regardless of inheritance. Distance is measured in base pairs. For the human genome, the lowest-resolution physical map is the banding patterns on the 24 different chromosomes; the highest-resolution map would be the complete nucleotide sequence of the chromosomes

Plasmid Autonomously replicating, extrachromosomal circular DNA molecules, distinct from the normal bacterial genome and non-essential for cell survival under non-selective conditions. Some plasmids are capable of integrating into the host genome. A number of artificially constructed plasmids are used as cloning vectors

Pleiotropic A gene is pleiotropic if it affects more than one, seemingly unrelated, characteristic of the phenotype

Polygenic disorders Genetic disorders resulting from the combined action of alleles of more than one gene (e.g. heart disease, diabetes and some cancers). Although such disorders are inherited, they depend on the simultaneous presence of several alleles; thus the hereditary patterns are usually more complex than those of single-gene disorders. *Compare* single-gene disorders

Polymerase chain reaction (PCR) A method for amplifying a DNA base sequence using a heat-stable polymerase and two 20-base primers, one complementary to the (+)-strand at one end of the sequence to be amplified and the other complementary to the (–)-strand at the other end. Because the newly synthesized DNA strands can subsequently serve as additional templates for the same primer sequences, successive rounds of primer annealing, strand elongation and dissociation produce rapid and highly specific amplification of the desired sequence. PCR also can be used to detect the existence of the defined sequence in a DNA sample

Polymerase, DNA or RNA Enzymes that catalyse the synthesis of nucleic acids on pre-existing nucleic acid templates, assembling RNA from ribonucleotides or DNA from deoxyribonucleotides

Polymorphism Difference in DNA sequence among individuals. Genetic variations occurring in more than 1% of a population would be considered useful polymorphisms for genetic linkage analysis. *Compare* mutation

Primer Short pre-existing polynucleotide chain to which new deoxyribonucleotides can be added by DNA polymerase

Proband A genetic-disease-affected individual around whom a family history of the disease is constructed

Probe Single-stranded DNA or RNA molecules of specific base sequence, labelled either radioactively or immunologically, that are used to detect the complementary base sequence by hybridization

Prokaryote Cell or organism lacking a membrane-bound, structurally discrete nucleus and other subcellular compartments. Bacteria are prokaryotes. *Compare* eukaryote; *See* chromosomes

Promoter A site on DNA to which RNA polymerase will bind and initiate transcription

Protein A large molecule composed of one or more chains of amino acids in a specific order; the order is determined by the base sequence of nucleotides in the gene coding for the protein. Proteins are required for the structure, function and regulation of the body's cells, tissues and organs, and each protein has unique functions. Examples are hormones, enzymes and antibodies

Purine A nitrogen-containing, single-ring, basic compound that occurs in nucleic acids. The purines in DNA and RNA are adenine and guanine

Pyrimidine A nitrogen-containing, double-ring, basic compound that occurs in nucleic acids. The pyrimidines in DNA are cytosine and thymine; in RNA, cytosine and uracil

Rare-cutter enzyme *See* restriction enzyme cutting site

Recombinant clones Clones containing recombinant DNA molecules. *See* recombinant DNA technologies

Recombinant DNA molecules A combination of DNA molecules of different origin that are joined using recombinant DNA technologies

Recombinant DNA technologies Procedures used to join together DNA segments in a cell-free system (an environment outside a cell or organism). Under appropriate conditions, a recombinant DNA molecule can enter a cell and replicate there, either autonomously or after it has become integrated into a cellular chromosome

Recombination The process by which progeny derive a combination of genes different from that of either parent. In higher organisms, this can occur by crossing over

Regulatory regions or sequences A DNA base sequence that controls gene expression

Resolution Degree of molecular detail on a physical map of DNA, ranging from low to high

Restriction enzyme cutting site A specific nucleotide sequence of DNA at which a particular restriction enzyme cuts the DNA. Some sites occur frequently in DNA (e.g. every several hundred base pairs), others much less frequently (rare-cutter, e.g. every 10 000 base pairs)

Restriction enzyme, endonuclease A protein that recognizes specific, short nucleotide sequences and cuts DNA at those sites. Bacteria contain over 400 such enzymes that recognize and cut over 100 different DNA sequences. *See* restriction enzyme cutting site

Restriction fragment A segment of DNA created from the cutting of a larger piece of DNA by a restriction enzyme

Restriction fragment length polymorphism (RFLP) Variation between individuals in DNA fragment sizes cut by specific restriction enzymes; polymorphic sequences that result in RFLPs are used as markers on both physical maps and genetic linkage maps. RFLPs are usually caused by mutation at a cutting site. *See* marker

Restriction map The delineation of specific restriction enzyme recognition sites along a segment of DNA; usually represented as a linear array of resulting restriction fragments

RFLP *See* restriction fragment length polymorphism

Ribonucleic acid (RNA) A chemical found in the nucleus and cytoplasm of cells; it plays an important role in protein synthesis and other chemical activities of the cell. The structure of RNA is similar to that of DNA. There are several classes of RNA molecules, including messenger RNA, transfer RNA, ribosomal RNA and other small RNAs, each serving a different purpose

Ribonucleotides *See* nucleotide

Ribosomal RNA (rRNA) A class of RNA found in the ribosomes of cells

Ribosomes Small cellular components composed of specialized ribosomal RNA and protein; site of protein synthesis. *See* ribonucleic acid (RNA)

RNA *See* ribonucleic acid

Sequence *See* base sequence

Sequence tagged site (STS) Short (200 to 500 bp) DNA sequence that has a single occurrence in the human genome and whose location and base sequence are known. Detectable by polymerase chain reaction, STSs are useful for localizing and orienting the mapping and sequence data reported from many different laboratories and serve as landmarks on the developing physical map of the human genome. Expressed sequence tags (ESTs) are STSs derived from complementary DNAs

Sequencing Determination of the order of nucleotides (base sequences) in a DNA or RNA molecule or the order of amino acids in a protein

Sex chromosomes The X and Y chromosomes in human beings that determine the sex of an individual. Females have two X chromosomes in diploid cells; males have an X and a Y chromosome. The sex chromosomes comprise the 23rd chromosome pair in a karyotype. *Compare* autosome

Shotgun method Cloning of DNA fragments randomly generated from a genome. *See* library, genomic library

Single-gene disorder Hereditary disorder caused by a mutant allele of a single gene (e.g. Duchenne muscular dystrophy, retinoblastoma, sickle-cell disease). *Compare* polygenic disorders

Somatic cells Any cell in the body except gametes and their precursors

Southern blotting Transfer by absorption of DNA fragments separated in electrophoretic gels to membrane filters for detection of specific base sequences by radiolabelled complementary probes

STS *See* sequence tagged site

Tandem repeat sequences Multiple copies of the same base sequence on a chromosome; used as a marker in physical mapping

Technology transfer The process of converting scientific findings from research laboratories into useful products by the commercial sector

tel Abbreviation for chromosome telomere

Telomere The ends of chromosomes. These specialized structures are involved in the replication and stability of linear DNA molecules. *See* DNA replication

Thymine (T) A nitrogenous base, one member of the base pair A–T (adenine–thymine)

Transcription The synthesis of an RNA copy from a sequence of DNA (a gene); the first step in gene expression. *Compare* translation

Transfer RNA (t-RNA) A class of RNA having structures with triplet nucleotide sequences that are complementary to the triplet nucleotide coding sequences of messenger RNA. The role of t-RNAs in protein synthesis is to bind with amino acids and transfer them to the ribosomes, where proteins are assembled according to the genetic code carried by messengerRNA

Transformation A process by which the genetic material carried by an individual cell is altered by incorporation of exogenous DNA into its genome

Translation The process in which the genetic code carried by messenger RNA directs the synthesis of proteins from amino acids. *Compare* transcription

Translocation The breaking and joining of a chromosomal fragment to a different chromosome

t-RNA *See* transfer RNA

Uracil A nitrogenous base normally found in RNA but not DNA; uracil is capable of forming a base pair with adenine

Vector *See* cloning vector

Virus A non-cellular biological entity that can reproduce only within a host cell. Viruses consist of nucleic acid covered by protein; some animal viruses are also surrounded by membrane. Inside the infected cell, the virus uses the synthetic capability of the host to produce progeny virus

VLSI Very large-scale integration, allowing over 100 000 transistors on a chip

YAC *See* yeast artificial chromosome

Yeast artificial chromosome (YAC) A vector used to clone DNA fragments (up to 400 kb); it is constructed from the telomeric, centromeric and replication origin sequences needed for replication in yeast cells. *Compare* cloning vector, cosmid

Index

References to figures and tables are *italicized*